The Author

David Zimmerman has been writing for and about Americans' health for 30 years. He writes for consumers, and also for doctors and other health professionals.

Mr. Zimmerman conducted the "Your Family's Health" column in the *Ladies' Home Journal* for a dozen years. His byline has appeared on health articles in *Woman's Day*, *Family Circle*, *Good Housekeeping*, *Red Book* and *McCalls*. His articles on scientific topics—particularly the conservation of peregrine falcons and other endangered species—have appeared in *Smithsonian*, the *New York Times Magazine*, *Audubon*, and many other magazines.

When he is not writing books, Mr. Zimmerman is an investigative reporter and analyst of the shifting, volatile relations between science, media, public policy, and personal health. He publishes this work in his newsletter PROBE.

A midwesterner by birth, Mr. Zimmerman now lives in Manhattan with his wife, who is a physician, their grown-up sons (from time to time), three cats, two turtles, and three hybrid rats named Hortense, Gretchen and Matilda.

Also by the Author

Rh, The Intimate History of a Disease and Its Conquest

To Save a Bird in Peril

ZIMMERMAN'S
Complete Guide to
NONPRESCRIPTION
DRUGS

Always for my Tobias

ZIMMERMAN'S
Complete Guide to
NONPRESCRIPTION
DRUGS

SECOND EDITION

David R. Zimmerman

(FORMERLY: *The Essential Guide to Nonprescription Drugs*)

DETROIT • WASHINGTON, D.C. • LONDON

Zimmerman's Complete Guide to Nonprescription Drugs (formerly: The Essential Guide to Nonprescription Drugs)

Published by **Visible Ink Press**™
a division of Gale Research Inc.
835 Penobscot Bldg.
Detroit MI 48226-4094

Visible Ink Press™ is a trademark of Gale Research Inc.

ISBN 0-8103-9421-9

Art Director: Cynthia Baldwin
Designer: Mary Krzewinski
David Zimmerman Inc. *Production Manager:* Angela M. Darling
Typesetting: The Graphix Group

Printed in the United States of America

10 9 8 7 6 5 4 3 2 1
Second Edition

How to Use This Guide

Zimmerman's Complete Guide to Nonprescription Drugs answers many questions about over-the-counter (OTC) drugs, so this book can be used in several ways. The column on the left gives some of the questions that you may have turned to this Guide to answer. The column on the right tells you how to find these answers.

You are—or someone else in the family is—distressed by a symptom or ailment. You want to know more about OTC drugs you can use to treat it, and their active ingredients. (The *active ingredients* are what make a drug work—or not work.)

Scan the **Contents** (pp. xiii-xxiv). The Unit titles tell you what groups—based on their purpose—are included in this Guide (examples: *Acne Medications* and *Reducing Aids*). Or: Check the **Symptoms Index**, on p. lv.

You've decided what your ailment is, and you have bought, or are thinking of buying, a nonprescription drug product that you think may help. How can you be sure that it will?

Check the product label to find out what the active ingredients are. Examples: the active ingredient in *Datril* (Bristol-Myers Squibb) is acetaminophen; in *Pepto-Bismol* (Procter & Gamble) it is bismuth subsalicylate. Then turn to the **Index**, beginning on page 1054, to find where you can read about the ingredient. *Or*: Find the ingredient in the Safety and Effectiveness of Active

Ingredients table near the end of each Unit. Many widely sold products, such as *Pepto-Bismol*, are evaluated in the Product Ratings tables that conclude most Units. Even if the product is not listed, if you know the active ingredient(s)—which should be listed on the label—you can judge the product's value using the Safety and Effectiveness of Active Ingredients table in the Unit. All safe and effective active ingredients, and most if not all that are not safe and effective, are evaluated in these tables.

You've checked the Guide, and have found you have a condition that is self-treatable with nonprescription drugs. You're on your way to the drugstore. Which product do you buy?

Check the Safety and Effectiveness table near the end of the appropriate Unit. In most cases only a handful of ingredients are safe and effective. Jot them down or jot down the names of one or two "A"-rated products from the Product Rating tables.

You think you know which product you want to use, because you've seen an ad on television, or you've used it before. Is it all it's cracked up to be?

Check the Product Ratings table that concludes most Units. If the product is not listed, check the active ingredient(s) in the Safety and Effectiveness table of the same unit in order to determine the safety and effectiveness of the product.

You want to upgrade your medicine chest.

Use this Guide to evaluate every nonprescription drug you have on hand. Discard those that are not evaluated "safe and effective" or "A."

You want to know more about nonprescription drugs in general. Can they really help? How do they work? Isn't it always better to go to a doctor?

The main text of this Guide explains in everyday language many symptoms and ailments. The Guide tells how nonprescription drugs can be effective, when a doctor should be consulted, and when and why experts say that self-medication often is useful and appropriate.

Unit Finders

The Unit titles in this Guide are arranged alphabetically. If you are looking for help with a toothache, simply turn to the Unit TOOTHACHE RELIEVERS in the *T*s. However, you may also want to know which other over-the-counter remedies are available for dental problems. In the following list, the Unit titles are grouped under general headings. For a complete list of Unit titles, see the Contents.

Baby-Care

Cradle-Cap Removers
Diaper-Rash Relievers
Teething Easers
Unguents and Powders for the Skin

Body-Odor Control

Antiperspirants
Deodorants for Ostomies and Incontinence
Germ-Killing Soaps

Eye- and Ear-Care

Ear-Care Aids
Eye Drops and Ointments
Eyes: Artificial Tears
Eyes: Corneal Edema
Eyewash

Gastrointestinal Discomfort

Antacids
Anti-Gas Agents
Diarrhea Remedies
Digestive Aids
Hangover and Overindulgence Remedies
Hemorrhoid Medications and Other Anorectal Applications
Kidney and Bladder Drugs
Laxatives
Motion-Sickness Medicines
Pancreatic Enzyme Supplements

Hair-Care

Dandruff and Seborrheic Scale Shampoos and Other Treatments
Hair-Growth Stimulants and Baldness Preventives

Hand-, Foot-, and Nail-Care

Corn and Callus Removers
Ingrown-Toenail Relievers
Jock Itch, Athlete's Foot, and Ringworm Cures
Nail-Biting and Thumb-Sucking Deterrents
Wart Paints

Men's Health Care

Hair-Growth Stimulants and Baldness Preventives
Jock Itch, Athlete's Foot, and Ringworm Cures and Other Treatments
Premature Ejaculation Retardants
Contraceptives

Nutrition

Reducing Aids
Salt Supplements and Substitutes
Vitamins and Minerals

Plant-and-Animal Poisons

Insect Repellents and Bite and Sting Treatments
Louse Poisons
Poison Ivy-Oak-Sumac Preventives and Palliatives
Worm-Killers for Pinworm Infestation

Respiratory Problems

Allergy Drugs
Asthma Drugs
Cold and Cough Medications
Smelling Salts
Smoking Deterrents

Sex

Aphrodisiacs
Contraceptives
Douches and Other Vaginal Drugs
Premature Ejaculation Retardants

Skin Care

Acne Medications
Bleaches for Skin Blemishes

Boil Ointments
Corn and Callus Removers
First Aid Antibiotics
First-Aid Antiseptics
Germ-Killing Soaps
Hormone Skin Creams and Oils
Insect Repellents and Bite and Sting Treatments
Itch and Pain Remedies Applied to the Skin
Jock Itch, Athlete's Foot, and Ringworm Cures
Liniments and Poultices for Aches and Pains
Poison Ivy-Oak-Sumac Preventives and Palliatives
Psoriasis Lotions
Styptic Pencils and Other Astringents
Sunscreens
Unguents and Powders to Protect the Skin
Wart Paints

Stimulants and Relaxants

Sleep Aids
Smelling Salts
Stimulants

Teeth and Mouth

Cold-Sore Balms
Fluoride Toothpastes and Rinses for Cavity Prevention
Medicaments for Sore Gums, Mouths, and Throats
Mouthwash for Oral Hygiene
Teeth: Anti-Plaque Products
Teeth: Desensitizers
Teething Easers
Toothache Relievers

Women's Health Care

Contraceptives
Douches and Other Vaginal Drugs
Menstrual-Distress Preparations
"Yeast" Killers for Feminine Itching

Contents

How This Guide Will Save You Money—And More than Pay for Itself

The main purpose of *Zimmerman's Complete Guide to Nonprescription Drugs* is to help you obtain better health care for yourself and your family.

Nonprescription drugs are among the most economical health resources. But researching and writing about them has brought to light some simple ways to save additional money—methods that will help this Guide to more than pay for itself during each year that you use it.

Here are a few of these cost-saving benefits:

• *Reduce medical appointments*—Millions of Americans now treat poison ivy, skin allergies, and other itchy rashes using safe and effective 1 percent hydrocortisone creams and ointments. Millions of women recently began self-treating recurrent 'yeast' infections with the effective anti-fungal drugs clotrimazole (*Vaginal Gyne-lotrimin*, Schering-Plough) and miconazole nitrate (*Monistat 7*, Ortho). These drugs have been switched from prescription (℞) to nonprescription status.

These switches save consumers the cost of going to the doctor, and then obtaining and filling a prescription for a drug such as hydrocortisone or a 'yeast'-stopping drug, which in many cases cannot have been less than about $50. And this estimate does not even include the cost of transportation and lost work time for the doctor's visit and a stop-off at the pharmacist's.

Whether you use a nonprescription drug that is a recent "switch" from ℞ status or an older, equally effective nonprescription drug, like the pain-reliever *lidocaine*, if this Guide helps you self-treat just one problem that previously would have taken you—or you and a child—to a doctor, you have saved about $40.

• *Buy only worthwhile drugs*—This Guide facilitates a second major cost saving: Many nonprescription drug products can be described as worthless, or of dubious value at best, on the basis of the FDA's *Over-the-Counter Drug Review*. The Guide allows you to purchase *only* products that are safe and effective. If you purchase two safe and effective products in a year in place of doubtful ones, and assuming a $4 cost savings for each item purchased, you have saved $8.

• *Find less-costly generics*—Drugs that are sold generically under their chemical names—*Acetaminophen*, instead of *Tylenol* (McNeil-CPC), for example—usually are significantly less expensive. This Guide allows you to identify the medically active ingredient, or ingredients, in brand-name products, so that you can find an equivalent generic product on the drugstore shelf. (If you can't find one, ask the pharmacist or clerk to help you.) The savings will be substantial:

Generic 325-mg *Acetaminophen* tablets can be purchased for one-sixth or less the cost of *Tylenol Regular Strength Tablets*, an analysis of wholesale prices in *drug facts and comparisons* 1992 suggests. The differences may be even greater among aspirins: Generic aspirin, in 325-mg tablets, may be less than a tenth as costly as the leading brand name, *Genuine Bayer Aspirin Tablets* (Glenbrook); however, the brand-name product does have a thin coating that prevents the tablets from dissolving during swallowing. By the same token, *Consumer Reports* (June 1992) analyzed the price of the new, half-strength (165 mg) enteric coated aspirin tablets *Halfprin* (Kramer); this dose, when recommended by a doctor, may be the most appropriate one for preventing heart attacks. The magazine reported that *Halfprin* is "12 times the price of generic aspirin," albeit easier to tolerate and a little more convenient to use. The same 165 mg dose can be obtained by taking two 81 mg baby aspirin tablets, or by breaking a standard aspirin tablet (325 mg) in half.

The price differences among other types of drugs may be less dramatic. But it seems reasonable to say that you can save half the cost of a brand name by buying a medicinally equivalent generic product, using the *Ingredient Tables* and *Product Ratings* Tables in this book for guidance. Five such generic purchases in a year, facilitated by this information, should save you $10, assuming a $2 savings on each purchase.

You will find other ways to use this Guide to enhance your health and also save money, for example, by avoiding products that the FDA says—as reported here—have not been shown to safely and effectively relieve the specific type of distress that you feel. In a time of tight budgets for most Americans, a dollar saved is a dollar that can be well spent on other daily expenses.

Tip-off: How You May Be Able to Protect Yourself from a Drug Price Rip-off

Consumers may often pay more for nonprescription drugs than they ought to, because of a tax ruse.

A tin of *Sucrets* sore throat lozenges (SmithKline Beecham) was purchased in New York City as part of the research for this Guide. It carries a price sticker ($4.49 TX) indicating that it is a taxable item. The New York State sales tax of 8¼ percent thus adds 37 cents to the $4.49 purchase price.

But *Sucrets* lozenges—which contain the medically active pain-relieving ingredient hexylresorcinol—are tax free, as indicated in a New York State Department of Taxation and Finance document (Publication 820).

The tax code in New York (Publication 840) specifically exempts from taxes "drugs and medicines intended for use internally or externally, in the cure, mitigation, treatment or prevention of illness or disease... . Products consumed... for the preservation of health are also exempt."

The document cites aspirin, lip balms, and medicated dandruff shampoos as tax exempt. Safe and effective sunscreens "a PABA rating of at least 5 percent" are, or should be, tax free, too.

It is not clear whether the retailer or the state profits from erroneous taxation of nonprescription drugs. It is clear that you, the consumer, are paying taxes for no good reason.

These overcharges occurred frequently when I purchased nonprescription drug products for this Guide. One discount store manager rang eight out of ten items as taxable, then grudgingly refunded two or three dollars when his error was called to his attention.

Besides New York, the other states that specifically exempt nonprescription drugs from sales tax are Florida, Maryland, Minnesota, New Jersey, Pennsylvania, and Rhode Island, as well as the District of Columbia (according to the Council of State Governments, in Lexington, Kentucky). In Illinois, the Council says, the nonprescription drugs tax is only 1 percent.

If you live in one of the non-tax states, what can you do to avoid paying illegal sales tax on nonprescription drug products?

If the product contains an active ingredient described in this Guide or has an active ingredient designated on the label, challenge the cashier if he or she rings it as a taxable item. Cashiers and clerks often don't know the "right ring" for these items. Their bosses, however, often do. They will re-ring the item as tax exempt when an error is called to their attention.

A family of four, which spends $200 (average) on nonprescription drugs each year, may save $5 to $10 annually by keeping a sharp eye out for inappropriately taxed nonprescription drugs.

Acknowledgments

One person has kept faith with me on this book project since its inception, fifteen years ago: my wife, Veva, to whom I am deeply grateful!

This Guide derives from a federally sponsored, decades-long review of nonprescription drugs. My principal source is the many FDA reports that have been published in the *Federal Register*, the official record of government actions. Therefore, I am especially indebted to the two hundred medical and scientific advisors who participated in the OTC Drug Review (Panel members are listed on pages 1043 to 1048); the FDA administrators, editors, and writers who prepared the various reports; and any number of other federal employees who skillfully shaped and guided the Review.

Particularly, I want to thank again Gerald M. Rachanow, P.D., J.D., Deputy Director of the Monograph Review staff, Office of Over-the-Counter Drug Evaluations, and his associate, Carol Doyle. Other FDA officials and staff people, particularly in the Press Office, have also helped.

Jack Walden and his associates at the Nonprescription Drug Manufacturers Association (NMDA) in Washington, D.C., have provided helpful information and answered many questions through the years.

At the National Institutes of Health (NIH) in Bethesda, Maryland, Marc Stern, Chief of the News Branch, has helped significantly to ensure the accuracy of this Guide: Through his good offices, the completed text was read and checked for factual accuracy by NIH information specialists. It is important to note, however, that these experts were not asked to read—and did not read—the Product Ratings that conclude most Units.

At HarperCollins, my original publisher for this Guide, I am particularly grateful to James Fox for his sense of fair play.

John Schmittroth was the first at Gale Research Inc. to sense promise in this venture.

It has been a writer's dream—of professional competence, skill, and steadfast support—to work with editor Rebecca Nelson in preparing the Gale and Visible Ink Press editions of this Guide. Theresa Murray copyedited the manuscript.

Peg Bessette, Christa Brelin, and Martin Connors helped put the Guide through its editorial paces. Ably assisting in the proofreading were Jacqueline Gural, Allison McNeill, Matthew Merta, David Oblender, LouAnn Shelton, Kelle Sisung, and Rita Skirpan.

Marco Di Vita of the Graphix Group skillfully typeset the many elements of this Guide.

Writing is a tough game, and collegiality is one of its saving graces. I am therefore grateful to my good colleague Dodi Schultz for suggesting that I bring this project to Gale. By the same token, Dodi's suggestion was prompted by a Gale executive's talk to members of the American Society of Journalists and Authors, of which Dodi and I both are members.

My colleague Tom Watkins has kindly contributed a wholly new Unit, on insulin for diabetics—an area in which he possesses special expertise.

John Heuston came through with a pinch hit in the bottom of the ninth. Hilda Greenbaum and many others have helped. I thank them all!

Angela Darling has earned her editor's stripes, and a row of bars and stars as well, for her unyielding and level-headed competence in typing and organizing this project and keeping it on schedule.

Words cannot express my thanks to all of my family—Veva, J.B., Toby—for their patience with me and with this endeavor. Truly, many years have gone by!

revised 10-day and 5-day warnings for analgesic drug products in § 343.50(c)(1)(i), (2)(i), and (3) in this tentative final monograph adequate to warn consumers to obtain professional help if symptoms persist or get worse or if new symptoms occur.

22. Two comments objected to the 5-day limitation of use of analgesic and antipyretic drug products by children under 12 years of age in the Panel's recommended warning statement in § 343.50(c)(1)(ii). The comments agreed with the Panel that the period of OTC use of analgesic and antipyretic drugs in children under 12 years of age should be limited, but disagreed over the length of time. Suggested alternatives were 2 or 3 days. One comment argued that this warning implies that OTC analgesic drug products are unsafe or toxic if used longer than 5 days.

The agency is proposing the following revised warning for children 2 years to under 12 years of age in § 343.50(c)(2)(i): "Do not give this product for pain for more than 5 days or for fever for more than 3 days unless directed by a doctor. If pain or fever persists or gets worse, if new symptoms occur, or if redness or swelling is present, consult a doctor because these could be signs of a serious condition." (see comment 18 above).

The comments submitted no data to support their suggestions for shorter time limitations. The Internal Analgesic Panel based its recommendation of a 5-day limitation for children on reports from poison control center data and on computer simulations that demonstrated that the plasma salicylate level could exceed 20 milligrams per 100 milliliters (mg/mL) (a toxic level) "among some smaller children of a particular age category following the recommended dosage schedule after 5 days" (42 FR 35368). The agency believes these data provide sufficient reason to propose the Panel's recommended 5-day use limitation for children.

23. Several comments opposed the number and length of warning statements the Panel recommended for OTC analgesic and antipyretic drug products. One comment expressed concern that an extensive list of warnings for products containing aspirin, compared to a shorter list for acetaminophen drug products, will lead consumers to conclude that aspirin drug products are more toxic and less useful than acetaminophen drug products. Other comments urged FDA to limit warning statements to those that are scientifically documented, clinically significant, and important to the appropriate use of the products by the average consumer. These comments

further urged that the statements be combined and condensed for ease of consumer understanding and to avoid label clutter that may cause consumers to ignore cautions and warnings in the labeling. One comment suggested the use of supplementary circulars, etc.

FDA agrees that the warning statements for OTC drug products should be limited to those that are scientifically documented, clinically significant, and important for the safe and effective use of the products by consumers. The agency is requiring warning statements for each ingredient on this basis, not on the basis of a comparable number of warnings for each ingredient. Warning statements are also being combined and condensed whenever possible for ease of consumer understanding. In addition, manufacturers are free to design ways of incorporating all required information in labeling, e.g., using flap labels, redesigning packages, or using a package insert.

24. Many comments opposed warnings that cite organs of the body as possible sites of damage by internal analgesic drug products, with some comments referring specifically to the Panel's recommended liver warning for acetaminophen in § 343.50(c)(5)(i). These comments argued that naming an organ that may be injured from an acute overdose or from excessive use of an analgesic drug would place the responsibility of recognizing organ damage on the consumer, who would then be assuming the role of a physician. The comments further argued that this kind of label warning may be misunderstood and may either alarm or cause anxiety in consumers who use drugs rationally. On the other hand, the comments added, such labeling may provide information that may induce individuals to harm themselves.

The comments favored a single, more general warning for all OTC internal analgesic drug products, such as the following: "Do not take this product for more than 10 days unless directed by a physician. Excessive use over a long period of time may cause permanent injury." One comment suggested that, if such a general warning is not adopted, all OTC drug products should bear labeling which fully discloses the conditions under which damage may occur.

The agency is not proposing to include the general warning suggested by the comments in this tentative final monograph. FDA believes that the self-medicating consumer should be made aware of potential risks of a particular OTC drug product through label warnings. As discussed in comment 25

below, the agency agrees that the warnings need not specify the toxic effects on particular organs of the body that can be caused by acute overdose of a drug, as in a suicide attempt, and is not proposing the Panel's recommended liver warning for acetaminophen in this tentative final monograph. However, the agency concludes that the warnings should include specific information on the known side effects or adverse reactions that may occur from use of the drug according to labeled directions, as well as potential dangers that may occur if the labeled directions are exceeded.

The agency concludes that when medical evidence shows that toxicity is associated with the use of an OTC drug, either within its recommended dosage or when used beyond its recommended time limit or dosage (except for acute overdose), it is appropriate to warn consumers of the potential toxicity. In such cases it may be necessary to include organ-specific warnings as well as general labeling statements.

25. Many comments opposed the liver warning recommended by the Panel for acetaminophen drug products in § 343.50(c)(5)(i), "Do not exceed recommended dosage because severe liver damage may occur." Some comments argued that acetaminophen taken in recommended OTC dosage ranges shows no evidence of hepatotoxicity and that the labeling required in § 330.1(g), "Keep this and all drugs out of the reach of children. In case of accidental overdose, seek professional assistance or contact a poison control center immediately," provides sufficient warning to consumers. The comments expressed concern that the liver warning recommended by the Panel may discourage consumers from ever using acetaminophen and that this warning may also encourage suicidal persons to abuse acetaminophen drug products. The comments also argued that the liver warning is especially inappropriate for children's acetaminophen drug products because there is a lack of documented fatalities and serious liver damage in children from acute acetaminophen overdose. The comments stated there may be differences between the metabolism and pharmacokinetics of acetaminophen in children and adults that would cause children to be less vulnerable to acetaminophen toxicity.

Other comments endorsed the recommended liver warning and pointed out that there are no unique signs of acetaminophen toxicity, such as ringing in the ears (tinnitus), and that symptoms of acetaminophen toxicity do not appear until a few days after the overdose.

A *Federal Register* page—one among thousands—from the U.S. Food and Drug Administration's Over-the-Counter Drug Review. The page is from the *Tentative Final Monograph* on pain, fever, and anti-inflammatory drugs taken internally. It records the FDA's reaction to letters, or "comments," from manufacturers and others on *warnings* that will be required on drug product labels. The comments oppose recommendations by a panel of independent experts to provide a warning telling parents how long a child should be given pain-relieving drugs before being taken to a doctor. The panel had proposed a limit of five days' nonprescription drug treatment before a doctor's help should be sought. The comments argued against this limit. The FDA agreed with the panel, disagreed with the comments, and kept the five-day warning. Other comments described on the page deal with possibly serious side effects of acetaminophen and other nonprescription pain-relieving drugs.

Introduction

Zimmerman's Complete Guide to Nonprescription Drugs is the only complete—and authoritative—key to the safety and the effectiveness of *all* nonprescription drug products sold in the United States. No other such guide exists.

The questions that the Guide will help you answer, about *all* active ingredients in *all* legitimate nonprescription drugs, include:

"Are they appropriate for the symptom or condition I am suffering?"

"Are they effective?"

"Are they safe?"

"What warning signs should I watch for?"

"Are they safe for my children?"

"How much should I take—and how often?"

"How long should I treat myself with a nonprescription product before seeing a doctor?"

Nonprescription Drugs as a Health Resource

Nobody really knows how many different nonprescription drug *products*—that is to say medicines that can be purchased *without* a doctor's prescription—are currently marketed in the United States. Estimates run to the hundreds of thousands. These nonprescription drugs also are called *over-the-counter drugs* or *OTC drugs*. In earlier days they were called *patent medicines*, or, less kindly, *"snake oils."*

The medicinally active ingredients in some of these products are traditional remedies: plant extracts, for example. Others—such as phenol and sulfur—are old standbys, now being pushed aside in the medicine cabinet, purse, pocket, and glove compartment by newer, stronger, safer drugs.

Some nonprescription drugs—and this is a growing and important group of them—are modern pharmaceutical inventions that have been switched from prescription (℞) to nonprescription legal status at the manufacturer's request. Nonprescription, or over-the-counter (OTC) sale *means*, to reiterate, that consumers can purchase and use these drugs without first obtaining a doctor's prescription.

Until very recently there was no way for the consumer to know, except by trial and error, which nonprescription drugs worked and which did not, which were safe and effective and which were not, which were possibly useful and which were worthless.

Nonprescription drugs were poorly regulated by the U.S. Food and Drug Administration (FDA). There was no requirement that they be rigorously assessed—and no one did so.

Tragedy Brings Change

A tragedy changed this: About 1960, in several countries, a sudden upsurge occurred in the number of babies born with severe, crippling birth defects. Some babies were born without one or more limbs. Or, instead of a normal limb, the babies had a small, distorted appendage that looked like a seal's flipper (*phocomelia*).

The cause of this disaster soon was traced: The mothers of these unfortunate babies all had used a new—and in the U.S., still experimental—sleeping medication called *thalidomide*. A prescient FDA drug expert, Frances O. Kelsey, M.D., had worried about this drug and managed to stall its approval in this country. But some *"thalidomide* babies" nevertheless were born to American mothers who had obtained the drug from Canada or abroad.

Congress reacted. The early 1960s was an era of consumerism and of strong public belief in the powers of science and medicine—and the law. In legislation passed in 1962, as amendments to the federal Food, Drug and Cosmetic Act—which is the basic American drug law—Congress told the FDA to make sure that *all* drugs, ℞ *and* OTC, are safe and effective.

FDA Fulfills Congressional Mandate

This Guide is concerned only with nonprescription drugs; there are other consumer reference sources for prescription (℞) medicines.

An ℞ drug usually is selected—*prescribed*—by a physician, dentist, or other licensed doctor, and it is used under his or her supervision. An OTC drug, by contrast, usually is selected by the consumer, the person who feels ill or who seeks relief, or by a parent, spouse, or other family member. In order to use a nonprescription drug, the individual or family member has to decide *something* is wrong; has to decide *what* is wrong; and then has to select an *appropriate* treatment. This Guide is written for the explicit purpose of help-ing consumers—which means all of us—make these informed, therapeutic decisions.

The medical rationale for selling medicines on a nonprescription basis was stated very clearly by then commissioner of the FDA, cardiologist Alexander M. Schmidt, M.D., in 1974: "An underlying premise ... of the sale of drugs over-the-counter, rather than on prescription, is that the consumer is capable of making an intelligent choice of a drug product if he [or she] pos-sesses adequate information about the products offered for treatment of specif-ic conditions or symptoms."

Nonprescription drugs differ from prescription medicines in several important ways, besides easier availability: they tend to be weaker—and safer. With a few exceptions, detailed in the text, they are not intended to treat seri-ous disease; also, with a few exceptions, they are not intended to treat major organs or organ systems.

A few nonprescription drugs—the antifungal agents used to treat ath-lete's foot and 'yeast' infections, for example—are *curative*: They actively kill funguses and so resolve the problem. Most nonprescription drugs, however, pro-vide *symptomatic* relief: They control pain, inflammation, itching, or some other condition, temporarily, while the body's natural recuperative powers cure the condition, or until a doctor's help can be obtained for more definitive therapy.

Nonprescription drugs have the advantage of being inexpensive. A small or medium-sized package or bottle of most of these products still can be purchased for about $4; few cost more than $10 and some cost less than $2. Nonprescription drugs thus are a valuable health resource in an era when med-ical costs are rising and budgets, for most families, continue to be quite tight.

OTC drugs account for less than 2 percent of Americans' health expen-ditures, according to industry sources, or a little more than a dime per person, per day. When the drugs work, they are a bargain.

Surveys have shown that virtually everybody uses OTC drugs. Retail sales are about $11.6 billion annually, according to the industry trade group, the Nonprescription Drug Manufacturers Association (NDMA), in Washington, D.C. These sales are projected to rise.

How Information Was Obtained

The problem is, where can the consumer find authoritative information on these products' safety, efficacy, and appropriate use?

The answer: *The FDA's Over-the-Counter Drug Review*.

This OTC Drug Review, as it is usually called, is a formal governmen-tal evaluation of all nonprescription drugs. It also provides the substance of this Guide. The OTC Drug Review was the FDA's answer to Congress' man-date that it guarantee the safety and efficacy of all nonprescription drugs.

Legally, the OTC Drug Review is a *regulatory process* to decide which non-prescription drugs should be kicked off the market, and which should stay—and on what conditions.

It took the FDA, its medical consultants, consumerists, and the drug industry several years to figure out how to conduct this regulatory process. The key was the discovery that while there are tens (or maybe hundreds) of thousands of different OTC drug products on pharmacy, discount, and grocery store shelves, they contain a far smaller number of medicinally *active ingredients*. Take, as an example, one high-selling category, pain relievers that are taken internally for headaches and other aches and pains: While there may be dozens of brand-name products, and hundreds or thousands of less well known house brands and generic labels, it turns out that they all contain only a few pain-relieving active ingredients. Most contain acetaminophen or aspirin or, more recently, ibuprofen. (Most other OTC pain relievers are close chemical relatives of aspirin.)

The same situation exists for other categories of OTC drugs: a myriad of products containing few active ingredients, and for most categories only a handful have been shown in the scientific literature—or could be so shown—to safely and effectively relieve the symptom(s) for which they are sold.

This understanding guided the FDA in organizing its OTC Drug Review. All products initially were divided into seventeen broad categories, which later were further subdivided into about fifty more specific groups. The FDA-appointed Advisory Review Panels of doctors, pharmacologists, nurses, and other authorities in each of the seventeen main areas. The Panels' members are listed on pp. 1043-1048.

Great care was taken in selecting the panelists: Most were distinguished academic medical specialists, including deans of medical or pharmacology schools, department heads, and other medical educators. Panels also included private practitioners—doctors and dentists who provide care in their private offices for many people who are suffering from ordinary, aggravating, day-to-day health problems. These practitioners were familiar with the common, nagging complaints that rarely are referred to hospital-based specialists. These are the kinds of medical and dental problems for which self-treatment with nonprescription drugs may be especially appropriate.

Each Panel further included a pharmacist (the individual who fills prescriptions at the drugstore and often advises health consumers on the choice and use of nonprescription drugs), and either a pharmacologist (an expert on drugs) or a toxicologist (a specialist in drugs' adverse effects). Every Panel benefited from at least one expert on the design and interpretation of scientific studies.

Consumers and the drug industry were both represented on all the Panels by non-voting members. The Consumer Federation of America nominated consumer representatives. The NDMA and other manufacturers' groups nominated the industry representatives.

The Panels were assisted in their work by special consultants hired by the FDA, and by FDA staff workers. These experts provided information from the agency's files and from exhaustive searches into the medical, drug, and chemical literatures available through federal research libraries. Staff work was done by FDA officials and employees.

Considerable information came from interested parties. For example, drug manufacturers and their Washington lawyers and lobbyists presented evidence to the Panels in support of various active ingredients—and, thus, the products that contain them. Doctors and consumer advocates also contributed information and points of view. The FDA states that everyone who asked to present data or suggestions to a Panel was able to do so.

The initial estimate was that there might be 750 active ingredients. Recent FDA status reports indicate there are almost 1,000 active ingredients, for which 1,500 to 2,000 different uses, or *indications*, have been claimed. (Each different medical use for a drug is a separate *indication*. Pain, fever, and inflammation are three different indications for aspirin.)

The Enemy: Time

Clearly, the OTC Drug Review was a massive undertaking—much more massive, in fact, than anybody anticipated when it finally got underway in the early 1970s. The original estimate was that the whole job might take three years. *Twenty years* now have gone by, and the OTC Review, according to current estimates, is only about three-quarters finished. At present, it looks like it will take a quarter of a century (a third of a century from passage of the directive Federal legislation) to complete it.

Many explanations, all probably partly correct, have been suggested for the apparent delays: There are a greater number of active ingredients and uses for them than was originally anticipated. There is a larger—and growing—literature to search, and rising mountains of data to be sifted. Maneuvers and appeals by drug makers who are trying to keep their products on the market certainly also have played a role. So, too, have twelve years of pro-business administrations in Washington. They have slowed the OTC Review and other regulatory activities, most notably by keeping the FDA short-staffed and fearful of high-level displeasure and intervention.

This stalling, however, has not yet stopped or seriously compromised the OTC Review. Republicans and Democrats alike understand that Americans, whether they are philosophically for or against government control, *want* to be assured that the drugs they use when ill are as safe and effective as science and government can make them.

The AIDS (Acquired Immune Deficiency Syndrome) epidemic, of course, has been a priority effort at the FDA, as at other federal health agencies. Anti-AIDS medications and powerful new life-or-death prescription drugs for other diseases obviously take precedence, in time and in human effort, over the fine print on a laxative bottle. The OTC Drug Review relies on a staff of fifteen to twenty people. Nevertheless, while the bureaucratic wheels at the FDA grind slowly, they also grind exceedingly small, and the OTC Review creaks onward.

The Review's ultimate goal, of course, is to ban all active ingredients that have not been shown to be safe and effective, and to permit the others to be marketed only in safe and effective dosages, in accurately labeled containers. Eventually, this will happen. Though consumers then will have far fewer types of products to choose from, they will be allowed a greater certainty that these products are safe and effective.

If the OTC Review had been completed quickly, there would have been less need, or perhaps no need at all, for this Guide as it is presently constructed. The huge lags were the spur: This Guide provides the experts' analyses in advance of the FDA's regulatory action. Consumers thus can use this information—*right now*—to enhance their health and well-being. Of course, the OTC Review judgments are tentative until a final decision is published for each ingredient and usage. But these preliminary judgments are the most prudent and authoritative ones available anywhere for consumers who must buy and use medicines *now*.

Stages of the OTC Review

The OTC Drug Review requires these stages for each group of drugs:

1. Evaluation by the expert panels, which write one or more reports. These reports are edited by the FDA, approved by the Panel chairman, and published in the *Federal Register*, the official record of U.S. government transactions. All of the Panel reports now have been published, the last in 1983.

   The Panel reports range in length from a few to hundreds of pages of medico-bureaucratic fine print. The scientific and medical background for each use of each active ingredient is summarized, and the Panel decides if the ingredient is safe, perhaps safe, or unsafe for each purpose for which it is marketed. The Panel also decides if the ingredient is effective, possibly effective, or ineffective for each marketed purpose.

2. Following publication of the *Panel Reports*, as they are called, drug makers, doctors, consumers, and anyone else who cares to, can write to the FDA to comment on each or every decision. Public participation is encouraged. The agency then sifts through these comments, and its staff experts decide, on the basis of scientific evidence, whether they agree or disagree with the comments. These FDA

staffers, from the agency's Center for Drug Evaluation and Research in Rockville, Maryland, then prepare a second-stage document, called (among other names) a *Tentative Final Monograph* (TFM).

The TFMs, of which all but five so far have been published, also appear in the *Federal Register*. They provide the FDA's evaluation of the Panels' decisions. The agency's views may be different, based on new information from the literature, data supplied by drug manufacturers to support their products and claims, and the FDA's re-analysis of the previous data. Legal guidelines for the regulatory process also play an important role. The TFMs are shorter than Panel reports. Each publication contains the FDA's draft of the Federal regulation that eventually will control the marketing of each active ingredient that it anticipates will stay on the market.

3. A second period of commentary and review follows. The FDA then publishes its *Final Monograph* (FM). This document contains a succinct summary and review of changes; and the FDA's explanation for them; and a final version of the new regulation. So far, thirty-six Final Monographs have been published in the *Federal Register*.

4. One year after the *Final Monograph* is published, it becomes effective. This means that all active ingredients that have not been included are banned from interstate commerce. Only the approved dosages of each drug can then be sold, and only approved labeling is permitted. A manufacturer cannot claim that a product relieves a condition that is not listed in the *Final Monograph*.

5. The *Final Monograph* is published in the *Code of Federal Regulations*, the compilation of rules that govern much of Americans' commerce and life. The OTC Drug Review *is* a federal regulatory effort.

Accomplishments of the OTC Review

What has the OTC Review achieved thus far?

In a 1992 report to Congress, FDA officials listed these major advances:

- Many indications for large numbers of ingredients have been banned because no data existed to support them. An additional 415 active ingredients also were due to be banned as this Guide went to press.

- Several types of OTC drugs are already wholly banned. They include aphrodisiacs, drugs to treat non-cancerous prostate conditions, camphorated oil, daytime sedatives, hair growers, hexachlorophene products, wound-healing products used in the mouth, stomach acidifiers, sweet spirits of nitre, and antiperspirant aerosols containing zirconium. These drugs were ruled to be hazardous, useless, or both.

• Companies have been forced to reformulate and/or relabel many brand-name and generic products to conform to the Review's new rules for the safety and effectiveness of commonly used active ingredients. Improvements have been made in drugs for acne, anorectal disorders, antacids, cough medicines, dandruff prevention, expectorants, sleep-aids, and others. "Consumers are, thereby, being provided better-labeled, safer, and more effective products," the Deputy Director of the FDA's Center for Drug Evaluation and Research, Gerald F. Meyer, has told Congress.

• As older, dangerous, and worthless drugs have been removed from druggists' shelves, a number of modern prescription drugs have been re-categorized by the FDA as nonprescription drugs. So far, there have been forty of these "℞ to OTC switches," as they are called in the business. They are an important new health resource.

℞ to OTC Switches

The reclassification of prescription (℞) drugs to nonprescription, or *over-the-counter*, legal status has been a major development associated with the OTC Drug Review. The forty active ingredients that have been recategorized in this way now are formulated into several hundred or more drug products.

In 1992, the Nonprescription Drug Manufacturers Association (NDMA) released a national survey of consumers' attitudes toward these "switch" products. It said that 27 percent of OTC Drug consumers use switch drugs. Half of the respondents said they would select a switch product, if available, over a traditional nonprescription product for the symptom or condition they needed to treat. More than one-third of the respondents cited switch drugs as their first choice for a nonprescription drug.

The active ingredients switched from ℞ to OTC since 1976 are listed in the table on the next page. To assist consumers who may wish to choose switched OTC drugs over more traditional products, the designation "℞ to OTC switch" appears next to them in the *Comments* column of the Product Ratings tables in Units throughout this Guide.

More is known about the switched drugs than about most standard OTC products, since they all have been assessed and monitored for fifteen or twenty years, or longer, under the stringent rules that the FDA applies to prescription drugs. These switch drugs also are more powerful than many traditional remedies. As a result, they may have a greater propensity to cause adverse effects—and consumers who use them should carefully read and follow label directions.

Ingredients Transferred from ℞ to OTC Status by the FDA Since 1976[1]

Ingredient	Purpose
acidulated phosphate fluoride rinse	prevents dental cavities
brompheniramine maleate	dries runny nose, relieves hay fever symptoms
chlophedianol hydrochloride	cough control
chlorpheniramine maleate	dries runny nose, relieves hay fever symptoms
clotrimazole	antifungal;combats yeast infections
dexbrompheniramine maleate	dries runny nose, relieves hay fever symptoms
diphenhydramine hydrochloride	cough control; sleep aid; controls nausea; dries runny nose, relieves hay fever symptoms
diphenhydramine monocitrate	sleep aid
doxylamine succinate	sleep aid; dries runny nose, hay fever
dyclonine hydrochloride	oral anesthetic
ephedrine sulfate	relief of anal itching and pain
epinephrine hydrochloride	relief of anal itching and pain
haloprogin	antifungal
hydrocortisone	relief of itching
hydrocortisone acetate	relief of itching
ibuprofen	relief of pain and fever; anti-inflammatory
loperamide	combats diarrhea
methoxyphenamine hydrochloride	relief of wheezing and shortness of breath in asthma
miconazole nitrate	antifungal; combats yeast infections
oxymetazoline hydrochloride	nasal decongestant; ocular vasoconstrictor
permethrin	kills head lice
phenylephrine hydrochloride	relief of anal itching and pain
phenylpropanolamine hydrochloride	nasal decongestant
potassium iodide	protects thyroid gland in nuclear emergencies
pseudoephedrine hydrochloride	nasal decongestant
pseudoephedrine sulfate	nasal decongestant
pyrantel pamoate	pinworm remedy
sodium fluoride rinse	prevents dental cavities
stannous fluoride gel	prevents dental cavities
stannous fluoride rinse	prevents dental cavities
tioconazole	antifungal
triprolidine hydrochloride	dries runny nose, relieves hay fever symptoms
xylometazoline hydrochloride	nasal decongestant

Sources: Federal Drug Administration, Nonprescription Drug Manufacturers Association

[1]These ingredients are not all currently available in OTC drug products.

A Word About Brand Names and Generics

Many consumers favor brand-name products—the ones advertised on radio, TV, and other media. These consumers of course are *paying* for these ads, which is one reason why brand-name products cost more—sometimes *ten times more*—than medicinally equivalent generic products.

For simple and relatively safe medicines, generic products are as safe and effective as brand-name products, according to the FDA. (In fact, many of the generic medicines are manufactured by brand-name companies or suppliers, and sold in bulk to generic distributing companies.)

This said, many people still prefer to buy drugs from the companies they know. This impulse may have some merit with regard to nonprescription drugs, because it is our impression that the big makers are coming into compliance with the proposed rules formulated by the FDA more quickly than some generic companies and other small, non-brand-name firms. Many of the more outlandish combination products still being marketed at this stage of the OTC Review carry generic labels or relatively obscure brand names.

The brand-name manufacturers probably feel they have better things to do than quibble about questionably safe or questionably effective ingredients, unless of course they are big money-makers, such as the decongestant and weight-loss aid *phenylpropanolamine hydrochloride*, about which safety questions persist.

By the same token, large manufacturers have the research staffs and resources to pay for clinical studies that will bring their products into compliance with the OTC Drug Review rules; they also retain lawyers and regulatory-affairs experts with time and skills to wear down FDA officials, and win some disputed points over the conference table. The big manufacturers also muster political clout; from time to time they appear to be able to use their clout successfully to shape some regulatory decisions to their advantage.

Brand-name manufacturers also can, and do, confuse consumers: One major way they do this is to interchange different ingredients under a single brand-name. Among cough, cold, and pain products, in particular, ingredients shift continually beneath brand names. Many brand names cover several or more significantly, *different* products.

The result is that you must read labels with extreme care to be sure you find the *product* that you set out to buy—the one you specifically need for the symptoms for which you seek relief. Under these circumstances, the purchase of single-ingredient products, and of generic products that are sold under the name of the specific active ingredient(s)—as described and evaluated in this Guide—can lead to more accurate and correct purchases and dosages.

Shortcomings Sketched

What about the OTC Review's and the FDA's shortcomings with regard to OTC drugs?

The major criticism, of course, has been the slow pace of the Review. In their trip up to Capitol Hill in 1992, administrator Meyer and his associates forecast publication of all Final Monographs by January 1, 1995. Similar forecasts have frequently been made in the past.

The pace, of course, is not wholly in the FDA's hands. Final clearance for each step must come from higher-ups in the Department of Health and Human Services (HHS)—who are highly subject to political pressures. Through his efforts with the President's Council on Competitiveness, Vice President Dan Quayle was able to slow the publication of new Federal Regulations early in 1992. One result was that publication of OTC Drug Review Tentative Final and *Final Monographs* in the *Federal Register* came to a virtual standstill. FDA administrator Meyer told Congress that twenty Monographs were due to be published in 1992. By mid-year, only four had appeared.

The OTC Drug Review has been strongly criticized by many drug manufacturers because of its often negative effects on some products—and on costs and sales. Nevertheless, the industry's trade group, the NDMA, supports the broad scope of this drug reform, even as it hotly contests many of the FDA's specific decisions.

Consumers, and consumer-oriented congressmen and organizations, have criticized some specific decisions that seem to favor drug makers over consumers. The actions that have caused greatest concern are: the preliminary decision to allow antihistamines to be sold in cough-cold remedies, the FDA's failure to limit or ban the use of *phenylpropanolamine* (PPA) as a nasal decongestant and an appetite suppressant, and the long delay in banning guar gum products that were promoted as weight-loss aids. Some guar gum users suffered blocked food pipes (esophagi) from these products, and at least one person eventually died of complications.

Reasons for This Guide

This Guide was conceived in 1977, when the huge *Panel Report* on OTC pain-relievers such as aspirin and acetaminophen had just been published. The first edition was published by Harper & Row, in 1983, as *The Essential Guide to Nonprescription Drugs*.

The aim was to update it fairly frequently, to keep consumers abreast of developments and changes as the OTC Review progressed. Unfortunately, this agenda could not be met. A decade has passed since the first edition appeared.

Now, in preparing this new, second edition, under a new title, for Gale Research Inc. and Visible Ink Press, much catch-up work has been necessary. This edition is identical in concept to the first, but the passage of time and progress in the OTC Review have wrought some changes.

What the Guide Contains

The Guide is constructed by digging out and rearranging the data in the OTC
Review, as presented in FDA documents published in the *Federal Register*.
Here, these data are strictly organized in *Units*—which also can be thought of
as *chapters*—on groups of drugs that can be purchased to prevent or relieve
specific conditions such as acne, headache and other pain, constipation, and
sunburn. After a brief introduction to each condition and an explanation of
methods to self-diagnose it, the available nonprescription drugs are described
generally. Then the specific uses or *indications* for these drugs, as defined by
the FDA, are given, along with the principal warnings that the agency has or
soon will require on the product labels. Not all *warnings* are listed in this text.
A consumer who purchases an OTC product should *always* carefully read—
and heed—all warnings on the label.

The individual active ingredients in the drugs and products covered in
the Unit are then briefly described; major attention is directed to their safety
and their effectiveness—the two criteria upon which FDA approval (or disap-
proval) is based. All active ingredients are arranged in three categories:
Approved, which means that the active ingredient is safe and effective at the
approved dosage(s); *Conditionally approved*, which means that the active
ingredients' safety or effectiveness, or both, have not been proved; or, finally,
a *Disapproved* category. Ingredients in this last group are unsafe, ineffective,
or both. The FDA plans to ban these disapproved ingredients from interstate
commerce unless manufacturers or others quickly produce convincing scientific evidence that would lead the agency's drug evaluators to change their minds.

The categorization of all active ingredients in the text of each Unit, and
in the summary tables such as *Safety and Effectiveness: Active Ingredients in
Over-the-Counter Drugs for Pain, Fever and Rheumatic Symptoms*, are based
strictly on the most recent assessment of each ingredient in the OTC Drug
Review. This Guide contains the current FDA assessment for each use of each
over-the-counter active ingredient that is being assessed in the OTC Review,
insofar as I have been able to locate and present the assessment.

How Products Are Rated

Product labels do not carry evaluations; the only sources of this information
are the FDA and this Guide. It should be added that while the *safe and effective* ingredients are fairly clear cut, some confusion exists as to whether a few
lower-rated ingredients belong in the "conditionally approved" or "disapproved" categories.

Certainly every consumer will want to purchase only medications that
contain safe and effective active ingredients. The purpose of this Guide is to
facilitate the choice of a safe and effective product every time a nonprescription drug is purchased.

To this end, a selection of drug products is evaluated at the end of most Units in Product Ratings tables. These Ratings directly reflect the OTC Drug Review evaluations of these products' ingredients. They also reflect my *interpretation* of these FDA evaluations.

The Product Ratings are based on the ingredients and on the product's intended uses. The accuracy of the label claims, which also is of concern to the FDA in the OTC Review, has *not* been considered in these ratings. (But products that do not make medicinal claims on the label have not been rated, *even if they contain medicinally active ingredients*. This applies particularly to some cosmetics.)

For most OTC drug products, the FDA requires or eventually will require an accurate listing of the dosage or concentration of each active ingredient. The "strength" is also required on labels by state pharmacy laws in 46 of the 50 states. Neither the federal nor state laws are fully enforced. (A few drug products, particularly fluoride toothpastes, may be exempt from this requirement under federal law.)

The NDMA, whose 72 active member companies account for about 95 percent of all OTC sales, also favors specific dosage information. "We do that voluntarily," NDMA Public Relations Director John T. Walden said.

My belief is that consumers need to know both the active ingredients and their dosages or concentrations in order to make informed decisions on whether to buy and how to use a nonprescription drug product. Therefore, products that fail to provide this information will be downgraded one rank because of the deficit.

The ratings are as follows:

A   means the product is safe and effective according to my interpretation of the OTC Review evaluation of its active ingredient(s).

B   means the active ingredient(s) is/are possibly safe and effective, according to my interpretation, but that the data to prove either safety or efficacy still are wanting.

C   means the product is not safe and effective, according to OTC Review criteria, based on its active ingredient(s).

Some groups of drugs—for example, anti-plaque dental products—have not yet been assessed by the FDA, so no Product Ratings are possible as yet. Generally speaking, however, the Food, Drug and Cosmetic Act assigns manufacturers the obligation of providing positive evidence that a product, or the ingredient(s) upon which it is based, is or are safe and effective. Lacking this evidence, the FDA categorizes a product or ingredient as *not generally recognized as safe and effective*, and sooner or later the FDA will ban it. Reciprocally, a manufacturer cannot legally market a product that has not won FDA approval, except under certain specific—and complex—conditions.

Single Ingredient *vs.* Combination Products

Nonprescription drug products can be divided into two major classes: *single-ingredient products*, which contain one active ingredient (an aspirin tablet, for example) and *combination products* that contain two or more such ingredients (*Excedrin P.M.* [Bristol-Myers], for example, which contains both the pain and fever reliever acetaminophen and the antihistamine and cough reliever *diphenhydramine hydrochloride).*

The philosophy of the OTC Drug Review has been—and to a significant degree still is—that, generally speaking, fewer is better, and a single active ingredient is best. Single-ingredient products are safer because they carry the risk of only one set of side effects. They also are safer because they help consumers identify the lowest effective dose of one drug that is capable of relieving the distress that they feel.

Nonprescription drug makers, however, maintain a different outlook: Hundreds, perhaps thousands of them are using the same, limited group of active ingredients in their products. So there is an understandable tendency to mix some of this and some of that in order to create an identifiable, reliable—and promotable—combination of these common ingredients.

Under the OTC Drug Review procedures, manufacturers are required to show that *each* ingredient in a combination is safe and effective, by itself, and that each makes a clear therapeutic contribution to the combination product, without negating the others or unduly enhancing their risks. These rules have cut back on the number of active ingredients in many types of products. If the goals of the physicians and other medical specialists who made up the expert panels are realized (and it is not yet clear that they will be) the OTC marketplace will shift significantly in the direction of single-ingredient products as the Review moves toward completion.

Reflecting this trend in the OTC Review, an effort has been made to list single-ingredient products in the *Product Ratings*, particularly for ingredients the FDA says are safe and effective. The hope is to list the name or indicate the existence of one or more single-ingredient brand-name or generic products for each safe and effective active ingredient. (Some safe and effective ingredients are not currently available in OTC products, however.)

Combination products continue to be useful and appealing to many consumers, so an effort has also been made to identify combinations that meet the FDA's criteria for safety and efficacy. These criteria are described in the texts of some Units, and in other Units are summarized in tables such as the one **Safety and Effectiveness: Combination Products Sold Over-the-Counter for the Care of the Eyes**. It should be noted, however, that while the specifications for Approved (safe and effective) products are fairly clear, the OTC Review guidelines that differentiate **Conditionally Safe and Effective** from **Unsafe or Ineffective** combinations are less so. One reason is that the FDA plans to ban combination products in both categories and so is not paying its greatest attention to the differences between them. This lack of clarity could result in misinterpretations in the *Product Ratings* for combination products, although I have tried to avoid them.

Note: For combinations, as well as for single-ingredient products that are rated B or C, at least one reason for the down-rating is provided in the adjacent column, under *Comment*.

More than 900 brand-name products and types of generic products are listed, with single-ingredient products favored, for the reasons cited previously. A large percentage of the products are taken from the original edition of this Guide, and all have been checked against current reference sources (*see* Sources). Additionally, an effort has been made to list and assess the most popular and widely sold brand-name products. This has been done by including "best-sellers" listed by the trade publication *Chain Drug Review* (January 1, 1992) as a source for the highest-earning products in major categories, as determined in market research by Racher Press and by Towne Oller & Associates. Since a brand-name, such as *Mylanta* (Johnson & Johnson-Merck) or *Tylenol* (McNeil-CPC), may cover a variety of *different* formulations in a variety of dosage forms (tablets, liquids, and others), an effort has been made to list two or three products—but by no means all of them—for the best-sellers.

A major thrust in OTC drug marketing is in the newer, R̨-to-OTC switch products. Using data from the NDMA and from the FDA "Orange Book" (*Approved Drug Products*, 12th edition, with updates through March, 1992), an effort has been made to include one or more examples of all R̨-to-OTC switch drugs.

I purchased, retail, approximately one hundred individual OTC drug products during the first half of 1992, and I have used the label information in the Product Ratings. I scanned advertisements in consumer and medical publications for new and unusual products. The effort has been to provide a representative selection of products available on the OTC marketplace.

A word needs to be said about the *inactive* ingredients in nonprescription drugs: A nonprescription drug label may list a half dozen or more ingredients, most of which have no medicinal benefit, even though they have long and imposing-sounding names. Only the *active ingredients* (the ones that have a medicinal effect) count in assessing a drug's safety and effectiveness.

Labels should give active ingredients first, and should designate them as "active ingredient(s)." In my view, consumers are best served—and should purchase when possible—products that list them in a larger type or in some other distinctive way so that there is no mistaking what the active ingredients are.

When the first edition of this Guide was published in 1983, most classes of drugs still were in the Advisory Review Panel stage. Today, many Final Monographs have been published as the last step in the regulatory process, pending later amendments. Thousands of hours of work and deliberation are crystallized in these regulations.

This constitutes progress in the OTC Drug Review. It has one downside: The Panel Reports, beyond their immediate purpose of providing regulatory recommendations to the FDA, are filled with interesting facts about drugs and diseases and much information. Each new step of the OTC Review—from *Panel Report* to *Tentative Final* to *Final Monograph* and entry of the *Final Rule* into the *Code of Federal Regulations*—eliminates non-regulatory information until, finally, none is left. For this reason, the present edition of this Guide, more than the first, has been supplemented with fresh health information from other authoritative sources—principally government reports and medical journals—as well as some late updates from journalistic sources, including interviews. My aim was to keep the book interesting, as well as informative. It must be stressed, however, that the judgments of active ingredients and their combinations strictly follow the OTC Review insofar as is possible.

In a few places where the Guide's advisors, particularly research physicians, or I disagree with the FDA's current stance on an ingredient, we provide dissenting views. But the judgments rendered—*safe and effective* or not—are strictly the FDA's.

(The FDA's second thoughts about phenylpropanolamine hydrochloride [PPA] as a nasal decongestant, as indicated in its long-deferred tentative ruling on this ingredient, is interpreted here as meaning that the agency now has doubts about this drug's safety. Accordingly, it will be treated here as only conditionally approved—with its safety still to be determined.)

One additional change has been made: A short section has been added at the end of many Units to suggest alternative avenues through which you can seek relief—usually through doctors—if nonprescription drugs fail to satisfactorily resolve a given condition. This section is called **When Further Relief Is Needed**.

This Guide does not cover homeopathic medications that are sold over-the-counter, unless they were submitted to the OTC Drug Review. The FDA has developed a special, looser set of rules for homeopathic preparations, few—if any—of which are likely to meet the OTC Review's standards. Hence, unless and until they are evaluated in this way, they are not safe and effective according to the FDA's definitions upon which this Guide is based.

A handful of nonprescription drugs appears to have escaped OTC review scrutiny. These drugs are not safe and effective, according to OTC Review criteria, and it can be assumed that sooner or later the FDA will ban them. By the same token, the wide variety of natural, herbal, and nutritional preparations that are outside the FDA's regulatory purview for OTC Drugs can only be considered as *not safe and effective*.

Consumers, of course, are free to buy and use them. But they must understand that in so doing they are ignoring the regulatory safeguards that, more and more, are assuring the safety and effectiveness of nonprescription drugs that are assessed in the OTC Drug Review.

Assessing the OTC Review

The question will inevitably come to mind: How successful has the OTC Drug Review been? Has it justified its cost to taxpayers of some $40 million, and of $125 million to manufacturers—which they may have passed on to consumers?

Many of the benefits are described above. I also can see a few unfortunate consequences:

One is that while regulatory assurances of safety and effectiveness now are being extended from prescription drugs to nonprescription ones, a third class of still-unregulated products is showing significant strength and growth. This includes folk remedies, herbal medicines, and vitamins and other nutrients that are widely promoted and sold through health food stores, vitamin stores, catalogues, and other retail outlets.

This marketing is done through loopholes in the FD&C Act; for example, extravagant medicinal claims are made that vitamins prevent or cure cancer, heart disease, and other serious illness. But these claims are not made on the product labels themselves. This makes it difficult for the FDA to take legal action to stop these sales.

By making traditional nonprescription drugs into products that must meet medical and scientific regulatory standards, the FDA and its supporters may be encouraging the growth of this rogue third group of products. Many Americans presently distrust science, medicine, and government. Many suppliers and health gurus stand ready to exploit these feelings by providing "drug" products that have not been shown to be safe and effective for the purposes for which they are sold.

The OTC Drug Review has forced nonprescription drugs into the pharmacologic mainstream. Major companies that have the resources to provide the studies the FDA demands on safety and efficacy certainly are playing an ever-increasing role in this market, to the exclusion of small and less well-heeled start-ups and privately owned companies. The safety, efficacy, and quality control of OTC products is likely to be improving as the result. But the little guy, the small company, has a far more difficult road to travel to get a product into the market. It is hard to count this as an advantage in a country that values individual initiative.

Many drugs now winning large market share in the OTC field are the "switch" drugs that major pharmaceutical makers sold for seventeen years or longer as ℞ items—until their patents ran out. "Switching" may provide some additional, extended patent protection. But there may be this rub to it: In order to market OTC, the companies may redefine the indications for these drugs, since the FDA does not allow treatments for major organs and organ systems to be marketed OTC (exceptions include bronchodilators for asthma; insulin for diabetes).

This means "switch" drug makers may have to find less serious conditions for which to sell the switch drugs OTC. To take one example, manufacturers hope to convert several special antihistamine drugs (H_2 blockers), that long have been used—profitably and with some medicinal success—to treat ulcers in the stomach and small intestine, into OTC remedies for heartburn. They can conduct clinical trials that probably will convince the FDA that these drugs do, in fact, relieve heartburn. But my skeptical view is that if the switch drugs in fact are useful for a new nonprescription purpose, then they should have been marketed explicitly for that purpose years ago, as prescription drugs. The fact that they were not raises my index of suspicion about late efforts to convert them to OTC's based on new indications.

In short, I think there is some cause for concern that Ŗ-to-OTC switches encourage recycling of older drugs, often at lower doses. If the buyers and users of nonprescription drugs are to be well served by drug makers, I think the industry and the FDA ought to find ways to facilitate development and marketing of *wholly new* drugs specifically for self-treatment. It does not seem right that consumers must wait 17 or 20 years, or longer, for prescriptions to be spun off as OTC's in order to buy and use them in treating their self-diagnosable symptoms and illnesses.

With these caveats, it is my belief that the OTC Drug Review—summarized here in what I hope is consumer-friendly fashion (*See* **How to Use This Guide**, pp. vii-xi)—benefits the American public.

A number of years ago, the publishers of the *Physicians Desk Reference for Nonprescription Drugs*—which is an industry-supported drug guide prepared principally for doctors—wrote:

"The FDA's OTC Drug Review is unprecedented—for this or any other industry—in its scope, its thoroughness and its openness. It is probably the most extensive scrutiny of an industry's product ever conducted."

I agree.

New York, NY
August 1992
David R. Zimmerman

WARNING FOR PREGNANT WOMEN AND NURSING MOTHERS

Women who are pregnant, believe they may be pregnant, or are nursing a baby should not take many kinds of nonprescription drugs, or should use them only under a doctor's direction. Note that specific warnings for pregnant and nursing women have not been included in many entries in this Guide.

If you are pregnant, or think that you may be, or if you are nursing, always read carefully the WARNING section on the label of any nonprescription drug product before you take it, or ask your doctor.

LABELS ON NONPRESCRIPTION DRUGS

The labels on R drugs provide very little information. The FDA requires that OTC drug labels be much more detailed and informative so that consumers can properly use these products without a health professional's advice. For this reason, explains the Nonprescription Drug Manufacturers Association (NMDA), the industry trade group and the companies it represents have been working with the government for half a century "to assure adequate labeling of OTC [drug]s." The NDMA says labels include (or should include) this information:

- Product name and statement of identity
- Active ingredients
- Inactive ingredients
- Name and location of manufacturer, distributor, or packer
- Net quantity of contents
- Description of tamper-resistant features
- Indications for use
- Directions and dosage instructions
- Warnings, cautionary statements, and drug interaction precautions (if any)
- Expiration date and lot or batch code

The following label contains consumer information required by the FDA and/or included under the industry's voluntary regulation program, according to NDMA.

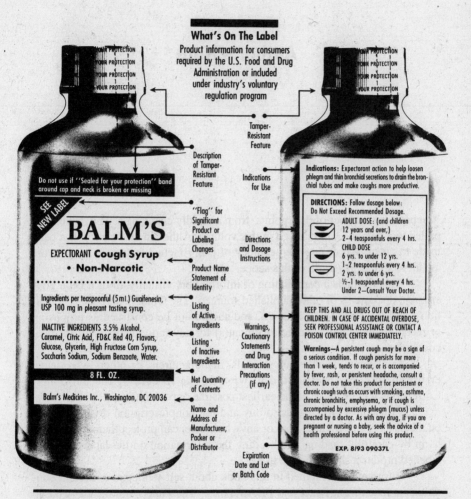

What's On The Label
Product information for consumers required by the U.S. Food and Drug Administration or included under industry's voluntary regulation program

Tamper-Resistant Feature

Do not use if "Sealed for your protection" band around cap and neck is broken or missing

SEE NEW LABEL

BALM'S

EXPECTORANT Cough Syrup
• Non-Narcotic

Ingredients per teaspoonful (5 ml.) Guaifenesin, USP 100 mg in pleasant tasting syrup.

INACTIVE INGREDIENTS 3.5% Alcohol, Caramel, Citric Acid, FD&C Red 40, Flavors, Glucose, Glycerin, High Fructose Corn Syrup, Saccharin Sodium, Sodium Benzoate, Water.

8 FL. OZ.

Balm's Medicines Inc., Washington, DC 20036

Description of Tamper-Resistant Feature

Indications for Use

"Flag" for Significant Product or Labeling Changes

Product Name Statement of Identity

Listing of Active Ingredients

Listing of Inactive Ingredients

Net Quantity of Contents

Name and Address of Manufacturer, Packer or Distributor

Directions and Dosage Instructions

Warnings, Cautionary Statements and Drug Interaction Precautions (if any)

Expiration Date and Lot or Batch Code

Indications: Expectorant action to help loosen phlegm and thin bronchial secretions to drain the bronchial tubes and make coughs more productive.

DIRECTIONS: Follow dosage below: Do Not Exceed Recommended Dosage.
ADULT DOSE: (and children 12 years and over,)
2–4 teaspoonfuls every 4 hrs.
CHILD DOSE
6 yrs. to under 12 yrs.
1–2 teaspoonfuls every 4 hrs.
2 yrs. to under 6 yrs.
½–1 teaspoonful every 4 hrs.
Under 2—Consult Your Doctor.

KEEP THIS AND ALL DRUGS OUT OF REACH OF CHILDREN. IN CASE OF ACCIDENTAL OVERDOSE, SEEK PROFESSIONAL ASSISTANCE OR CONTACT A POISON CONTROL CENTER IMMEDIATELY.

Warnings—A persistent cough may be a sign of a serious condition. If cough persists for more than 1 week, tends to recur, or is accompanied by fever, rash, or persistent headache, consult a doctor. Do not take this product for persistent or chronic cough such as occurs with smoking, asthma, chronic bronchitis, emphysema, or if cough is accompanied by excessive phlegm (mucus) unless directed by a doctor. As with any drug, if you are pregnant or nursing a baby, seek the advice of a health professional before using this product.

EXP. 8/93 09037L

Whereas prescription drug labels for the patient carry minimal information, FDA requires that OTC labels be much more detailed so that consumers can properly use the products without the advice of a health professional.

Source: NDMA, with permission.

Author's Note

An enormous number of data points, from a rapidly changing screen, have been pulled together and summarized in this volume. Although every effort has been made to check and ensure the accuracy of every factual statement here, errors are inevitable in any work of this scope.

This Guide is a compilation of information, virtually all of it from government documents or other published sources. The Guide's purpose is educational and informational. It is not, and should not be construed as proposing or recommending any specific treatment(s) for any individuals or for medical conditions.

Consumers, health professionals, manufacturers, or others who detect errors in this text are invited to write to me in care of the publisher. Corrections will be made at the earliest possible opportunity.

Consumers who decide to buy and use nonprescription drugs, whether on the basis of information here or anywhere else, can protect themselves from harm by carefully reading and heeding the information on the labels. Poorly labelled products should not be used.

Information contained in this book about self-treatment of certain conditions is taken from Panel and FDA reports. The Panels and the FDA based their recommendations on what is generally suitable for the average individual. Before using the information in this book you should take into account your personal medical history and be aware of the basis on which the recommendations have been made. Also be aware that some individuals have idiosyncratic (that is to say, out of the ordinary) reactions to some medication. In addition, any individual should carefully monitor self-treatment of any condition, keeping in mind that over-the-counter drugs are *medicines* and should be used with care and according to label directions. If any condition for which you are treating yourself persists, professional care should be sought.

Finally, an individual who has a chronic condition or who is taking medication under a doctor's direction for any reason should always seek medical advice before engaging in any course of self-treatment.

I have chosen, in as random a manner as I could devise, the brand name and generic products for evaluation in the Product Ratings that conclude most Units. These products were also selected in an effort to represent products from a variety of manufacturers.

These ratings represent my own opinion of individual brand-name and generic products, based on the latest findings of the independent OTC Review Panels and the FDA about the active ingredients and combinations of active ingredients contained in these products.

I have no interest in any company that manufactures, distributes, or sells over-the-counter drugs.

D.R. Zimmerman

Symptoms Index

• a 't' appearing next to a page number denotes table

N

Nasal congestion, in allergy, 24-25; during a cold, 131t, 132
Nausea, 298, 467; dysmenorrhea and, 711; and motion sickness, 733

O

Odor, of breath, 742; of ostomy, 271; of underarm, 85; vaginal, 330
Overindulgence, in food and drink, 466

P

Pain, abdominal, 318; anorectal, 483t; of arthritis, 780; burning, in lower throat and chest, 58; chronic, 790; dull, 640; during ear care, 355; fever, and inflammation, 759-760; of fungal infections, 580; menstrual, 710; of skin, 550-552; in tooth, 956-957
Perspiration, 84-86; severe, 92
Phlegm, 148; and asthma, 102; and cough, 135
Pimple, acne, 5; of herpes, 211
Pink eye, 367
Poison ivy-oak-sumac, 821
Premenstrual distress, 710
Pressure, abdominal, 318; intestinal, 78
Prickly heat, 273
Psoriasis, 847

R

Rash, bright red, irritating, 273; with cough, 140; diaper, 273; in fungal infection, 580; itching of, 551; of poison-ivy-oak-sumac, 813; of

seborrheic dermatitis, 259
Red eye, 365

S

Scalp, inflammation, of cradle cap, 247; scales 251-252; sores, 654
Shortness of breath, and asthma, 102
Sinus congestion, 131, 132
Skin, chafed, cracked, or windburned, 967t; darkened patches of, 113; eruption, 119; irritation, 550-551; sunburned, 909; wrinkled, 522, 909; wounds, 415, 427
Sleeplessness, in children, 1029; persistent, 875
Sneezing, 151; during a cold, 131t, 132
Sore, anal, 480; corneal, 368; at edge of mouth or nose, 210; inside mouth, 212; on scalp, 654
Sore gums, 661, 662
Sore joints, 765
Sore throat, 132
Sour stomach, 54, 58, 79, 320t
Stomachache, 316, 467
Stuffed-up nose, in allergy, 24-25; during a cold, 133, 162-163; in rhinitis, 135
Sunburn, 909; minor, 967t; pain of, 552; severe, 925
Sweating, *see also* Perspiration; excessive, 85, 91; heavy, 1014; and shock, 415
Swelling, anorectal, 479, 480, 483t; around toenail, 525; on big toe, 240; of bite or sting, 531; of cornea, 396; of nasal tissues, 163

T

Tear insufficiency, 364, 388-389
Tearing, 365

Acne Medications

There is no single disease which causes more emotional injury, more maladjustment between parents and children, more general insecurity and feelings of inferiority, and greater sums of emotional suffering than does acne.
—Marion B. Sulzberger, M.D.

The principal sufferers of acne are teenagers, for whom, in particular, this report on nonprescription acne medications is written.

Older persons with deep, pitting acne that will not go away by now know most of the simple facts about this disease. They should be under a dermatologist's care, as should any younger person who is or thinks he or she is suffering from severe acne. Women in their twenties and thirties who develop patches of tiny but unsightly red raised bumps on their chins and foreheads probably can blame the cosmetics they use. If a change from oil-based to water-based products and the avoidance of face creams does not bring relief after six or eight weeks, these

ACNE MEDICATIONS is based on the report "Topical Acne Drug Products for OTC Human Use," by the FDA's Advisory Review Panel on OTC Antimicrobial Drug Products (Antimicrobial II Panel); on the FDA's two Tentative Final Monographs, Notice(s) of Proposed Rulemaking; and on FDA's Final Rule and Monograph on these products.

women too should probably see a dermatologist.

There are few teenagers who have not been bothered—indeed, mortified—by the sudden emergence of a pimple or another blemish before an important social event. The Panel and the FDA have important news for them. Unfortunately not all of it is good news.

Bad news: Acne cannot be cured.

Good news: It can be effectively treated in most individuals.

Bad news: Treatment can be long and costly: Many effective medications work slowly and are available only by prescription, and their use must be monitored by a doctor.

Good news: Simple self-care steps and one or two nonprescription drugs can be used to clear up or significantly improve many cases of acne.

Bad news: No method is effective against all acne cases. Each young person needs individualized treatment, which may consist of nonprescription drugs, prescription drugs, other measures, or a combination of all available remedies.

Good news: Many of the old myths about what causes acne have no basis in fact, and so no longer need to concern adolescents.

Bad news: Many of the drugs that have been heavily promoted for self-treatment of acne are worthless. Some may even be dangerous and should be crossed off the list by teenagers who are deciding which products to buy. The following discussion should help them assess the products available.

Claims

Accurate

- "For the treatment (or management) of acne"
- "Dries and clears acne blemishes"
- "Clears blackheads"
- "Clears up most whiteheads"
- "Helps clear acne pimples"
- "Penetrates pores to eliminate most blackheads and acne pimples"
- "Helps keep skin clear of new acne whiteheads"
- "Helps prevent new blackheads and acne pimples"
- "Helps prevent new acne pimples"

Unproved

- "Antibacterial" (germ-killing activity not yet proved)
- "Kills acne bacteria and helps clear acne pimples"
- "Penetrates follicles [or pores] to kill bacteria associated with acne"
- "Reduces the bacterial products associated with the irritation of acne"

False or Misleading

- Modifiers such as "prompt" or "fast"
- "Clears up more pimples faster"
- "Works fast against surface pimples"
- "Clinically proven for prompt effective relief of acne"
- "Makes externally caused skin flareups look better while they're getting better"
- "Helps involute inflamed pustules"
- "Fights acne pimples"
- "Kills facial germs"
- "Strips away oils and waxy buildup that can lead to pimples and blackheads"
- "Helps prevent the reinfection of pimples"
- "Hypoallergenic"
- "An effective antimicrobial against a wide variety of both gram negative and gram positive bacteria and fungi"
- "Helps heal and clear acne by molecular action"
- "Produces a soft, light peeling of the skin"
- "Contains time-proved ingredients"

WARNING:

 All over-the-counter acne medications are for external use only. None are to be taken by mouth. Using other topical acne products at the same time or immediately following use of this product may increase dryness or irritation of the skin. If this occurs, only one medication should be used unless directed by a doctor.

Myths and Facts About Acne

A lot has been learned about acne in recent years. So it is time to squelch some of the myths about the disorder, on the basis of research cited by the Panel. Here are the facts:

- Chocolate and "junk foods" do not cause acne nor make it worse, and for the most part other foods do not either. New theories about diet and skin blemishes pop up all the time and then, after a few years, are shot down by scientific studies. Unless there is some food that you, individually, find will routinely cause your face to break out, you should stop worrying about your choice of foods. On the other hand, one study suggests that either overeating or undereating—in terms of *quantity*—may cause acne in boys, though it seems not to in girls.

- Neither too little nor too much sex is responsible for acne. Neither does it matter what kind of sex you are getting—or not getting.

- Soap and water will not cure acne. Adults may tell adolescents it will, but the Panel sides with kids who say, "No, it won't!" Simply leaving acne alone is no better. Treatment with drugs, which may have to continue for many months, will probably be needed.

- Three out of four teenagers have some acne, and in one in every four the condition is moderate to severe.

- Facial acne is as common in teenaged girls as it is in boys. It starts earlier in girls, but is less severe.

- Half of the teenagers who have acne say they are bothered by it, and more than half treat their faces in one way or another. But only one in ten teenagers has consulted a doctor.

- Moderate to severe acne is more common in white adolescents than in black adolescents. But mild acne—that is, blackheads and whiteheads but no inflammation—is more common in blacks.

- The more "nervous" an adolescent is, the more likely it is that he or she will suffer from acne. Moments of high stress—when a teenager wants things under control—tend to be just those moments when, infuriatingly, a blemish appears.

Why Acne Develops

The increased production of sex hormones in adolescence is the principal stimulus for acne. Androgens (male sex hormones), particularly testosterone, are to blame.

The androgens circulate through the body in the bloodstream, in both males and females, and act upon tiny glands in the pores (or hair follicles) of the skin. These are called the *sebaceous glands*, and their principal function is to secrete the oily substance called *sebum*. Sebum naturally softens and lubricates the skin. When the sebaceous glands are stimulated by testosterone, they produce more sebum—which is discharged through a duct into the hair follicle and then moved outward to the skin's surface. Sebaceous glands are most numerous on the face, shoulders, and upper back—areas where acne tends to develop. People with acne may have larger sebaceous glands than persons whose skins remains clear. It has also been shown that the more sebum the glands secrete, the more severe the acne.

If sebum simply flowed on outward to the skin, where it could be wiped away, it would pose no problems. But there are complicating factors. A "plug" can form in the pore. The plug consists of sebum and dead skin cells and may also contain bacteria, hair fragments, and other debris. As more material accumulates, these plugs swell into *pimples*, which are small, inflamed bumps.

In this initial stage, as a small, white bump, this plug is called a *whitehead*. If some of the accumulated material pushes outward and develops a black tip, the plug is called a *blackhead*. The black color appears to come from the skin pigment *melanin*.

Blackheads and whiteheads are bad enough, but there may be worse to come. Enter here several species of microorganisms, the best known of which is called *Propionibacterium acnes*, or *P. acnes* for short. The microorganism *P. acnes* lives on the skin and seems to dote upon sebum, which it eats. It releases enzymes that break sebum down into greasy substances called *free fatty acids*.

These acids are extremely irritating. When these acids leak or burst out of whiteheads or blackheads into surrounding tissues, the acids provoke an inflammatory reaction. The tissue reddens, and red-colored blemishes—flaws—appear in the skin. Affected areas may feel painful, irritated, or itchy. Swelling occurs. Rubbing, pushing, or scratching the blemish only increases the inflammation.

Because *P. acnes* bacteria are infectious organisms, the body mobilizes its defense forces—including white blood cells—to fight them. Many white blood cells die in combat; their remains are pus. This explains why many pimples develop greenish-white heads before they finally break open and drain or recede gradually back into the body.

In some cases the inflammation fails to subside. Then irregular red blemishes called *nodules* develop on the face and form scars. Cosmetic surgery may be required to remove or reduce them.

This, in brief, is how Panel members and other experts believe acne starts and progresses. But many questions remain unanswered, and these theories will change as new information becomes available.

Treatments for Acne

Early treatment may reduce the severity of the disease. But, reviewers caution, there is no evidence that any treatment program built around scrubs or soaps and other nonprescription products—or anything else— can wholly prevent acne.

Left alone, most blemishes will vanish within two to four weeks. A drug that shortens this recovery time is, according to the experts, effective in *treating* acne. A drug that reduces the number of new eruptions between week four and eight of the treatment is *protectively* beneficial as well. Evaluators say that drugs that are effective in treating acne will also prevent new eruptions.

Effective acne treatment slows the cellular turnover rate and the accumulation of cellular debris in the pores; slows the production of sebum; and kills or inhibits *P. acnes* and other microorganisms in the pores. These actions stifle the inflammatory activity of the enzymes they produce.

There are several safe and effective methods now used in efforts to treat acne:

Applying these nonprescription drugs to the skin:

- SALICYLIC ACID 0.5 to 2 percent in a cream, gel, lotion or ointment
- SULFUR 3 to 10 percent
- SULFUR-RESORCINOL COMBINATIONS

Applying these prescription drugs to the skin:

- ANTIBIOTICS (clindamycin, erythromycin, tetracycline)

- *TRETINOIN* (vitamin A acid)

Taking these prescription drugs internally:

- *ANTIBIOTICS* (tetracycline, erythromycin, minocycline)
- *CORTICOSTEROIDS*
- *ESTROGENS*
- *13-CIS RETINOIC ACID*, sold by prescription as *Accutane* (Roche Dermatologics), for severe cystic acne, if used with *scrupulous* care, as directed by a physician

Using these skin treatments:

- *ACNE SURGERY* (comedo extraction and lancing of pimples)
- *DERMABRASION* (skin peeling)
- *FIBRIN INJECTIONS TO BUILD UP CONCAVE SCARS*
- *FREEZING* (cryotherapy with carbon dioxide in the form of dry ice or slush, or with liquid nitrogen)
- *STEROID INJECTIONS INTO ACNE NODULES AND CYSTS*

Only nonprescription drug treatments are assessed here. If such a product does not work satisfactorily, or if you feel you might do better with more intensive therapy, then the person to see is your pediatrician or adolescent-medicine specialist, your family doctor, or, preferably, a dermatologist. The key thing to remember is that many of the methods discussed here do work, but only if you adhere religiously to the treatment plan that you—or you and your doctor—have decided to try. Then, you must give the program enough time (weeks or even months) to become effective.

First Aid for Pimples

A few methods are available to provide fast clearance of one or two large, ugly pimples or of large blackheads or whiteheads. The bad stuff can often be forced out by using a tool called a *comedo extractor*. It can be bought at a drugstore.

Dermatologists are of two minds about this pimple-squeezing tool. Some warn that it is dangerous, because the infected material may be forced back into the bloodstream and carried to other parts of the body. They particularly warn against squeezing pimples that erupt in the triangular area between the top of the nose and the corners of the mouth, because some of the underlying blood vessels drain directly into the brain.

Not all dermatologists take this dire view, however. At least one nationally known skin doctor has said it is safe to carefully drain these lesions using a comedo extractor. The middle course—if a really important social event looms—is to schedule an emergency visit with a dermatologist, and let him "squeeze" the pimple for you. Another alternative is temporarily covering up the blemish with special cover-up makeup that is available for this purpose.

Abrasive Scrubs

A wide variety of anti-acne soaps, pastes, and cleansers contain mildly abrasive substances such as *polyethylene granules*. These abrasives are very popular, perhaps because they provide something one can *do* about acne: scrub out clogged pores.

The studies that have been conducted on these ingredients are inconclusive, however. One researcher found in a 10-year study of 1000 patients that aluminum oxide fused to soap paste was the most effective of several abrasives. But he failed to keep accurate blemish counts between those patients who used this abrasive system and those who didn't. The researcher said that scrubbing with an abrasive replaces the urge to pick and squeeze the pimples, which could be an advantage.

Two other highly regarded acne specialists carefully tested five abrasive preparations in patients with moderate to conspicuous whiteheads and blackheads. None of the abrasives provided a clinically significant benefit. The abrasives all reduced the number of pimples, whiteheads, and blackheads in the first weeks of treatment. But some test subjects ended up with *more* of these blemishes after eight weeks than they had when they started.

Because acne sufferers' skin is sensitive to physical injury, the researchers warned against use of abrasives.

The Panel's view is that abrasives such as polyethylene "do not have an effect on acne lesions." The FDA agrees that they are not safe and effective drugs. Products that claim to remove oil or cleanse the skin now are judged by the FDA (and by federal law) to be cosmetics, *not* drugs—and so fall outside the purview of the OTC Drug Review, which is summarized in this book.

Will Zinc Supplements Help?

One popular self-treatment for acne is zinc tablets taken by mouth. These tablets can be obtained from drug- or health-food stores. Zinc is an essential trace element; the body needs about 15 mg per day, and most people get at least this amount in their diets.

A person who takes three 220-mg tablets of zinc sulfate daily to treat acne is getting 150 mg of elemental zinc, or 10 times the daily requirement. This may lead to unpleasant side effects, including nausea, vomiting, stomach cramps, and diarrhea.

Although a dietary deficiency of zinc has been shown to cause acne, Panel members doubt that large numbers of teenage Americans are zinc-deficient, and there is no good explanation of how zinc supplements relieve this condition, if in fact they do.

A number of scientifically controlled, double-blind studies have been conducted on oral zinc therapy; these are studies in which neither the researcher nor the experimental subjects know who is getting which drug until the study is completed. Some show significant improvement that is not duplicated either by dummy medication or by other acne treatments. Other results are equivocal. Until more conclusive evidence emerges, the Panel said, oral zinc could not be recommended as a treatment for acne.

Problems in Judging Products

Two problems bedevil efforts to assess anti-acne active ingredients and products. The first problem is that the vehicle (base) in which the active ingredient is formulated may influence its effectiveness. The Panel did not offer any suggestions on which bases to choose. The second problem, also difficult—for scientists trying to rate acne medications as well as for sufferers who use them—is the method of evaluating test results.

Some scientists—and some sufferers—count the blemishes before and after treatment. Others break down the blemishes into types before counting. Still others grade the severity of each blemish, whereas an alternative method is to venture an over all estimate of how well the treatment has worked. As yet there is no universally accepted way to measure acne's severity or to assess treatment benefits.

Combination Products

For the most part, the fewer active ingredients in a drug product, the safer it is. Based on this philosophy, the Panel judged most combination products unfavorably and, generally speaking, would require that each be proved more effective—yet not more toxic—than the single active ingredients used alone.

Panel members found few well-run clinical studies that demonstrate a clear advantage to combination preparations. So the Panel approved, and the FDA ruled to be safe and effective only one combination, and one close variant:

> The combination of sulfur 3 to 8 percent + resorcinol 2 percent, and the equivalent combination of sulfur 3 to 8 percent + resorcinol monoacetate 3 percent.

APPROVED ACTIVE INGREDIENTS IN ACNE PREPARATIONS

• RESORCINOL 2 PERCENT OR RESORCINOL MONOACETATE 3 PERCENT IN COMBINATION WITH SULFUR: Resorcinol is a skin-peeling agent. The Panel had some doubts about its safety, and stronger doubts about its effectiveness, and proposed that resorcinol and resorcinol acetate not be used as single-ingredient products. (*See* p. 15.) The FDA concurs with this judgment.

Despite this, resorcinol and resorcinol acetate have long been used in combination anti-acne medications, particularly with sulfur, and there is some evidence that they enhance sulfur's effectiveness. On this basis, the Panel gave an unenthusiastic evaluation of "safe and effective" to 2 percent resorcinol and 3 percent resorcinol monoacetate when used in combination with sulfur. The FDA, also without much enthusiasm, approved 2 percent resorcinol and 3 percent resorcinol acetate as safe and effective when combined with 3 percent to 8 percent sulfur.

WARNING:

 Apply to affected skin areas only. Do not use on broken skin or apply to large areas of the body.

• SALICYLIC ACID: A skin-peeling agent that is chemically related to aspirin, salicylic acid has been used to treat acne and other skin disorders for more than a century. But as the Panel noted, the way it works has never been precisely explained.

In one of the better studies, 2 percent salicylic acid lotion was compared with a non-medicated bar soap. The 109 subjects all had mild acne. After two weeks' treatment, the salicylic-acid lotion proved to be far superior in reducing blackheads, but no significant difference appeared between the two groups in terms of pimple counts, frequency of new blemishes, or over all improvement.

The researchers decided that 14 days was too short a time to measure improvement, so they ran a second, 3-month test on 177 acne sufferers. Three-quarters of the participants treated with the salicylic-acid lotion had good to excellent results, compared with only 10 percent in those who used the soap. The treatment group had fewer blackheads and pimples, and their faces were significantly less oily.

This study, and several others in which supplemental treatments were used in addition to salicylic acid, led the evaluators to believe that salicylic acid may be an effective ingredient. But it was decided that definitive tests must be done to confirm this belief.

Definitive tests have now been performed to the FDA's satisfaction. In one 12-week clinical trial, 180 patients with acne were studied. Forty percent of them had good or excellent reduction in pimples and other acne blemishes. But only 5 percent had comparable results when they used the liquid vehicle alone, without the active drug. Benzoyl peroxide, which also was tested, was even less effective: It yielded good to excellent reduction in pimples and other blemishes in only 2 percent of test subjects. (*See* Benzoyl Peroxide, further on.) The salicylic acid was particularly effective against angry, red (inflammatory) pimples and whiteheads and blackheads.

In the second study, salicylic acid 2 percent yielded good to excellent results for 98 percent of patients with a variety of acne blemishes. A much milder dose, salicylic acid 0.5 percent, was almost as good: It was effective for 90 percent of the patients. By contrast, the liquid vehicle, without the active drug, produced comparable benefit for only 11 percent of the subjects. Based on these findings, it might be wise to start treatment with a lower (0.5 or 1 percent) dose of salicylic acid.

Based on these recent studies, FDA judged salicylic acid 0.5 to 2 percent to be safe and effective for the self-medication of acne.

WARNING:

 Do not get [salicylic acid products] into eyes. If excessive skin irritation develops, or if irritation increases, discontinue use and consult a doctor.

• *SULFUR:* For thousands of years people have used this pungent yellow element medicinally for acne and other purposes. Yet sulfur's safety and effectiveness in controlling acne had not been well-studied, scientifically, the Panel said. Sulfur is believed to act by causing the outer layer of dead and dying skin to peel away; it also may kill microorganisms like *P. acnes*.

The Panel judged sulfur to be safe, largely on the basis of its years of use, its acceptance by dermatologists, and the scarcity of reports of severe side effects.

The evaluators said that too few controlled tests have been conducted with sulfur. Nevertheless, the handful of studies that are available show that sulfur, usually in combination with one or more other ingredients, is superior to dummy drugs. In one study, 3 percent sulfur, twice daily, cut blemish counts by half or more in 12 weeks in one-third of those treated. Only 10 percent of patients treated with a dummy mixture had comparable benefit. The conclusion: Sulfur is a safe and effective acne treatment at concentrations of 3 to 10 percent.

WARNING:

 Do not get [sulfur products] into eyes. If excessive skin irritation develops, or if irritation increases, discontinue use and consult a doctor.

CONDITIONALLY APPROVED ACTIVE INGREDIENT IN ACNE PREPARATIONS

Only one ingredient remains in this category.

• *BENZOYL PEROXIDE:* This compound has been used in a variety of medicines since the 1920s. It appears to act in two ways, which are possibly related. The drug mildly irritates the blemished outer layer of skin and causes it to peel away. It then kills underlying microorganisms—particularly *P. acnes*—perhaps by overwhelming their environment with oxygen, which they cannot tolerate.

Many studies have been conducted to determine whether benzoyl peroxide is effective. After evaluating these test results, the

Panel concluded that the chemical decreases counts of all types of acne blemish—including blackheads, whiteheads, and other pimples—in a much greater percentage of users than do dummy medications. In one study, for example, benzoyl peroxide was tested in patients with moderate to severe acne. The number of facial blemishes dropped from an average of 11 to an average of 7 blemishes per person in the group that used a 5.5 percent benzoyl peroxide preparation one or more times daily. By comparison, in a control group who treated themselves with the dummy preparation, blemish counts *rose*, from 10 to 11 blemlishes per person. In another study, two-thirds of persons using the active ingredient improved, whereas only one-third of the control individuals showed improvement.

A few studies indicate that a weaker 2.5 percent concentration of benzoyl peroxide, which is relatively non-irritating to the skin, is almost as effective as a more potent 10 percent concentration. So the Panel decided that concentrations of 2.5 to 10 percent are safe and effective for self-treating acne.

The FDA initially agreed. Then, the agency learned of two studies in the scientific literature that its experts had previously overlooked. Both studies showed that application of benzoyl peroxide to the skin of mice promoted the growth of tumors. Several additional such experiments then were performed. They showed that benzoyl peroxide promoted the development of benign skin tumors and also skin cancers in a high proportion of mice from genetic strains that are used for these experiments because they are very susceptible to cancer.

The FDA decided, in 1991, that "the evidence…is substantial to establish benzoyl peroxide as a potent skin tumor promoter in more than one strain of mice and other laboratory animals tested. . . . It appears that benzoyl peroxide shares a spectrum of features with the true (complete cancer-causing) initiators of cancer."

The FDA wrote to the Nonprescription Drug Manufacturers Association (NMDA), expressing its concern about benzoyl peroxide's safety. The NMDA disagreed with the FDA, saying that, in its view, benzoyl peroxide meets the FDA's tests for safety and efficacy. Human studies, it said, showed no link between the use of benzoyl peroxide and the development of cancer.

The FDA demanded additional safety studies on this ingredient, and has retained it in an intermediary category—as *effective* but *not proved safe*—pending the outcome of these studies.

WARNING:

 Do not use this medication if you have very sensitive skin or if you are sensitive to benzoyl peroxide. This product may cause irritation, characterized by redness, burning, itching, peeling, or possibly swelling. More frequent use or higher concentrations may aggravate such irritation. Mild irritation may be reduced by using the product less frequently or in a lower concentration. If irritation becomes severe, discontinue use; if irritation still continues, consult a doctor. Keep away from eyes, lips, and mouth.

DISAPPROVED ACTIVE INGREDIENTS IN ACNE PREPARATIONS

Until recently, many acne products contained ingredients that didn't work or were unsafe. The FDA banned their manufacture and sale in interstate commerce, effective May 1992. Some of these ingredients may still be made and sold, legally, within a state. Some may still be present in products in the medicine cabinet. These should be discarded. The banned ingredients are listed in the table Safety and Effectiveness: Active Ingredients in Over-the-Counter Acne Medications.

INACTIVE INGREDIENTS

Many impressive-sounding chemicals are formulated into acne products, but in reality they play no active role in clearing skin. They are used to provide bulk, as preservatives, or to lend the product cosmetic appeal. Some of these inactive ingredients are

alcohol
allantoin
aluminum oxide
bentonite
benzalkonium chloride
benzethonium chloride
calcium phosphate
carbomer 940

carboxyvinyl polymer
cetyl alcohol
citric acid
colloidal alumina
cosmetic colors
dioctyl sodium
  sulfosuccinate
edetate disodium

glycerin
glyceryl monostearate
hydrocarbon hydrotropes
isopropyl alcohol
isopropyl palmitate
laureth-4 (polyoxyethylene
  lauryl ether)
menthol
methylbenzethonium
  chloride
methylparaben (methyl
  parasept)
methyl salicylate
polyethylene

polyethylene glycol
  monostearate
polyethylene glycol 1000
  monostearate
propylene glycol
propylparaben (propyl
  parasept)
purified water
soapless cleansers
sodium hydroxide
sodium lauryl sulfate
stearic acid
sulfated surfactants
sulfonated alkyl benzenes
wetting agents

Safety and Effectiveness: Active Ingredients in Over-the-Counter Acne Medications

Active Ingredient	Assessment
alkyl isoquinolinium bromide	not safe and effective
aluminum compounds: alcloxa, aluminum chlorohydrex, aluminum hydroxide, and magnesium aluminum silicate	not safe and effective
benzocaine	not safe and effective
benzoic acid	not safe and effective
benzoyl peroxide	effective but not proved safe
boron compounds: boric acid and sodium	not safe and effective
calcium polysulfide	not safe and effective
calcium thiosulfate	not safe and effective
camphor	not safe and effective
chlorhydroxyquinoline	not safe and effective

Safety and Effectiveness: Active Ingredients in Over-the-Counter Acne Medications (contd)

Active Ingredient	Assessment
chloroxylenol	not safe and effective
coal tar	not safe and effective
dibenzothiophene	not safe and effective
estrone	not safe and effective
magnesium sulfate	not safe and effective
phenolates: phenol and phenolate sodium	not safe and effective
phenyl salicylate	not safe and effective
povidone-iodine	not safe and effective
pyrilamine maleate	not safe and effective
resorcinol 2% and resorcinol monoacetate 3% in combination with sulfur 3%-8%	safe and effective
resorcinol and resorcinol monoacetate as single ingredients	not safe and effective
resorcinol and resorcinol monoacetate in combination with salicylic acid	not safe and effective
salicylic acid 0.5%-2%	safe and effective
sodium thiosulfate	not safe and effective
sulfur 3%-10%	safe and effective
tetracaine hydrochloride	not safe and effective
thymol	not safe and effective
vitamin E	not safe and effective
zinc compounds: zinc oxide, zinc stearate, and zinc sulfide	not safe and effective

Acne Medications: Product Ratings

SINGLE-INGREDIENT PRODUCTS

Product and Distributor	Dosage of Active Ingredients	Rating*	Comment
benzoyl peroxide preparations: (products listed by dosage form and strength)			
Benoxyl 5 (Stiefel)	**lotion:** 5%	B	concern persists that this ingredient could cause cancer
Benzoyl peroxide (generic)		B	
Cuticura Acne (DEP Corp.)		B	
Dry and Clear (Whitehall)		B	
Oxy 5 (Norcliff Thayer)		B	
Neutrogena Acne Mask (Neutrogena)	**mask:** 5%	B	concern persists that this ingredient could cause cancer
Del Aqua-5 (Del-Ray)	**gel:** 5%	B	concern persists that this ingredient could cause cancer
Fostex 5% BPO (Westwood)		B	
Ben-Aqua 10	**lotion:** 10%	B	concern persists that this ingredient could cause cancer
Benoxyl 10 (Stiefel)		B	
Benzoyl peroxide (generic)		B	

Acne Medications: Product Ratings (contd)

Product and Distributor	Dosage of Active Ingredients	Rating*	Comment
Clearasil 10% (Vicks Personal Care)		B	
Oxy 10 (Norcliff Thayer)		B	
Clearasil Maximum Strength Acne Treatment (Vicks Personal Care)	cream: 10%	B	concern persists that this ingredient could cause cancer
Fostex 10% BPO Tinted (Westwood)		B	
pHisoAc BP (Winthrop Pharmaceutical)		B	
salicyclic acid preparations			
Acne Cream (Commerce)	gel: 5%	A	
Clearasil Double Clear (Richardson-Vicks)	medicated pads: 1.25%		
Regular strength		A	
Maximum strength	2%	A	
Listerex Scrub (Warner-Lambert)	lotion: 2%	A	

Oxy Clean Medicated Cleanser
and Pads (Norcliff Thayer)
Regular Strength — **medicated pads: 0.5%** — A
Maximum Strength — 2% — A

Oxy Night Watch (S.K. Beecham) — **lotion: 1%** — A

Propa P.H. Medicated — **cream: 2%** — A

Salicylic Acid Soap (Stiefel) — **soap: 3.5%** — C — too much salicylic acid

Saligel Acne Gel (Stiefel) — **gel: 5%** — A

sulfur preparations

Acne Aid (Stiefel) — **cream: 10%** — A

Acno (Baker-Cummins) — **lotion: 3% sulfur + 2% salicylic acid** — C — disapproved combination

Fostex Medicated Cover-Up (Westwood) — **cream: 2%** — C — not enough sulfur

Liquimat (Owen-Allercreme) — **lotion: 5%** — A

Sulfur Soap (Stiefel) — **soap: 10%** — A

Sulpho-Lac (Bradley) — **soap: 5%** — A

Xerac (Person & Covey) — **gel: 4% (microcrystalline)** — A

Acne Medications: Product Ratings (contd)

Product and Distributor	Dosage of Active Ingredients	Rating*	Comment
	COMBINATION PRODUCTS		
Acnomel (SmithKline Beecham)	**cream:** 8% sulfur + 2% resorcinol	A	
Acnotex (C & M Pharm.)	**lotion:** 8% sulfur + 2.25% salicylic acid	C	disapproved combination
Clearasil (Vicks Personal Care)	**stick:** 8% sulfur + 1% resorcinol	C	not enough resorcinol
Fostril (Westwood)	**lotion:** 2% sulfur + zinc oxide	C	less-than-effective dose of sulfur; combination not approved
Komed Mild (Barnes-Hind)	**lotion:** 2% sodium thiosulfate + 2% salicylic acid	C	sodium thiosulfate not effective; combination not approved
RA (Medco Labs)	**lotion:** 3% resorcinol + 6% calamine	C	too much resorcinol; calamine not effective
Rezamid (Summers)	**lotion:** 5% sulfur + 2% resorcinol	A	
Sulforcin (Owen)	**lotion:** 5% sulfur + 2% resorcinol	A	

Product and Distributor	Dosage of Active Ingredients	Rating*	Comment
	MEDICATED BAR SOAPS		
Aveeno Cleansing Bar (Rydelle)	**soap:** 2% sulfur + 2% salicylic acid + 50% colloidal oatmeal	C	colloidal oatmeal not submitted for Panel's assessment; too little sulfur

Product and Distributor	Dosage of Active Ingredients	Rating*	Comment
Buf-Bar (3M Personal Care)	soap: 3% sulfur	A	
Clearasil Antibacterial Soap (Vicks Personal Care)	soap: 0.75% triclosan	C	not proved safe or effective; antibacterial drugs disapproved for acne
Fostex Medicated Cleansing Bar (Westwood)	soap: 2% sulfur + 2% salicylic acid	C	not enough sulfur; combination is not approved
Salicylic Acid and Sulfur (Stiefel)	soap: 10% precipitated sulfur + 3% salicylic acid	C	disapproved combination
Sastid (Stiefel)	soap: 10% precipitated sulfur + 3% salicylic acid	C	disapproved combination
Sulfur Soap (Stiefel)	soap: 10% precipitated sulfur	A	

LIQUID CLEANSERS

Product and Distributor	Dosage of Active Ingredients	Rating*	Comment
Acno Cleanser (Baker-Cummins)	liquid: no active anti-acne ingredients	C	contains no active anti-acne ingredients
Drytex Lotion (C & M Pharm.)	lotion: 10% salicylic acid	C	too strong
d-SEB Gel Skin Cleanser (Cooper Care)	gel: 2% chloroxylenol	C	not an approved ingredient for self-care products
Neutrogena Cleansing Wash (Neutrogena)	liquid: no active anti-acne ingredients	C	contains no active anti-acne ingredients

Acne Medications: Product Ratings (contd)

Product and Distributor	Dosage of Active Ingredients	Rating*	Comment
Tyrosum Liquid (Summers)	**liquid:** no active anti-acne ingredients	C	not safe or effective as an anti-acne drug, since it contains no medicinal ingredients

---

*Author's interpretation of FDA criteria. Based on contents, not claims.

Allergy Drugs

Hay fever and other forms of respiratory allergies—also called *allergic rhinitis*—afflict 25 to 30 million Americans. These sufferers' seasonal allergies may be caused by hay, hence the name "hay fever," or grass. But pollens from ragweed, trees, and a wide range of other plants can cause the sneezing and wheezing, the itchy, runny, reddened eyes, and itchiness around the face, and in the mouth and throat that afflict many people at certain, fixed times each year. Other allergy sufferers may experience such symptoms at any time of the year.

These chronic upper respiratory allergies are not all caused by plants and plant products. People can be allergic to the saliva or dander of cats, horses, or other animals. Others suffer allergic attacks when exposed to air pollutants, cigarette smoke, mold spores, household dust, or certain foods.

Some allergies are simply a nuisance. Others are far more severe and can merge into serious pulmonary disorders like bronchitis and asthma. (*See* ASTHMA DRUGS.) Allergies may be similar to, and

---

ALLERGY DRUGS is based on the report of the FDA's Advisory Review Panel on OTC Cold, Cough, Allergy, and Bronchodilator and Anti-Asthmatic Products, and on the FDA's Tentative Final Monographs on antihistamines, nasal decongestants, and combination products.

difficult to distinguish from common colds. If the symptoms continue for more than a week or seem never to stop, an allergy, not a cold, is the probable cause. Reappearance of the sneezing and wheezing at a particular season each year, or in a particular locale, also indicates a diagnosis of allergy, not common cold.

Causes of Allergy

Allergy is a form of *immune reaction*, in which the individual becomes hypersensitive to a particular substance (an allergen) that may be touched, swallowed, or carried by air into the lungs.

The allergen triggers the production of a reactive substance (an antibody) that attaches itself to certain types of body cells: mast cells in the blood and basophils in other tissues. The allergens become stuck to these complexes.

This reaction prompts the cells to secrete *histamine*, which acts as an irritant that causes itchiness, tear formation, and other allergic symptoms. As their name implies, *antihistamines* interrupt the allergic process by blocking histamine's access to the secretory cells. These drugs thus provide direct relief for allergic symptoms.

Antihistamines also have a mild *drying effect* (technically, an *anticholinergic* effect) on mucous membranes and other body tissues. This effect accounts in part for these drugs' ability to relieve the runny eyes and noses that characterize upper respiratory allergic reactions.

The best way to relieve allergic complaints is to have an allergist identify the offending substance or substances and then, if possible, avoid it or them. But when avoidance is impossible, nonprescription antihistamines will often provide substantial relief. If they fail, stronger drugs—including injections of epinephrine and corticosteroids—can be provided by a doctor. It now is possible to tame certain allergies—including those caused by some pollens and by bee stings—with the use of desensitizing injections (preparations that dampen the person's sensitivity to the allergen).

One respiratory allergy symptom that antihistamines do not relieve very well is stuffed-up nose, or, technically, *nasal congestion*. Nonprescription drugs that can relieve congestion by shrinking the inflamed small blood vessels along the nasal passages are called *nasal decongestants*. Several have been evaluated by the Panel and FDA as safe and effective, with the important proviso that they be used for a limited period of just a few days. The reason is that continuing use, and even stopping after several days' use, can cause the nose to become stopped up again, a condition called *rebound congestion*. If this occurs, one should stop using these drugs completely, except as advised by a physician.

Single Ingredient versus Combination Products

Because the symptoms and some of the drug treatments are the same, manufacturers place allergy drugs and drugs to relieve coughs and colds in a single category, *cough-cold-allergy drugs*. Some of these products are effective for allergies; some for coughs and colds; and some for allergies *and* coughs and colds.

This can confuse consumers. They may, as a result, purchase expensive combination products, designed to treat a variety of symptoms, when they suffer just one or a few of these symptoms, and so require only simple medication.

The safest way out of this dilemma is to purchase and use single-ingredient products. For allergies, single-ingredient antihistamines are likely to be the most useful. If the major symptom is stuffed-up nose, then a single-ingredient nasal decongestant might be tried. However, the one type of combination product that may be appropriate for allergy sufferers is an antihistamine plus a decongestant. The problem with these combinations is that while allergy-sufferers require relief that continues over several days, or even weeks, decongestants should only be taken for a few days at a time. So again, it may be preferable to use separate, single-ingredient products.

The combination products that are prominently displayed in stores and advertised on TV may contain ingredients that allergy sufferers probably do not need: cough relievers, pain-fever relievers, expectorants. It is futile and potentially hazardous to take medicinal ingredients that you do not need—and it is a waste of money as well. Therefore, for allergic symptoms, consider a single-ingredient antihistamine, or a single-ingredient decongestant if a stuffy nose is your one bothersome symptom, or an antihistamine plus a decongestant. Note, however, that some of these combinations are safe and effective, while others are not. *See* the table Safety and Effectiveness: Combination Products Sold Over-the-Counter for Allergy Symptoms.

Antihistamines

 Claims for Antihistamines

Accurate

- "Temporarily relieves runny nose and decreases sneezing, itching of the nose or throat, and itchy, watery eyes due to hay fever or other upper respiratory allergies"

- "Temporarily dries runny nose and alleviates sneezing, itching of the nose or throat, and itchy, watery eyes due to upper respiratory allergy (allergic rhinitis)"

WARNINGS:

 Do not take [an antihistamine] product if you have asthma, glaucoma, lung disease, shortness of breath, difficulty in breathing, or difficulty in urination due to ... prostate ... enlargement unless directed by a doctor

May cause drowsiness; alcohol, sedatives and tranquilizers may increase the drowsiness effect. Avoid alcoholic beverages. Do not take this product if you are taking sedatives or tranquilizers without first consulting your doctor.... Use caution when driving a motor vehicle or operating machinery.

Some antihistamines cause "marked drowsiness" rather than just plain "drowsiness." Those drugs that carry this additional risk are identified in the following descriptions.

APPROVED ANTIHISTAMINE ACTIVE INGREDIENTS

The FDA currently lists a dozen antihistamines as safe and effective treatments for sneezing and runny nose associated with allergic rhinitis. Most, if not all, were used for many years in prescription drug products, then switched to nonprescription status as their patents ran out. Their safety generally speaking was established in this earlier period.

Antihistamines are powerful, sometimes useful drugs—but they are not very interesting except, perhaps, to pharmacologists and the companies that produce them. So the following descriptions will be brief.

- *BROMPHENIRAMINE MALEATE:* A half-billion dosage units of this antihistamine were sold annually, on a prescription basis. Very few serious adverse effects were reported. Brompheniramine is rated by the American Medical Association as having only a low risk of drowsiness. Verdict: safe and effective. (*See* the table Recommended Dosage for Over-the-Counter Antihistamines.)

- *CHLORCYCLIZINE HYDROCHLORIDE:* This antihistamine was introduced in 1949. Chlorcyclizine has passed numerous safety checks and raised few complaints from consumers or others through the years. It was not reviewed by the FDA's panel of outside experts on these drugs. Based on its record of use, the agency switched the drug to over-the-counter status. (*See* the table Recommended Dosage for Over-the-Counter Antihistamines.)

- *CHLORPHENIRAMINE MALEATE:* In one recent year, two billion tablets and capsules of this drug were sold. There were fewer than 2000 reports of side effects, none fatal. Therefore, the Panel ruled that chlorpheniramine is safe, and the FDA agrees that it is safe and effective and also effective against allergic runny nose and sneezing. (*See* the table Recommended Dosage for Over-the-Counter Antihistamines.)

- *DEXBROMPHENIRAMINE MALEATE:* This chemical element of brompheniramine maleate long had been sold in prescription (℞) allergy-cold relief products. It is believed to be the most medicinally active form of the drug, and it is stronger—so doses are lower. The FDA switched it to nonprescription status in 1987. (*See* the table Recommended Dosage for Over-the-Counter Antihistamines.)

- *DIPHENHYDRAMINE HYDROCHLORIDE:* This is an old and unquestionably effective antihistamine. It is widely used as a prescription and as a nonprescription drug.

  The main and serious problem with it is its pronounced sedative effect: It makes people sleepy. Up to half of people who take the standard 50-mg dose may experience this effect. Because of this, diphenhydramine is sold over-the-counter for helping people go to sleep. (*See* SLEEP AIDS.) (*See* the table Recommended Dosage for Over-the-Counter Antihistamines.)

  The FDA warns that "marked drowsiness" may occur when this antihistamine is used, and it cautions consumers against operating a motor vehicle or machinery while taking it.

- *DOXYLAMINE SUCCINATE:* This is an effective antihistamine whose major liability is that, in the FDA's words, it can cause "marked drowsiness." So people who take it should use caution if they drive or operate machinery. The FDA evaluated, at great length, several epidemiologic studies that suggest this drug may cause birth defects. After extensive review of the medical literature, the FDA concluded "that it is unlikely that this ingredient is a teratogen [causes birth defects]." But the agency could not absolutely rule out this possibility. So it warns:

 "If you are pregnant or nursing a baby, seek the advice of a health professional before using this [drug]."

(*See* the table Recommended Dosage for Over-the-Counter Antihistamines.)

• *PHENINDRAMINE TARTRATE:* This is a fast-acting antihistamine that has been shown to provide effective relief to allergy sufferers. FDA has approved its use to relieve allergy symptoms, on the basis of tests on another chemically unrelated antihistamine, chlorpheniramine. (*See* Chlorpheniramine.) The Panel said that reports in the literature over a thirty-year period suggest that phenindramine tartrate produces more side effects than some other antihistamines, including dry mouth and overstimulation and excitation—particularly in children—as well as, paradoxically, both drowsiness and insomnia. (*See* the table Recommended Dosage for Over-the-Counter Antihistamines.)

• *PHENIRAMINE MALEATE:* This is a widely used and very safe antihistamine. In one recent year in which 291 million dosage units were sold, 358 suspected toxic reactions were reported; half a dozen of these people required hospitalization but there were no deaths. This is an "old" drug—it was introduced more than three decades ago—and it has not been studied as rigorously as some newer ones. But both clinical experience and animal studies indicate that it is effective against hay fever and other allergic symptoms. (*See* Recommended Dosage for Over-the-Counter Antihistamines.)

• *PYRILAMINE MALEATE:* Compared with several other approved antihistamines, this one produces many side effects, although usually mild ones. These reactions include drowsiness, listlessness, irritability, and loss of appetite. Some users experience nausea and vomiting. On the other hand, even large overdose appears not to have fatal consequences. About two-thirds of hay fever sufferers who use pyrilamine maleate obtain symptomatic relief. (*See* the table Recommended Dosage for Over-the-Counter Antihistamines.)

• *THONZYLAMINE HYDROCHLORIDE:* Some studies of this drug, which is more than 30 years old, indicate that it is among the least toxic of its type. In one recent period, during which approximately 80 million dosage units were sold annually, no suspected poisonings with thonzylamine hydrochloride were reported to the FDA. The other side of the coin is that this drug has been studied less rigorously than some newer antihistamines.

• *TRIPROLIDINE HYDROCHLORIDE:* This antihistamine had been sold on prescription (℞) for a quarter century. The FDA decided it is safe and effective for nonprescription sales and self-medication. The American Medical Association, in its 1991 *Drug Evaluations*, says the incidence of side effects is low; the most common is drowsiness. (*See* the table Recommended Dosage for Over-the-Counter Antihistamines.)

CONDITIONALLY APPROVED ANTIHISTAMINE ACTIVE INGREDIENTS

One antihistamine was conditionally approved for lack of scientifically sound studies to clearly establish its effectiveness.

• *PHENYLTOLOXAMINE DIHYDROGEN CITRATE:* Data from animal experiments and human trials suggest that this is one of the safest antihistamines currently marketed. The FDA received only one report of an adverse reaction during a recent five-year period, in which there were sales of between one-third and one-half billion tablets and other dosage units each year. But, despite these huge sales, there is surprisingly little rigorous experimental data to prove the drug's effectiveness or establish the minimum effective dosage level.

DISAPPROVED ANTIHISTAMINE ACTIVE INGREDIENTS

None.

Recommended Dosage for Over-the-Counter Antihistamines

Active Ingredient	Adults and children over 12 years old	Children 6 to 12 years old	Children under 6 years old
brompheniramine maleate	4 mg every 4 to 6 hr (24 mg daily maximum)	2 mg every 4 to 6 hr (12 mg daily maximum), or as directed by a doctor	consult a doctor
chlorcyclizine hydrochloride	25 mg every 6 to 8 hr (75 mg daily maximum)	consult a doctor	consult a doctor
chlorpheniramine maleate	4 mg every 4 to 6 hr (24 mg daily maximum)	2 mg every 4 to 6 hr (12 mg daily maximum), or as directed by a doctor	consult a doctor
dexbrompheniramine maleate	2 mg every 4 to 6 hr (12 mg daily maximum)	1 mg every 4 to 6 hr (6 mg daily maximum), or as directed by a doctor	consult a doctor
diphenhydramine hydrochloride	25 to 50 mg every 4 to 6 hr (300 mg daily maximum)	12.5 to 25 mg every 4 to 6 hr (150 mg daily maximum), or as directed by a doctor	consult a doctor
doxylamine succinate	7.5 to 12.5 mg every 4 to 6 hr (75 mg daily maximum)	3.75 to 6.25 mg every 4 to 6 hr (37.5 mg daily maximum), or as directed by a doctor	consult a doctor

phenindamine tartrate	25 mg every 4 to 6 hr (150 mg daily maximum)	12.5 mg every 4 to 6 hr (75 mg daily maximum), or as directed by a doctor	consult a doctor
pheniramine maleate	12.5 to 25 mg every 4 to 6 hr (150 mg daily maximum)	6.25 to 12.5 mg every 4 to 6 hr (75 mg daily maximum), or as directed by a doctor	consult a doctor
pyrilamine maleate	25 to 50 mg every 6 to 8 hr (200 mg daily maximum)	12.5 to 25 mg every 6 to 8 hr (100 mg daily maximum), or as directed by a doctor	consult a doctor
thonzylamine hydrochloride	50 to 100 mg every 4 to 6 hrs (600 mg daily maximum)	25 to 50 mg every 4 to 6 hr (300 mg daily maximum), or as directed by adoctor	consult a doctor
triprolidine hydrochloride	2.5 mg every 4 to 6 hrs (10 mg daily maximum)	1.25 mg every 4 to 6 hr (daily maximum 5 mg), or as directed by a doctor	consult a doctor

Nasal Decongestants

A number of drugs called nasal decongestants will effectively relieve nasal stuffiness and improve breathing in allergy sufferers. They do this *not* by drying up nasal discharge —which is what antihistamines in part may do—but by significantly *constricting*, or narrowing, swollen blood vessels in the mucosal lining of the nose and sinuses. It is the swelling and inflammation of these tissues that are largely to blame for stuffy noses.

The remarkable constrictive effect these drugs can have on blood vessels has one unfortunate result: rebound congestion as the drug wears off. The mucosal blood vessels may swell out more than before, so that the nose may feel even more stuffed up than it was. The risk can be reduced by using these drugs no more often than the label advises, and for no more than three or seven days at a time. (Oral forms, while less effective, are less likely to produce rebound congestion than nasal sprays.)

Nasal decongestants are formulated for (1) *topical application* as nose drops, sprays and jellies; (2) *inhalation* from inhalers or in steam vapors; and (3) *oral ingestion* in liquid or tablets.

When these potent compounds are put directly into the nose—rather than being swallowed—very little drug is absorbed into the bloodstream and carried to the rest of the body. So inhaled decongestants and nasal jellies are remarkably free from systemic side effects, unlike decongestants that are taken orally. Decongestants that are taken orally are carried throughout the body and can affect major organ systems. Persons with high blood pressure, heart disease, diabetes, or thyroid disease should not take decongestants orally except on a doctor's orders.

 Claims for Nasal Decongestants

Certain claims can legitimately be made for safe and effective nasal decongestants. Unlike some other drugs, decongestants can be tested objectively: The resistance to airflow through the stuffed-up nasal passage can be measured. In that way, the amount of air flowing through medicated nostrils can easily be compared with the amount passing through nostrils not exposed to the drug.

Accurate

- "For the temporary relief of nasal congestion due to hay fever or other upper respiratory allergies"

- "For the temporary relief of stopped-up nose"

•"Helps clear nasal passages"

•"Promotes nasal and sinus drainage"

•"Decongests nasal passages; shrinks swollen membranes"

These warnings are applicable to all safe and effective nasal decongestants *except* desoxyephedrine-L and proplylhexedrine inhalers, which carry less risk:

WARNINGS:

 Do not exceed recommended dosage because at higher doses nervousness, dizziness, or sleeplessness may occur.

Do not take this [decongestant] if you have heart disease, high blood pressure, thyroid disease, diabetes or difficulty in urination due to enlargement of the prostate gland, unless directed by a doctor.

Do not take this drug if you are taking a prescription drug for high blood pressure or depression, without first consulting your doctor.

APPROVED NASAL DECONGESTANT ACTIVE INGREDIENTS

- **DESOXYEPHEDRINE-L (TOPICAL):** Nose drops and sprays containing this substance caused burning, stinging, sneezing, and runny nose in up to one out of five test subjects. But no serious side effects have been reported, so the Panel considers the drug safe.

  Fresh data from four scientific studies that confirmed the effectiveness of desoxyephedrine-L inhalers were submitted to the FDA. They satisfied the agency that the drug is effective. The new data also indicate that this drug can be used for up to seven days without risk of rebound congestion. (*See* the table Recommended Dosage of Nasal Decongestants.)

- **EPHEDRINE PREPARATIONS (TOPICAL):** Ephedrine preparations include ephedrine, ephedrine hydrochloride, ephedrine sulfate, and racephedrine hydrochloride. Ephedrine has been available in the United States for more than half a century. Numerous tests have shown it to be safe and effective when applied as a nasal spray, as drops, or as jelly in concentrations of 0.5 to 1 percent. Rebound congestion is unlikely at those low doses if the drug is not used longer than three days. Ephedrine acts quickly, reaching its maximal decongestant effect within one hour. It loses its effectiveness after four hours. (*See* the table, Recommended Dosage of Nasal Decongestants.)

• NAPHAZOLINE HYDROCHLORIDE (TOPICAL): This drug has some notable advantages and some notable disadvantages. It is effective, and it produces a noticeable decongestant effect within 10 minutes. Relief continues for up to five or six hours. Tests suggest that most people who use it experience some relief from their symptoms. The disadvantages are that rebound congestion sometimes occurs after even a single treatment; it is fairly likely to occur after repeated use. What is more, naphazoline can be habit-forming. If accidentally swallowed, it can cause marked drowsiness. It should not be used by children under 12 years of age. But, despite these problems, naphazoline was evaluated as safe and effective as a nasal decongestant. (*See* the table Recommended Dosage of Nasal Decongestants.)

• OXYMETAZOLINE HYDROCHLORIDE (TOPICAL): This drug is a long-acting decongestant. Its effect begins to wane only after five or six hours. Twice-a-day doses should provide adequate relief without causing rebound congestion. The drug has been shown to be safe and effective in double-blind trials. In one, the nasal airways of 7 out of 14 children treated with the preparation twice daily were completely open for 9 to 12 hours each day. In another study, in 30 children, three drops in each nostril three times daily provided persistently effective clearance of the nasal passages for two weeks. (*See* the table Recommended Dosage of Nasal Decongestants.)

• PHENYLEPHRINE HYDROCHLORIDE (TOPICAL OR ORAL): While potent, this decongestant is both safe and effective. Tests show statistically significant decongestive effect when the drug is administered orally. In one study, for example, a 10-mg dose yielded an average reduction of 11 percent in airway resistance at 15 minutes; a 21 percent reduction was shown at one and two hours. Similar benefit has been reported when the drug is administered in nasal drops and sprays. Oral phenylephrine can raise blood pressure and increase heart rate, but at the low doses taken to clear stuffed-up noses, such effects are unlikely to occur. However, persons taking prescription drugs that contain substances called monoamine oxidase (MAO) inhibitors may experience serious cardiovascular effects when they take even the approved oral over-the-counter dose of phenylephrine. The FDA warns, too, that the 1-percent preparations of this drug are especially likely to cause rebound congestion and other side effects. (*See* the table Recommended Dosage of Nasal Decongestants.)

- *PROPYLHEXEDRINE (INHALED):* This drug has a wide margin of safety and relative freedom from toxic effects. So it can be used—for up to seven days—by persons who cannot use ephedrine and similar decongestants. (*See* the table Recommended Dosage of Nasal Decongestants.)

- *PSEUDOEPHEDRINE PREPARATIONS (TAKEN ORALLY):* The safety and effectiveness of pseudoephedrine hydrochloride and pseudoephedrine sulfate, given orally, have been demonstrated clinically and in scientific studies on cold sufferers. Side effects are minimal; they include drowsiness, headache, and insomnia. In the recommended dosage, pseudoephedrine appears unlikely to cause significant elevations of blood pressure in hypertensive persons. Persons taking MAO inhibitors, however, should avoid this drug. (Anyone who is not sure whether his prescribed medication is an MAO inhibitor should check with his or her doctor.) (*See* the table Recommended Dosage of Nasal Decongestants.)

- *XYLOMETAZOLINE (TOPICAL):* This is a potent decongestant that was moved from prescription to nonprescription status after the Panel determined that it is safe and effective for nonprescription use. It is long-acting: A single dose may provide relief for more than five hours. Rebound congestion is less of a problem than with some other nasal decongestants. Tests have shown that xylometazoline produces an objective increase in airflow through the nasal passages and a subjective sense of relief from the stuffed-up feeling. (*See* the table Recommended Dosage of Nasal Decongestants.)

CONDITIONALLY APPROVED NASAL DECONGESTANT ACTIVE INGREDIENTS

Many agents are conditionally approved as nasal decongestants pending further testing.

- *BORNYL ACETATE (TOPICAL):* The safety of bornyl acetate, an aromatic substance, is attested to by long clinical use. But there is no well-documented study to show its effectiveness as a nasal decongestant and evaluators could not even determine a suitable dosage for testing purposes.

- *CAMPHOR (INHALED):* Camphor is judged by this Panel to be safe in customary dosages. But studies on its effectiveness as a decongestant have been in multi-ingredient products, so camphor's contribution, if any, is difficult to determine.

• *CEDAR-LEAF OIL (TOPICAL):* This is a turpentine-like volatile oil that is steam-distilled from the fresh leaves of the cedar tree *Thuja occidentalis.* It is dangerous if eaten, but safe when applied to the chest, neck, and back in the dose used in a widely marketed ointment. Compared with an inert preparation, combination products that include cedar-leaf oil significantly reduced congestion over a period of several hours. However, the role of cedar-leaf oil needs to be determined by suitably testing it as an individual ingredient. The Panel could not determine a dosage for this substance.

• *EPHEDRINE PREPARATIONS (TAKEN ORALLY):* Ephedrine preparations are safe when taken orally, as they are when inhaled. They can, however, cause tension, nervousness, tremor, and sleeplessness. In high doses they appear to work as nasal decongestants. But no studies have been submitted to show that they are effective for this purpose at the dosage levels recommended for use without prescription.

• *PEPPERMINT OIL (MENTHOL) (TOPICAL OR INHALED):* Some combination products containing this aromatic substance have been shown to make breathing easier. But peppermint oil's contribution to this therapeutic effect has not been established.

• *PHENYLPROPANOLAMINE PREPARATIONS: PHENYLPROPANOLAMINE BITARTRATE, PHENYLPROPANOLAMINE HYDROCHLORIDE, PHENYLPROPANOLAMINE MALEATE (TOPICAL OR ORAL):* Forms of phenylpropanolamine are among the most frequently used nasal decongestants. Several well-monitored studies have demonstrated their effectiveness.

The Panel decided that the oral forms, but not inhaled forms of this drug were safe. But subsequently a number of studies were published showing that phenylpropanolamine can cause significant—perhaps dangerous—rises in blood pressure, as well as other side effects. Many doctors said it should not be sold over-the-counter, either as a nasal decongestant or as an appetite suppressant—for which it is also widely used. (*See* REDUCING AIDS.) Because of these concerns, the FDA has given phenylpropanolamine a tentative equivocal status—technically neither approved, conditionally approved, or disapproved—until it makes up its administrative mind whether to permit it or ban it in over-the-counter preparations.

DISAPPROVED NASAL DECONGESTANT ACTIVE INGREDIENTS

None.

Recommended Dosage for Over-the-Counter Nasal Decongestants Taken Through the Nose (Drops, Sprays, Jellies, or Inhalations)

Active Ingredient	Adults and children over 12 years old	Children 6 to 12 years old	Children under 6 years old*
desoxyephedrine-L	2 inhalations per nostril not oftener than every 2 hr	1 inhalation per nostril not oftener than every 2 hr with adult supervision	consult a doctor
ephedrine 0.5%	2 to 3 drops or sprays per nostril every 4 or more hr, or 1 application of jelly per nostril	1 to 2 drops or sprays per nostril every 4 or more hr, or 1 application of jelly per nostril with adult supervision	consult a doctor
naphazoline hydrochloride 0.05%	1 to 2 drops or sprays per nostril not oftener than every 6 hr, or 1 application of jelly per nostril	consult a doctor	consult a doctor
0.025%		1 or 2 drops or sprays per nostril not oftener than every 6 hr, or 1 application of jelly per nostril with adult supervision	consult a doctor

Recommended Dosage for Over-the-Counter Nasal Decongestants Taken Through the Nose (Drops, Sprays, Jellies, or Inhalations) (contd)

Active Ingredient	Adults and children over 12 years old	Children 6 to 12 years old	Children under 6 years old*
oxymetazoline hydrochloride 0.05%	2 to 3 drops or sprays per nostril not oftener than twice daily, or 1 to 2 applications of jelly per nostril	2 or 3 drops or sprays per nostril not oftener than twice daily, or 1 to 2 applications of jelly per nostril, with adult supervision	consult a doctor
phenylephrine hydrochloride 1%	2 or 3 drops or sprays per nostril not oftener than every 4 hr, or 1 application of jelly per nostril	consult a doctor	consult a doctor
0.5%	2 to 3 drops or sprays per nostril not oftener than every 4 hr, or 1 application of jelly per nostril	consult a doctor	consult a doctor
0.25%	2 to 3 drops or sprays per nostril not oftener than every 4 hr, or 1 application of jelly per nostril	2 to 3 drops or sprays per nostril not oftener than every 4 hr, or 1 application of jelly per nostril, with adult supervision	consult a doctor

Active Ingredient	Adults and Children Over 12 years	Children 6 to 12 years	Children 2 to 6 years
0.125%			for children 2 to 6, 2 to 3 drops or sprays per nostril, not oftener than every 4 hr, with adult supervision; for children under 2, consult a doctor
propylhexedrine (inhaler)	2 inhalations per nostril not oftener than once every 2 hr	1 inhalation per nostril no oftener than once every 2 hr, with adult supervision	consult a doctor
xylometazoline 0.1%	2 or 3 drops or sprays per nostril not oftener than every 8 to 10 hr, or 1 application of jelly per nostril	consult a doctor	consult a doctor
0.05%		2 or 3 drops or sprays per nostril not oftener than every 8 to 10 hr, or 1 application of jelly, with adult supervision	consult a doctor

Recommended Dosage for Over-the-Counter Nasal Decongestants Taken by Mouth

Active Ingredient	Adults and Children Over 12 years	Children 6 to 12 years	Children 2 to 6 years*
phenylephrine hydrochloride	10 mg every 4 hr (60 mg daily maximum)	5 mg every 4 hr (30 mg daily maximum)	2.5 mg every 4 hr (15 mg daily maximum)

Recommended Dosage for Over-the-Counter Nasal Decongestants Taken by Mouth (contd)

Active Ingredient	Adults and Children Over 12 years	Children 6 to 12 years	Children 2 to 6 years*
pseudoephedrine	60 mg every 4 to 6 hr (240 mg daily maximum)	30 mg every 4 to 6 hr (120 mg daily maximum)	15 mg every 4 to 6 hr (60 mg daily maximum)

* For children under 2: consult a doctor.

Safety and Effectiveness:
Antihistamines in Over-the-Counter Allergy Medications

Active Ingredient	Assessment
brompheniramine maleate	safe and effective
chlorcyclizine hydrochloride	safe and effective
chlorpheniramine maleate	safe and effective
dexbrompheniramine maleate	safe and effective
diphenhydramine hydrochloride	safe and effective
doxylamine succinate	safe and effective
phenindamine tartrate	safe and effective
pheniramine maleate	safe and effective
phenyltoloxamine dihydrogen citrate	safe but not proved effective
pyrilamine maleate	safe and effective
thonzylamine hydrochloride	safe and effective
triprolidine hydrochloride	safe and effective

Safety and Effectiveness: Active Ingredients
in Over-the-Counter Nasal Decongestants

Active Ingredient	Assessment
bornyl acetate	
inhalant	safe but not proved effective
camphor	
inhalant	safe but not proved effective*
ointment	safe but not proved effective
cedar-leaf oil	
ointment	safe but not proved effective
desoxyephedrine-L	
inhalant	safe and effective

Safety and Effectiveness: Active Ingredients
in Over-the-Counter Nasal Decongestants (contd)

Active Ingredient	Assessment
ephedrine preparations: ephedrine, ephedrine hydrochloride, ephedrine sulfate, and racephedrine hydrochloride	
nose drops, sprays, jellies	safe and effective
oral	safe but not proved effective
eucalyptol and eucalyptus oil	
inhalant, ointment	safe but not proved effective*
naphazoline hydrochloride	
nose drops, sprays, jellies	safe and effective
oxymetazoline hydrochloride	
nose drops, sprays, jellies	safe and effective
menthol	
inhalant	safe and effective*
lozenge	safe but not proved effective
ointment	safe but not proved effective
phenylephrine hydrochloride	
nose drops, sprays, jellies	safe and effective
oral	safe and effective
phenylpropanolamine preparations: phenylpropanolamine bitartrate, phenylpropanolamine hydrochloride, and phenylpropanolamine maleate	
nose drops, sprays, oral	not proved safe and effective
propylhexedrine	
inhalant	safe and effective
pseudoephedrine preparations: pseudoephedrine hydrochloride and pseudoephedrine sulfate	
oral	safe and effective

Safety and Effectiveness: Active Ingredients in Over-the-Counter Nasal Decongestants (contd)

Active Ingredient	Assessment
xylometazoline	
nose drops, sprays, nasal jellies	safe and effective

---

*These ingredients safe and effective in combination with desoxyephedrine-L.

Safety and Effectiveness: Combination Products Sold Over-the-Counter for Allergy Symptoms

Safe and Effective Combinations

Each individual ingredient must be safe and effective, except as noted.

1 antihistamine + 1 nasal decongestant taken by mouth

desoxyephedrine-L + aromatics (camphor, eucalyptol, menthol) in an inhaler as a nasal decongestant taken through the nose. (Note: The aromatic ingredients are not safe and effective individually, or in any combination as decongestants, except when combined with desoxyephedrine-L in an inhaler.)

Conditionally Safe or Conditionally Effective Combinations

1 or more conditionally approved ingredients or conditionally approved labeling but no disapproved ingredient or labeling less than minimally effective dosage in 1 or more ingredients claimed to relieve the same symptom

2 approved ingredients from the same drug group

combinations containing small amounts of a conditionally approved active ingredient intended to counteract side effects of other ingredient(s) — e.g., caffeine combinations containing an antihistamine for which a sleep-aid claim is made

combinations containing several claimed active ingredients that are mixtures of volatile substances, with overlapping pharmacologic activities for which a minimum effective dose cannot be established for 1 or more ingredient(s) (exception: desoxyephedrine-L + aromatics are safe and effective)

Unsafe or Ineffective Combinations

a combination with any disapproved ingredient or disapproved labeling

a combination of approved ingredients from different groups, each for a different symptom, if any ingredient is present at less than the minimum effective dose

Allergy Drugs: Product Ratings

ANTIHISTAMINES

Product and Distributor	Dosage of Active Ingredients	Rating*	Comment
brompheniramine maleate			
Brompheniramine (generic)	**elixir:** 2 mg per teaspoonful **tablets:** 4 mg	A	℞ to OTC switch
Dimetane (Robins)	**elixir:** 2 mg per teaspoonful **tablets:** 4 mg **timed-release tablets:** 8 mg, 12 mg	A	℞ to OTC switch
chlorpheniramine maleate			
Alla-Chlor (Rugby)	**syrup:** 2 mg per teaspoonful	A	℞ to OTC switch
Chlo-Amine (Hollister-Stier)	**chewable tablets:** 2 mg	A	children's dosage, ℞ to OTC switch
Chlorpheniramine (generic)	**tablets:** 4 mg	A	℞ to OTC switch
Chlor-Trimeton (Schering-Plough)	**syrup:** 2 mg per teaspoonful	A	℞ to OTC switch
Chlor-Trimeton (Schering-Plough)	**tablets:** 4 mg	A	℞ to OTC switch
Chlor-Trimeton Repetabs (Schering-Plough)	**tablets, timed-release:** 8 mg	A	℞ to OTC switch

Teldrin (SmithKline Beecham)	capsules, timed-release: 12 mg	A	℞ to OTC switch
diphenhydramine hydrochloride			
Belix (Halsey)	elixir: 12.5 mg per teaspoonful	A	℞ to OTC switch
Benadryl 25 (Parke-Davis Consumer)	capsules; tablets: 25 mg	A	℞ to OTC switch
Benylin (Parke-Davis Consumer)	syrup: 12.5 mg per teaspoonful	A	℞ to OTC switch
Diphenhydramine (generic)	capsules; tablets: 25 mg	A	℞ to OTC switch
Diphenhydramine (generic)	elixir, syrup: 12.5 mg per teaspoonful	A	℞ to OTC switch
pyrilamine maleate			
Pyrilamine maleate (generic)	tablets: 25 mg	A	
triprolidine hydrochloride			
Actidil (Burroughs Wellcome)	tablets: 2.5 mg	A	℞ to OTC switch
	syrup: 1.25 mg per teaspoonful	A	℞ to OTC switch

Allergy Drugs: Product Ratings (contd)

DECONGESTANTS

Product and Distributor	Dosage of Active Ingredients	Rating*	Comment
desoxyephedrine-l			
Vicks Inhaler (Vicks Health Care)	**inhaler:** 50 mg + menthol, camphor, eucalyptus	C	but a recently purchased Vicks Inhaler does *not* list desoxyephedrine-l on the container; it would not be effective: C
ephedrine hydrochloride			
Efedron Nasal (Hyrex)	**jelly:** 0.6%	A	
ephedrine sulfate			
Ephedrine sulfate (generic)	**capsules:** 25 mg	B	not proved effective
Vatronol (Vicks Health Care)	**nose drops:** 0.5%	A	
epinephrine hydrochloride			
Adrenalin Chloride (Parke-Davis)	**nose-drops:** 0.1%	C	not submitted to or approved by Panel as an over-the-counter nasal decongestant
naphazoline hydrochloride			

Privine (Ciba Consumer)	**nose drops:** 0.05% **nasal spray:** 0.05%	A A	
oxymetazoline hydrochloride			
Afrin (Schering-Plough)	**pediatric nose drops:** 0.025% **nose drops:** 0.05%	A A	for children, R̶ to OTC switch R̶ to OTC switch
Allerest 12-Hour Nasal (Pharmacraft)			
Dristan Long Lasting (Whitehall)	**nasal spray:** 0.05%	A	R̶ to OTC switch
Duration (Schering-Plough)		A	R̶ to OTC switch
4-Way Long-Lasting Nasal Spray (Bristol-Meyers)		A	R̶ to OTC switch
Neo-Synephrine 12 Hour (Winthrop Consumer)			
Oxymetazolone (generic)		A	R̶ to OTC switch
Sinex Long-Acting (Vicks Health Care)		A	R̶ to OTC switch
phenylephrine hydrochloride (products listed in order of increasing strength)			
Alconefrin 25 (Webcon)	**nose-drops:** 0.25%	A	dosage for older children, adults
Alconefrin 50 (Webcon)	**nose drops:** 0.5%	A	adult dosage
Doktors (Scherer)	**nose drops:** 0.25%	A	

Allergy Drugs: Product Ratings (contd)

Product and Distributor	Dosage of Active Ingredients	Rating*	Comment
Duration (Plough)	nasal spray: 0.5%	A	
Neo-Synephrine (Sanofi Winthrop)	nose drops: 0.125%	A	dosage for children
	nose drops: 1%	A	
	nasal spray: 0.25%	A	
	nasal spray: 0.25%	A	
	nasal spray, nasal drops, and	A	
	nasal jelly: 0.5%	A	
Nostril (Boehringer-I)	nasal spray: 0.5%	A	
Phenylephrine hydrochloride (generic)	solution: 1%	A	
Rhinall (Scherer)	nasal spray: 0.25%	A	
phenylpropanolamine hydrochloride			
Phenylpropanolamine hydrochloride (generic)	tablets: 25 mg, 50 mg, 75 mg (timed release)	A	℞ to OTC switch
Propagest (Carnrick)	tablets: 25 mg	A	℞ to OTC switch
propylhexedrine			
Benzedrex (SmithKline Beecham)	inhaler: 250 mg + menthol	A	
pseudoephedrine hydrochloride			

Dorcol Children's Decongestant (Sandoz)	liquid: 15 mg per teaspoonful	A	children's dosage, ℞ to OTC switch
Pseudoephedrine hydrochloride (generic)		A	children's dosage, ℞ to OTC switch
Sudafed (Burroughs Wellcome)	tablets: 30 mg, 60mg	A	℞ to OTC switch
Cenafed Syrup (Century Pharm.)	liquid: 30 mg per teaspoonful	A	℞ to OTC switch
Children's Sudafed (Burroughs Wellcome)	liquid: 30 mg per teaspoonful	A	children's dosage, ℞ to OTC switch
Pseudo Syrup (Major)		A	℞ to OTC switch
Pseudoephedrine hydrochloride (generic)		A	℞ to OTC switch
pseudoephedrine sulfate			
Afrinol Repetabs (Schering-Plough)	tablets, timed action: 120 mg	A	℞ to OTC switch
xylometazoline hydrochloride			
Otrivin Pediatric Nasal Drops (Ciba Consumer)	pediatric nose drops: 0.05%	A	children's dosage, ℞ to OTC switch
Otrivin (Ciba Consumer)	spray: 0.1%	A	℞ to OTC switch
Xylometazaloine hydrochloride (generic)		A	℞ to OTC switch

Allergy Drugs: Product Ratings (contd)

COMBINATION PRODUCTS

Product and Distributor	Dosage of Active Ingredients	Rating*	Comment
Dristan Nasal (Whitehall)	**spray:** 0.5% phenylephrine hydrochloride + 0.2% pheniramine maleate	C	This combination has not been shown to be safe and effective — and FDA has said it is not clear which symptoms it is indicated for.
Myci-Spray (Misemer)	**spray:** 0.25% phenylephrine + 0.2% pheniramine maleate	C	This combination has not been shown to be safe.
4-Way Fast Acting (Bristol-Myers)	**nasal spray:** 0.5% phenylephrine hydrochloride + 0.05% naphazoline hydrochloride + 0.2% pyrilamine maleate	B	2 approved ingredients from same category (decongestants)
Vicks VapoRub (Richardson-Vicks)	**ointment:** 4.7% camphor + 2.6% menthol + 1.2% eucalyptus oil	A	
Vicks VapoStream (Richardson-Vicks)	**liquid for vaporizers:** menthol 3.2% + camphor 6.2% + eucalyptus oil 1.5%	B	FDA not convinced this combination is safe and effective

*Author's interpretation of FDA criteria. Based on contents, not claims.

Antacids

Millions of people use over-the-counter antacids—liquids, gels, tablets, capsules, chewing gums, and powders—to relieve symptoms of upper gastrointestinal distress. An antacid neutralizes *hydrochloric acid*. When a person smells, tastes, chews, or swallows food—or sometimes even thinks about it—hydrochloric acid is produced. This is a potent gastric acid that is secreted by glands in the lining of the stomach to aid in the digestion of food. Why the same amount of acid plagues some people but not others remains unclear.

The only symptoms that can be safely and effectively self-diagnosed and self-treated with nonprescription antacids are those that are caused by excess stomach acid. These symptoms have been described as a burning distress that is felt in the upper abdomen, behind the chest, and as high up as the throat.

Antacids are used, often in high doses, to relieve the pain of ulcers in the stomach or *duodenum* (first part of the small intestine). This usage should be recommended and monitored by a doctor. (*See* p. 57.)

ANTACIDS is based on the report of the FDA's Advisory Review Panel on OTC Antacid Drugs, the FDA's Tentative Final Order for Antacid Products, the FDA's Final Order for Antacid and Antiflatulent Products Generally Recognized as Safe and Effective and Not Misbranded, and official addenda of the OTC Drug Review.

Claims

Accurate

For relief of any of the following:

• "Heartburn"

• "Sour stomach"

• "Acid indigestion"

• "Upset stomach" that occurs in association with any of the previous symptoms

False or Misleading

• For the relief of any of the following:

• "Gas"

• "Upper abdominal pressure"

• "Full feeling"

• "Nausea"

• "Excessive eructations [belching]"

• "Sour breath"

• "Nervous and emotional disturbances"

• "Excessive smoking"

• "Food intolerance"

• "Consumption of alcoholic beverages"

• "Nervous-tension headaches"

• "Cold symptoms"

• "Morning sickness of pregnancy"

How They Work

Antacids do *not* act by forming a protective, physical "coating" to keep acid away from the stomach wall. (But: *See* Heartburn Special, further on.) They work by means that are well-described in the old saying, "opposites attract." That is, the antacid's negatively charged particles (negative ions) link with the positively charged hydrogen particles (ions) in the molecules of hydrochloric acid. Neutralization results.

In terms of *acidity* and its opposite, *alkalinity*, the chemical scale, called *pH*, ranges from 0 to 14. A pH of 7 is neutral. A substance that has a pH lower than 7 is acid. The lower the pH, the greater the acidity. The higher the pH above 7, the greater the alkalinity.

The stomach's normal pH is acidic to begin with. But in persons with gastric acidity, the pH may be somewhat below normal. There is also an increase in the *amount* of acid in the stomach.

Antacids raise the pH in the direction of pH 7, but they do not—and need not—completely neutralize the acids. An antacid that raises the stomach contents from pH 1.5 to pH 3.5 has produced a hundred-fold reduction in the concentration of acid. In other words, 99 percent of the acid has been neutralized. This in turn inhibits *pepsin*, another potent component of the digestive juices. Pepsin's potentially irritating effect on the stomach lining has been largely stopped when the stomach contents reach a pH of 3.5.

Potency and Palatability

The Panel stipulated that one dose of an antacid product must be able to neutralize the amount of gastric juice found in a normal person's stomach at rest between meals: about 1 to 2 ounces of gastric juice. This is measured in a lab test, in which a comparable amount of pure hydrochloric acid must be raised to pH 3.5 within 10 minutes. The tight time requirement was set because antacids must act rapidly to be of value. When taken between meals, most of a standard dose of an antacid has passed out of the stomach in 15 minutes.

The neutralizing capacity of the added substance (the antacid) is expressed in milliequivalents (meq) of hydrochloric acid. Every antacid product must have a total neutralizing capacity of at least 5 meq of hydrochloric acid per dosage unit. This is roughly enough to raise the pH in an essentially empty stomach to 3.5. The more potent a product is, the more acid it will neutralize. A product that neutralizes 7.5 meq acid per dose is half again as potent as one that neutralizes 5 meq; one that neutralizes 10 meq is twice as potent.

The FDA requires manufacturers to test their antacids, and that potency information must be included on product information intended for doctors. But manufacturers are *not* allowed to list the neutralizing capacity on labels of products sold over-the-counter to consumers. The reason? Publicizing this information, FDA believes, might lead users to place undue reliance on an antacid's potency when there are other important considerations in choosing a product — for example, its constipating effect, sodium content, and suitability for use over a certain length of time. (These subjects are discussed throughout this unit.)

Nevertheless, consumers may wish to know this information since the more potent the antacid, the less one has to take —and, by and large, the cheaper an effective dose is. The *acid-neutralizing capacity*, or ANC, for a number of antacid products is listed further on. The data reveal significant disparity in potency between antacid products.

These differences become more dramatic if one considers the antacid dose required to neutralize the acid present between meals in the stomach of a person with highly acidic digestive juices. The dose that will usually relieve pain in a person with a gastric ulcer must provide an ANC of roughly 152. If one uses *Riopan Extra Strength* (Whitehall), 5 teaspoonfuls of antacid would be required. With *Titralac Plus* (3M Personal Care), 13 teaspoonfuls of the product would be required. Similarly, it would take 20 *Rolaids* tablets (Warner-Lambet), ANC 7.5, or 15 teaspoons of *Amphojel* (Wyeth-Ayerst), ANC 10, to achieve this result.

In using antacids to treat ulcers, there clearly is a major advantage in selecting a more potent antacid—one with a high ANC. By and large, the more potent the antacid, the *less* expensive an effective dose will be, which is also an advantage.

These potency differences also present a challenge to individuals who use antacids to self-treat heartburn, sour stomach, and other less-serious symptoms that appear to be related to acid. Many manufacturers recommend doses of 1 to 3 teaspoonfuls of liquid antacid, which would provide very different acid-neutralizing capacity, depending on the product. At these doses, which are approved by the FDA, the weaker antacids may deliver precious little neutralizing capacity. This suggests that relatively insignificant neutralizing will suffice to quell these symptoms or, alternatively, as the Panel maintained, that acid and its neutralization may not be the whole story in the appearance or the relief of these symptoms.

Potency is not the only factor to consider in selecting an antacid. Palatability may be even more important. Antacids taste bad to many people, who thus may tend to take too little rather than too much of a product. The way to circumvent this problem is to choose the product that you, as an individual, find most palatable.

Safety and Effectiveness

There is great variability in the dosage needs for antacids, since acid secretion varies widely from person to person and it also varies in the same person from time to time. Antacids are relatively nontoxic and have a low potential for abuse. For these reasons the Panel decided not to set a maximum daily dosage limit based on effectiveness. Some ingredients, however, are potentially more toxic than others, and dosage limits *were* set in terms of safety. Sodium, for example, promotes water retention and high blood pressure—particularly in older persons and in those whose kidneys may be failing. The sodium content of antacids now must appear on product labels.

An officially required label warning cautions users not to exceed the maximum daily dose and not to use the product for more than two weeks unless under a doctor's direction.

Antacids have one other potentially serious problem: They interfere with the absorption of other drugs from the intestinal tract into the bloodstream and body. Therefore, the FDA warns:

 "If you are presently taking a prescription drug, do not take an antacid without checking with your doctor."

Acid-Neutralizing Capacity of Liquid Antacids

Product	Acid-Neutralizing Capacity in Meq Acid/Tsp Antacid	Standard Dose (to Neutralize 152 Meq Acid)
ALternaGEL (J & J-Merck)	16	9½ tsp
Aludrox (Wyeth-Ayerst)	12	13 tsp
Amphojel (Wyeth-Ayerst)	10	15 tsp
Camalox (Rorer)	18.5	8 tsp
Di-Gel (Plough)	10.5	14 tsp
Gelusil (Parke-Davis)	12	13 tsp
Gelusil M (Parke-Davis)	15	10 tsp

Acid-Neutralizing Capacity of Liquid Antacids (contd)

Product	Acid-Neutralizing Capacity in Meq Acid/Tsp Antacid	Standard Dose (to Neutralize 152 Meq Acid)
Maalox (Rorer)	13.3	11 tsp
Maalox Therapeutic Concentrate (Rorer)	27.2	5 tsp
Mylanta (J & J-Merck)	12.7	12 tsp
Mylanta-II (J & J-Merck)	25.4	6 tsp
Riopan (Whitehall)	15	10 tsp
Riopan Extra Strength (Whitehall)	30	5 tsp
Titralac Plus (3M Personal Care)	11	14 tsp

Acid-Neutralizing Capacity of Antacids in Tablets

Product	Acid-Neutralizing Capacity in Meq Acid/Tablet	Number of Tablets (To Neutralize 152 Meq Acid)
Alka-Seltzer (Miles)	10.6	15
Amphojel Tablets (0.6 grams) (Wyeth-Ayerst)	16	9
Camalox Tablets (Rorer)	18	9
Gelusil Tablets (Parke-Davis)	12	13
Gelusil-II Tablets (Parke-Davis)	21	7
Mylanta-II Tablets (J & J-Merck)	23	7
Riopan Tablets (Whitehall)	13.5	12
Rolaids (Warner-Lambert)	7.5	20
Tums (Norcliff Thayer)	10	15

Antacids and Peptic Ulcers

Evaluators did not try to relate gastric-acid symptoms to underlying causes or disease states. They did note, however, that the over-the-counter antacid products used for the self-treatment of acid indigestion also are prescribed—often in much higher dosages—to treat peptic ulcers. Peptic ulcers are serious, often painful, erosions into the wall of the stomach or upper small intestine (duodenum). These disorders are believed to be caused, in part at least, by excessive gastric acid.

A clinical study published in 1977 demonstrated that extremely large dosages—up to seven 1-ounce doses of antacid products containing aluminum hydroxide or a combination of aluminum hydroxide and magnesium hydroxide each day—will heal most duodenal ulcers within seven weeks. This therapy was found equal in effectiveness to the use of a potent prescription drug (*Tagamet*, SmithKline Beecham).

However, these investigators concurred with the Panel's earlier conclusion that ulcers should not be self-treated. Persons with diagnosed or presumed ulcer disease, or any other acid-related gastrointestinal disorders, should be under the care and supervision of a physician, even if the medication they are taking is a nonprescription antacid. What is more, now there are several drugs for treating ulcers that are at least as effective and certainly easier to take than antacids for treating an ulcer.

Combination Products

The four principal types of neutralizing ingredients in antacids are sodium bicarbonate, calcium carbonate, aluminum compounds, and magnesium compounds. Almost all antacid products contain at least one of the four; most contain at least two. The ingredients and the products into which they are formulated vary considerably in potency. Sodium bicarbonate and calcium carbonate are more potent than the magnesium compounds, which in turn tend to be more potent than the aluminum ones.

Some combination products treat acid indigestion and closely related symptoms. Others are intended to simultaneously treat gastric acidity and other problems, such as headache (*See* Approved Combinations, further on).

Antacids Combined with Other Antacids

The FDA permits up to four antacid active ingredients to be combined, provided that each contributes at least 25 percent of the product's acid-neutralizing capacity. (A number of inactive ingredients are used in formulating the products, but they were outside the reviewers' purview.)

A modest amount of a laxative that has been categorized as safe and effective can be added to an antacid product to correct its constipating effect. But no laxative effect can be claimed for such a product. Nor can a substance like mineral oil be used, since too few people experience acid indigestion and constipation (for which mineral oil may be helpful) at the same time.

Antacids Combined with Other Active Ingredients

Approved combinations

A drug that safely and effectively relieves symptoms of intestinal gas (flatulence) can be combined with an antacid. This antacid-antiflatulent combination is to be used—and must be labeled—only for the relief of gas that is experienced with heartburn, sour stomach, or acid indigestion. One drug, simethicone, is approved as a safe and effective over-the-counter drug for treating gas pains, and so it may be combined with antacids. (*See* ANTI-GAS AGENTS.)

The FDA also permits the combination of antacid ingredients with the safe and effective pain-killing ingredients (analgesics) aspirin and acetaminophen. The antacid-acetaminophen combinations are approved only for when acid indigestion and headache occur together. The antacid-aspirin combinations may be labeled for pain symptoms alone or for pain *and* acid indigestion.

Heartburn Special

One group of antacids may be especially useful for *heartburn*, which in fact has nothing to do with the heart. Rather, this sharp burning pain in the lower throat and chest, which some people experience often, particularly after eating a spicy-hot meal, is due to the reverse movement of stomach contents up past the muscular ring, or valve, that separates the stomach from the *esophagus*, or food pipe. The reason this heartburn-producing *gastro-esophageal reflux* occurs is unclear; but some individuals suffer several or more such episodes each day.

Recent surveys indicate that between 7 and 10 percent of presumably healthy subjects in the United States experience heartburn on a daily basis; as many as 40 percent have it at least once a month. So this condition, which usually is mild and passing, but occasionally can be severe enough to require surgical intervention, is gaining new attention in the medical community.

In part, this is because gastro-enterologists now are beginning to think that many of the "ulcer" cases that they have been treating with prescription drugs in fact are gastro-esophageal reflux, a recent editorial in the *New England Journal of Medicine* (vol. 326, pp. 825-27, 1992) suggests. In part, this fresh attention derives from new promotional campaigns for antacids, according to "The Pink Sheet" (February 24, 1992).

Besides drugs, the *New England Journal* editorialist, University of Alabama gastro-enterologist Joel E. Richter, M.D., suggests these steps to help relieve mild heartburn:

• Raise the head of the bed at night.

• Eat smaller meals.

• Don't eat just before bedtime.

• Avoid foods that aggravate your heartburn.

• Cut down on smoking and alcoholic beverages.

One currently marketed type of antacid preparation has been developed particularly to meet this problem. The FDA's OTC Drug Review staff and advisors were not convinced of its efficacy, but the original manufacturer submitted a New Drug Application and so won continuing approval for the preparation; other makers since have produced similar products. (The original brand is *Gaviscon* [Marion Merrell Dow].)

These products contain an inactive ingredient, *alginic acid*, or the sodium salt *sodium alginate*, in addition to two standard antacid ingredients, *aluminum carbonate* and *magnesium carbonate*. These products also contain sodium bicarbonate as an inactive ingredient. The alginic acid and sodium bicarbonate react to create a floating foam that rises in the stomach. This foam bathes the top of the stomach and lower esophagus with the two antacids. The original manufacturer claims the product "is effective because of its unique ability to foam and float on the top of stomach contents, protecting the esophagus from acid irritation." The FDA allows, but does not vouch for this claim.

APPROVED ANTACID ACTIVE INGREDIENTS

Most traditional antacid ingredients have been approved for over-the-counter use in the FDA's OTC review process. They are judged to be effective on the basis of reports in the scientific literature and on tests showing that each tablet, capsule, or other dosage unit has the capacity to neutralize the acid present between meals in an essentially empty stomach. A few combinations that flunked the OTC Review have since been approved by the FDA as new drugs.

Compared with other groups of drugs, like pain-killers, antacids are considered very safe. Nevertheless, they may pose a threat to some persons, particularly if taken in large amounts for extended periods of time.

• *ALUMINUM COMPOUNDS:* The compounds that contain aluminum tend to be very safe as antacid ingredients because very little aluminum is absorbed from the gastrointestinal tract into the body. So no dosage limits have been established—except for aluminum phosphate (8 grams per day), because phosphate intake should be limited.

The complications that do occur when taking aluminum-containing antacids usually are the result of their obstructive effect in the intestines. These products tend to be viscous, and since they are relatively weak as antacids, large doses may be required, which could induce intestinal blockage. Simple constipation, however, is the more common occurrence. Some manufacturers counteract the constipating tendency of aluminum antacid ingredients by combining them with magnesium ingredients or other substances that have the opposite (laxative) effect.

WARNING:

 Aluminum interferes with the absorption of some prescription drugs, most notably the antibiotic tetracycline. It should not be taken by patients for whom tetracycline has been prescribed by a doctor.

Even though the FDA concurred with the Panel in approving

aluminum-containing compounds as safe and effective, more recent studies indicate that they could be risky for individuals with kidney problems and for persons on kidney dialysis, in whom they can cause a severe neurologic disturbance called dialysis dementia. Of wider concern is recent evidence that suggests that heavy use of aluminum-containing antacids may adversely affect the metabolism of the minerals phosphorus, calcium, and fluoride in the body and cause or intensify bone abnormalities. Some evidence also suggests that aluminum may cause or contribute to the development of *Alzheimer's disease*. This has not been proved, and may not be true.

• *BICARBONATE COMPOUNDS:* The bicarbonate compounds used as antacids include sodium bicarbonate (ordinary baking soda) and potassium bicarbonate. Both are potent neutralizers of stomach acid. So are sodium carbonate and potassium carbonate, which are used in effervescent preparations that are drunk as bubbling liquids.

The bicarbonates' principal drawback is that they are readily absorbed into the body. There they can measurably increase the alkalinity of blood plasma and other body tissues. They probably cannot raise the pH of plasma beyond the normal range, but the effects of their prolonged use are largely unknown. Bicarbonates can be particularly risky for persons with impaired kidney function. When carbonate is taken as sodium bicarbonate, the sodium is absorbed from the intestine into the body. For people with defective kidneys who have trouble ridding their bodies of sodium, this buildup can be a hazard.

Sodium bicarbonate—which is widely used as a food product, tooth cleanser, and mouthwash, as well as an antacid—has an extremely low potential for causing injury by overdose. But the suggested upper dosage limit is 10 grams per day for persons up to age 60; 5 grams per day for persons over 60 years of age.

• *BISMUTH COMPOUNDS:* The bismuth-containing compounds marketed as antacids are considered safe in the amounts commonly used. The oral dose for adults is 1 gram, and the usual daily dosage is 4 grams, so 4 doses (a total of 16 grams) can be taken each day.

• *CALCIUM COMPOUNDS:* The two approved ingredients—calcium carbonate and calcium phosphate—are fast-acting neutralizers of gastric acid. They also are quite potent. Very small doses are as effective as far larger amounts of other antacid ingredients.

However, safety considerations suggest limiting one's intake of calcium. It can cause constipation. It also is readily absorbed from the gastrointestinal tract into the body and may form calcium kidney stones or trigger other toxic consequences. For these reasons, the Panel recommended that no more than 8 grams of calcium carbonate be taken daily. The limit for calcium phosphate is 13.1 grams (about half an ounce).

Consumers should also be aware of a somewhat puzzling dual action. While calcium-containing antacid ingredients relieve acidity, they can also stimulate the secretion of stomach acids, which is the opposite effect of that sought. Some experts say, therefore, that calcium-containing compounds should not be used as antacids. But the information thus far available does not warrant such a restriction. So these active ingredients are fully approved as safe and effective for self-treatment.

- *CITRATES:* Neither the Panel nor the FDA has much to say about citrate-containing antacid ingredients like citric acid, except that they are safe and effective. The recommended maximum daily dosage is 8 grams, a bit less than a third of an ounce.

- *GLYCINE (AMINOACETIC ACID):* This amino acid is practically nontoxic. It is judged safe without dosage restriction for nonprescription use as an antacid for use up to two weeks. Research studies indicate that amino acids like glycine are quite effective in initially neutralizing sour stomach contents, but they are less effective in providing further neutralization after a pH of 2.5 has been achieved.

- *MAGNESIUM COMPOUNDS:* For the most part, the magnesium antacid substances are less potent than calcium or sodium carbonates. When magnesium compounds neutralize hydrochloric acid, the compound magnesium chloride is formed. Some of it is absorbed into the body, but then it is rapidly and safely excreted by the kidneys, except in people whose kidney function is impaired.

WARNING:

 For those persons whose kidney function is impaired, lowered blood pressure, nausea, vomiting, respiratory distress, and even coma may follow ingestion of these magnesium compounds.

Magnesium is an essential nutrient that is contained in food. About one-third of dietary magnesium is absorbed. Even less of the magnesium in antacids is absorbed. This unabsorbed magnesium has the effect of pulling water into the intestine, causing diarrhea. To counteract this effect, materials that have the opposite (or constipating) effect—particularly calcium or aluminum—are often mixed with magnesium in antacid products.

Panel reviewers said that magnesium-containing antacids are, in commonly used dosages, unlikely to cause other side effects. No restriction has been placed on daily intake, and they may be used for up to two weeks. However, products that contain relatively large amounts of magnesium should not be used by persons with kidney problems except under medical supervision.

- *MILK SOLIDS, DRIED:* Milk solids are used as antacid active ingredients. They are safe for this purpose in the amounts usually taken in antacid products, so no dosage limit has been set on their use.
- *PHOSPHATE COMPOUNDS:* The amounts of phosphates usually taken orally for antacid purposes are relatively low and safe. Products formulated with mono- or dibasic calcium phosphate as the phosphate source usually contain 200 mg per tablet; the customary dosage is up to 8 tablets per day. Products that contain aluminum phosphate are formulated with up to 2 grams per tablet, with a recommended dosage of up to 4 tablets daily. When the phosphate source is tricalcium phosphate, each tablet contains 1 to 4 grams, and the package directions suggest up to 6 tablets daily. All these dosages are safe, provided the product is not used longer than two weeks without the individual's seeing a doctor.
- *POTASSIUM COMPOUNDS:* Several antacids contain potassium, usually in the form of sodium potassium tartrate or potassium citrate. While the buildup of potassium in the body can be dangerous, it is a rare problem that tends to occur only in people with inadequate kidney function. There is no evidence that healthy persons risk potassium toxicity (*hyperkalemia*) when they use the popular antacids that contain this ingredient. No maximum daily intake level has been set, but products that contain relatively large amounts of potassium must carry the warning that persons with kidney disease should take them only under the advice and care of a physician.
- *SILICATES:* Antacid active ingredients that carry silicates—including magnesium aluminosilicates and magnesium trisilicate—appear relatively safe. While there are reports of patients' developing kidney stones, there is insufficient evidence to conclude that a maximum daily dosage must be set.

Magnesium trisilicate, however, may interfere with the absorption of some other drugs. Persons who are taking other medications should consult their doctor.
- *SODIUM COMPOUNDS:* The problem with sodium, which principally con-

cerns older persons, is that it triggers and exacerbates high blood pressure. This risk is increased when a person has poor kidney function and cannot quickly excrete sodium from the body. Thus, limits have been set on the amount that should be taken each day in nonprescription antacid products, including sodium bicarbonate (baking soda), sodium carbonate, and sodium potassium carbonate. If one were taking pure sodium bicarbonate powder—baking soda—this limit would be 2 to 2½ teaspoonfuls for persons over age 60, and 4½ teaspoonfuls for younger persons.

• TARTRATE COMPOUNDS: Although tartrates, which include tartaric acid and its salts, are found in baking powder and a variety of other foods, and seem safe, the effect of their repeated day-to-day medicinal use in antacids has not been adequately studied. In high doses, they conceivably could cause kidney problems.

It still is not clear whether tartrate is absorbed into the body; tartrate metabolism is poorly defined. Balancing both this lack of knowledge and possible risk against traditional usage, evaluators set a maximum daily dose limit of 15 grams—just over half an ounce—even though tartrate and its equivalents are assessed as safe and effective.

CONDITIONALLY APPROVED ANTACID ACTIVE INGREDIENTS
None.

DISAPPROVED ANTACID ACTIVE INGREDIENTS
None.

Safety and Effectiveness:
Active Ingredients in Over-the-Counter Antacids

Neutralizing Agent	Assessment
aluminum compounds aluminum carbonate	safe and effective
aluminum hydroxide	safe and effective

Safety and Effectiveness:
Active Ingredients in Over-the-Counter Antacids (contd)

Neutralizing Agent	Assessment
aluminum hydroxide-hexitol, stabilized polymer	safe and effective
aluminum hydroxide-magnesium carbonate, co-dried gel	safe and effective
aluminum hydroxide-magnesium trisilicate, co-dried gel	safe and effective
aluminum hydroxide-sucrose powder, hydrated	safe and effective
aluminum phosphate gel	safe and effective
dihydroxyaluminum aminoacetate	safe and effective
dihydroxyaluminum aminoacetic acid	safe and effective
dihydroxyaluminum sodium carbonate	safe and effective
bismuth compounds bismuth aluminate	safe and effective
bismuth carbonate	safe and effective
bismuth subcarbonate	safe and effective
bismuth subgallate	safe and effective
bismuth subnitrate	safe and effective
calcium compounds calcium carbonate	safe and effective
calcium phosphate	safe and effective
citrate compounds citric acid	safe and effective
citric salts	safe and effective
glycine (aminoacetic acid)	safe and effective
magnesium compounds hydrated magnesium aluminate, activated sulfate	safe and effective

Safety and Effectiveness:
Active Ingredients in Over-the-Counter Antacids (contd)

Neutralizing Agent	Assessment
magaldrate	safe and effective
magnesium aluminosilicate	safe and effective
magnesium carbonate	safe and effective
magnesium glycinate	safe and effective
magnesium hydroxide	safe and effective
magnesium oxide	safe and effective
magnesium trisilicate	safe and effective
milk solids, dried	safe and effective
phosphate compounds aluminum phosphate	safe and effective
mono- or dibasic calcium salt	safe and effective
tricalcium phosphate	safe and effective
potassium compounds potassium bicarbonate	safe and effective
potassium carbonate	safe and effective
sodium potassium tartrate	safe and effective
silicates magnesium aluminosilicate	safe and effective
magnesium trisilicate	safe and effective
sodium compounds sodium bicarbonate	safe and effective
sodium carbonate	safe and effective
sodium potassium tartrate	safe and effective
tartrate compounds sodium potassium tartrate	safe and effective
tartaric acid	safe and effective
tartrate	safe and effective

Antacids: Product Ratings

Product and Distributor	Dosage of Active Ingredients	Rating *	Comment
SINGLE-INGREDIENT PRODUCTS			
aluminum carbonate gel, basic			
Basaljel (Wyeth-Ayerst)	**capsules and swallow tablets:** dried basic aluminum carbonate gel equivalent to 608 mg dried aluminum hydroxide gel or 500 mg aluminum hydroxide	A	
aluminum hydroxide gel			
Alternagel (Stuart)	**liquid:** 600 mg per teaspoonful	A	
Alu-Cap (Riker)	**capsules:** 475 mg	A	
Aluminum Hydroxide Gel (generic)	**suspension:** 320 mg, 600 mg per teaspoonful	A	
Amphojel (Wyeth-Ayerst)	**tablets:** 300 mg, 600 mg	A	
	suspension: 320 mg per teaspoonful	A	
aluminum phosphate gel			
Phosphaljel (Wyeth-Ayerst)	**suspension:** 233 mg per teaspoonful	A	

Antacids: Product Ratings (contd)

Product and Distributor	Dosage of Active Ingredients	Rating*	Comment
calcium carbonate			
Alka-Mints (Miles Labs.)	**chewable tablets:** 850 mg	A	
Amitone (SmithKline Beecham)	**chewable tablets:** 350 mg	A	
Calcium carbonate (generic)	**tablets:** 500 mg, 650 mg	A	
Chooz (Schering Plough)	**chewable tablets:** 500 mg	A	
Mallamint (Hauck)	**chewable tablets:** 420 mg	A	
Tums (SmithKline Beecham)	**chewable tablets:** 500 mg	A	
Tums Extra Strength Liquid (SmithKline Beecham)	**liquid:** 1000 mg per teaspoonful	A	
dihydroxyaluminum sodium carbonate			
Rolaids (Warner-Lambert)	**chewable tablets:** 334 mg	A	
magaldrate (hydroxymagnesium aluminate)			
Riopan (Whitehall)	**swallow tablets:** 480 mg	A	
	chewable tablets: 480 mg	A	
	suspension: 540 mg per teaspoonful	A	
Riopan Extra Strength (Whitehall)	**suspension:** 1080 mg per teaspoonful	A	

magnesium carbonate			
Magnesium carbonate (generic)	**powder**	A	
magnesium hydroxide (magnesia)			
Milk of magnesia (generic)	**liquid:** 390 mg per teaspoonful	A	
	tablets: 325 mg	A	
Phillips' Milk of Magnesia (Sterling Health)	**suspension:** approx. 400 mg per teaspoonful	A	
magnesium oxide			
Mag Ox 400 (Blaine)	**tablets:** 400 mg	A	
Maox (Kenneth Manne)	**tablets:** 420 mg	A	
Uro-Mag (Blaine)	**capsules:** 140 mg	A	
magnesium trisilicate			
Magnesium trisilicate (generic)	**tablets:** 488 mg	A	
sodium bicarbonate (contains 27% sodium)			
Arm & Hammer Baking Soda (Church & Dwight)	**powder:** bicarbonate of soda, USP	A	grocery store item
Soda Mint (generic)	**tablets:** 325 mg	A	
Sodium bicarbonate (generic)	**tablets:** 325 mg, 650 mg	A	

Antacids: Product Ratings (contd)

COMBINATION PRODUCTS

Product and Distributor	aluminum hydroxide	magnesium hydroxide	calcium carbonate	magnesium trisilicate	Other Content†	Rating*	Comment
Capsules and Tablets							
Alkets Tablets (Upjohn)			780 mg		130 mg magnesium carbonate + 65 mg magnesium oxide	A	
Alma-Mag #4 Improved Tablets (Rugby)	200 mg	200 mg		488 mg	25 mg simethicone	A	also relieves gas
Bisodol Tablets (Whitehall)		178 mg	194 mg			A	
Calcilac Tablets (Schein)			420 mg		180 mg glycine	A	
Di-Gel Tablets (Schering-Plough)		128 mg	280 mg		20 mg simethicone	A	also relieves gas

Product						
Gaviscon Tablets (Marion Merrell Dow)	80 mg			20 mg		A
Gelusil Tablets (Parke-Davis)	200 mg	200 mg			25 mg simethicone	A	also relieves gas
Gelusil II Tablets Parke-Davis)	400 mg	400 mg			30 mg simethicone	A	also relieves gas
Glycate Tablets (Forest)			300 mg		150 mg glycine	A
Maalox Extra Strength Tablets (Rhone-Poulenc Rorer)	400 mg	400 mg				A
Maalox Plus Tablets (Rhone-Poulenc Rorer)	200 mg	200 mg			25 mg simethicone	A	also relieves gas
Maalox Tablets (Rhone-Poulenc Rorer)	200 mg	200 mg				A
Mylanta Tablets (Stuart)	200 mg	200 mg			20 mg simethicone	A	also relieves gas

Antacids: Product Ratings (contd)

Product and Distributor	aluminum hydroxide	magnesium hydroxide	calcium carbonate	magnesium trisilicate	Other Content[†]	Rating*	Comment
Mylanta-II Tablets (Stuart)	400 mg	400 mg			40 mg simethicone	A	also relieves gas
Riopan Plus Tablets (Whitehall)					480 mg magaldrate + 20 mg simethicone	A	also relieves gas
Spastosed Tablets (Vortech)			226 mg		162 mg magnesium carbonate + tartrazine	A	
Titralac Tablets (3M Personal Care)			420 mg				

Product and Distributor	aluminum hydroxide	magnesium hydroxide	calcium carbonate	magnesium trisilicate	Other Content[†]	Rating*	Comment

Liquids and Suspensions: contents given mg per teaspoonful (5 ml)

Almacone II Suspension (Rugby)	400 mg	400 mg			40 mg simethicone	A	also relieves gas

Aludrox Suspension (Wyeth-Ayerst)	307 mg	103 mg		A	
Camalox Suspension (Rhone-Poulenc Rorer)	225 mg	200 mg	250 mg	A	
Gaviscon Extra Strength Relief Formula (Marion Merrill Dow)	32 mg		119 mg magnesium carbonate + alginic acid	A	specially formulated for heartburn relief
Di-Gel Liquid (Schering-Plough)	200 mg	200 mg	20 mg simethicone	A	also relieves gas
Maalox Heartburn Relif Formula (Rhone-Poulenc Rorer)	350 mg		140 mg aluminum hydroxide-magnesium carbonate co-dried gel + 175 mg magnesium carbonate	A	

Antacids: Product Ratings (contd)

Product and Distributor	aluminum hydroxide	magnesium hydroxide	calcium carbonate	magnesium trisilicate	Other Content†	Rating*	Comment
Extra Strength Maalox Plus Suspension (Rhone-Poulenc Rorer)	500 mg	450 mg			40 mg simethicone	A	also relieves gas
Mylanta Liquid (Stuart)	200 mg	200 mg			20 mg simethicone	A	also relieves gas
Mylanta-II Liquid (Stuart)	400 mg	400 mg			40 mg simethicone	A	also relieves gas
Riopan Plus Suspension (Whitehall)					540 mg magaldrate + 20 mg simethicone	A	also relieves gas
Tums Extra Strength Liquid w/ simethicone (SmithKline Beecham)			1000 mg		30 mg simethicone	A	also relieves gas

WinGel Liquid (Sanofi Winthrop)   180 mg   160 mg   A

POWDERS AND EFFERVESCENT TABLETS

Product and Distributor	Dosage of Active Ingredients	Rating*	Comment
Alka-Seltzer (Miles Labs.)	**effervescent tablets:** 958 mg sodium bicarbonate + 832 mg citric acid + 312 mg potassium bicarbonate + 311 mg sodium	A	
Alka-Seltzer with Aspirin (Miles Labs.)	**effervescent tablets:** 1916 mg sodium bicarbonate + 1000 mg citric acid + 325 mg aspirin + 567 mg sodium	A	also relieves headache
Bisodol (Whitehall)	**powder:** 716 mg sodium bicarbonate + 528 mg magnesium carbonate + 196 mg sodium per 5 ml	A	
Bromo Seltzer (Warner-Lambert)	**effervescent granules:** 325 mg acetaminophen + 2781 mg sodium bicarbonate + 2224 mg citric acid per dosage measure	A	also relieves headache

Antacids: Product Ratings (contd)

Product and Distributor	Dosage of Active Ingredients	Rating*	Comment
Citrocarbonate (Upjohn)	**effervescent granules:** 1820 mg sodium citrate + 780 mg sodium bicarbonate + 700 mg sodium per 3.9 g dose	A	
ENO (Beecham)	**powder:** 1620 mg sodium tartrate + 1172 mg sodium citrate + 819 mg sodium per teaspoonful	A	

*Author's interpretation of FDA criteria. Based on contents, not claims.
†All currently marketed antacid products are required to meet final standards of the Over the Counter Drug Review.

Anti-Gas Agents

A drug that expels gas from the stomach and intestines is often called an *antiflatulent*, since *flatus* is the technical—and polite—word for gastrointestinal-tract gas.

One active ingredient, simethicone, is approved as safe and effective for evacuating gastrointestinal gas. It appears to lower the surface tension of small gas bubbles in the stomach and intestines. This appears to cause the bubbles to combine into larger ones that are more easily expelled, according to FDA.

The causes of gastrointestinal gas, which also are discussed in the unit DIGESTIVE AIDS, include swallowing air during chewing and eating. Some people swallow air at other times, particularly when they are nervous. The chewing of chewing gum or the wearing of dentures also may contribute to this problem.

The foods one eats influence the gas content of the gut. The FDA identifies these foods as *flatuogenic*, or "gassers":

ANTI-GAS AGENTS is based on the report of the FDA's Advisory Review Panel on OTC Antacid Drugs, the FDA's Tentative Final Order for Antacid Products, the FDA's Final Order for Antacid and Antiflatulent Products Generally Recognized as Safe and Effective and Not Misbranded, the report of the OTC Advisory Review Panel on Miscellaneous Internal Drug Products entitled "Digestive Aid Drug Products for OTC Human Use," the FDA's Tentative Final Monograph for these products, and official addenda of the OTC Drug Review process.

Highly flatuogenic: beans, bagels, bran, broccoli, brussels sprouts, cabbage, cauliflower, onions, and, for people who are lactose intolerant, milk and milk products.

Moderately flatuogenic: bread and pastries, radishes, apples, prune juice, raisins, carrots, bananas, apricots, celery, citrus fruits, let- tuce, eggplant.

For people who drink a lot of them, FDA adds to the list of flatuogenics beer and soft drinks, which of course have gas added for *fizz* (*FDA Consumer*, April 1987).

 Claims

Accurate
- "Antiflatulent"
- "Antigas"
- "Relieves the symptoms of gas"
- "Alleviates bloating, pressure, fullness or stuffed feeling, commonly referred to as gas"

False or Misleading
- References to "belching" and "colic"

- SIMETHICONE: Simethicone has been marketed for a number of years, often in combination with antacid ingredients. Antacid panelists assessed it as safe but raised questions about its effectiveness. They believed it rea- sonably certain that the surface action causes small gas bubbles to coa- lesce, forming larger ones, but they had reservations about whether this action is truly beneficial. The Panel wondered if the sensations that con- sumers complain of really result from accumulations of gas.

    These doubts were allayed by two studies in which neither patients nor doctors knew whether the preparation being used con- tained simethicone or was a similar-tasting dummy substance (place- bo). Participants in one study were primed with gas-inducing meals. "In both studies," the FDA reported, "the patients showed a statisti- cally significant preference for simethicone" in treating gas.

    Meanwhile, however, a second OTC Advisory Review Panel— this one on OTC Miscellaneous Internal Drug Products—had looked at simethicone and had raised doubts about its effectiveness. Even if simethicone is effective, this Panel of experts said, it is not at all clear that this relief has much to do with evacuating gas from the gut. This Panel suggested that simethicone had not been proven to be effective as an anti-gas agent.

The FDA then was between a rock and a hard place, since it had told manufacturers that, once it approved an ingredient in a final monograph—as it had done for simethicone—the decision (in this case, approval) would stand. The agency therefore issued the following statement to extricate itself from this regulatory impasse on simethicone:

"The [FDA] agrees...that the final monograph for OTC anti-flatulent drug products should not be revoked or modified based on the [Miscellaneous Internal Drug Products] Panel's recommendations. Although the agency agrees with [that] Panel that data are insufficient to demonstrate that excessive gas actually causes the symptoms of bloating, pressure, and fullness [for which people take simethicone products], data are available to demonstrate that 'gas' is a word used by consumers to describe these symptoms...Therefore...evidence need not be available demonstrating the cause of a symptom as long as there is sufficient evidence to show that an ingredient provides relief from the symptom."

This double-talk suggests that the FDA-approved "anti-gas" claim for simethicone should be taken with a grain of salt—a view bolstered by researchers at Our Lady of Mercy Medical Center, in the Bronx, N.Y.: They fed a half pound of baked beans each to healthy volunteers. Simethicone (160 mg) did not significantly reduce hydrogen sulfide—which is gas from undigested food—on the breath, or symptoms of bloating or abdominal discomfort, compared to look-alike dummy medication (placebo). However activated charcoal tablets (2080 mg) did significantly reduce hydrogen sulfide excretion and the abdominal symptoms (*Annals of Internal Medicine,* vol. 105, pp. 61-2, 1986).

Simethicone can be combined with safe and effective antacids, provided the product is labeled both for the relief of "gas" and concurrent symptoms of sour stomach, heartburn, or acid indigestion, and accompanying upset stomach. The maximum daily dosage recommended in over-the-counter preparations is 500 mg. (Higher dosages can be prescribed by doctors.)

Safety and Effectiveness:
Active Ingredient in Over-the-Counter Anti-Gas Agents

Ingredient	Assessment
simethicone	safe and effective

Anti-Gas Products: Ratings

SINGLE INGREDIENT PRODUCTS

Product and Distributor	Dosage of Active Ingredients	Rating*	Comment
simethicone			
Mylicon (Stuart)	**chewable tablets:** 40 mg; **drops:** 40 mg per 0.6 ml	A	
Mylicon-80 (Stuart)	**chewable tablets:** 80 mg	A	
Phazyme 125 (Reed and Carnrick)	**capsules:** 125 mg	A	
Silain (Robins)	**tablets:** 50 mg	A	

COMBINATION PRODUCTS

Product and Distributor	Dosage of Active Ingredients	Rating*	Comment
Flatulex (Dayton Laboratories)	**dual-coated tablets:** 80 mg simethicone + 250 mg activated charcoal	B	activated charcoal not proved effective

Products containing antacids + simethicone appear on pp. 70–75 (Antacids Combination Product Ratings). They are identified under Comment by the notation "also relieves gas."

*Author's interpretation of FDA criteria. Based on contents, not claims.

Antiperspirants

Body odor is not new. Neither are efforts to subdue it. Early Egyptian, Greek, and Roman literatures record efforts to control it through bathing, grooming, and perfuming practices. The French of the seventeenth century, who rarely bathed, raised to an art the use of perfumed oils and waters to disguise the smell of their unclean bodies.

The link between sweat and odor began to be more clearly understood when the sweat glands were discovered in the nineteenth century. The first product marketed specifically for underarm odor was *Mum*, introduced in 1888. This preparation used zinc oxide in a cream base. *Everdry* in 1902 and *Hush* in 1908 were the first to use aluminum chloride solutions. In 1914, *Odo-Ro-No* was the first product to be launched with national magazine advertising that claimed it would remedy excessive perspiration and keep dresses "clean and dainty." Five years later, *Odo-Ro-No* advertising again led the way: It was the first to assert that perspiration and body odor—or "B.O." as it later came to be called—are socially shocking and offensive.

ANTIPERSPIRANTS is based on the preliminary and final reports of the FDA Advisory Review Panel on OTC Antiperspirant Drug Products, the FDA's Tentative Final Monograph on these products, and on the FDA final regulation on aerosol drug and cosmetic products containing zirconium.

In the first 50 years, antiperspirants were used mainly by women, who came to consider them almost as essential as soap. In recent decades, however, more and more men have begun to use antiperspirants, which is why sales continue to rise. Sale of these products is spurred by highly competitive advertising, which creates a strong sense of need for these products in the consumer's mind.

Underarm antiperspirant preparations actually perform two functions: They reduce the amount of perspiration secreted under the arms and they mask or control odor. The same ingredients in the products can, and do, perform both functions. The FDA evaluators were faced with a peculiar problem in judging these two functions. Products that affect, or are claimed to affect body secretions, are defined as *drugs* under the federal Food, Drug and Cosmetic Act; they are called *antiperspirants*. Products that simply mask or control odor (deodorants) or are claimed to perform only these functions, are defined as *cosmetics*. As such, the latter are not considered in the Over-the-Counter (OTC) Drug Review, and they—and the claims made for them—are much less stringently regulated than drugs are. The result is that consumers are denied a rigorous scientific evaluation of the deodorant effect of these products. This is unfortunate because many people believe the products' anti-odor function is the most important one. Confoundingly, some antiperspirant active ingredients are sold as deodorants, but without antiperspirant claims on the labels, which can only contribute to consumers' confusion. The more circumspect choice for consumers probably is to purchase these compounds as *antiperspirants*.

 ### Claims

Accurate
- "Reduces underarm wetness"
- "Decreases underarm dampness"
- "Diminishes underarm perspiration"

False, Misleading, or Unproved
- "Completely guards your family"
- "Helps stop wetness"
- "Really helps keep you dry"
- "Stops," "halts," or "ends" underarm perspiration
- "Dry formula"

- "Dry"
- "Extra-strength"
- References to "problem" or "especially troublesome" sweat
- References to "longer-lasting" or "24-hour" protection or to "emotional" sweating

---

 WARNING:
Do not apply to broken skin. If rash or irritation develops, discontinue use. For spray products, avoid excessive inhalation.

Perspiration

Sources

Human perspiration is produced by two kinds of sweat glands, the apocrine and the eccrine.

Apocrine glands These structures lie close to the hair follicles and are found all over the body's surface at birth. Most of them gradually disappear. In adults, the remaining apocrine glands are concentrated in the armpits (axilla) and around the anus and the nipples.

These glands are inactive during childhood. They develop and begin to function during puberty—apparently due to sex-hormone stimulation—and then tend to *atrophy,* or wither, in old age. Their exact function remains unknown.

Sweat secretion from the apocrine glands is scant and slow. After an apocrine gland produces a single small droplet of sweat, a long period follows before the same gland is ready to secrete another droplet. Droplets dry into glue-like granules that stick to the underarm skin and hairs. They are normally odorless.

Eccrine glands Most of the body's sweat is produced by the eccrine glands. These glands appear in abundance on all body surfaces except on the lips and on parts of the sexual organs. Since babies have much smaller skin surfaces than adults, their eccrine glands are much more closely spaced, which may be why they seem to sweat more freely.

Eccrine sweat is copious and consists mostly of water. But it also contains small amounts of salt, potassium, urea, lactate, and glucose. In extreme heat and with high water intake, human subjects have been reported to secrete up to 3 gallons of sweat in 24 hours, most of it through the eccrine glands.

The eccrine glands have a clear physiological role: they regulate body heat. (The popular notion that people need to sweat to "purify" their bodies is mistaken.) Evaporation of eccrine sweat from the skin rapidly cools the body. Persons who are unable to sweat cannot tolerate ambient temperatures much above 80° F; neither can they easily endure the heat generated by vigorous physical exercise.

The eccrine glands function in response to nerve impulses. They can be stimulated by external heat or fever, by eating spicy foods, and by emotional stress. Sweating induced by emotional reactions is particularly noticeable in the armpits and on the palms of the hands and the soles of the feet.

Excessive sweating—technically called *hyperhidrosis*—principally involves the eccrine glands. The condition is most common from early adolescence to the mid-twenties. Most heavy sweating follows over-heating, or fear and embarrassment, or other emotional responses. However, it also may accompany conditions such as shock, diabetes, hyperthyroidism, nausea, or overconsumption of alcohol.

It takes several minutes or longer for physical heat to produce perspiration. But heated emotions can generate an almost instantaneous sweat response!

Armpit Odor

Because the armpits are normally warm and moist, they create a hospitable environment for bacteria. Convincing scientific evidence exists to show that armpit odor arises from bacteria that grow in secretions of the apocrine glands. One research group collected fresh apocrine sweat from unwashed armpits and showed that it was odorless. When kept for six hours at room temperature, however, the bacteria in it multiplied rapidly, and the sweat acquired a characteristically rank "armpit" odor. When sweat from the same source was refrigerated, no odor developed.

Apocrine sweat collected from armpits that had been shaved and disinfected with alcohol developed no odor at room temperature. In other tests, armpits treated with an antibacterial cleanser remained odor-free for 18 hours longer than untreated armpits.

The copious moisture provided by the eccrine glands facilitates the growth of the bacteria and contributes to the dispersal of odor. The hair tuft under the arm acts as a kind of wick from which mixed eccrine and bacterially decomposed apocrine sweat evaporates into one's personal environment.

Few attempts have been made to discover exactly which bacteria cause underarm odor and how many of them need to be present for the odor to be detectable, even though, as the Panel pointedly commented, "the American public spends hundreds of millions of dollars annually to combat these bacteria."

In 1990, however, a breakthrough was claimed by chemist George Preti and several colleagues at the Monell Chemical Senses Center in Philadelphia. They said they had isolated more than 100 different chemicals from several men's unwashed armpits. They then sniffed the isolated compounds one at a time, and found that *hexonic acid* is the principal source of armpit odor.

If this report is confirmed, antiperspirant and deodorant makers obviously will try to develop and market products that specifically neutralize hexonic acid. To date (1992), no such product has emerged into view.

What purpose these odors may serve in human beings is only beginning to be investigated. The currently favored view is that apocrine-gland secretions function as chemical signals—pheromones—that activate specific behavioral responses in other members of the same species. If we believe antiperspirant and deodorant advertisements, we are repelled by underarm odor, particularly when it emanates from a member of the opposite sex. But it is possible that at an unconscious (or perhaps even at a conscious) level these odors serve as sexual attractants.

How Antiperspirants Work

These products reduce underarm wetness. This reduction in turn retards bacterial growth. Decreased wetness and fewer bacteria probably account for how antiperspirants prevent or decrease armpit odor for meaningful periods of time when they are applied once or twice daily on a fairly regular basis. Although antiperspirants reduce underarm wetness so that it is more difficult for bacteria to grow, their effectiveness against odor may *also* depend on their ability to kill bacteria. But the evidence for such a direct antibacterial action is fragmentary.

The manner in which aluminum compounds, the principal components of antiperspirants, act on sweat glands is unknown. One theory maintains that they penetrate some distance into the sweat duct and bind to the duct wall to block the passage of water. Pressure then builds up in the duct. This action, through a biofeedback mechanism, stops further sweat secretion. A competing theory suggests that the sweat duct is made more permeable to water. In this way, like a leaky hose, moisture is dispersed back into the surrounding skin rather than emerging from it in large droplets. A third view holds that aluminum chloride and comparable chemicals block transmission of the nerve impulses that turn on the sweat glands. Finally, one industry representative claims that his product acts like glue to block up the sweat duct—a concept that was received skeptically by the reviewers.

Whatever the mechanism, antiperspirants act only on the eccrine glands. They have no effect on the apocrine glands, whose bacterially altered secretions are the principal source of underarm odor. In fact, no known nonprescription product can halt or control apocrine sweat, and *antiperspirants were not specifically evaluated on their ability to quell underarm odor since this is technically a cosmetic action, not a drug action.* But the evaluators were satisfied by industry "sniff tests" and other evidence that aluminum and zirconium salts—the ingredients in antiperspirants that reduce underarm moisture—also reduce underarm odor.

Antiperspirant Effectiveness

Antiperspirant effectiveness is often tested by applying the product to one armpit, and the base alone—that is, the cream, liquid, or spray in which the active ingredient is formulated—to the other. A dozen or more persons may participate in each test. Cotton pads are placed in each armpit, and the subjects either go about their daily routines or are put into a hot, humid room. Some testers challenge subjects with mental puzzles or try to upset them to enhance sweating. After a set time the pads are collected and weighed. If the pads in the treated armpit weigh less than the others, the ingredient is judged to have antiperspirant activity. The greater the difference in weight between the two pads, the more effective the ingredient. Most antiperspirants reduce wetness by 20 to 40 percent.

Reviewers considered this a low over-all level of effectiveness. But when tests showed that a reduction of less than 20 percent cannot be detected, they chose that figure as a standard: To be considered effective, a product must provide at least a 20-percent reduction in underarm perspiration in at least half of the users who apply it once a day.

The effectiveness of antiperspirants depends on regular use.

They do not usually become effective immediately. Some take hours; others require even more time and repeated applications. To achieve maximal levels of effectiveness, they must be used at least once daily.

A few antiperspirant products are marketed to reduce sweat on body surfaces other than the armpits, particularly for the feet and hands. The decreases they produced were too small to be noticed by the user, and the Panel regarded these products as no more than conditionally effective. The FDA agrees.

Forms of Antiperspirants

Test results submitted for review showed that, as a class, aerosol products are the *least* effective and lotions the *most* effective. The ranges in average sweat reduction in tests with various types of underarm products are as shown.

aerosols	20 to 33 percent
liquids	15 to 54 percent
sticks	35 to 40 percent
creams	35 to 47 percent
roll-ons	14 to 70 percent
lotions	38 to 62 percent

Most products reduce sweat by 20 percent or more in the majority of users. But consumers may have to try out several different products for themselves. People vary greatly in their responses to antiperspirants, and a person's response may vary from time to time. To make matters more confusing, unnoted changes in manufacturers' formulations, even in an inactive ingredient, can significantly change a product's effectiveness. So the Panel suggests that consumers would do well to try out several products and change brands from time to time if they are not fully satisfied.

Combination Products

Many antiperspirants contain substances with jawbreaking names that seem to be combinations of two or more active ingredients. These are, however, considered to be single ingredients. No product submitted for review contained more than one active ingredient for the reduction of perspiration.

The only combination containing antiperspirants and other types of drugs that were submitted for review are combinations of antifungal active ingredients + an antiperspirant for the prevention and treatment of athlete's foot. The Panel and the FDA agree that, in principle, this could be a safe and effective combination. But supportive data are sparse, and the Panel did not approve any specific antiperspirant ingredient as safe and effective for this purpose. Rather, it granted them only conditional approval. Of the few such products currently marketed, the FDA adds, none can as yet be rated as safe and effective; so these combinations for now are at best only conditionally approved.

APPROVED ANTIPERSPIRANT ACTIVE INGREDIENTS

Many active ingredients are approved as safe and effective for reducing underarm wetness. All are aluminum compounds or aluminum-and-zirconium compounds. (*See* the table Safety and Effectiveness: Active Ingredients in Over-the-Counter Antiperspirants, to determine which category a particular product belongs to.)

• ALUMINUM CHLORIDE: Antiperspirant products containing aluminum chloride in a water-based (aqueous) solution are potent inhibitors of underarm moisture. But they tend to be more irritating to the skin and more damaging to clothing than aluminum chlorohydrate products (*see* further on).

In one comparative test, under everyday conditions, a 13.3 percent aluminum chloride preparation was compared with a 22 percent aluminum chlorohydrate preparation. The latter was more effective an hour after application. But after 12 hours, the aluminum chloride had reduced sweat production by half, compared with only a one-third reduction by the aluminum chlorohydrate. After 3½ days and several applications, the aluminum chloride still provided a 49 percent reduction in sweat, compared with a barely effective 22 percent reduction with aluminum chlorohydrate.

The Panel concluded from this and other tests that up to 15 percent solutions of aluminum chloride are more effective in reducing perspiration than other antiperspirant compounds. But a significantly greater potential exists for producing skin irritation. The FDA concurs; consumers are forewarned.

• ALUMINUM CHLOROHYDRATES: Many aluminum chlorohydrate ingredients are approved as safe and effective when formulated in liquids, creams, sprays, and other products that are applied directly to the skin. Although these forms vary chemically, their effect on the skin is much the same, so they are discussed here as a group.

The safety of the aluminum chlorohydrates has been demonstrated by skin tests in animals and humans as well as by marketing experience. Manufacturers receive about six complaints of adverse reactions for every million product units sold, a very low complaint rate for skin products. A concentration of up to 25-percent aluminum chlorohydrate in the base is safe.

The effectiveness of aluminum chlorohydrate has been established by hot-room tests. Some tests were conducted under emotionally stressful conditions that enhance sweating. The tests were designed to produce tension, fear, frustration, and embarrassment. Sweat reductions were in the range of 26 to 46 percent. Tests also showed that different formulations of the same ingredient can produce significantly different levels of sweat inhibition. In some instances formulations that contained a relatively high percentage of an aluminum chlorhydrate were less effective than those of lower concentration. Assessment: safe and effective.

• *ALUMINUM SULFATE, BUFFERED:* Used by itself, aluminum sulfate is highly irritating. But the addition of *sodium aluminum lactate* provides a buffer against irritation. A product that contains 8 percent of each of these aluminum ingredients—*Arrid Extra Dry Cream* (Carter)—has been widely used for years. Test results with buffered aluminum sulfate show that this ingredient produces neither irritation nor allergic responses. In one allergy test of 204 subjects, reactions to it were milder than reactions to a widely marketed mild soap.

Hot-room tests showed that buffered aluminum preparations are effective, reducing underarm wetness by 25 to 31 percent.

However, because various inactive ingredients can change a preparation's effectiveness, evaluators recommended that the final formulation of buffered aluminum sulfate products be tested further.

• *ALUMINUM ZIRCONIUM CHLOROHYDRATES:* These compounds are safe and effective antiperspirant ingredients when applied directly to the underarm skin. Bumps and other irritant reactions occur in a small number of people, but these minor problems are easily recognized, and disappear when the product is discontinued.

CONDITIONALLY APPROVED ANTIPERSPIRANT ACTIVE INGREDIENTS

None.

DISAPPROVED ANTIPERSPIRANT ACTIVE INGREDIENTS

None.

When Greater Relief Is Needed

People who sweat copiously (*hyperphydrosis*) probably cannot obtain adequate relief from nonprescription antiperspirants. Doctors, and particularly skin specialists (dermatologists), have a number of alternative methods to help them.

The doctors can, for example, prescribe an alcohol-based aluminum-chloride solution that penetrates the skin more effectively than water-base nonprescription products and so may be much more effective. One or two treatments weekly may be all that is needed. Several other applications also have proved helpful to some heavy sweaters.

As a last resort, surgical methods have been used to deaden the nerves or eliminate sweat glands from the armpits. For most people, fortunately, these extreme measures are not necessary. Some sufferers are relieved to find that their super sweating diminishes significantly as they get older.

Ways to Dry Sweaty Feet

Antiperspirants are not intended to be used on—and probably are not effective on—sweaty feet. Here are some alternative suggestions from a podiatrist (foot specialist), as reported in the magazine *FDA Consumer* (Dec. 1985):

- Wear only leather or fabric shoes or sandals, and be sure they are specially made to "breathe."

- Switch shoes daily, or more often, so that each pair will have ample time to dry out.

- Wear cotton socks, and change them at noon.

- Use a powder—but not cornstarch—to dry the feet.

See Unguents and Powders for the Skin.

Safety and Effectiveness: Active Ingredients in Over-the-Counter Antiperspirants

Active Ingredient	Assessment: In Nonaerosol Dosage Form	Assessment: In Aerosol Dosage Form
aluminum chlorohydrates (dosage: up to 25% in the base)	safe and effective	safe and effective
aluminum chlorohydrex PEG*	safe and effective	safe and effective
aluminum chlorohydrex PG†	safe and effective	safe and effective
aluminum dichlorohydrate	safe and effective	safe and effective
aluminum dichlorohydrex PEG	safe and effective	safe and effective
aluminum dichlorohydrex PG	safe and effective	safe and effective
aluminum sesquichlorohydrex PEG	safe and effective	safe and effective
aluminum sesquichlorohydrex PG	safe and effective	safe and effective
aluminum chloride (dosage: up to 15% in aqueous solution)	safe and effective	
aluminum sulfate, buffered	safe and effective	
aluminum zirconium chlorohydrates (dosage: up to 20% in the base)		
aluminum zirconium octachlorohydrate	safe and effective	

aluminum zirconium octachlorohydrex Gly‡	safe and effective
aluminum zirconium pentachlorohydrate	safe and effective
aluminum zirconium pentachlorohydrex Gly	safe and effective
aluminum zirconium tetrachlorohydrate	safe and effective
aluminum zirconium tetrachlorohydrex Gly	safe and effective
aluminum zirconium trichlorohydrate	safe and effective
aluminum zirconium trichlorohydrex Gly	safe and effective

* PEG = polyethylene glycol complex
† PG = propylene glycol complex
‡ Gly = glycine complex

Antiperspirants: Product Ratings

Product and Distributor	Dosage of Active Ingredients	Rating*	Comment

All active ingredients listed in the previous table are safe and effective, and so, presumably, are all products that contain them. They all would be rated "A." The other side of the coin is that many of these products fail to list the concentration of the antiperspirant active ingredient. Any such product should be designated "B," because consumers have the right—and it may be a legal right—to know the *dosage* or *concentration* of every medicinally active ingredient found in a product.

*Authors interpretation of FDA criteria. Based on contents, not claims.

Aphrodisiacs

Aphrodisiacs or love potions are at least as old as the Bible. They live on in folklore and also are produced today commercially in bottles with labels that may describe them, more prosaically, as "energizers" or "tonics."

Since no manufacturer submitted an aphrodisiac or sexual tonic for review, the Panel (with the FDA's help) drew up its own list from medical and folkloric literature. Then the Panel evaluated these drugs. Subsequently, the FDA obtained or was sent several published scientific papers that describe clinical trials in impotent men using preparations that contain one of these drugs, yohimbine.

The Panel and more recent FDA evaluations of these findings are not encouraging. Some prescription preparations do influence sexual desire and performance. But the dried plants and insects and other substances long believed to be erotic stimulants all are ineffective, unsafe, or both. Moreover, they are inappropriate therapy for persons with sexual problems—those who will be most tempted to use them.

APHRODISIACS is based on the report "OTC Aphrodisiac Drug Products" by the FDA's Advisory Review Panel on OTC Miscellaneous Internal Drug Products, and on FDA's Tentative Final Rule and Final Rule on these products.

What Do Love Potions Do?

An aphrodisiac is defined by the Panel as a drug that is claimed to arouse or increase sexual desire or improve sexual performance. Wanting and doing are, of course, two very different functions. It is the *doing,* or the inability to do, that appears most often to drive people to seek medicinal assistance. Aphrodisiacs are likely to be sought by persons troubled by frigidity, impotence, or some other sexual problem. These conditions, however, are not amenable to self-treatment. Panel reviewers and the FDA say the better recourse is psychotherapy, which very often can provide significant help, or medical therapy with a urologist, gynecologist, endocrinologist, or other physician who specializes in the treatment of sexual problems.

Sex hormones, available by prescription but not over-the-counter, can affect sexual behavior. Women who are given the male sex hormone testosterone as a treatment for breast cancer, for example, often experience a stepped-up sex drive. (However, side effects include facial hair growth or other signs of masculinization.) In men who have an actual deficiency of testosterone, hormonal supplements can be effective. But men with normal testosterone levels show few if any changes in feelings or behavior when these supplements are administered. Estrogen, the female sex hormone, does not increase a woman's sexual desire (libido). It is experienced as a powerful turn-off by men, who sometimes are given the substance as a treatment for prostatic cancers.

Thus both male and female sex hormones can have powerful effects—negative and positive—on libido. But the Panel warns that they are not safe to use except under a physician's supervision.

Few individuals who believe in or sell drugs that are supposed to be aphrodisiacs seem willing to put them to the test of science. These true-believers also, almost surely, lack the tens or hundreds of millions of dollars that this testing may cost. As the result, no specific ingredient is listed as safe and effective, or even conditionally so, for want of the requisite evidence. Also, because the reviewers believe that people who suffer from sexual problems are best helped by seeking professional advice, *all* claims for aphrodisiacs are disapproved.

 Claims

False or Misleading
• "Acts as an aphrodisiac"

- "Arouses or increases sexual desire and improves sexual performance"
- "Helps restore sexual vigor, potency, and performance"
- "Improves performance, staying power, and sexual potency"
- "Builds virility and sexual potency"
- "Creates an uncontrollable desire for immediate sexual gratification"
- "Expands nature's gift of love"

APPROVED ACTIVE INGREDIENTS

None.

CONDITIONALLY APPROVED ACTIVE INGREDIENTS

None.

DISAPPROVED ACTIVE INGREDIENTS

The FDA banned the sale of all aphrodisiacs in interstate commerce in 1990. But desperate hope springs eternal, and where there is a market, manufacturers and vendors can usually be found to meet it. Aphrodisiacs, whether or not they are labeled as such, will probably continue to be widely sold as food products or herbs or as illicit drugs that are outside the regular trade channels monitored by FDA.

For these reasons, the several disapproved ingredients that have been promoted, marketed, and used as aphrodisiacs in the past are briefly described and evaluated in this Unit. Consumers who encounter aphrodisiacs, in whatever guise, thus may be better informed about their dubious value.

Yohimbine, it should be noted, continues to be available as a prescription drug, although neither its effectiveness nor its safety has been well established. A variety of other and probably better drugs and techniques are now available to assist men and women with sexual problems, who previously had only recourse to unproved and poorly regulated products. Sexual dysfunction is now recognized and can be treated within medicine's mainstream.

- **CANTHARIDES PREPARATIONS: CANTHARIDES, SPANISH FLY, CANTHARIDIN:** These are dried, ground-up insects of the genus *Cantharides*. Cantharidin is the pharmacologically active ingredient in these drugs, which are popularly called "Spanish fly." When swallowed, they cause extreme irritation of the genito-urinary tract. This may bring blood to the clitoris, or to the penis, causing an erection. But the Panel says it has found no evidence that this effect is accompanied either by increased sexual desire or by improved sexual performance.

  These irritants, what is more, have been reported to cause serious damage to the genitourinary tract. The severe gastroenteritis that may occur as a result of taking these substances has even resulted in death. So the result of evaluation is obvious: not safe and not effective.

- **DON QUAL:** Finding no mention of this substance in any medical or scientific index in the previous 20 years, reviewers judged it not safe and effective as an over-the-counter aphrodisiac.

- **ESTROGENS:** While estrogens (female sex hormones) are prescribed for various medical reasons, they do not enhance women's sexuality and they decidedly decrease responses when given to men. Therefore, in addition to being ineffective they also are unsafe as aphrodisiacs.

- **GINSENG:** The root of this plant is highly acclaimed in Eastern folklore as an aphrodisiac. Ginseng contains substances called *panaxosides* that have a weak masculinizing effect. But the Panel could find no medical or scientific reports to show that ginseng enhances men's libido or sexual performance. Conclusion: not safe and effective when used as a drug.

- **GOLDEN SEAL:** This plant was classified as ineffective because reviewers could find no information on its use as an aphrodisiac.

- **GOTU KOLA:** An Asian plant, gotu kola contains *tritarpenes*, substances that have mildly masculinizing properties like the panaxosides in ginseng. However, no data could be found to support the notion that these chemicals arouse desire or improve sexual performance, or are safe. So gotu kola was judged not safe and effective.

- **KOREAN GINSENG:** *See* Ginseng.

- **LICORICE:** This extract from *Glycyrrhiza*, a type of sweet-root plant that is used in candies, contains tritarpenes. There is no evidence of aphrodisiac qualities. Conclusion: ineffective.

- **METHYLTESTOSTERONE:** This is a potent masculinizing hormone. As a prescription drug, it can be of value in some instances where a man's lack of desire stems from inadequate levels of natural testosterone. However, because both diagnosis and treatment require medical expertise, reviewers list methyltestosterone as unsafe for over-the-counter sales and self-medication.

- **NUX VOMICA:** The seeds of the Indian tree *Strychnos nux vomica* are used as a sexual tonic, often in combination with other substances. The bitter-tasting active ingredient is the poison strychnine, which has been claimed, on the basis of users' testimonials, to act as a sexual stimulant. But no scientific studies support this belief, and the Panel and FDA's judgment is that nux vomica is ineffective as well as unsafe.

- **PEGA PALO:** This is one of the few aphrodisiacs that have been tested, with findings reported, a long while ago, in a medical publication, in this case the *Journal of the National Medical Association* (Vol. 52, pp. 25-28, 1960). An alcoholic extract of pega palo plant (*Rhynchosia pyramidalis*) was used to treat 50 men with sexual impotence related to partial or complete loss of sexual desire and erections. The researchers claimed the pega palo enhanced sexual desire in 41 of the men and restored 16 of them to normal sexual activity during the period of the test. Dummy medication was used for comparative purposes. But the doctors knew who was getting the active drug and who the dummy. This single-blind testing may have biased the reporting of results. Further, the outcome of treatment with the dummy drug was not given. So Panel reviewers concluded that the study did not meet the criteria for a properly controlled scientific investigation. Pega palo cannot be considered safe and effective.

- **SARSAPARILLA:** This root extract from *Smilax* plants contains, among other chemicals, tritarpenes. These substances have not been shown to act as an aphrodisiac, so sarsaparilla is judged ineffective.

- **STRYCHNINE:** *See* Nux vomica.

- **YOHIMBINE:** A plant alkaloid derived from the bark of the tree *Coryanthe johimbe*, yohimbine has been used for centuries as an aphrodisiac. But there is little acceptable medical evidence that yohimbine bolsters either desire or performance.

In one recent report, published in *The Lancet* (Vol. 2, pp. 421-23, 1987), medical researchers at Queens University in Kingston, Ontario, in Canada studied 48 men whose impotence clearly was psychological in origin. The investigators gave capsules containing yohimbine to 29 of the men, who took it three times a day. The other 19 men took capsules that contained a placebo (dummy medication). The men and their wives reported back to the researchers on how well the men penetrated the wives during sexual intercourse.

After 10 weeks, 9 of the 29 men taking the active drug achieved "complete improvement," and 9 others had "partial improvement." The rest did not improve. But among the 19 men taking the dummy drug, only 1 man had complete improvement and 2 others partial improvement.

These were encouraging results. But when the researchers switched the 18 poor-responders among the men taking the dummy drug onto yohimbine, only 3 men showed any improvement; the other 15 had no improvement at all—a discouraging finding.

The researchers said these findings, over all, showed that yohimbine is effective. But the FDA argues that the poor results in the 19 crossover subjects temper the positive findings. The study, as a whole, shows that "some suggestive evidence that yohimbine may be useful in treating male impotence," the FDA says. But the study was too small and too inconclusive to establish its effectiveness as a self-treatment drug. The FDA said, too, that yohimbine can have serious side effects (it stimulates anxiety for example) and so should be used only under medical supervision, as a prescription drug, if it is used at all. It is not safe and effective for self-medication.

Safety and Effectiveness:
Aphrodisiacs That May be Sold Illegally Over-the-Counter

Active Ingredient	Assessment
cantharides preparations: cantharides, Spanish fly, and cantharidin	not safe and effective
don qual	not safe and effective
estrogens	not safe and effective
ginseng	not safe and effective
golden seal	not safe and effective
gotu kola	not safe and effective

Safety and Effectiveness:
Aphrodisiacs That May Be Sold Illegally Over-the-Counter (contd)

Active Ingredient	Assessment
Korean ginseng (*see* Ginseng)	
licorice	not safe and effective
methyltestosterone	not safe and effective
nux vomica	not safe and effective
pega palo	not safe and effective
sarsaparilla	not safe and effective
Spanish fly (*see* Cantharides Preparations)	
strychnine (*see* Nux Vomica)	
yohimbine	not safe and effective

Aphrodisiacs: Product Ratings

All products marketed over-the-counter as aphrodisiacs are not safe and effective, as stipulated by FDA, and are banned in interstate commerce. They continue to be sold— "Hope springs eternal in the human breast . . ." (Alexander Pope).

Asthma Drugs

Asthma—which means *panting* in Greek—is a common, often serious disease in which the smooth muscles that line the bronchial airway to the lungs tighten and go into spasms, narrowing and even obstructing the airway. Tightness in the chest, wheezing, coughing, and shortness of breath are the principal symptoms that result. A frightening choking feeling occurs as breathing becomes more difficult. The sufferer may look pale or even blue. At first the cough is dry; later, thick phlegm may be produced. During an attack, an asthmatic person often feels a sense of impending doom.

Asthma usually (but not always) starts in childhood. Pollens, dust, and other allergy-producing substances have been implicated as causes. However, both hereditary factors (e.g., a family history of hay fever and the like) and an individual's emotional or psychological state are thought to play important roles.

The incidence of asthma and of asthma deaths has been increasing since the early 1980s, particularly among blacks. The poor health

ASTHMA DRUGS is based on the report of the FDA's Advisory Review Panel on OTC Cold, Cough, Allergy, Bronchodilator, and Anti-Asthmatic Drug Products; on the FDA's Tentative Final and Final Monographs on OTC Bronchodilator Drug Products; on FDA's Tentative Final Monograph on Cold, Cough, Allergy, Bronchodilator and Antihistaminic Combination Drug Products; and on related OTC Drug Review documents.

care that results from poverty during economic hard times may be part of the reason. Cramped living conditions, in which many people live together in close quarters also may be a contributing factor to this increase. There is evidence, too, that recent building-construction trends, in which apartments and houses are largely sealed off from the outside and from fresh air—so that people must breathe recirculated air—may increase the incidence of asthma.

Asthma thus is a persistent and also a very serious condition. No one should try to treat himself or herself for asthma except in close and continuing cooperation with a physician.

Very potent and effective drugs are available for asthma on a prescription basis. Some of the nonprescription drugs that are marketed for asthmatic self-medication also are very strong, and therefore their use carries some risk. A major reason they retain their nonprescription status is that, as with insulin for diabetics, the FDA and doctors want asthma sufferers to have fast recourse to drug therapy in case they suffer an attack away from home and cannot reach a doctor or a hospital to obtain a prescription drug and other care. Also, asthmatics have demonstrated to the FDA's satisfaction that they can treat minor attacks safely and effectively using these OTC medications.

Bronchodilators

In asthma, the muscle spasms that cause the narrowing of air passages often abate of their own accord. When the airway is reopened, normal breathing is restored. Drugs that relax these muscles, and relieve wheezing and shortness of breath, are called *bronchodilators* (bronchial muscle relaxers). They are administered as tablets, liquids, sprays, or inhalants. Several are quite effective and work quickly.

Because of their potency and potential for severe side effects, these drugs should be used only in dosages approved by a doctor. Bronchodilators can make the heart race and seem to pound noisily in the chest. They can also elevate blood pressure and blood sugar to dangerous levels. Nervousness, sleeplessness, nausea, and vomiting are other possible side effects. Therefore, bronchodilators must be used carefully and treated with extraordinary respect. They must be kept away from small children, who can be seriously hurt by swallowing or inhaling the drugs.

WARNING:
If these products do not provide good, rapid relief—within 20 minutes to an hour at most—the Panel urges asthmatics to call a doctor or go (or be taken) to a hospital emergency room. This is imperative because drugs that are providing only slight relief may be masking a severe and worsening attack that could prove fatal if not treated by a doctor.

Two principal groups of drugs are used as nonprescription bronchodilators: The *sympathomimetics* stimulate the production of an enzyme that relaxes smooth muscle in the bronchial tubes, thus dilating (widening) the air passages. The *theophyllines* inhibit a different enzyme that otherwise prevents smooth muscle from relaxing.

The FDA has different views of these two classes of drugs: Used as directed, the sympathomimetics are safe and effective. The theophyllines, while effective, are however only marginally safe, if that. For these reasons, the FDA discarded the Panel's recommendation and has not allowed theophylline preparations to be sold over-the-counter as single-ingredient products. What is more, the FDA also has said that it plans to ban theophylline in combination nonprescription asthma relief products.

 ## Claims for Bronchodilators

Accurate

- "For temporary relief of bronchial asthma"

- "For symptomatic relief of bronchial asthma"

- "For eas[ing] breathing for asthma patients by reducing spasms of bronchial muscles"

WARNINGS:
Do not use a bronchodilator product unless a diagnosis of asthma has been made by a doctor.

Do not use a bronchodilator product if you have heart disease, high blood pressure, thyroid disease, diabetes, or difficulty in urination due to enlargement of the prostate gland, unless directed by a doctor.

Do not use a bronchodilator product if you have ever been hospitalized for asthma, or if you are taking any prescription drug for asthma, unless directed by a doctor.

Do not use if you are currently taking a prescription drug for high blood pressure or depression, without first consulting your doctor.

Do not continue to use a bronchodilator product, but seek medical assistance immediately if symptoms are not relieved within 1 hour, or become worse.

Some users of a bronchodilator may experience nervousness, tremor, sleeplessness, nausea, and loss of appetite. If these symptoms persist or become worse, consult your doctor.

APPROVED BRONCHODILATOR ACTIVE INGREDIENTS

• *EPHEDRINE PREPARATIONS:* Ephedrine, ephedrine hydrochloride, ephedrine sulfate, and racephedrine hydrochloride are taken orally. They ease breathing rather slowly—after 15 to 60 minutes. Relief may last 3 to 5 hours. Studies show that these preparations significantly diminish airway constrictions and improve airflow to the lungs. One study showed 10 to 25 percent improvement.

Ephedrine's side effects—on the heartbeat, nervous system, and urinary flow—discourage abuse of these preparations. Persons taking prescription drugs that are monoamine oxidase (MAO) inhibitors—potent drugs used principally as antidepressants—can experience a dangerous rise in blood pressure when they take ephedrine and so should not use it.

Although the Panel considered ephedrine safe and effective, it also cautioned that its usefulness is limited to milder cases of asthma.

 WARNING:
Do not continue to use an ephedrine product, but seek medical assistance immediately if symptoms are not relieved within 1 hour, or become worse.

• *EPINEPHRINE PREPARATIONS:* These include epinephrine, epinephrine bitartrate, and racepinephrine hydrochloride.

Epinephrine, a hormone secreted by the adrenal gland, is popularly known as *adrenalin*. It stimulates the heart and other organ systems. The familiar increase in heart rate you experience when faced with physical danger or emotional stress comes from an increase of epinephrine released into the bloodstream.

Epinephrine, epinephrine bitartrate, and epinephrine hydrochloride tend to be safer, faster-acting, and more effective than ephedrine preparations for treating asthma. But the benefits are of much shorter duration. In clinical use and in scientifically controlled trials, epinephrine provided significant relief within 5 minutes. Measurable improvements in bronchial air flow soon followed. Such benefits are likely to wane within an hour or so, however. These drugs must be taken as inhalants because they are largely destroyed by stomach acid when swallowed.

A few years ago there was considerable concern about epinephrine's safety because it is chemically related to isoproterenol, a more potent bronchodilator that caused a number of deaths in England. Severe side effects, however, do not appear to occur with epinephrine, possibly because epinephrine is inhaled in more dilute solutions; only a small amount of the drug is absorbed into the bloodstream. Also, by contracting the blood vessels that pass through the lungs, epinephrine may limit its own distribution through the bloodstream to other parts of the body.

 WARNINGS:
This safe and effective drug can be overused or abused by children and adolescents for the "high" it produces; therefore, its use should be monitored by an adult. Epinephrine should not be taken by persons using prescription drugs that are MAO inhibitors.

Do not use this bronchodilator unless a diagnosis of asthma has been made by a doctor.

Do not use more frequently or at higher doses than recommended unless directed by a doctor. Excessive use may cause nervousness and rapid heart beat, and possibly, adverse effects on the heart.

Do not continue to use this product, but seek medical assistance immediately if symptoms are not relieved within 20 minutes or if they become worse.

Dosage Recommendations for Safe and Effective Over-the-Counter Bronchodilators Dosage (Maximum Daily Dosage)

Active Ingredient	Adults	Children
ephedrine oral prepra-tions (ephedrine, ephedrine hydrochloride, ephedrine sulfate, racephedrine hydrocholoride)	12.5 to 25 mg not more often than every 4 hours (150 mg, or as directed by a doctor)	consult doctor
epinephrine inhalant preparations (epinephrine, epinephrine bitartrate, racepinephrine hydrochloride)	1 to 3 inhalations of 1% aqueous solution not more often than once every 3 hours from hand-held rubber bulb nebulizer, or 1 or 2 inhalations of 0.16 to 0.25 mg from a pressurized, metered dose aerosol container every 3 hours	over age 4, same as adults; under age 4, consult doctor

CONDITIONALLY APPROVED BRONCHODILATOR ACTIVE INGREDIENTS

None.

DISAPPROVED BRONCHODILATOR ACTIVE INGREDIENT

• THEOPHYLLINE PREPARATIONS: These include aminophylline, theophylline calcium salicylate and theophylline sodium glycinate. These potent bronchial muscle relaxants are chemically similar to caffeine.

The most common side effects of theophylline—loss of appetite, nausea, and vomiting—are unlikely to occur (or to be severe) in asthmatics who take the low doses found in nonprescription preparations.

 WARNING:
However, overdose of theophylline—especially in children—may lead to very serious consequences including convulsions and death.

Because of these risks, FDA classifies theophylline as not safe and effective for use in nonprescription combination drug products to relieve asthma.

The most appropriate dosage should be determined by a doctor, because the amount of theophylline needed varies widely from one individual to the next. One carefully conducted study showed the effective dosage to range from 300 mg to as high as 3200 mg per 24 hours. Fortunately, each person's effective dose remains fairly constant, so when a doctor determines an appropriate dose, the person with asthma can be reasonably sure of using the correct quantity in over-the-counter products.

At this stage, in the early 1990s, experts outside the FDA remain divided on the question of whether or not theophylline should be removed from all over-the-counter products, as the FDA plans. Many experts are in agreement, however, that better medications than fixed-dosage nonprescription combination tablets are available, on prescription, for treating asthmatic emergencies.

Theophylline preparations sold over-the-counter for asthma all are combination products, as required by the FDA. They typically contain 100 to 130 mg of theophylline combined with 24 mg of an ephedrine. Small amounts of the sedative phenobarbital may be formulated into theophylline preparations to counteract the caffeine-like stimulating effect of the theophyllines. The phenobarbital also is categorized as not safe and effective in these combination products.

Combination Products

The FDA disapproves of most of the combination anti-asthmatic drug products that remain on the market today. In combination products labeled for the treatment of asthma, the only combination it approves as safe and effective is:

> 1 safe and effective bronchodilator + guaifenesin

This type of product is useful for relieving the coughing that often is a symptom in asthma. (*See* p. 149.)

Conditionally Approved by FDA:

combinations that might include one safe and effective
bronchodilator + caffeine as a corrective substance

Disapproved by the FDA:

any combination containing theophylline
any combination containing phenobarbital
any combination containing a stimulant dose (100 mg) of caffeine

Safety and Effectiveness: Bronchodilators Sold
Over-the-Counter for Asthma

Active Ingredient	Assessment
aminophylline in a combination product	not safe and effective*
ephedrine	safe and effective
ephedrine hydrochloride	safe and effective
ephedrine sulfate	safe and effective
epinephrine	safe and effective
epinephrine bitartrate	safe and effective
racephedrine hydrochloride	safe and effective
racepinephrine hydrochloride	safe and effective
theophylline, anhydrous, in a combination product	not safe and effective*
theophylline calcium salicylate in a combination product	not safe and effective*
theophylline sodium glycinate in a combination product	not safe and effective*

*Available without prescription in combination products only.

Asthma Drugs: Product Ratings

SINGLE-INGREDIENT PRODUCTS

Product and Distributor	Dosage of Active Ingredients	Rating*	Comment
ephedrine sulfate			
Ephedrine sulfate (generic)	**capsules:** 25 mg	A	
epinephrine			
Adrenalin Chloride (Parke-Davis)	**solution for nebulization:** 1:100	A	
AsthmaHaler Mist (Menley & James)	**aerosol:** 0.3 mg epinephrine bitartrate (equivalent to 0.16 mg epinephrine base) per spray	A	
AsthmaNefrin (Menley & James)	**solution for nebulization:** 2.25% racepinephrine (equivalent to 1.125% epinephrine base)	A	
Bronitin Mist (Whitehall)	**aerosol:** 0.3 mg epinephrine bitartrate (equivalent to 0.16 mg epinephrine base) per spray	A	
Bronkaid Mist (Sanofi Winthrop)	**aerosol:** 0.25 mg epinephrine per spray	A	

Product and Distributor	Dosage of Active Ingredients	Rating*	Comment
Primatene Mist Suspension (Whitehall)	aerosol: 0.3 mg epinephrine bitartrate (equivalent to 0.16 mg epinephrine base) per spray	A	

COMBINATION PRODUCTS

Product and Distributor	Dosage of Active Ingredients	Rating*	Comment
Capsules and Tablets			
Bronkaid Tablets (Sanofi Winthrop)	tablets: 100 mg theophylline + 24 mg ephedrine sulfate + 100 mg guaifenesin	C	theophylline combinations disapproved
Bronkotabs Tablets (Sanofi Winthrop)	tablets: 100 mg theophylline + 24 mg ephedrine sulfate + 100 mg guaifenesin + 8 mg phenobarbital	C	both theophylline and phenobarbital disapproved
Bronitin Tablets (Whitehall)	tablets: 118 mg theophylline + 24 mg ephedrine hydrochloride + 100 mg guaifenesin + 16.6 mg pyrilamine maleate	C	theophylline combinations disapproved
Congestac Caplets (Menley & James)	caplets: 60 mg pseudoephedrine hydrochloride + 400 mg guaifenesin	A	
Primatene Tablets (Whitehall)	tablets: 130 mg theophylline + 24 mg ephedrine hydrochloride	C	theophylline combinations disapproved

Asthma Drugs: Product Ratings (contd)

Product and Distributor	Dosage of Active Ingredients	Rating*	Comment
Liquids			
Bronkolixir Elixir (Winthrop)	**liquid:** 45 mg theophylline + 36 mg ephedrine sulfate + 150 mg guaifenesin + 12 mg phenobarbital per 2 teaspoonfuls	C	theophylline and phenobarbital make this unsafe
Fedahist Expectorant (generic)	**syrup:** 30 mg pseudoephedrine hydrochloride + 200 mg guaifenesin	A	
Tedral Suspension (Parke-Davis)	**liquid:** 177 mg theophylline + 36 mg ephedrine hydrochloride	C	theophylline combinations disapproved

*Author's interpretation of FDA criteria. Based on contents, not claims.

Bleaches for Skin Blemishes

An Industrial Mishap

Where: a leather tannery. When: 1939. Who: Black American working men and women. Problem: White, depigmented spots appear on the workers' hands. Explanation: The problem was traced to a variant form of the chemical *hydroquinone*—a constituent of the protective rubber work-gloves the workers were wearing.

Based on this mishap, hydroquinone now is formulated into over-the-counter preparations used for bleaching small darkened patches of skin. These defects can be freckles, age spots, or the facial pigmentation that sometimes results from pregnancy or the use of oral contraceptives. Hydroquinone is the only chemical used in these preparations, and it is safe and effective at low concentrations.

Meanwhile, in recent decades black Africans have started using hydroquinone skin bleaches, sometimes in higher concentrations than

BLEACHES FOR SKIN BLEMISHES is based on the report "Skin Bleaching Products" by the FDA's Advisory Review Panel on OTC Miscellaneous External Drug Products and the FDA's Tentative Final Monograph on these products.

the nonprescription drugs usually sold in the United States. A blotchy, disfiguring skin condition called *ochronosis* occasionally results. A cancer risk has not been ruled out. "Fade creams" also are used by some black Americans. Consumer affairs officials in New York City have asked FDA to consider banning these products in the United States. An agency spokeswoman says this request is being studied (*New York Times*, Feb. 26, 1992).

 Claims

Accurate

- "Lightens dark (brownish) pigment in the skin"
- "For the gradual fading of blotches in the skin such as age and liver spots, freckles, or pigment in the skin that may occur in pregnancy, or from the use of oral contraceptives"

 WARNINGS:
Products must be kept away from the eyes.

Bleaches should not be used on children under 12 years unless directed by a doctor.

Some users may experience a mild skin irritation. If skin irritation becomes severe, stop use and see a doctor. If no improvement is seen after three months, stop the treatment. Lightening effect may not be noticeable when used on very dark skin.

Sun exposure should be limited by using a sunscreen agent, a sunblocking agent, or protective clothing to cover bleached skin during and after use of these products.

Why Dark Spots Arise

The normal hues of human skin are due to the dark pigment *melanin* produced by skin cells. (Black people simply have more melanin than white people do.)

Freckles appear naturally on many light-skinned young persons, particularly if they spend much time in the sun. Of greater concern to many persons are the larger "age spots" or "liver spots" that develop in middle age on sun-exposed body surfaces. They affect both men and women. The candid, albeit unpleasant, technical name for these spots is *senile lentigines*: freckles of old age.

Hormonal imbalances caused by pregnancy or by the so-called "false pregnancy" created by oral contraceptives can create widespread facial hyperpigmentation. Also, a number of diseases may unevenly darken the skin. Endocrine disorders like Addison's disease and hyperthyroidism cause changes in skin color, as do liver conditions and rheumatoid arthritis. Some drugs used to treat serious illness—cancer, mental illness, and malaria—may discolor the skin, too. Rubbing the skin, overexposure to the sun, industrial chemicals, and a host of other environmental factors also may darken small skin areas.

Because of these problems, the Panel said that "there is valid reason for some people to use skin bleaches" because of the emotional and social problems that can compound the cosmetic disfiguration.

APPROVED ACTIVE INGREDIENT IN SKIN-BLEACHING AGENTS

• **HYDROQUINONE:** This is the only active ingredient evaluated safe and effective as a skin bleach. It is an industrial chemical, a dihydroxybenzene. Chemicals in this group have a variety of uses. For example, they inhibit oxidation and are therefore mixed into fats to keep them from becoming rancid. Hydroquinone is a principal ingredient of photographic developer.

Although concentrations of 5 percent hydroquinone may seriously and permanently damage human skin when used for prolonged periods of time, the 1.5 to 2 percent concentrations allowed in bleach creams have not been reported to cause damage. A mild, temporary inflammation may initially arise on the treatment site—but this may foretell success, rather than failure, for the treatment.

Tests in animals and in humans show that this ingredient can be ingested in fairly high amounts without risk—it is not a systemic poison.

The question of *how* hydroquinone fades skin spots has been studied by a number of scientists, but the answer remains unclear. Apparently the compound inhibits or injures melanin-producing skin cells or the melanin granules within them.

Consumers should know that hydroquinone bleach creams produce only a partial change; they lighten dark spots by about 50 percent at best. This means that they are more effective on relatively light spots than they are on relatively dark ones, for which some remaining overpigmentation can be anticipated even after treatment. In either case, treatment takes three weeks to three months of daily (and nightly) applications to produce results.

The results of skin-bleaching with hydroquinone are likely not to last. Depigmented areas will darken again when exposed to the sun, which is why users are cautioned to cover up in the sun or apply a sunscreen. (The only type of skin-bleach combination product approved is a mixture of hydroquinone and a sunscreen.)

The approved dosage is a thin layer of the medication on the affected area twice daily, or use as directed by a doctor.

CONDITIONALLY APPROVED ACTIVE INGREDIENTS IN SKIN-BLEACHING AGENTS

None.

DISAPPROVED ACTIVE INGREDIENTS IN SKIN-BLEACHING AGENTS

None.

When Greater Relief Is Needed

Dermatologists have several methods for removing or fading small skin blemishes. One is careful tattooing of the blemished area with a pigment that is normal skin color.

Significant lightening of liver spots *without* the skin depigmentation that can occur during treatment with hydroquinone, has been reported using the prescription (℞) drug tretinoin (*Retin-A*, Ortho). Skin doctors at the University of Michigan Medical Center, in Ann Arbor reported (*New England Journal of Medicine*, February 6, 1992, pp. 368-74) that tretinoin "significantly improves...liver spots." In their very persuasive report, they add that the blemishes "do not return for at least six months after therapy is discontinued."

Safety and Effectiveness:
Active Ingredient in Over-the-Counter Skin Bleaches

Active Ingredient	Assessment
hydroquinone (1.5 to 2%)	safe and effective

Bleaches for Skin Blemishes: Product Ratings

SINGLE INGREDIENT PRODUCTS

Product and Distributor	Dosage of Active Ingredient	Rating*	Comment
hydroquinone			
Eldoquin (ICN)	cream: 2%	A	
	lotion: 2%	A	
Porcelana (DEP)	cream: 2%	A	

COMBINATION PRODUCTS

Product and Distributor	Dosage of Active Ingredients	Rating*	Comment
hydroquinone + sunscreen or sunblock			
Eldopaque (ICN)	cream: 2% + sunblock opaque base	A	
Esoterica Facial (Medicis)	cream: 2% + 3.3% padimate O + 2.5% oxybenzone	A	
Porcelana with Sunscreen (DEP)	cream: 2% + 2.5% padimate O	A	

*Author's interpretation of Panel criteria. Based on contents, not claims.

Boil Ointments

A red, angry-looking, pus-filled eruption on the skin is apt to be a boil (furuncle). These abscesses are usually caused by bacteria, of which *Staphylococcus aureus* is the most common culprit, and they seem to bedevil some people much more often than others.

Several nonprescription drug products are sold for treating boils. They sometimes are called *drawing ointments*, because they are intended to help draw the pus together in a raised, pointed bump that will open and drain of its own accord, or that can easily be opened with a sterile needle or blade. The Panel that reviewed these preparations came to the conclusion that it is unwise to self-treat a boil with over-the-counter drugs, since the pus, if not carefully contained, can spread the infection over the skin surface, and into the bloodstream and brain—which could be lethal. The Panel also worried that self-treating boils could spread the germs to others. The Panel's decision: Boils should be treated only by a doctor.

The FDA, prompted in part by a boil-ointment maker, who said

BOIL OINTMENTS is based on the report "Boil Ointment Drug Products for OTC Human Use," by the FDA's Advisory Review Panel on OTC Miscellaneous External Drug Products, and FDA's Tentative Final Monograph on these products.

he had sold millions of containers of his product over a quarter century, with only a few, mild problems, decided to re-examine the issue. The FDA reviewed the recent medical literature. Agency drug evaluators found that boils rarely lead to serious wider infections in the original sufferers—or in others with whom they are in contact.

Boils *are* painful, the agency confirmed. But most sufferers do not take the problem to a doctor. So, removing all self-medication for boils from the market, as the Panel proposed, simply would add to the burden of these people's suffering. (Sufferers who have several or more boils during a year, however, do tend to seek medical care. This reassured FDA that people can and do care for themselves *responsibly* when they suffer this problem.)

The FDA decided, therefore, that there is a place in boil sufferers' medicine cabinets, and in the OTC drug marketplace, for boil ointments.

None of the existing ingredients or products as yet meet the test of science for safety and effectiveness, the agency declared. But to encourage manufacturers, including the one who stepped forward to report his long marketing success with a product, the FDA awarded a conditional approval—*not proved safe and effective*—to the ingredients in this maker's preparation and to one other single ingredient. The agency asked manufacturers to come back with the evidence required for approval.

 Claim

The FDA will approve this claim and these warnings for boil ointment products *if* one or more active ingredients is shown to be safe and effective.

Accurate
• "For temporary relief of pain and discomfort of boils"

 WARNINGS:
Do not use on boils on the lips, nose, cheeks, or forehead. Consult a doctor for treatment of boils in these areas.

For external use only.

Avoid contact with the eyes.

Do not use this [boil ointment] for more than 7 days. If condition worsens, or does not improve, if fever occurs, or if redness develops around the boil, consult a doctor.

Boil Care

Very small boils sometimes recede without any specific treatment. Soaking a boil in hot water or covering it periodically with hot cloths will help bring it to a "point" so that it will drain spontaneously or can be pricked with a needle point sterilized in a flame or with any other sharp, sterile instrument.

The several ingredients in over-the-counter boil ointments are intended to relieve the itching, inflammation, and pain including, perhaps, the pain of lancing the boil. These ingredients also are intended to kill or curtail microorganisms that escape onto the skin surface, preventing the spread of infection. These products may also help bring the boil to a point, so that drainage can more readily occur.

Large, serious, or persistent boils or boils that are spreading across the skin *do* require medical care. The doctor can lance a boil more skillfully and safely than you can yourself—even with the help of a family member or a friend. The doctor can send a pus sample to the laboratory to identify the microorganism that is causing the boil and then prescribe a topical or systemic antibiotic that will effectively kill it. Not all boils, the Panel pointed out, are caused by *Staphylococcus*.

The warning against self-treating boils on the face reflects that blood vessels that serve facial areas also serve the brain. Doctors should treat these boils to prevent secondary brain infections.

APPROVED ACTIVE INGREDIENTS IN BOIL OINTMENTS
None.

CONDITIONALLY APPROVED ACTIVE INGREDIENTS IN BOIL OINTMENTS

- BENZOCAINE: This is a pain-reliever that is safe and effective for cuts, scrapes, and other minor skin injuries in concentrations of 5 to 20 percent. *See* pp. 557-558, Benzocaine in ITCH AND PAIN REMEDIES

APPLIED TO THE SKIN.

• *ICHTHAMMOL:* Ichthammol is a weak, old drug that is used to treat a number of skin disorders. It reduces redness (inflammation) and constricts small blood vessels. It is an astringent and anti-irritant that purportedly soothes the skin as well as kills some germs. Ichthammol also, on the negative side, can cause the skin to thicken in an unsightly way where it is applied.

This drug long has been used as a "drawing salve" for boils, FDA says. But there is no evidence that it is medicinally safe or effective in the concentration of 19 percent in which it currently is formulated into a self-treatment product for boils.

• *SULFUR:* This bright yellow elemental substance has been used medicinally since at least the time of the ancient Egyptians. It has a mild antiseptic (germ-killing) effect. Sulfur is a safe and effective drug for the self-treatment of acne in concentrations of 3 to 10 percent. (*See* ACNE MEDICATIONS.) But there is little evidence that the 0.44 percent sulfur in the successfully marketed boil ointment product that the FDA is evaluating is either safe or effective.

DISAPPROVED ACTIVE INGREDIENTS IN BOIL OINTMENTS

None.

Safety and Effectiveness:
Active Ingredients in Over-the-Counter Boil Ointments

Active Ingredient	Panel's Assessment
benzocaine	not proved safe and effective
ichthammol	not proved safe and effective
sulfur	not proved safe and effective

Boil Ointments: Product Ratings

Product and Distributor	Dosage of Active Ingredients	Rating *	Comment
Boil-Ease (Commerce)	salve: 5% benzocaine + 1.9% ichthammol + 0.44% sulfur	B	this combination gets FDA's conditional approval while the agency studies it more closely
Boyol Salve (Pfeiffer)	salve: 10% ichthammol + benzocaine + lanolin + petrolatum	C	ichthammol not proved safe or effective; this combination not approved

*Author's interpretation of FDA criteria. Based on contents, not claims.

Camphor: Special Note

Camphor has been used medicinally for thousands of years, for a variety of purposes. This may be surprising, given the evaluators' declaration—backed by the FDA and other medical authorities—that it "appears to have little, if any, therapeutic benefit."

Perhaps camphor's popularity rests on its sensory effects on the body: It has a pungent odor, associated with healing, which may be particularly appreciated by a person who has been cut off from smells by a cold or a stuffed-up nose. Camphor creates feelings of both coolness and warmth when applied to the skin. It is irritating enough to cause visible reddening of the skin when it is applied as a liniment or a rub. This latter effect appears to have been the principal use for the strong preparation called *camphor liniment*—which FDA has banned as hazardous.

Over-the-counter drugs that contain high concentrations of camphor are dangerous. Furthermore, they are of little or no medicinal value. For this reason, they have been banned. Less concentrated cam-

CAMPHOR: SPECIAL NOTE is based on the report "Camphorated Oil and Camphor-Containing Drug Products" by the FDA's Advisory Review Panel on OTC Miscellaneous External Drug Products; on the Panel's "Statement Concerning OTC Drug Products Containing Camphor"; on the FDA's Preambles to these documents; and on the FDA's Final Order on Camphorated Oil.

phor products continue to be marketed, and some are safe and effective for the purposes for which they are labeled.

These conclusions from the Panel and the FDA are outlined here, in terms of three levels of risk:

- Products containing more than 11 percent camphor are *extremely dangerous*. The FDA, acting on the Panel's recommendation, already has banned them in interstate commerce.

- Most products containing 2.5 to 11 percent camphor are *unsafe* and appear to have no appreciable therapeutic value. The Panel believed that these products also should be banned, and the FDA is evaluating this recommendation as part of the Over-the-Counter Drug Review. Many products containing 2.5 to 11 percent camphor already are gone. Others may follow.

- Products containing 2.5 percent or less camphor are *safe*, even if of doubtful effectiveness, if each container holds no more than 360 mg of camphor. This amount probably would not be lethal if eaten by a child (*see* Safe Camphor Preparations, further on). Even so, the Panel recommended that these products be marketed in containers with child-resistant lids. One manufacturer said this packaging restriction is absurd; the company points out that it would limit camphor products to containers holding no more than about one-half ounce.

Extremely Dangerous Camphor Preparations

The extremely dangerous camphor drugs removed by the FDA from the over-the-counter market contain camphor at concentrations of 11 percent or greater. The FDA asked manufacturers to recall stock of these preparations, and it banned further sales of camphorated oil. These highly dangerous substances may be labeled with any of the names that follow or with names like them:

  camphor 11 percent (or above)
  camphorated oil
  camphor liniment

Note: Camphorated oil is 20 percent camphor in cottonseed oil. *Camphor liniment* is another name for camphorated oil.

The symptoms of camphor poisoning may appear within minutes or they may be delayed several hours if the victim has just eaten food. These symptoms include a feeling of warmth, headache, dizziness, mental confusion, restlessness, delirium, and hallucinations. They may be accompanied by increased muscular excitability, tremors, jerky movements, convulsions, central nervous system depression, and coma. In severe poisoning, respiratory failure or extreme convulsions are usually the cause of death.

If you suspect someone has ingested camphor, smell his or her breath, mouth, and saliva. If you believe camphor may have been taken, phone your doctor, hospital, or poison control center. (*See* p. 829, where you should write down these important emergency phone numbers.)

Banning camphor products containing 11 percent or more camphor represented little therapeutic loss. The American Pharmaceutical Association, which represents the nation's pharmacists, testified that not once in camphor's long history (it was officially noted in the first *United States Pharmacopeia*, published in 1820) has the literature shown a single reference concerning the drug's effectiveness.

Conclusion: The hazards outweigh by far any medicinal value, and camphorated oil by any name, as well as all other products with greater than 11 percent camphor, are neither safe nor effective.

Unsafe Camphor Preparations

A wide variety of single and combination products have been marketed containing concentrations of camphor between 2.5 percent and 11 percent. They have been (and some still may be) used as cough suppressors, nasal decongestants, and itch and pain remedies and are formulated as steam inhalants as well as liniments and rubs.

The Panel was particularly concerned about a camphor preparation called *camphor spirit*. It consists of 9 to 11 percent camphor in alcohol. The evaluators were worried that when camphorated oil (20 percent camphor) disappeared from the nonprescription market, camphor spirit—which also is hazardous—might replace it on druggists' shelves.

Many camphor-containing drug products for external use were submitted for evaluation. Reviewers found little scientific evidence of medicinal value, but discovered much data to support the viewpoint that camphor products of 2.5 to 11 percent concentration pose a hazard to health. A past president of the National Clearinghouse for Poison Control Centers recommended that any nonprescription medication containing camphor be limited to 2.5 percent concentration to reduce the risk of accidental poisoning. The American Academy of Pediatrics Committee on Drugs maintained that even relatively small amounts of camphor taken orally have resulted in deaths. This professional group also emphasized the significance of camphor's rapid absorption through the skin or by inhalation, and noted that when it is used by a pregnant woman, it can cross the placenta and poison a fetus.

The Panel concluded that camphor spirit and all other camphor preparations with concentrations between 2.5 and 11 percent are unsafe and ineffective. It has recommended to the FDA that such products should be removed from the over-the-counter market. The FDA is assessing this recommendation within the guidelines of the whole over-the-counter drug-review program, and if it concurs, most of these products will be banned from interstate commerce under penalty of law.

Safe Camphor Preparations

One important exception must be noted to the condemnation of products with up to 11 percent camphor: A manufacturer presented data that persuaded the FDA that when camphor is combined with another old medicinal remedy, *phenol*, at a ratio of approximately 2.3 camphor to 1 part phenol, in a light mineral oil base (rather than in alcohol or water as is usually the case), the two active ingredients and the oil serve to modulate the untoward effects. This combination of camphor 10.8 percent + phenol 4.7 percent in light mineral oil has been shown—to the FDA's satisfaction—to be safe and effective as an *analgesic* (itch-pain reliever) and *antiseptic* (germ killer) when applied, carefully and in small amounts, to cuts, scrapes, minor burns, insect bites, and other minor skin injuries.

These Panel-FDA assessments of camphor extend to *camphorated metacresol*, a closely related compound; *metacresol* is a phenol-like substance. Camphorated metacresol is safe and effective as an itch-pain remedy at concentrations of three parts camphor to one part metacresol up to 10.8 percent camphor + 3.6 percent metacresol.

Although the Panel and the FDA were skeptical that camphor has any beneficial value, judgments on products containing concentrations of less than 2.5 percent camphor were referred to the Panels considering various types of products in which camphor has been used. Several safe and effective uses for camphor have emerged from this process. The following are currently approved uses for camphor, *not* combined with phenol, and for camphorated metacresol:

Camphor 0.1 to 2.5 percent for itching and pain and as an anesthetic. (*See* p. 559.)

Camphor 4.7 to 5.3 percent in a salve or 6.2 percent in a steam inhalant for relief of coughing. (*See* p. 141.)

Camphor up to 2.5 percent in liniments for aches and pains. (*See* pp. 650-651.)

Camphor up to 2.5 percent for cold sores. (*See* pp. 215, 220.)

Camphor 0.1 to 2.5 percent for poison ivy-oak-sumac. (*See* p. 817.)

Camphorated metacresol (camphor 3 to 10.8 percent, metacresol 1 to 3.6 percent in a 3 to 1 ratio) for itching, pain, and as an antiseptic. (*See* p. 559.)

Camphorated metacresol (same dosage), for poison ivy-oak-sumac. (*See* p. 817.)

Camphorated metacresol (same dosage) for cold sores. (*See* pp. 215, 220.)

Safety and Effectiveness:
Active Ingredients in Over-the-Counter Camphor Products

Active Ingredient	Assessment
camphor under 2.5%	safe, and effective for some uses
camphor 2.5 to 11%	not safe or effective
camphor 10.8% + phenol 4.7% in light mineral oil base	safe, and effective for some uses
camphor 11 to 20%	not safe or effective
camphor spirits	not safe or effective
camphorated metacresol (camphor 3 to 10.8% + metacresol 1 to 3.6% in a 3 to 1 ratio)	safe, and effective for some uses
camphorated oil (camphorated liniment)	not safe or effective

Camphor: Product Ratings – Rated for Safety Only *

Product and Distributor	Dosage of Active Ingredients	Rating†	Comment
Caladryl Lotion (Parke-Davis)	2%	A	
Campho-Phenique Liquid (Sterling Health)	10.8%	A	
Deep-Down (SmithKline Beecham)	0.5%	A	
Double-Ice Arthri-Care Gel (Commerce)	3.1%	C	
Heet Liniment	3.6%	C	
Heet Spray (Whitehall)	3%	C	
Rhuli Spray (Rydelle)	0.7%	A	
Rhuli Cream (Rydelle)	0.3%	A	

*Based on *drugs facts & comparisons* and industry sources.
†Author's interpretation of FDA criteria. Based on contents, not claims.

Cold and Cough Medicines

Americans buy a billion dollars' worth of cold, cough, and allergy drugs over-the-counter annually. Many of the 50,000 products sold for this purpose are complex combinations of several active ingredients for which a puzzling variety of claims are made. This variety can be confusing for the person who is ill as well as for the pharmacist who may be asked to help.

By sorting out the specific symptoms for which people buy and use these products, identifying the group or groups of drugs that could be expected to relieve each type of symptom, and evaluating the safety and effectiveness of the drugs' active ingredients in each of these groups, the reviewing Panel has set criteria by which consumers can choose their medications more wisely. So armed, consumers will be in a better position to assess which drug ingredients actually are needed —singly or in combination form. They can spare themselves the risk and cost of cold and cough drugs they do not need.

COLD AND COUGH MEDICINES is based on the report of the FDA's Advisory Review Panel on OTC Cold, Cough, Allergy, Bronchodilator, and Anti-Asthmatic Products; the FDA's Tentative Final Order on OTC Anticholinergic and Expectorant Drug Products; and on these additional FDA documents: Final Order on Anticholinergic Drug Products, Final Order on Expectorant Drug Products, two Tentative Final Orders on Antihistaminic Drug Products, Tentative Final Order on Nasal Decongestant Drug Products, Tentative and Final Orders on Bronchodilator Drug Products, and Tentative Final Order on Combination Drug Products for these uses.

How to Find the Drugs that Relieve Specific Symptoms

The Symptom Key to Drugs for Colds and Coughs gives the general group of medicines that offers relief for specific symptoms, and tells where these medications are described.

Symptom Key to Drugs for Colds and Coughs

Symptom	*Drug Group*	*See Page*
aches (generalized)	pain, fever, inflammation relievers	132
bronchospasm	bronchial muscle relaxers (bronchodilators)	168
cough	cough suppressors	139
	expectorants	148
fever	pain, fever, inflammation relievers	132
nasal congestion	nasal decongestants	162
runny nose	antihistamines	150
sinus congestion	nasal decongestants	162
	pain, fever, inflammation relievers	132
sneezing	antihistamines	150
sore throat	pain, fever, inflammation relievers	132
	sore-throat and mouth medicines	132

Tables at the end of this Unit are set up to help consumers select safe and effective drugs to meet their specific needs of the moment. The prospective purchaser must keep in mind what these drugs can and cannot do. They cannot cure the common cold, or any other condition. But they can—and do—partially relieve some of the distressing symptoms associated with colds and other upper respiratory infections. Some also can relieve symptoms caused by hay fever and other allergies. (*See* ALLERGY DRUGS.)

The Panel was concerned that the consumer clearly understand that these remedies can relieve some symptoms but *cannot* cure colds.

Aches and Pains

Colds and other viral infections, such as flu, generate aches, pains, and generalized malaise. These miseries can be relieved to a significant degree with over-the-counter pain, fever, and inflammation medications, which also, of course, reduce the fever that accompanies infections. The most commonly used of these drugs are acetaminophen, aspirin, and ibuprofen. They often are combined with ingredients that relieve other cold and cough symptoms. (*See* PAIN, FEVER, AND ANTI-INFLAMMATORY DRUGS TAKEN INTERNALLY.)

Fever

See Aches and Pains.

Sore Throat

A sore throat frequently accompanies cough, nasal congestion, and other cold symptoms. It can be treated with aspirin and other pain relievers that are taken internally, and with drugs specifically designed for use in the mouth and throat. (*See* MEDICAMENTS FOR SORE GUMS, MOUTHS, AND THROATS and PAIN, FEVER, AND ANTI-INFLAMMATORY DRUGS TAKEN INTERNALLY.)

The Common Cold

Common colds, or, simply *colds*, are respiratory infections that are *self-limiting*—sooner or later they get better all by themselves. Colds rarely are serious illnesses; but they can be quite annoying and unpleasant.

A cold often starts abruptly with a sore throat, sneezing, and runny nose, followed by a stuffy nose. The nasal discharge then may become thick and uncomfortable, and may have a disagreeable odor. The eyes begin to water; the voice becomes husky; the nose feels increasingly blocked up. The senses of smell and taste vanish temporarily; and the cold may spread to the sinuses, producing headache. A wide variety of aches and pains, as well as fever and lethargy, may follow. This misery can continue for a week or two, with coughing and other symptoms coming and going. Discouraging though it may be, the Panel says there is "no generally accepted treatment that can prevent, cure, or shorten the course of the 'common cold.' Treatments which are available only relieve symptoms."

Once over, cold miseries may soon return, because of reinfection by exposure to other people. Many individuals suffer several colds a year. Debate has long raged as to whether emotional factors, particularly *stress*, contribute to or cause colds. The answer now appears to be yes.

For Flu, Too...

Several major over-the-counter drug-makers have begun renaming standard cold-cough products for "flu relief." The thrust of their promotions is that these preparations—which usually contain a pain reliever, an antihistamine, a decongestant, and sometimes a cough suppressor—are different, stronger formulations: "for more than a cold—for flu."

But they are not medicinally different.

A marketing analyst, Kathryn Greengrove Griffe, of Kline & Company, a consulting firm in Fairfield, N.J., told the *New York Times* (Feb. 3, 1992):

> "The contents of the flu remedies are the same as the multi-symptom cold medicines. It's the marketing that's different."

One difference, besides the product name, is the price:

> "Usually," the *Times* says, summing matters up, the new flu products contain "the same ingredients as cold medicine—often at higher prices."

Researchers recently conducted psychological tests on 400 volunteers at the British Medical Research Council's Common Cold Unit in Salisbury, England. The Unit is one of the few live-in facilities in the world where volunteers are deliberately infected with cold viruses for experimental purposes. The subjects in the psychological experiment were exposed to cold viruses. Three quarters of the volunteers who were only minimally stressed in their everyday lives became infected. But nine out of ten who were highly stressed showed signs of infections, psychologist Sheldon Cohen, Ph.D. and his co-workers reported (*New England Journal of Medicine*, Vol. 325, Aug. 29, 1991).

More dramatically: Only a quarter of the low-stress individuals developed symptoms. But half of the highly stressed men and women developed cold symptoms. "Psychological stress was associated . . . with increased risk of acute infectious respiratory illness [common colds]," the researchers reported.

The researchers say they do not yet know how to translate their findings into a practical method to prevent or relieve common colds in people living stressful lives.

Coughing

A cough's main purpose is to clear the airway to the lungs. It is a protective physiological reflex—part voluntary, part involuntary—that occurs often in healthy people as well as in sick ones. Infections, chemical irritants, retained body secretions, and foreign bodies that block the airway, all cause coughing by stimulating the nerve endings in the respiratory tract. (Curiously, tickling the outer ear also sets some people to coughing.)

Drugs that reduce the number and intensity of coughs are called *cough suppressors* or, technically, *antitussives*. A few of them are safe and very effective. But because coughing is one of the ways that the body fights illness, it is not always wise to suppress it with drugs. The Panel offered some guidance.

Irritative Cough

A *dry* cough, which may be caused by colds or by inhalation of irritating dust or gases, is readily recognizable. It is a hacking kind of cough that produces no sputum or other discharge. Consumers can effectively self-treat these coughs with nonprescription products.

Productive Cough

This sputum- or exudate-producing cough is often associated with asthma or bronchitis. It indicates that phlegm and other secretions are being retained in the airways to the lung. Suppressing this kind of cough is a bad, even dangerous, idea because the body needs to rid itself of the phlegm: The Panel went so far as to warn against cough suppressants, but it suggests that an *expectorant* may be helpful. Evaluators also reiterate this time-honored rule: *Any cough that persists more than a week should be investigated by a physician to rule out the possibility of a serious underlying illness.*

Sinus Congestion

The paranasal sinuses (so called because they connect with the nasal cavity) are mucous membrane-lined air cavities in the bony structure of the skull. When the nose becomes congested, drainage of the sinuses is impaired. The sinus membranes become inflamed—a condition called *sinusitis*—and may become infected. This produces headache, facial pain, and tenderness over the affected sinuses.

Nasal decongestants relieve congested sinuses by opening up the nasal passages so they can drain. Pain relievers like aspirin will reduce the discomfort. If the symptoms persist or are accompanied by fever, a doctor should be consulted.

Rhinitis

Rhinitis is nasal inflammation. Marked by a reddening of the nose, it characteristically occurs when you are suffering a cold, but it can occur under some other circumstances.

Allergic Rhinitis

This is one of the commonest allergic responses; it tends to recur at the same season each year. The symptoms include sneezy, watery nasal discharge that may become thicker if a respiratory infection sets in, and an itchy, stuffed-up feeling. The eyes may itch, redden, and water. Puffy eyelids and headaches are less common consequences. The sinuses may fill with mucus.

People who frequently suffer these symptoms usually begin to have some sense of what allergen they are responding to. Their suspicions often can be confirmed by an allergist using standard tests.

The most effective nonprescription drugs for treating allergic rhinitis are antihistamines. Nasal decongestants may be of some help, too. (*See* ALLERGY DRUGS.)

Vasomotor Rhinitis

This is a non-seasonal problem, unlike many forms of allergic rhinitis, but it tends to recur. The blood vessels of the nasal lining appear to become extremely sensitive and reactive for reasons that remain unclear. The symptoms are like those of allergic rhinitis, but allergen testing yields no clear-cut categorization. Antihistamines are less effective against vasomotor rhinitis than they are allergic rhinitis; nasal decongestants may bring some relief.

Single versus Combination Products

The Panel took a dim view of the shotgun approach of treating colds and related ailments with combination products containing two or more active ingredients. The Panel's wariness is remarkable when you consider that the vast majority of cold, cough, and allergy products in fact contain two or more medicinal ingredients.

When drug firms submitted product data for review, they included information on 152 active ingredients. Yet only 24 of these 152 were formulated as single-ingredient products.

Single-ingredient products were considered preferable by the Panel, because they are safer. They allow you to vary the dose of each ingredient individually, and they also give you an opportunity to select a single drug for a specific symptom. This way you can more easily recognize a specific drug's action on the body and learn to adjust the dosage as necessary. Gaining this experience in using a drug can be very useful if the symptom returns.

Commenting on the apparent shortage of such single-ingredient medications, the Panel strongly recommended that all components of combination products be made readily available as single ingredients to allow consumers the opportunity to make more discriminating selections.

However, despite reservations about combining ingredients, the Panel states that, at demonstrably safe and effective doses, combinations "may offer a convenient and rational approach for [relieving] concurrent symptoms." The FDA, subsequently, has been much more lenient than the Panel in giving its official, albeit still-tentative nod of approval to combination products containing three or more active ingredients.

The FDA says it "agrees [with the Panel] that single ingredient products are desirable and should be available. However, [it] recognizes that a significant target population exists for some over-the-counter combination products to treat concurrent symptoms."

Acceptable and unacceptable combinations are summarized in the table Safety and Effectiveness: Combination Products Sold Over-the-Counter for Colds and Coughs at the end of this Unit.

Timed-Release Products

Cold-cough drugs and other medicines taken orally dissolve in the stomach and intestines. They then are absorbed through the gut wall and into the bloodstream, which carries them to the head, lungs, nose, and other target organs. This action generally occurs within an hour or two. So a drug's peak activity, as defined by its maximal levels in the bloodstream, typically occurs about one or two hours after ingestion. A drug may continue to be present and active for several more hours—up to about six hours after it is taken.

Many cold-cough remedies now are formulated as timed-release products to spread out and delay absorption of the drug from the gastrointestinal tract. The aim is to provide effective drug action for up to eight to twelve hours, rather than the three to six hours obtainable from ordinary medication. Timed-release drugs have the advantage of being easier to take, since fewer doses are necessary. They may provide longer-acting relief and also entail fewer and less-severe side effects because blood levels of the drug can be kept fairly constant.

Unfortunately, it is hard to manufacture uniformly effective timed-release products. The capsules or pills tend to dissolve irregularly, depending in part on the acidity of the user's stomach. They may dissolve too slowly and travel too far down into the gut to be effective, or they may dissolve too rapidly to be wholly safe.

Nevertheless, with the exception of *guaifenesin*, all the cold and cough drugs reviewed were assessed as suitable for timed-release formulation. Initially, timed-release drugs used for cold and cough products were granted only *conditional* approval from the standpoint of safety and effectiveness, pending submission of more satisfactory evidence.

The Schering Corporation subsequently obtained approval from the FDA for a repeat-action tablet of *chlorpheniramine maleate* (*Chlor-Trimeton*), an antihistamine. Similar approval was granted Menley and James Laboratories for chlorpheniramine maleate sustained-release capsules. Other timed-release products have been approved in a similar way by the FDA. All timed-release cold-cough preparations therefore are safe and effective.

Alcohol

Alcohol—a fairly stiff dose of it—is formulated into some over-the-counter cold-cough medicines. Some contain 25 percent alcohol. Since 25 percent alcohol equals *50 proof*, users may not need the shot-glass-like dispensers provided with some of these products to remind them that the medicine has an alcoholic potency midway between wine and whiskey.

One "deadly" risk of this "polypharmacy" was described by a Dallas doctor in a letter to the *New England Journal of Medicine* (July 4, 1985, p. 48). His patient, a heavy drinker, tapered off his usual two-to-three cases of beer daily and switched to *NyQuil* (Vicks) instead. It is 25 percent alcohol. This man drank most of a 12-ounce bottle of the medicine and experienced severe liver poisoning, probably because he also consumed almost 7 grams (7000 mg) of acetaminophen that was also in this preparation.

Technically, alcohol appears to be an inactive ingredient in these preparations and so is outside the FDA's present regulatory purview. But the agency "urges manufacturers to use the least possible amount of alcohol to achieve solubility [of the active ingredients], stability, and palatability for all cough-cold drug products."

Dosage of Cold and Cough Medicines

Dosage recommendations for approved active ingredients in cough suppressors, expectorants, antihistamines, and nasal decongestants are found in the discussions for each of these drug groups in the following section.

Dosage of Cold and Cough Medicines for Children

Children are commonly given cold-cough preparations. Yet very little is known about how they react to these drugs or how much they should take. With the help of an *ad hoc* committee of pediatric drug specialists, the Panel established these general guidelines for children:

under age 2 years	dosage to be determined by a physician
ages 2 to 6 years	one-quarter the adult dose
ages 6 to 12 years	one-half the adult dose
over 12 years	adult dosage

Some ingredients should not be taken by children. For example, nonprescription products that contain more than 10 percent alcohol by weight should not be given to youngsters under the age of 6 years, except under a doctor's supervision.

The question has been raised whether children, who suffer repeatedly from colds and other minor respiratory infections, need cold remedies. One negative view comes from pediatrician Nancy Hutton of the Johns Hopkins University School of Medicine in Baltimore.

She treated a group of five-year-olds newly symptomatic with colds with one of three regimens: an antihistamine-decongestant combination product, a dummy tablet (placebo) containing no active drugs, or, simply, nothing. Two days later, Dr. Hutton asked the parents how their kids were doing. She reports that over half the youngsters in *all* groups already were feeling better, and it made no difference whether they were on the active drugs, the dummy drugs, or no drugs at all (*Journal of Pediatrics* Vol. 118, January, 1991).

Dr. Hutton's advice: Skip the medication. "If a child just has a runny nose and is feeling a little cranky," she adds, "the best thing to give him is a box of Kleenex."

For more severe symptoms, or if in doubt: Phone the pediatrician!

Cough Suppressors (Antitussives)

As its name implies, an antitussive (a cough suppressant) suppresses or inhibits the act of coughing. Some of these agents act in the brain, on the cough center in the medulla, to suppress the impulse to cough. The narcotic *codeine*, and *dextromethorphan*, which is a potent non-narcotic, both act in this way.

A second group of cough suppressors act on the throat and bronchial passages. They deaden or lessen pain, relax the smooth muscles that are involved in coughing, or thin out sticky phlegm deposits so that fewer coughs are required to expel them.

Claims for Cough Suppressors

Approved

- "temporarily alleviates cough due to minor bronchial irritation"
- "temporarily calms cough associated with the common cold"
- "temporarily quiets cough as may occur with a cold or inhaled irritants"
- "relieves the impulse to cough"
- "temporarily helps you cough less"
- "temporarily suppresses the impulse to cough to help you get to sleep"

Cough suppressors sold over-the-counter are intended—and should be used—to diminish coughs that arise suddenly, owing to bronchial irritation. They should not be used for more than one week. Once again, coughs that last longer or are accompanied by high fever, rash, or persistent headache may signal the presence of serious disease; they should be investigated by a doctor.

Persons with asthma, emphysema, and other diseases characterized by overproduction of bronchial secretions need to cough to keep their airways clear. They should not take cough suppressors except under medical supervision. Similarly, coughs caused by smoking should not be treated with these agents. (The better medicine would be to stop smoking.)

Cough suppressors are tested by the straightforward method of comparing the number of coughs that subjects emit when they are using the drug with when they are using a dummy drug. These tests are more scientifically reliable in blind studies; that is, when the subjects (and preferably the testers, too) do not know whether the active drug or the dummy is being used. In these experiments, a number of throat irritants, including ammonia vapor and sprays of peppermint water and citric acid, are used to stimulate coughing so that the efficacy of the drug can be quickly and conveniently assessed.

APPROVED ANTITUSSIVE ACTIVE INGREDIENTS

Several antitussives are approved as safe and effective by the FDA. A few are taken internally. Others are sucked as *lozenges*, or cough drops, to soothe the inflamed membranes of the throat or are inhaled from medicated steam or an aromatic ointment spread on the skin.

• CAMPHOR: Camphor, like peppermint oil (*see* further on), has long been used to relieve coughing and perhaps also to relax and relieve other cold symptoms with its pungent medicinal aroma; its value for these latter purposes, however, has not been proved. A number of studies by manufacturers and others convinced the FDA that camphor is safe and effective for relieving cough when applied topically in ointment or steam. The agency agreed with drug makers that camphor either reduces the sensitivity of cough-receptor nerve endings in the throat or soothes and calms irritated or inflamed tissues in the throat. Camphor may act both directly and indirectly.

Dosage of Camphor

The approved dosage in an ointment is 4.7 to 5.3 percent. Adults, and children as young as two years old, can use such an ointment up to three times a day. Spread it on the chest and throat, so the fumes can be easily inhaled. For children under two years old, use only as instructed by a doctor.

The approved dosage of camphor for application in medicated steam is 6.2 percent; add the medication to a vaporizer or other hot or boiling water as directed on the label. Adults and children over age two years may use the medication up to three times daily. For children under two years, use only as directed by a doctor.

 WARNING:
For external use only. Do not take by mouth.

• CHLOPHEDIANOL HYDROCHLORIDE: This ingredient had been marketed as a prescription (℞) cough-suppressor for more than a quarter century when the FDA switched it in 1987 to nonprescription status. The agency said the medical record shows it to be safe and effective. It is not a narcotic, and it appears to act directly on the cough control center in the brain in relieving coughing. However, a search of several standard drug compendia in the early 1990s failed to disclose a nonprescription product that contains chlophedianol hydrochloride.

• *CODEINE PREPARATIONS: CODEINE, CODEINEPHOSPHATE, AND CODEINE SULFATE:* Whether in healthy volunteers who are subjected to cough-inducing agents or in patients with chronic coughs, codeine's effectiveness in suppressing coughs has been demonstrated time and again. It is an extremely effective drug. But since most clinical tests have been in adults with chronic coughs, its effectiveness against acute coughs, in colds or for coughs in children, is not nearly as well documented, though it was judged effective for this use.

Codeine may be formulated in nonprescription cough preparations as codeine, codeine phosphate, or codeine sulfate. They are of essentially equal potency, and all are judged to be safe and effective by the FDA.

The major issue that surrounds codeine's use is its safety. It is a narcotic drug, and when large amounts are taken it can be addictive. But the Panel and the FDA believe the potential for abuse is negligible and that the drug has a low risk of inducing dependency in the small doses in which—under regulation of the Federal Drug Enforcement Agency—it is formulated in over-the-counter cough remedies. Nonetheless, in an attempt to regulate this narcotic drug, purchasers now must sign a special register in the drugstore when they buy a codeine cough preparation, and in many states consumers cannot buy any codeine preparations without a prescription.

The states in which codeine cough products can be purchased over-the-counter—meaning *without* a doctor's prescription—as of 1991 are as follows (according to the National Association of Boards of Pharmacy, Park Ridge, Illinois):

Alaska	Kansas
Arizona	Kentucky (by pharmacist only)
Arkansas	Maine
Connecticut (some jurisdictions)	Massachusetts (some jurisdictions)
Florida	Michigan
Georgia (unclear)	Mississippi
Hawaii	Nevada (by pharmacist only)
Idaho (by pharmacist only)	New Jersey (unclear) (by pharmacist only)
Illinois (by pharmacist only)	New Mexico
Indiana	North Carolina
Iowa	Ohio

Oklahoma	Washington
Rhode Island (unclear)	West Virginia
South Carolina	Wisconsin
Tennessee	Wyoming
Virginia	District of Columbia

Because it *suppresses* coughing, codeine should not be taken by people with thick, wet coughs who need to clear their respiratory passages. Neither should it be taken by those with chronic lung disorders or shortness of breath, except under medical supervision. Codeine's side effects are drowsiness and the aggravation of constipation.

Claim for Codeine Preparations

Accurate
• "Calms the cough control center and relieves coughing"

• *DEXTROMETHORPHAN AND DEXTROMETHORPHAN HYDROBROMIDE:* These variants of morphine lack morphine's pain-killing and addictive traits. But they are highly effective cough suppressants and are used in cough medicines as nonnarcotic alternatives to codeine.

Overdoses of dextromethorphan have produced bizarre behavior and other symptoms such as drowsiness and respiratory depression, but not physical dependence or death. Because of the drug's low order of toxicity, it was assessed as being possibly the safest nonprescription cough suppressor available, although the FDA is investigating its possible abuse as a hallucinogen. The AMA says, in its *Drug Evaluation* 1991, "Dextromethorphan is the safest antitussive available..." It is commonly supplied in a liquid cough syrup or elixir but also is formulated into "cough drops."

Claims for Dextromethorphan

Accurate
• "Calms cough impulses without narcotics"
• "Non-narcotic cough suppressant for the temporary control of coughs"

Recommended Dosage for Over-the-Counter Oral Cough Suppressors

Active Ingredient	Adults and Children Over 12	Children 6 to 12	Children 2 to 6
codeine	10 to 20 mg every 4 to 6 hr (120 mg daily maximum)	5 to 10 mg every 4 to 6 hr (60 mg daily maximum)	consult a doctor
dextromethorphan, dextromethorphan hydrobromide	10 to 20 mg every 4 hr or 30 mg every 6 to 8 hr (120 mg daily maximum)	5 to 10 mg every 4 hr or 15 mg every 6 to 8 hr (60 mg daily maximum)	2.5 to 5 mg every 4 hr or 7.5 mg every 6 to 8 hr (30 mg daily maximum)
diphenhydramine hydrochloride	25 mg every 4 hr (150 mg daily maximum)	12.5 mg every 4 hr (75 mg daily maximum)	only as recommended by a doctor

WARNING:
Do not use [dextromethorphan] if you are taking a monoamine oxidase (MAO) inhibitor. Consult your doctor.

• *DIPHENHYDRAMINE HYDROCHLORIDE:* This antihistamine was introduced clinically in the United States as a prescription drug more than three decades ago. The Panel found that it is as effective a cough suppressor as codeine, but the FDA disagreed, saying there was inadequate evidence to show that it acts directly on the cough center in the brain, as an approved antitussive of its type is required to do. The FDA also questioned the safety of diphenhydramine hydrochloride, noting that drowsiness is a side effect in thirty percent or more of those who use this drug. This side effect is particularly dangerous in people who take this drug and then drive a car or operate heavy machinery.

On the basis of fresh studies, supplied predominantly by the drug manufacturer, Parke-Davis Consumer Health Products, the FDA reversed its view in the 1980s and approved the company's *Benylin Cough Syrup,* in which diphenhydramine hydrochloride is the cough-suppressing active ingredient, as a safe and effective new drug. Other makers' products containing this ingredient have been approved since then.

 WARNING:
The FDA mandates the important warning: "May cause marked drowsiness; alcohol may increase the drowsiness effect. Avoid alcoholic beverages…Do not take if you are taking sedatives or tranquilizers without first consulting your doctor. Use caution when driving a motor vehicle or operating machinery."

A note about confusing names: Parke-Davis's *Benylin Cough Syrup* has diphenhydramine as its active ingredient. The same maker's *Benylin DM* contains dextromethorphan. The former has a sedative side effect, which could be dangerous if you are driving a truck or a car, while the latter does not. So there may be risk if a consumer mistakenly buys the diphenhydramine product, thinking it is the non-sedating dextromethorphan product. Read labels carefully when buying these cough suppressants.

• *PEPPERMINT OIL:* Peppermint oil, a very old drug, is also called *menthol.*

A century ago, a physician, Dr. Frank H. Potter, reported in the *Journal of the American Medical Association* (Vol. 14, p. 147, 1890) that peppermint oil "seems to be a drug with a future of great usefulness" in treating inflammation of the airways and other cold symptoms.

Peppermint oil preparations are put into ointments and salves, inhalants, and lozenges. They are safe in customary dosages, although high doses and accidental overdoses are hazardous. Like camphor, peppermint oil produces a first-cool-then-warm feeling when it is applied to the skin and mucosal tissues.

In the low doses used to relieve coughing, the Panel and the FDA were initially convinced it was safe; effectiveness was another matter. But several studies, with varying results, have persuaded the

Cough Drops

These products ride a thin line between medicine and candy. They may be called *lozenges*, *troches*, or *pastils*, and they are sold in a variety of shapes and sizes. Cough drops are meant to be held in the mouth, and sucked. This allows the soothing medication, and the saliva that must be secreted to melt the cough drop to ooze down the throat.

One theory has it that it is the saliva called up by the sucking that does much of the soothing—so that the same benefit might be obtained by sucking a small, round stone. On the other hand, accidentally swallowing a cough drop is not any cause for concern—but swallowing a stone well might be!

Cough drops can be quite useful in some circumstances, particularly in a theater or concert hall. The concert hall in Amsterdam, Holland, has occasionally handed out cough drops at the door (with the request that concert-goers not crinkle the cellophane).
Most but not all cough drops now meet FDA standards, and the ones that fail to can hardly be very harmful. These products' labels *are* difficult to read, however. So cough drops are analyzed in the table on pp. 188-189 in the Product Ratings Section; the products are listed alphabetically, and their medicinally-active ingredients are indicated.

FDA that 2.8 percent peppermint oil in petrolatum is significantly more effective in quelling coughing than the petroleum alone. (Two studies showed this effect; a third failed to.)

Dosage of Peppermint Oil

The approved dosage is 2.6 to 2.8 percent peppermint oil, which can be used up to three times daily by adults and children over two years of age. Rub the preparation on the chest and throat in a thick layer, and leave clothing loose so fumes can reach the nostrils, the FDA says. Children under two years old should not be treated with this ointment except on a doctor's recommendation.

The FDA reviewed other studies in which 3.2 percent peppermint oil in a steam preparation, along with 6.2 camphor significantly relieved coughing, and on this basis, approved the combination of 3.2 percent peppermint oil + 6.2 percent camphor as an antitussive. Surprisingly, the data to support this approval is not summarized in the *Federal Register* (Aug. 12, 1987) in which the approval is granted, which might leave doubts in some consumers' minds.

Peppermint oil, in candy-like lozenges, will safely and effectively quell coughing, the FDA decided on the basis of manufacturers' studies. These products are very safe in the standard dosages of 5 to 10 mg. Lozenges and cough drops with less than 5 mg or more than 10 mg of peppermint oil are disapproved.

CONDITIONALLY APPROVED ANTITUSSIVE ACTIVE INGREDIENTS

None.

DISAPPROVED ANTITUSSIVE ACTIVE INGREDIENTS

The FDA has disapproved—finally—a number of ingredients that long had been listed as active ingredients in nonprescription cough suppressant products. But, instead of removing these ingredients from their products, some manufacturers have kept them on as *inactive* ingredients—and no doubt also continue to charge for them. They may include small amounts of peppermint oil, camphor, pine extracts, horehound, eucalyptus, or thymol. The FDA appears to be allowing them to do so. This practice may be deceptive, as well as costly for consumers, since some of these ingredients are highly aromatic. They provide the smell if not the substance of medicinal value.

Expectorants

An expectorant is a drug used to promote or facilitate the removal of thick and excessive secretions from the bronchial airways. This may temporarily relieve coughs due to minor throat and bronchial irritations that commonly occur with a cold.

The secretions that expectorants are claimed to act on are the thick respiratory-tract fluids, saliva and postnasal drip, which may be referred to as *phlegm*, *sputum*, or *mucus*.

An expectorant may reduce the thickness of impacted bronchial secretions or dilute them so that they are looser and are more easily evacuated. Some expectorants act directly on nerve endings in the bronchial airways. Others irritate the stomach, triggering a secretory reflex that increases fluid discharges into the stomach and respiratory tract. Still other expectorants stimulate the vomiting center of the brain and other brain areas that are involved in the movement of these thick fluids. When the irritating—sometimes choking—accumulations are gone, the need to cough is diminished.

Expectorants should be useful in relieving irritative, nonproductive coughs or thick, dry coughs in which little sputum is being expelled. Persons who already are coughing up copious amounts of loose phlegm would be less likely to need these drugs.

Many over-the-counter expectorant drugs have been sold for decades. They have a good safety record and their continued popularity suggests that they are effective. But there has been little objective, scientific evidence to confirm their efficacy. Because of this lack of reliable findings, the Panel did not approve any expectorants as safe and effective. Most were granted conditional approval.

The FDA essentially sustained these judgments in 1982 and noted that to the best of its knowledge only one expectorant ingredient, guaifenesin, was undergoing tests that could qualify it for a "safe and effective" designation. This research now has been completed to the FDA's satisfaction, and guaifenesin is the one—and only—approved nonprescription expectorant. The others all have been or will be banned as active ingredients in over-the-counter medications.

Claims for Expectorants

Accurate

- "Helps loosen phlegm and thin [out] bronchial secretions to rid the bronchial passageways of bothersome mucus"
- "Helps loosen sputum and thin [out] bronchial secretions to drain bronchial tubes"
- "Helps loosen phlegm and thin [out] bronchial secretions to make coughs more productive"

Inappropriate

- "Helps you cough less," or any other cough-relief claim that does not include the explanation that this relief is due to loosening of phlegm and drainage of the bronchial airways.

APPROVED EXPECTORANT ACTIVE INGREDIENT

- **GUAIFENESIN (GLYCEROL GUIACOLATE):** Guaifenesin, pronounced *gwy-uh-FIN-uh-sin*, is the only safe and effective nonprescription expectorant, the FDA has decided. It has been marketed for many years in a variety of products. Few complaints had been registered about this ingredient, and the Panel and the FDA agreed, early on, that it is safe. But they questioned its effectiveness, saying that the available clinical studies were inconclusive. The FDA asked for one additional, convincing clinical study, which subsequently was done.

  It was conducted on patients with chronic bronchitis, in an inpatient facility. The 40 subjects were given either guaifenesin cough syrup or the same syrup minus the active drug. Neither the subjects nor the doctors who administered the test knew who was getting which preparation while the two-week test was in progress.

  The subjects recorded their impressions of the treatments' effectiveness in helping them expectorate phlegm. The quantity produced and its stickiness were measured, the latter by timing the speed with which a glob of the stuff rolled down an inclined plane (a microscope slide set at a 45-degree angle).

  Patients who received the active drug initially produced more sputum, and then, after a week, began to produce less of it. At the end of two weeks, they were producing only one-third as much of it as patients taking the dummy preparation. Some of the patients taking guaifenesin "experienced a complete clearing of sputum production" the FDA says. None taking the dummy medication experienced comparable relief. The guaifenesin patients secreted significantly more sputum early on in the treatment than did the patients treated with the dummy medication. On this basis, the FDA concluded that this ingredient is effective, as well as safe, as an expectorant.

The safe and effective dosage for adults, including children over 12 years old, is 200 to 400 mg of guaifenesin every four hours, not to exceed 2400 mg per day. For children 6 to 12 years of age, it is 100 to 200 mg guaifenesin every four hours, not to exceed 1200 mg in a day. For children 2 to 6 years of age, the dosage is 50 to 100 mg every four hours, not to exceed 600 mg per day. This drug should not be given to children under 2 years without its having been recommended by a doctor.

CONDITIONALLY APPROVED EXPECTORANT ACTIVE INGREDIENTS

None.

DISAPPROVED EXPECTORANT ACTIVE INGREDIENTS

None.

Antihistamines

The antihistaminic drugs, developed in France, were first used medically in 1942. They were introduced into the United States a few years later. As a class of medication, they have proved to be extremely safe and extremely useful for several purposes. Fifty different antihistamines have been marketed in prescription and nonprescription products in the United States.

A principal use of antihistamines is to relieve allergic reactions caused by the release of *histamine*. This irritating body substance attaches itself to secretory cells of the nose, eyes, lungs, and skin, enhancing their fluid-making activity. Antihistamines counteract these distressing effects by blocking histamine receptor sites on the cells (*see* ALLERGY DRUGS).

The most controversial decision in the two-decade-old Over-the-Counter Drug Review almost certainly is the FDA's approval of antihistamines for the treatment of cold symptoms. Many widely sold cold remedies contain these drugs, mainly on the basis of a few pivotal—but also equivocal—studies. Cold medications containing antihistamines cost consumers close to $1 billion per year.

Careful recent studies have shown however, that colds do not increase *histamine* release. Yet, historically, allergies and colds have been treated in similar ways, and by the 1970s, many very popular products were promoted for the relief of *both* cold *and* allergy symptoms. The Panel of experts said, however, that antihistamines had never been proved, in credible, scientifically controlled studies, to be useful in relieving cold symptoms.

These drugs *did* affect people with colds, the Panel conceded. Antihistamines have as a side effect a moderate to pronounced sedative effect: They make people drowsy. For this reason, all over-the-counter *soporifics* (sleep-inducing agents) in fact are antihistamines (*see* SLEEP AIDS). When a person is cranky and irritable with a cold, a drug that will let him unwind and facilitate rest and sleep may be useful. But it would not pass the test of law, which says that to be promoted for relief of cold symptoms, a drug has to be shown to relieve one or more such specific symptoms.

Antihistamines have another, relatively mild drying effect (*anticholinergic* effect). They decrease the release of fluids from cells and body tissues. The Panel said this could, conceivably, help dry up a wet and annoying cold.

This possibility was put to the test in a study published in the *Journal of the American Medical Association* (*JAMA*) (Vol. 242, pp. 2414-17, 1979), which was sponsored by a major maker of antihistaminic cold medicines, Schering Corporation. Its antihistamine *chlorpheniramine maleate* is sold under the trade name *Chlor-Trimeton*. The study was conducted by doctors at three U.S. medical centers. A total of 271 patients with new colds participated.

They were treated—and closely studied—as in-patients for two days, and then followed for four additional days at home. Some patients received chlorpheniramine maleate. Others were given a look-alike placebo (dummy preparation). Neither doctors nor patients knew which patients were taking the active drug, and which ones the placebo.

Both groups of patients recovered quite rapidly from their colds; by week's end, most were much improved. In addition, the two groups' symptoms improved in strikingly similar ways: When the test codes were broken at the end of the study, so that analysts could compare the results, the course of recovery, on average, was very similar between the active drug and the dummy drug. Both in terms of patient-subjects' assessments of how they felt, as recorded in diaries that they kept, and the doctors' "objective" evaluation of their symptoms, the antihistamine-treated patients did feel a little bit better at any particular time-check during the treatment week. However, there was no statistically significant difference in patients' "over all evaluation" of the treatments between those on chlorpheniramine and those on the dummy drug. And, only at one of the doctors' time-check examinations, on the second treatment day, was the benefit from the antihistamine statistically better than that of the dummy drug from the doctors' point of view.

Nevertheless, by analyzing different symptoms—such as runny nose, sneezing, postnasal drip, cough and watery eyes—*separately*, and then adding up the scores, the investigators noted several time-checks when there was statistically significant benefit from the antihistamine. When the doctors' ratings of individual symptom improvement were added up, there was slight-to-moderate benefit from the antihistamine, but the benefit was statistically significant only at three checkpoints during the week-long study.

Examination of the improvement curves, as published in *JAMA*, — *See* pp. 161-162 — shows that the two cold-relief curves are almost identical. What is more, in most instances even a significant improvement in the drug-treated subjects was attained by the placebo-treated patients within a few hours to a day later.

Based on its analyses of these data, and data from several similar studies, the FDA concluded that the evidence does *not* prove that chlorpheniramine is effective against itching of the nose or throat or itchy or watering eyes. But the FDA did conclude that "chlorpheniramine is effective in treating runny nose and sneezing associated with the common cold."

It is noteworthy that while the FDA often goes on for page after page of small type in the *Federal Register* (where OTC Drug Review findings are published) this fairly momentous decision was announced in a single paragraph. What is more, the FDA did not include its analysis of the data. Then, going a giant step further—but still in the same paragraph—the agency declared that "because the pharmacologic actions of the various [safe and effective] antihistamines are similar, the agency believes that the data submitted for chlorpheniramine allow safe and effective status for these claims to be extended to *all* safe and effective antihistamine active ingredients" (emphasis added).

The chlorpheniramine studies, in other words, were interpreted by the FDA to mean that similar claims for relieving runny nose and sneezing can be made for the dozen other antihistamines that are sold over-the-counter. This generalizing of results seems to violate the spirit, if not the intent of the OTC Drug Review procedures, which require *each* separate ingredient to be shown, scientifically, to fulfill any specific claim that is made for it.

Weighed against the limited benefits antihistamines provide in controlling sneezing and drying up runny nose, antihistamines can have a number of troublesome side effects, the most prominent of which is *drowsiness*. This effect makes it dangerous for people taking them to drive motor vehicles or operate machines. The use of alcohol or tranquilizing drugs may aggravate this drug-induced loss of alertness and propensity for sleep.

In short, many observers do not believe that the decision to approve cold-relief claims for antihistamines is good medicine or beneficial to consumers.

After the FDA announced its tentative decision, in 1985, a symposium of ear, nose, and throat specialists listened to fresh evidence from three controlled clinical studies. In describing these findings, *Consumer Reports* (January 1989, p. 8), says:

> "In contrast to the Schering studies…none of the [three new] studies found antihistamines significantly more effective than a placebo in relieving cold symptoms."

This summary, unfortunately, is not quite accurate: In one study, chlorpheniramine did significantly reduce sneezing, compared with controls, confirming the Schering studies. The drug-treated patients also secreted less mucus. There was some reduction in the outbreak of colds and cold symptoms.

Nevertheless, the several panelists, who met at Children's Hospital in Pittsburgh in 1987, to present and discuss these data, concluded, in the *Pediatric Infectious Disease Journal* (Vol. 7, pp. 215-42, 1988):

> "The data appear to be conclusive that antihistamines do *not* have a place in the management of upper respiratory infections" (emphasis added).

Consumer Reports adds:

> "It's time for the FDA to oust antihistamines from cold remedies."

Thus far, the agency has not done so. But, prodded by Congress, FDA officials said early in 1992 that they are re-thinking their decision.

 ## Claims for Antihistamines

Accurate

- "Temporarily relieves runny nose and sneezing associated with the common cold"
- "Temporarily dries runny nose and decreases sneezing..."
- "Temporarily reduces runny nose and sneezing . . ."

False or Misleading

- "Temporarily relieves itching of the nose and throat associated with the common cold"
- "Temporarily relieves itchy, watery eyes associated with the common cold"

 WARNINGS:
"Do not take [an antihistamine] product if you have asthma, glaucoma, lung disease, shortness of breath, difficulty in breathing, or difficulty in urination due to... prostate...unless directed by a doctor."

"May cause drowsiness; alcohol, sedative, and tranquilizers may increase the drowsiness effect. Avoid alcoholic beverages. Do not take this product if you are taking sedatives or tranquilizers without first consulting your doctor. ...Use caution when driving a motor vehicle or operating machinery."

Some antihistamines cause "marked drowsiness," rather than just plain "drowsiness." Those that carry this additional risk are identified in the descriptions of these drugs in the following section.

APPROVED ANTIHISTAMINE ACTIVE INGREDIENTS

The FDA currently lists a dozen antihistamines as safe and effective treatments for sneezing and runny nose associated with colds. Most, if not all, were used for many years in prescription drug products, then switched to nonprescription status as their patents ran out. Generally speaking, their safety was established in this earlier period.

Antihistamines are powerful, sometimes useful drugs, but they are not very interesting except, perhaps, to pharmacologists and the companies that produce them. What is more, their dubious value in fighting cold symptoms is based largely, if not wholly on the chlorpheniramine studies, described previously. Therefore, the following descriptions therefore will be brief.

- *BROMPHENIRAMINE MALEATE:* A half billion dosage units of this antihistamine were sold annually, on a prescription basis. Very few serious adverse effects were reported. Brompheniramine is rated by the American Medical Association as having only a low risk of drowsiness. Verdict: safe and effective. (*See* the table Recommended Dosage for Over-the-Counter Antihistamines.)

- *CHLORCYCLIZINE HYDROCHLORIDE:* This antihistamine was introduced in 1949. Chlorcyclizine has passed numerous safety checks and raised few complaints from consumers or others through the year. It was not reviewed by the FDA's panel of outside experts on these drugs. Based on its record of use, the agency switched the drug to over-the-counter status. (*See* the table Recommended Dosage for Over-the-Counter Antihistamines.)

- *CHLORPHENIRAMINE MALEATE:* In one recent year, two billion tablets and capsules of this drug were sold. There were fewer than 2000 reports of side effects, none fatal. Therefore, the Panel ruled that chlorpheniramine is safe, and the FDA—in the disputed finding described under Antihistamines—ruled it effective against runny nose and sneezing. (*See* the table Recommended Dosage for Over-the-Counter Antihistamines.)

• *DEXBROMPHENIRAMINE MALEATE:* This chemical element of brompheniramine maleate long had been sold in prescription (℞) allergy-cold relief products. It is believed to be the most medicinally active form of the drug, and it is stronger, so doses are lower. The FDA switched it to nonprescription status in 1987. (*See* the table Recommended Dosage for Over-the-Counter Antihistamines.)

• *DIPHENHYDRAMINE HYDROCHLORIDE:* This drug is an old and unquestionably effective antihistamine. It is widely used as a prescription and a nonprescription drug.

The main and serious problem with it as an allergy or cold reliever is its pronounced sedative effect: It makes people sleepy. Up to half of people who take the standard 50-mg dose may experience this effect. Because of this, diphenhydramine is sold over-the-counter for helping people go to sleep (*See* SLEEP AIDS.) (*See* the table Recommended Dosage for Over-the-Counter Antihistamines.)

The FDA warns that "marked drowsiness" may occur when this antihistamine is used and cautions consumers against operating a motor vehicle or machinery while taking it.

• *DOXYLAMINE SUCCINATE:* The major liability of this effective antihistamine is that, in the FDA's words, it can cause "marked drowsiness." People who take it should use caution if they drive or operate machinery. The FDA evaluated, at great length, several epidemiological studies that suggest this drug may cause birth defects. After extensive review of the medical literature, the FDA concluded "that it is unlikely that this ingredient is a teratogen [causes birth defects]." But the agency could not absolutely rule out this possibility. So it gives this warning:

 "If you are pregnant or nursing a baby, seek the advice of a health professional before using this [drug]."

(*See* the table Recommended Dosage for Over-the-Counter Antihistamines.)

• *PHENIDRAMINE TARTRATE:* Phenidramine tartrate is a fast-acting antihistamine that has been shown to provide effective relief to allergy sufferers. The FDA has approved its use to relieve runny nose and sneezing in cold sufferers, on the basis of tests on another chemically unrelated antihistamine, chlorpheniramine (*see* previously). The Panel said that reports in the literature over a thirty-year period suggest that phenidramine tartrate produces more side effects than do some other antihistamines, including dry mouth and overstimulation and excitation—particularly in children—as well as, paradoxically, both drowsiness and insomnia. (*See* the table Recommended Dosage for Over-the-Counter Antihistamines.)

* PHENIRAMINE MALEATE: This is a widely used and very safe antihistamine. In one recent year in which 291 million dosage units were sold, 358 suspected toxic reactions were reported; half a dozen of these people required hospitalization but there were no deaths. This is an "old" drug (it was introduced more than three decades ago) and it has not been studied as rigorously as some newer ones. But both clinical experience and animal studies indicate that it is effective against hay fever and other allergic symptoms, and the FDA credits it with efficacy against runny nose and sneezing in cold sufferers. (*See* the table Recommended Dosage for Over-the-Counter Antihistamines.)

* PYRILAMINE MALEATE: Compared with several other approved antihistamines, this one produces many side effects, although usually mild ones. These reactions include drowsiness, listlessness, irritability, and loss of appetite. Some users experience nausea and vomiting. On the other hand, even large overdose appears not to have fatal consequences. About two-thirds of hay-fever sufferers who use pyrilamine maleate obtain symptomatic relief, and the FDA approves its use to relieve sneezy and runny nose in colds. (*See* the table Recommended Dosage for Over-the-Counter Antihistamines.)

* THONZYLAMINE HYDROCHLORIDE: Some studies of this drug, which is more than 30 years old, indicate that it is among the least toxic of its type. In one recent period, during which there were approximately 80 million dosage units sold annually, no suspected poisonings with thonzylamine hydrochloride were reported to the FDA. The other side of the coin is that this drug has been studied less rigorously than some newer antihistamines. (*See* the table Recommended Dosage for Over-the-Counter Antihistamines.)

* TRIPROLIDINE HYDROCHLORIDE: This antihistamine had been sold on prescription (℞) for a quarter century. The FDA decided it is safe and effective for nonprescription sales and self-medication. The American Medical Association, in its 1991 *Drug Evaluations*, says the incidence

of side effects is low; the most common is drowsiness. (*See* the table Recommended Dosage for Over-the-Counter Antihistamines.)

CONDITIONALLY APPROVED ANTIHISTAMINE ACTIVE INGREDIENTS

One antihistamine was conditionally approved for lack of scientifically sound studies to clearly establish its effectiveness.

• PHENYLTOLOXAMINE DIHYDROGEN CITRATE: Data from animal experiments and human trials suggest that this is one of the safest antihistamines currently marketed. The FDA received only one report of an adverse reaction during a recent five-year period, in which there were sales of between one-third and one-half-billion tablets and other dosage units each year. But, despite these huge sales, there is surprisingly little rigorous experimental data to prove the drug's effectiveness or establish the minimum effective dosage level.

DISAPPROVED ANTIHISTAMINE ACTIVE INGREDIENTS

None.

Recommended Dosage for Over-the-Counter Antihistamines

Active Ingredient	Adults and Children Over 12	Children 6 to 12	Children Under 6
brompheniramine maleate	4 mg every 4 to 6 hr (24 mg daily maximum)	2 mg every 4 to 6 hr (12 mg daily maximum), or as directed by a doctor	consult a doctor
chlorcyclizine hydrochloride	25 mg every 6 to 8 hr (75 mg daily maximum)	consult a doctor	consult a doctor
chlorpheniramine maleate	4 mg every 4 to 6 hr (24 mg daily maximum)	2 mg every 4 to 6 hr (12 mg daily maximum), or as directed by a doctor	consult a doctor
dexbrompheniramine maleate	2 mg every 4 to 6 hr (12 mg daily maximum)	1 mg every 4 to 6 hr (6 mg daily maximum), or as directed by a doctor	consult a doctor
diphenhydramine hydrochloride	25 to 50 mg every 4 to 6 hr (300 mg daily maximum)	12.5 to 25 mg every 4 to 6 hr (150 mg daily maximum), or as directed by adoctor	consult a doctor
doxylamine succinate	7.5 to 12.5 mg every 4 to 6 hr (75 mg daily maximum)	3.75 to 6.25 mg every 4 to 6 hr (37.5 mg daily maximum), or as directed by a doctor	consult a doctor

Recommended Dosage for Over-the-Counter Antihistamines (contd)

Active Ingredient	Adults and Children Over 12	Children 6 to 12	Children Under 6
phenindamine tartrate	25 mg every 4 to 6 hr (150 mg daily maximum)	12.5 mg every 4 to 6 hr (75 mg daily maximum), or as directed by a doctor	consult a doctor
pheniramine maleate	12.5 to 25 mg every 4 to 6 hr (150 mg daily maximum)	6.25 to 12.5 mg every 4 to 6 hr (75 mg daily maximum), or as directed by a doctor	consult a doctor
pyrilamine maleate	25 to 50 mg every 6 to 8 hr (200 mg daily maximum) 12.5 to 25 mg	every 6 to 8 hr (100 mg daily maximum), or as directed by a doctor	consult a doctor
thonzylamine hydrochloride	50 to 100 mg every 4 to 6 hr (600 mg daily maximum)	25 to 50 mg every 4 to 6 hrs (300 mg daily maximum), or as directed by a doctor	consult a doctor
triprolidine hydrochloride	2.5 mg every 4 to 6 hr (10 mg daily maximum)	1.25 mg every 4 to 6 hr (5 mg daily maximum), or as directed by a doctor	consult a doctor

Do Antihistamines Help Kill Colds?

Charts like these, in a study published in the *Journal of the American Medical Association* (*JAMA*) (Nov. 30, 1979, pp. 2414-17) were used by makers of chlorpheniramine maleate to justify this antihistamine's inclusion in nonprescription cold preparations.

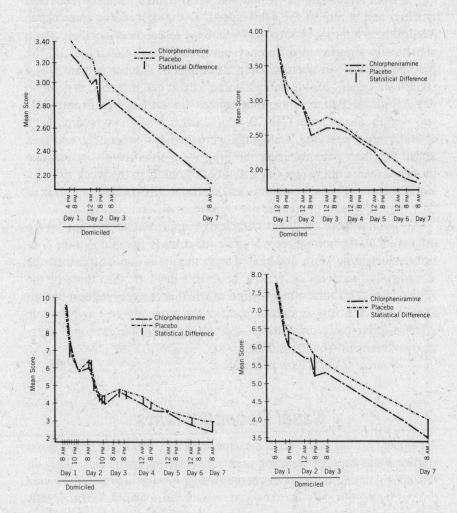

Vertical lines indicate severity of cold symptoms. Horizontal lines are time. Heavy diagonal lines represent changes in cold symptoms—as judged by research doctors or the subjects themselves—in persons who took the antihistamine. Lighter lines are condition of subjects who took a dummy medication, without the antihistamine. Neither the subjects nor their doctors knew whether a particular individual was taking the active drug or the placebo (dummy medication) during the treatment week.

Both antihistamine-treated and sham-treated subjects recovered quickly, and at almost the same speed, as the descending lines show. Vertical bars indicate checkpoints where the researchers say there was a statistically significant difference between the antihistamine and the placebo groups. In doctors' over all ratings of subjects', there was a significant benefit for the antihistamine only at one moment, at noon on day 2 (Fig. 1). Patients on antihistamines did not feel significantly better, over all, at any point (Fig. 2). But when individual symptoms, such as stuffy nose, sneezing, and cough were analyzed separately, and then added together, patients using the drug were significantly better than those who were not using it at a number of points in the week (Fig. 3). But depiction of nasal symptoms, as determined by the doctors, showed only three moments of statistically significant difference (Fig. 4).

Even if these small but statistically significant advantages for the drug are real, the normal recovery rate for colds is so rapid that the control subjects who were not treated with the antihistamine reached the same level of recovery only a few hours to a day later than those on the active drug. This raises the question of whether the very modest benefit seen in this, and similar studies, justifies the monetary cost and the side effects—principally drowsiness—of putting antihistamines into over-theo-counter cold-cough products.

Source: *JAMA*, with permission.

Nasal Decongestants

A number of drugs called *nasal decongestants* will effectively relieve nasal stuffiness and improve breathing in persons suffering from colds. They do this *not* by drying up nasal discharge (which is what antihistamines may do) but by significantly narrowing, or *constricting*, swollen blood vessels in the mucosal lining of the nose and sinuses. It is the swelling and inflammation of these tissues that are largely to blame for stuffy noses.

The remarkable constrictive effect these drugs can have on blood vessels has one unfortunate result: rebound congestion as the drug wears off. The mucosal blood vessels may swell out more than before, so the nose may feel even more stuffed up than it was. The risk can be reduced by using these drugs no more often than the label advises and for no more than three or seven days at a time. (Oral forms, while less effective, are less likely to produce rebound congestion than nasal sprays.)

Nasal decongestants are formulated for (1) *topical application* as nose drops, sprays, and jellies, (2) *inhalation* from inhalers or in steam vapors, and (3) *oral ingestion* in liquid or tablets.

When these potent compounds are put directly into the nose—rather than being swallowed—very little drug is absorbed into the bloodstream and carried to the rest of the body. So inhaled decongestants and nasal jellies are remarkably free from systemic side effects, unlike decongestants that are taken orally. Decongestants that are taken orally are carried throughout the body and can affect major organ systems. Persons with high blood pressure, heart disease, diabetes, or thyroid disease should not take decongestants orally except on a doctor's orders.

There is a different risk for products that are introduced into the nose: the spread of infection via contaminated dispensers. In order to prevent the spread of germs, only one person should use each drug dispenser.

 ### Claims for Nasal Decongestants

Certain claims can legitimately be made for safe and effective nasal decongestants. Unlike some other cold and cough drugs, decongestants can be tested objectively: the resistance to airflow through the stuffed-up nasal passage can be measured. In that way, the amount of air flowing through medicated nostrils can easily be compared with the amount passing through nostrils not exposed to the drug.

Accurate
- "For the temporary relief of nasal congestion due to the common cold"
- "For the temporary relief of stopped-up nose"
- "Helps clear nasal passages"
- "Helps decongest sinus openings and passages; relieves sinus pressure"
- "Promotes nasal and sinus drainage"

• "Decongests nasal passages; shrinks swollen membranes"

 WARNINGS:
These warnings are applicable to all safe and effective nasal decongestants *except* desoxyephedrine-L and propyl-hexedrine inhalers, which carry less risk:

"Do not exceed recommended dosage because at higher doses nervousness, dizziness, or sleeplessness may occur."

"Do not take this [decongestant] if you have heart disease, high blood pressure, thyroid disease, diabetes, or difficulty in urination due to enlargement of the prostate gland, unless directed by a doctor."

"Do not take this drug if you are taking a prescription drug for high blood pressure or depression, without first consulting your doctor."

APPROVED NASAL DECONGESTANT ACTIVE INGREDIENTS

• *DESOXYEPHEDRINE-L (INHALER):* Inhalers that contained this substance caused burning, stinging, sneezing, and runny nose in up to one out of five test subjects. But no serious side effects have been reported, so the Panel considers the drug safe.

Fresh data from four scientific studies that confirmed the effectiveness of desoxyephedrine-L inhalers were submitted to the FDA. The data satisfied the agency that the drug is effective. The new data also indicate that this drug can be used for up to seven days without risk of rebound congestion. (*See* the table Recommended Dosage for Over-the-Counter Nasal Decongestants.)

• *EPHEDRINE PREPARATIONS (TOPICAL):* Ephedrine preparations include ephedrine, ephedrine hydrochloride, ephedrine sulfate, and racephedrine hydrochloride. Ephedrine has been available in the United States for more than half a century. Numerous tests have shown it to be safe and effective when applied as a nasal spray, drops, or jelly in concentrations of 0.5 to 1 percent. Rebound congestion is unlikely at those low doses if the drug is not used longer than three days.

Ephedrine acts quickly, reaching its maximal decongestant effect within one hour. It loses its effectiveness after four hours. (*See* the table Recommended Dosage for Over-the-Counter Nasal Decongestants.)

- *NAPHAZOLINE HYDROCHLORIDE (TOPICAL):* This drug has some notable advantages and some notable disadvantages. It is effective, and it produces a noticeable decongestant effect within 10 minutes. Relief continues for up to five or six hours. Tests suggest that most people who use it experience some relief from their symptoms. The disadvantages are that rebound congestion sometimes occurs after even a single treatment; it is fairly likely to occur after repeated use. What is more, naphazoline can be habit-forming. If accidentally swallowed, it can cause marked drowsiness. It should not be used by children under 12. But, despite these problems, naphazoline was evaluated as safe and effective as a nasal decongestant. (*See* the table Recommended Dosage for Over-the-Counter Nasal Decongestants.)

- *OXYMETAZOLINE HYDROCHLORIDE (TOPICAL):* This is a long-acting decongestant. The decongestant effect begins to decline only after five or six hours. Twice-a-day doses should provide adequate relief without causing rebound congestion. The drug has been shown to be safe and effective in double-blind trials. In one, the nasal airways of 7 out of 14 children treated with the preparation twice daily were completely open for 9 to 12 hours each day. In another study, in 30 children, three drops in each nostril three times daily provided persistently effective clearance of the nasal passages for two weeks. (*See* the table Recommended Dosage for Over-the-Counter Nasal Decongestants.)

- *PHENYLEPHRINE HYDROCHLORIDE (TOPICAL OR ORAL):* Although potent, this decongestant is both safe and effective. Tests show statistically significant decongestive effect when the drug is administered orally. In one study, for example, a 10-mg dose yielded an average reduction of 11 percent in airway resistance at 15 minutes; a 21 percent reduction was shown at one and two hours. Similar benefit has been reported when the drug is administered in nasal drops and sprays. Oral phenylephrine can raise blood pressure and increase heart rate, but at the low doses taken to clear stuffed-up noses, such effects are unlikely to occur. However, persons taking prescription drugs that contain substances called monoamine oxidase (MAO) inhibitors may experience serious cardiovascular effects when they take even the approved oral over-the-counter dose of phenylephrine. The FDA warns, too, that the 1 percent preparations of this drug are especially likely to cause rebound congestion and other side effects. (*See* the table

Recommended Dosage for Over-the-Counter Nasal Decongestants.)

- *PROPYLHEXEDRINE (INHALED):* This drug has a wide margin of safety and relative freedom from toxic effects. It can be used for up to seven days by persons who cannot use ephedrine and similar decongestants. (*See* the table Recommended Dosage for Over-the-Counter Nasal Decongestants.)

- *PSEUDOEPHEDRINE PREPARATIONS (TAKEN ORALLY):* The safety and effectiveness of pseudoephedrine hydrochloride and pseudoephedrine sulfate, given orally, have been demonstrated clinically and in scientific studies on cold sufferers. Side effects are minimal; they include drowsiness, headache, and insomnia. In the recommended dosage, pseudoephedrine appears unlikely to cause significant elevations of blood pressure in hypertensive persons. Persons taking MAO inhibitors, however, should avoid this drug. (Anyone who is not sure whether his prescribed medication is an MAO inhibitor should check with his or her doctor.) (*See* the table Recommended Dosage for Over-the-Counter Nasal Decongestants.)

- *XYLOMETAZOLINE (TOPICAL):* This is a potent decongestant that was moved from prescription (℞) to nonprescription status after the Panel determined that it is safe and effective for nonprescription use. It is long-acting: A single dose may provide relief for more than five hours. Rebound congestion is less of a problem than with some other nasal decongestants. Tests have shown that xylometazoline produces an objective increase in airflow through the nasal passages and subjective sense of relief from the stuffed-up feeling. (*See* the table Recommended Dosage for Over-the-Counter Nasal Decongestants.)

CONDITIONALLY APPROVED NASAL DECONGESTANT ACTIVE INGREDIENTS

Many agents are conditionally approved as nasal decongestants pending further testing.

- *BORNYL ACETATE (TOPICAL):* The safety of bornyl acetate, an aromatic substance, is attested to by long clinical use. But there is no well-documented study to show its effectiveness as a nasal decongestant and evaluators could not even determine a suitable dosage for testing purposes.

- *CAMPHOR (INHALED):* (Described earlier under Cough Suppressors, p. 141.) Camphor is judged to be safe in customary dosages. But studies on its effectiveness as a decongestant have been in multi-ingredient products, so camphor's contribution, if any, is difficult to determine.

- *CEDAR-LEAF OIL (TOPICAL):* This is a turpentine-like volatile oil that is steam-distilled from the fresh leaves of the cedar tree *Thuja occidentalis.* It is dangerous if eaten but safe when applied to the chest, neck, and back in the dose used in a widely-marketed ointment. Compared with an inert preparation, combination products that include cedar-leaf oil significantly reduced congestion over a period of several hours. However, the role of cedar-leaf oil must be determined by suitably testing it as an individual ingredient. The Panel could not determine a dosage for this substance.

- *EPHEDRINE PREPARATIONS (TAKEN ORALLY):* Ephedrine preparations are safe when taken orally, as they are when inhaled. They can, however, cause tension, nervousness, tremor, and sleeplessness. In high doses they appear to work as nasal decongestants. But no studies have been submitted to show that they are effective for this purpose at the dosage levels recommended for use without prescription (℞).

- *PEPPERMINT OIL (MENTHOL) (TOPICAL OR INHALED):* Some combination products containing this aromatic substance have been shown to make breathing easier. But menthol's contribution to this therapeutic effect has not been established.

- *PHENYLPROPANOLAMINE PREPARATIONS:* Including phenylpropanolamine bitartrate, phenylpropanolamine hydrochloride, phenylpropanolamine maleate (topical or oral): Forms of phenylpropanolamine are among the most frequently used nasal decongestants. Several well-monitored studies have demonstrated their effectiveness.

   The Panel decided that the oral forms but not inhaled forms of these drugs were safe. But subsequently a number of studies were published showing that phenylpropanolamine can cause significant—perhaps dangerous—rises in blood pressure, as well as other side effects. Many doctors said it should not be sold over-the-counter, either as a nasal decongestant or as an appetite suppressant, for which it is also widely used. (*See* REDUCING AIDS.)

   In the meanwhile, however, FDA had specifically approved several new phenylpropanolamine products as safe and effective, in a parallel approval process outside the OTC Drug Review. These include sustained release combination products for relieving colds and allergies that contain up to 75 mg of phenylpropanolamine hydrochloride, along with an antihistamine (brompheniramine maleate or chlorpheniramine maleate).

   Because of these concerns, the FDA has given phenylpropanolamine an equivocal status—technically neither approved, conditionally approved or disapproved—until it determines whether to permit it or ban it in over-the-counter preparations.

DISAPPROVED NASAL DECONGESTANT ACTIVE INGREDIENTS
None.

Bronchodilators

These drugs relax the smooth muscles lining the airways between the windpipe and the lungs. They relieve coughing and open the airways to facilitate normal breathing.

The bronchodilators (bronchial muscle relaxants) that are sold without prescription (℞) include ephedrine preparations and epinephrine preparations. They are very useful for asthma sufferers (*See* ASTHMA DRUGS).

The FDA disallows these agents as single-ingredient drugs for colds and for coughs not caused by asthma. It disapproves of their use for nonasthmatic symptoms.

A few combination drug products for coughs and colds still contain bronchodilators. They have not been proved safe and effective for this purpose. The likelihood is that they soon will be banned for sale for ordinary coughs due to colds.

APPROVED BRONCHODILATOR ACTIVE INGREDIENTS
None.

CONDITIONALLY APPROVED BRONCHODILATOR ACTIVE INGREDIENTS
None.

DISAPPROVED BRONCHODILATOR ACTIVE INGREDIENTS
• EPHEDRINE

- *Ephedrine hydrochloride*
- *Ephedrine sulfate*
- *Epinephrine*
- *Epinephrine bitartrate*
- *Racephedrine hydrochloride*

See also Asthma Drugs.

Miscellaneous Ingredients

A few ingredients that do not fall under the aforementioned categories are formulated into combination products used to treat colds and coughs. The Panel takes a dim view of their worth.

APPROVED MISCELLANEOUS INGREDIENTS

None.

CONDITIONALLY APPROVED MISCELLANEOUS INGREDIENTS

- *Ascorbic acid (vitamin C):* Few medical topics have stirred more comment and conversation than the question of whether vitamin C cures the common cold. The Panel says the evidence to show that it *does* remains inconclusive, so that any *label claim* for this effect is *misbranding*. Vitamin C appears to be essentially safe, even in the extremely high doses that some people take. But until it is proved to be effective, the Panel would grant only conditional approval to Vitamin C.
- *Caffeine:* The Panel "presumes" that caffeine is formulated into combination cold-cough remedies to counteract the soporific ("drowsiness causing") effects of antihistamines. In the customary low doses, caffeine is certainly safe. But there are no data to show that it is effective.

DISAPPROVED MISCELLANEOUS INGREDIENTS

None.

Recommended Dosage for Over-the-Counter Nasal Decongestants Taken Through the Nose (Drops, Sprays, Jellies, or Inhalations)

Active Ingredient	Adults and Children Over 12	Children 6 to 12	Children Under 6 years*
desoxyephedrine-L (inhaler) with camphor, eucalyptol, menthol	2 inhalations per nostril not oftener than every 2 hr	1 inhalation per nostril not oftener than every 2 hr with adult supervision	consult a doctor
ephedrine 0.5%	2 to 3 drops or sprays per nostril every 4 or more hr, or 1 application of jelly per nostril	1 to 2 drops or sprays per nostril every 4 or more hr, or 1 application of jelly per nostril with adult supervision	consult a doctor
naphazoline hydrochloride 0.05%	1 to 2 drops or sprays per nostril not oftener than every 6 hr, or 1 application of jelly per nostril	consult a doctor	consult a doctor
0.025%		1 or 2 drops or sprays per nostril not oftener than every 6 hr, or 1 application of jelly per nostril with adult supervision	consult a doctor
oxymetazoline hydrochloride 0.05%	2 to 3 drops or sprays per nostril not oftener than twice daily, or 1 to 2 applications of jelly per nostril	2 or 3 drops or sprays per nostril not oftener than twice daily, or 1 to 2 applications of jelly per nostril, with adult supervision	consult a doctor

phenylephrine hydrochloride 1%	2 or 3 drops or sprays per nostril not oftener than every 4 hr, or 1 application of jelly per nostril	consult a doctor	consult a doctor
0.5%	2 to 3 drops or sprays per nostril not oftener than every 4 hr, or 1 application of jelly per nostril	consult a doctor	consult a doctor
0.25%	2 to 3 drops or sprays per nostril not oftener than every 4 hr, or 1 application of jelly per nostril	2 to 3 drops or sprays per nostril not oftener than every 4 hr, or 1 application of jelly per nostril, with adult supervision	consult a doctor
0.125%			for children 2 to 6, 2 to 3 drops or sprays per nostril, not oftener than every 4 hrs, with adult supervision; for children under 2, consult a doctor
propylhexedrine (with menthol) inhaler	2 inhalations per nostril not oftener than once every 2 hrs	1 inhalation per nostril not oftener than once every 2 hr, with adult supervision	consult a doctor
xylometazoline 0.1%	2 or 3 drops or sprays per nostril not oftener than every 8 to 10 hr, or 1 application of jelly per nostril	consult a doctor	consult a doctor

Recommended Dosage for Over-the-Counter Nasal Decongestants Taken Through the Nose (Drops, Sprays, Jellies, or Inhalations) (contd)

Active Ingredient	Adults and Children Over 12 years	Children 6 to 12	Children Under 6 years*
xylometazoline 0.05%		2 or 3 drops or sprays per nostril not oftener than every 8 to 10 hr, or 1 application of jelly, with adult supervision	consult a doctor

Recommended Dosage for Over-the-Counter Nasal Decongestants Taken by Mouth

Active Ingredient	Adults and Children Over 12 years	Children 6 to 12 years	Children 2 to 6 years*
phenylephrine hydrochloride	10 mg every 4 hr (60 mg daily maximum)	5 mg every 4 hr (30 mg daily maximum)	2.5 mg every 4 hr (15 mg daily maximum)
pseudoephedrine	60 mg every 4 to 6 hr (240 mg daily maximum)	30 mg every 4 to 6 hr (120 mg daily maximum)	15 mg every 4 to 6 hr (60 mg daily maximum)

* For children under 2 years of age, consult a doctor.

Safety and Effectiveness: Active Ingredients in Over-the-Counter Cough Medicines

Active Ingredients	Cough Suppressor	Expectorant	Nasal Decongestant
bornyl acetate *inhalant*			safe but not proved effective
camphor *inhalant*	safe and effective		safe but not proved effective
ointment	safe and effective		safe but not proved effective
cedar-leaf oil *ointment*			safe but not proved effective
chlophedianol hydrochloride *oral*	safe and effective		
codeine preparations: codeine, codeine phosphate, and codeine sulfate *oral*	safe and effective		
desoxyephedrine-L *inhalant*			safe and effective
dextromethorphan *oral*	safe and effective		
dextromethorphan hydrobromide *oral*	safe and effective		
diphenhydramine hydrochloride *oral*	safe and effective		

Safety and Effectiveness: Active Ingredients in Over-the-Counter Cough Medicines (contd)

Active Ingredients	Cough Suppressor	Expectorant	Nasal Decongestant
ephedrine preparations: ephedrine, ephedrine hydrochloride, ephedrine sulfate, and racephedrine hydrochloride *nose drops, sprays, jellies*			safe and effective
oral			safe but not proved effective
eucalyptol and eucalyptus oil inhalant *ointment*			safe but not proved effective*
guaifenesin (glycerol guaiacol) *oral*		safe and effective	
naphazoline hydrochloride *nose drops, sprays, jellies*			safe and effective
oxymetazoline hydrochloride *nose drops, sprays, jellies*			safe and effective
peppermint oil (menthol) *inhalant*	safe and effective		safe but not proved effective
lozenge	safe and effective		safe but not proved effective
ointment	safe and effective		safe but not proved effective

phenylephrine hydrochloride
nose drops, sprays, jellies

oral

safe and effective

safe and effective

phenyl-propanolamine preparations: (phenylpropano-
lamine bitartrate, phenyl-
propanolam ine hydro-chlo-
ride, and phenylpropanolamine maleate *nose drops,
sprays, oral*

not proved safe and effective

safe and effective

propylhexedrine *inhalant*

pseudoephedrine preparations:
pseudoephedrine hydrochloride and pseudoephedrine
sulfate *oral*

safe and effective

xylometazoline *nose drops,
sprays, nasal jellies*

safe and effective

---

*These ingredients are safe and effective when formulated with desoxyephedrine-*L* in an inhalant product.

Safety and Effectiveness: Antihistamines in Over-the-Counter Cold and Cough Medications

Active Ingredient	Assessment
brompheniramine maleate	safe and effective
chloryclizine hydrochloride	safe and effective
chlorpheniramine maleate	safe and effective
dexbrompheniramine maleate	safe and effective
diphenhydramine hydrochloride	safe and effective
doxylamine succinate	safe and effective
phenindamine tartrate	safe and effective
pheniramine maleate	safe and effective
phenyltoloxamine citrate	safe but not proved effective
pyrilamine maleate	safe and effective
thonzylamine hydrochloride	safe and effective
triprolidine hydrochloride	safe and effective

Safety and Effectiveness: Combination Products Sold Over-the-Counter for Colds and Coughs

Safe and Effective Combinations

Each individual ingredient must be safe and effective, except as noted.
- 1 or more pain-fever relievers + 1 antihistamine
- 1 or more pain-fever relievers + 1 oral cough suppressor
- 1 or more pain-fever relievers + 1 expectorant
- 1 or more pain-fever relievers + 1 nasal decongestant taken internally
- 1 or more pain-fever relievers + 1 antihistamine + 1 nasal decongestant
- 1 or more pain-fever relievers + 1 oral cough suppressor + 1 nasal decongestant taken by mouth
- 1 or more pain-fever relievers + 1 oral cough suppressor + 1 antihistamine + 1 nasal decongestant taken by mouth
- 1 antihistamine + 1 cough suppressor (label must warn of possible "marked drowsiness")

Safety and Effectiveness:
Combination Products Sold Over-the-Counter
for Colds and Coughs (contd)

---

1 antihistamine + 1 nasal decongestant taken by mouth

1 antihistamine + 1 nasal decongestant taken by mouth + 1 cough suppressor

1 cough suppressor + 1 expectorant (labeled only for "nonproductive coughs")

1 cough suppressor + 1 nasal decongestant taken by mouth

1 cough suppressor + local anesthetic or pain-fever reliever (as lozenge only)

1 cough suppressor + 1 expectorant + 1 nasal decongestant taken by mouth
(labeled only for "nonproductive coughs")

1 expectorant + 1 nasal decongestant taken by mouth

1 nasal decongestant taken by mouth + 1 local anesthetic (as lozenge only)

1 oral cough suppressor + 1 throat soother (demulcent) (as lozenge only)

1 nasal decongestant taken by mouth + 1 throat soother (demulcent)
(as lozenge only)

1 nasal decongestant taken by mouth + 1 cough suppressor + 1 throat soother
(demulcent) (as lozenge only)

1 oral cough suppressor + 1 local anesthetic + 1 throat soother (demulcent) (as
lozenge only)

1 nasal decongestant taken by mouth + 1 local anesthetic + 1 throat soother
(demulcent) (as lozenge only)

1 nasal decongestant taken by mouth + 1 cough suppressor + 1 local pain
reliever + 1 throat soother (demulcent) (as lozenge only)

desoxyephedrine-L + aromatics (bornyl acetate, camphor, lavender oil, menthol,
methyl salicylate) in an inhaler as nasal decongestant taken through the nose.
(*Note:* The aromatic ingredients are not safe and effective individually, or in
any combination as decongestants, except when combined with
desoxyephedrine-L in an inhaler.)

peppermint oil + camphor + eucalyptus oil in a suitable ointment vehicle as an
inhaled cough suppressor. (*Note:* Eucalyptus oil is not safe and effective as
a single-ingredient cough suppressor.)

Conditionally Safe or Conditionally Effective Combinations

1 or more conditionally approved ingredients or conditionally approved
labeling but no disapproved ingredient or labeling

less-than-minimally effective dosage in 1 or more ingredients claimed to relieve
the same symptom

2 approved ingredients from the same drug group

2 antihistamines if one is also a safe and effective cough suppressor

1 safe and effective antihistamine + 1 additional antihistamine if it is a cough
suppressor

1 antihistamine + 1 local anesthetic

1 antihistamine + 1 throat soother (demulcent)

1 expectorant + 1 throat soother (demulcent)

Safety and Effectiveness:
Combination Products Sold Over-the-Counter
for Colds and Coughs (contd)

---

1 expectorant + 1 local anesthetic

1 antihistamine + 1 nasal decongestant as nose drops or spray (effectiveness not established)

1 cough suppressor + 1 bronchodilator, labeled only for "nonasthmatic cough" (effectiveness not established)

1 expectorant + 1 bronchodilator, labeled only for "nonasthmatic cough" (effectiveness not established)

1 cough suppressor + 1 expectorant, labeled only for "productive cough"

1 cough suppressor + 1 expectorant + 1 nasal decongestant, labeled only for "productive cough"

combinations containing 3 or more active ingredients from same group (e.g. nasal decongestants)

combinations containing small amounts of a conditionally approved active ingredient intended to counteract side effects of other ingredient—e.g., caffeine

combinations containing an antihistamine for which a sleep-aid claim is made

combinations containing several claimed active ingredients that are mixtures of volatile substances, with overlapping pharmacologic activities for which a minimum effective dose cannot be established for 1 or more ingredient(s) (exception: desoxyephedrine-L + aromatics are safe and effective)

1 or more pain-fever relievers + 1 cough suppressor + 1 expectorant + 1 nasal decongestant

all other combinations of 4 or more active ingredients (For the one exception, See Safe and Effective Combinations above.)

combinations containing vitamin C for which no claims of effectiveness against colds are made

peppermint oil + camphor + eucalyptus oil containing combinations for steam inhalation or topical use as nasal decongestant or a cough suppressor

peppermint oil + camphor (as lozenge, as cough suppressor)

Unsafe or Ineffective Combinations

a combination with any disapproved ingredient or disapproved labeling

a combination of approved ingredients from different groups, each for a different symptom, if any ingredient is present at less than the minimum effective dose

1 pain-fever reliever + 1 bronchodilator

1 antihistamine + 1 expectorant (ingredients counteract each other)

1 bronchodilator + 1 antihistamine

combinations containing more than 30 mg of caffeine

combinations containing 15 to 30 mg of caffeine "to combat lethargy" if they do not contain an antihistamine

Safety and Effectiveness:
Combination Products Sold Over-the-Counter
for Colds and Coughs (contd)

combinations containing 2 antihistamines, 1 of which is added and labeled
    exclusively as a sleep aid
combinations containing vitamin C or any other vitamin and labeled for
    prevention or treatment of colds
1 antihistamine + 1 debriding agent/wound cleanser
1 antihistamine + 1 astringent
1 cough suppressor + 1 astringent
phenylpropanolamine + ephedrine + caffeine
ephedrine + caffeine
phenylpropanolamine + caffeine
pseudoephedrine + caffeine

Cold and Cough Medicines: Product Ratings

SINGLE INGREDIENT PRODUCTS

COUGH SUPRESSORS

Product and Distributor	Dosage of Active Ingredients	Rating*	Comment
dextromethorphan hydrobromide			
Dextromethorphan hydrobromide (generic)	syrup: 10 mg per teaspoonful	A	
Pertussin CS (Pertussin)	liquid: 3.5 mg per teaspoonful	A	children's dosage
Robitussin Pediatric (Robins)	liquid: 7.5 mg per teaspoonful	A	children's dosage
diphenhydramine hydrochloride			
Benylin Cough Syrup (Parke-Davis)	syrup: 12.5 mg per teaspoonful	A	℞ to OTC switch
Diphenhydramine (generic)		A	℞ to OTC switch

EXPECTORANTS

Product and Distributor	Dosage of Active Ingredients	Rating*	Comment
guaifenesin			
Breonesin (Winthrop)	capsules: 200 mg	A	
Gee-Gee (Jones)	tablets: 200 mg	A	

Glycotuss (Pal-Pak)	tablets: 100 mg	A	
Glytuss (Mayrand)	tablets: 200 mg	A	
Guaifenesin (generic)	syrup: 100 mg per teaspoonful	A	
terpin hydrate			
Terpin hydrate (generic)	elixir: 85 mg per teaspoonful	C	not effective, and banned, but some may still be around in medicine cabinets and on drugstore shelves

ANTIHISTAMINES

Product and Distributor	Dosage of Active Ingredients	Rating*	Comment
brompheniramine maleate			
Brompheniramine (generic)	elixir: 2 mg per teaspoonful tablets: 4 mg	A	Rx to OTC switch
Dimetane (Robins)	elixir: 2 mg per teaspoonful tablets: 4 mg timed-release tablets: 8 mg, 12 mg	A	Rx to OTC switch

*Author's interpretation of FDA criteria. Based on contents, not claims.

Cold and Cough Medicines: Product Ratings (contd)

SINGLE INGREDIENT PRODUCTS

ANTIHISTAMINES

Product and Distributor	Dosage of Active Ingredients	Rating*	Comment
chlorpheniramine maleate			
Alla-Chlor (Rugby)	syrup: 2 mg per teaspoonful	A	℞ to OTC switch
Chlo-Amine (Hollister-Stier)	chewable tablets: 2 mg	A	children's dosage, ℞ to OTC switch
Chlorpheniramine (generic)	tablets: 4 mg	A	℞ to OTC switch
Chlor-Trimeton (Schering-Plough)	syrup: 2 mg per teaspoonful tablets: 4 mg	A A	℞ to OTC switch ℞ to OTC switch
Chlor-Trimeton Repetabs (Schering-Plough)	tablets, timed-release: 8 mg	A	℞ to OTC switch
Teldrin (SmithKline Beecham)	capsules, timed-release: 12 mg	A	℞ to OTC switch
diphenhydramine hydrochloride			
Belix (Halsey)	elixir: 12.5 mg per teaspoonful	A	℞ to OTC switch
Benadryl 25 (Parke-Davis Consumer)	capsules; tablets: 25 mg	A	℞ to OTC switch

Product and Distributor	Dosage of Active Ingredients	Rating*	Comment
Benylin (Parke-Davis Consumer)	syrup: 12.5 mg per teaspoonful	A	Rx to OTC switch
Diphenhydramine (generic)	capsules; tablets: 25 mg elixir, syrup: 12.5 mg per teaspoonful	A A	Rx to OTC switch / Rx to OTC switch
pyrilamine maleate			
Pyrilamine maleate (generic)	tablets: 25 mg	A	Rx to OTC switch
triprolidine hydrochloride			
Actidil (Burroughs Wellcome)	tablets: 2.5 mg syrup: 1.25 mg per teaspoonful	A A	Rx to OTC switch / Rx to OTC switch

DECONGESTANTS

Product and Distributor	Dosage of Active Ingredients	Rating*	Comment
desoxyephedrine-L			
Vicks Inhaler (Vicks Health Care)	inhaler: 50 mg + menthol, camphor, eucalyptus	A	but a recently purchased Vicks Inhaler does not list desoxyephedrine-L on the container; it is not effective: C
ephedrine sulfate			
Ephedrine sulfate (generic)	capsules: 25 mg	B	not proved effective
Vatronol (Vicks Health Care)	nose drops: 0.5%	A	

Cold and Cough Medicines: Product Ratings (contd)

SINGLE INGREDIENT PRODUCTS: ANTIHISTAMINES

Product and Distributor	Dosage of Active Ingredients	Rating*	Comment
ephedrine hydrochloride			
Efedron Nasal (Hyrex)	jelly: 0.6%	A	
naphazoline hydrochloride			
Privine (Ciba Consumer)	nose drops: 0.05% nasal spray: 0.05%	A A	
oxymetazoline hydrochloride			
Afrin (Schering-Plough)	pediatric nose drops: 0.025% nose drops: 0.05%	A A	for children, ℞ to OTC switch ℞ to OTC switch
Allerest 12-Hour Nasal (Pharmacraft)			
Dristan Long Lasting (Whitehall)	nasal spray: 0.05%	A	℞ to OTC switch
Duration (Schering-Plough)		A	℞ to OTC switch

Drug	Form/Strength		Notes
4-Way Long-Lasting Nasal Spray (Bristol-Meyers)		A	Rx to OTC switch
Neo-Synephrine 12 Hour (Winthrop Consumer)		A	Rx to OTC switch
Oxymetazolone (generic)		A	Rx to OTC switch
Sinex Long-Acting (Vicks Health Care)		A	Rx to OTC switch

phenylephrine hydrochloride (products listed in order of increasing strength)

Drug	Form/Strength		Notes
Alconefrin 25 (Webcon)	nose-drops: 0.25%	A	dosage for older children, adults
Alconefrin 50 (Webcon)	nose drops: 0.5%	A	adult dosage
Doktors (Scherer)	nose drops: 0.25%	A	
Duration (Plough)	nasal spray: 0.5%	A	
Neo-Synephrine (Sanofi Winthrop)	nose drops: 0.125%	A	dosage for children
	nose drops: 1%	A	
	nasal spray: 0.25%	A	
	nasal spray: 0.25%	A	
	nasal spray, nasal drops, and nasal jelly: 0.5%	A	
Nostril (Boehringer-I)	nasal spray: 0.5%	A	
Phenyephrine hydrochloride (generic)	solution: 1%	A	

Cold and Cough Medicines: Product Ratings (contd)

SINGLE INGREDIENT PRODUCTS

Product and Distributor	Dosage of Active Ingredients	Rating*	Comment
Rhinall (Scherer)	nasal spray: 0.25%	A	
phenylpropanolamine hydrochloride			
Phenylpropanolamine hydrochloride (generic)	**tablets:** 25 mg, 50 mg, 75 mg (timed release)	B	safety not confirmed; ℞ to OTC switch
Propagest (Carrick)	**tablets:** 25 mg	B	safety not confirmed; ℞ to OTC switch
propylhexedrine			
Benzedrex (SmithKline Beecham)	**inhaler:** 250 mg + menthol	A	
pseudoephedrine hydrochloride (products are listed in order of increasing strength)			
Dorcol Children's Decongestant (Sandoz)	**liquid:** 15 mg per teaspoonful	A	children's dosage, ℞ to OTC switch
Pseudoephedrine hydrochloride (generic)	**liquid:** 30 mg per teaspoonful	A	children's dosage, ℞ to OTC switch
Cenafed Syrup (Century Pharm.)	**liquid:** 30 mg per teaspoonful	A	℞ to OTC switch
Children's Sudafed (Burroughs Wellcome)	**liquid:** 30 mg per teaspoonful	A	children's dosage, ℞ to OTC switch

Pseudo Syrup (Major)		A	℞ to OTC switch
Pseudoephedrine hydrochloride (generic)		A	℞ to OTC switch
Sudafed (Burroughs Wellcome)	tablets: 30 mg, 60mg	A	℞ to OTC switch
pseudoephedrine sulfate			
Afrinol Repetabs (Schering-Plough)	tablets, timed action: 120 mg	A	℞ to OTC switch
xylometazoline hydrochloride			
Otrivin Pediatric Nasal Drops (Ciba Consumer)	pediatric nose drops: 0.05%	A	children's dosage, ℞ to OTC switch
Otrivin (Ciba Consumer)	spray: 0.1%	A	℞ to OTC switch
Xylometazoline hydrochloride (generic)		A	℞ to OTC switch

COMBINATION PRODUCTS

Product and Distributor	Dosage of Active Ingredients	Rating*	Comment
Topical Products			
Dristan Nasal (Whitehall)	spray: 0.5% phenylephrine hydrochloride + 0.2% pheniramine maleate	C	This combination has not been shown to be safe and effective — and FDA has said it is not clear which symptoms it is indicated for.

Cold and Cough Medicines: Product Ratings (contd)

COMBINATION PRODUCTS

Product and Distributor	Dosage of Active Ingredients	Rating*	Comment
Sprays, Steam Inhalers, Ointments			
4-Way Fast Acting (Bristol-Myers)	**nasal spray:** 0.5% phenylephrine hydrochloride + 0.05% naphazoline hydrochloride + 0.2% pyrilamine maleate	B	2 approved ingredients from same category (decongestants)
Myci-Spray (Misemer)	**spray:** 0.25% phenylephrine + 0.2% pheniramine maleate	C	This combination has not been shown to be safe.
Vicks VapoRub (Richardson-Vicks)	**ointment:** 4.7% camphor + 2.6% menthol + 1.2% eucalyptus oil	A	
Vicks VapoStream (Richardson-Vicks)	**liquid for vaporizers:** menthol 3.2% + camphor 6.2% + eucalyptus oil 1.5%	B	FDA not convinced this combination is safe and effective
Lozenges, Including Cough Drops, Troches & Tablets			
Halls Mentho-Lyptus Spearmint (Warner-Lambert)	5 mg menthol + 4 mg eucalyptus oil	C	eucalyptus not safe or effective
Hold DM (Menley & James)	5 mg dextromethorphan hydrobromide	A	

Product	Ingredients	Rating	Comment
Luden's Wild Cherry Throat Drops (Luden's)	pectin	A	
New Extra Strength Vicks Cherry Eucalyptus (Richardson-Vicks)	menthol: 10 mg	A	name is deceptive
Pine Bros. Wild Cherry Throat Drops (United)	glycerin	A	
Ricola Cherry Mint Herb Throat Drops (Ricola)	1.5 mg menthol	A	
Ricola Menthol-Eucalyptus Herb Throat Drops (Ricola)	4.5 mg menthol + 4.5 mg eucalyptusoil	C	eucalyptus not safe or effective
Smith Bros. Black Licorice (Smith Bros)	licorice + anethole	C	neither ingredient approved in OTC Review
Sucrets Cough Control (SmithKline-Beecham)	5 mg dextromethorphan hydrobromide	A	
Vicks Formula 44 Cough Control Discs (Richardson-Vicks)	5 mg dextromethorphan hydrobromide + 1.25 mg benzocaine	A	

*Author's interpretation of FDA criteria. Based on contents, not claims.

Cold and Cough Medicines: Product Ratings (contd)

COMBINATION PRODUCTS: DECONGESTANT + PAIN-RELIEVER

Product and Distributor	Dosage of Active Ingredients	Rating*	Comment
Advil Cold & Sinus (Whitehall)	**caplets:** 30 mg pseudoephedrine hydrochloride + 200 mg ibuprofen	A	R̶ to OTC switch (ibuprofen)
BC Cold Powder Non-Drowsy Formula (Block)	**powder:** 25 mg phenylpropanolamine hydrochloride + 650 mg aspirin + lactose	C	the decongestant may not be safe; combination of cold-cough ingredient with antacid (lactose) not approved
Congespirin for Children (Bristol-Myers Squibb)	**tablets:** 1.25 mg phenylephrine + 81 mg acetaminophen	A	dosage for children
Contac Non-Drowsy Formula Sinus Caplets (SmithKline-Beecham)	**caplets:** 30 mg pseudoephedrine + 500 mg acetaminophen	A	
Maximum Strength Sine-Aid Tablets and Caplets (McNeil-CPC)	**caplets, tablets:** 30 mg pseudoephedrine hydrochloride + 500 mg acetaminophen	A	
Maximum Strength Sinutab without Drowsiness Tablets and Caplets (Parke-Davis)		A	

| Ornex Caplets (Menley & James) | caplets: 30 mg pseudoephedrine + 325 mg acetaminophen | A | |
| Sinus Excedrin (Bristol Myers-Squibb) | caplets, tablets: 30 mg pseudoephedrine hydrochloride + 500 mg acetaminophen | A | |

ANTIHISTAMINE + PAIN-RELIEVER

Product and Distributor	*Dosage of Active Ingredients*	*Rating**	*Comment*
Coricidin Tablets (Schering-Plough)	tablets: 2 mg chlorpheniramine maleate + 325 mg acetaminophen	A	Rx to OTC switch (chlorpheniramine)
Percogesic Tablets (Richardson-Vicks)	tablets: 30 mg phenyltoloxamine citrate + 325 mg acetaminophen	B	this antihistamine not proved effective
Phenetron Compound Tablets (Lannett)	tablets: 2 mg chlorpheniramine maleate + 390 mg aspirin + 30 mg caffeine	A	Rx to OTC switch (chlorpheniramine)
Phenylgesic Tablets (Goldline)		B	

*Author's interpretation of FDA critera. Based on contents, not claims.

Cold and Cough Medicines: Product Ratings (contd)

COMBINATION PRODUCTS†

DECONGESTANT + ANTIHISTAMINE

Product and Distributor	Dosage of Active Ingredients	Rating*	Comment
Sustained-Release Capsules and Tablets (products listed by strength of active ingredients)			
Coltab Children's Tablets (Hauck)	**tablets:** 2.5 mg phenylephrine hydrochloride + 1 mg chlorpheniramine maleate	A	children's dosage ℞ to OTC switch (both ingredients)
Contac Continuous Action Nasal Decongestant/Antihistamine Capsules (SmithKline Beecham)	**capsules:** 75 mg phenylpropanolamine hydrochloride + 8 mg chlorpheniramine maleate	A?	approved by FDA on basis of New Drug Application, bypassing OTC Review, in which phenylpropanolamine's safety has been questioned; ℞ to OTC switch (both ingredients)
Phenylpropanolamine HCl/Chlorpheniramine Maleate (Generic)		A?	see previous comments
Contac Maximum Strength 12-Hour Caplets (SmithKline-Beecham)	**caplets:** 75 mg phenylpropanolamine hydrochloride + 12 mg chlorpheniramine maleate	A?	see previous comments
Phenylpropanolamine HCl Chlorpheniramine Maleate (generic)	**tablets:** 75 mg phenylpropanolamine hydrochloride + 12 mg chlorpheniramine maleate	A?	see previous comments

Product	Formulation		Comments
Triaminic-12 (Sandoz)	**tablets:** 75 mg phenyl-propanolamine hydrochloride + 12 mg chlorpheniramine maleate	A?	*see previous comments*
Bromatapp Extended Release Tablets (generic)	**tablets:** 75 mg phenyl-propanolamine hydrochloride + 12 mg brompheniramine maleate	A?	approved by FDA on basis of New Drug Application, bypassing OTC Review, in which phenyl-propanolamine's safety has been questioned; Rx to OTC switch (both ingredients)
Dimetapp Extentabs (Robins)		A?	*see previous comments*
Isoclor Timesules (Fisons)	**capsules:** 120 mg pseu-doephedrine hydrochloride + 8 mg chlorpheniramine maleate	A	Rx to OTC switch (both ingredients)
Allergy D Capsules (Laser)	**capsules:** 120 mg pseu-doephedrine hydrochloride + 12 mg chlorpheniramine maleate	A	Rx to OTC switch (both ingredients)
Actifed 12-Hour Capsules (Burroughs Wellcome)	**capsules:** 120 mg pseu-doephedrine hydrochloride + 5 mg triprolidine hydrochloride	A	Rx to OTC switch (both ingredients)
Disophrol Chronotabs (Schering-Plough)	**tablets:** 120 mg pseudoephedrine sulfate + 6 mg dexbrompheni-ramine maleate	A	Rx to OTC switch (both ingredients)

Cold and Cough Medicines: Product Ratings (contd)

COMBINATION PRODUCTS†

Product and Distributor	Dosage of Active Ingredients	Rating*	Comment
Drixoral Sustained-Action Tablets (Schering-Plough)	**tablets:** 120 mg pseudoephedrine sulfate + 6 mg dexbrompheniramine maleate	A	see previous comments
Resporal Tablets (Pioneer)		A	see previous comments
Tablets and Capsules (products listed by strength of active ingredients)			
Histatab Plus Tablets (Century)	**tablets:** 5 mg phenylephrine hydrochloride + 2 mg chlorpheniramine maleate	A	℞ to OTC switch (both ingredients)
A.R.M. Caplets (SmithKline Beecham)	**caplets:** 25 mg phenylpropanolamine hydrochloride + 4 mg chlorpheniramine maleate	B	phenylpropanolamine may not be safe; ℞ to OTC switch (both ingredients)
Triaminic Allergy Tablets (Sandoz)	**tablets**	B	see previous comments
Conex D.A. Tablets (Forest)	**tablets:** 37.5 mg phenylpropanolamine hydrochloride + 4 mg chlorpheniramine maleate	B	see previous comments

Product	Ingredients		Comments
Allerest Maximum Strength Tablets (Fisons)	**tablets:** 30 mg pseudoephedrine hydrochloride + 2 mg chlorpheniramine maleate	A	R to OTC switch (both ingredients)
Fedahist Tablets (generic)	**tablets:** 60 mg pseudoephedrine hydrochloride + 4 mg chlorpheniramine maleate	A	R to OTC switch (both ingredients)
Isoclor Tablets (Fisons)		A	*see previous comments*
Sudafed Plus Tablets (Burroughs Wellcome)		A	*see previous comments*
Benadryl Decongestant (Parke-Davis)	**capsules, tablets:** 60 mg pseudoephedrine hydrochloride + 25 mg diphenhydramine hydrochloride	A	R to OTC switch (both ingredients)
Actifed (Burroughs Wellcome)	**tablets, capsules:** 60 mg pseudoephedrine hydrochloride + 2.5 mg triprolidine hydrochloride	A	R to OTC switch (both ingredients)
Pseudoephedrine hydrochloride/triprolidine hydrochloride (generic)		A	R to OTC switch (both ingredients)
Chlor-Trimeton 4-Hour Relief Tablets (Schering-Plough)	**tablets:** 60 mg pseudoephedrine sulfate + 4 mg chlorpheniramine maleate	A	R to OTC switch (both ingredients)

Cold and Cough Medicines: Product Ratings (contd)

COMBINATION PRODUCTS

Liquids (all dosages per teaspoonful) (products listed by strength of active ingredients)

Product and Distributor	Dosage of Active Ingredients	Rating*	Comment
Dimetane Decongestant Elixer (Robins)	**liquid:** 5 mg phenylephrine hydrochloride + 2 mg brompheniramine maleate	A	℞ to OTC switch (brompheniramine maleate)
Demazin Syrup (Schering-Plough)	**syrup:** 12.5 mg phenylpropanolamine hydrochloride + 2 mg chlorpheniramine maleate	B	safety of phenylpropanolamine remains in doubt; ℞ to OTC switch (both ingredients)
Triaminic Syrup (Sandoz)		B	see previous comment
Dimetapp Elixir (Robins)	**liquid:** 12.5 mg phenylpropanolamine hydrochloride + 2 mg brompheniramine maleate	B	safety of phenylpropanolamine remains in doubt; ℞ to OTC switch (both ingredients)
Paratapp Elixer (Parmed)		B	see previous comments
Dorcol Pediatric Cold Formula Liquid (Sandoz)	**liquid:** 15 mg pseudoephedrine hydrochloride + 1 mg chlorpheniramine maleate	A	children's dosage; ℞ to OTC switch (both ingredients)
Fedahist (several makers)	**syrup:** 30 mg pseudoephedrine hydrochloride + 2 mg chlorpheniramine maleate	A	℞ to OTC switch (both ingredients)

Ryna Liquid (Wallace)	A	*see* previous comment
Sudafed Plus Liquid (Burroughs Wellcome)	A	*see* previous comment
Rhinosyn Syrup (Great Southern) **syrup:** 60 mg pseudoephedrine hydrochloride + 4 mg chlorpheniramine maleate	A	Rx to OTC switch (both ingredients)
Actifed Syrup (Burroughs Wellcome) **syrup:** 30 mg pseudoephedrine hydrochloride + 1.25 mg triprolidine	A	Rx to OTC switch (both ingredients)
Triprolidine Hydrochloride with Pseudoephedrine Hydrochloride Syrup (generic)	A	*see* previous comment
Drixoral Syrup (Schering-Plough) **syrup:** 30 mg pseudoephedrine sulfate + 2 mg brompheniramine maleate	A	Rx to OTC switch (both ingredients)

---

*Author's interpretation of FDA criteria. Based on contents, not claims.

Cold and Cough Medicines: Product Ratings (contd)

COMBINATION PRODUCTS

DECONGESTANT + ANTIHISTAMINE + PAIN-RELIEVER PRODUCTS

Product and Distributor	Decongestant	Antihistamine	Pain-Fever Reliever/Other	Rating*	Comment
Tablets and Caplets					
Alka-Seltzer Plus Cold Medicine Tablets (Miles Inc.)	24.08 mg phenyl-propanolamine bitartrate	2 mg chlorpheni-ramine maleate	325 mg aspirin	B	safety of phenyl-propanolamine not established; ℞ to OTC switch (first two ingredients)
Coricidin 'D' Decongestant Tablets (Schering-Plough)	12.5 mg phenyl-propanolamine hydrochloride	2 mg chlorpheni-ramine maleate	325 mg aceta-minophen	B	safety of phenyl-propanolamine not established; ℞ to OTC switch (first two ingredients)
Coricidin Demilets Tablets (Schering-Plough)	6.25 mg phenyl-propanolamine hydrochloride	1 mg chlorpheni-ramine maleate	80 mg aspirin	B	children's dosage; safety of phenyl-propanolamine not established; ℞ to OTC switch (first two ingredients)

Product					
Coricidin Max Strength-Sinus Headache Tablets (Schering-Plough)	12.5 mg phenyl-propanolamine hydrochloride	2 mg chlorpheni-ramine maleate	500 mg aceta-minophen	B	safety of phenyl-propanolamine not established; Rx to OTC switch (first two ingredients)
Dristan Tablets (Whitehall)	5 mg phenylephrine hydrochloride	2 mg chlorpheni-ramine maleate	325 mg aceta-minophen	A	correct formulation for children 6-12 (1 tablet) and adults (2 tablets); Rx to OTC switch (first two ingredients)
Dristan-AF Tablets (Whitehall)	5 mg phenylephrine hydrochloride	2 mg chlorpheni-ramine maleate	325 mg aceta-minophen + 16.2 mg caffeine	A	see previous comment
4-Way Cold Tablets (Bristol-Myers Squibb)	12.5 mg phenyl-propanolamine hydrochloride	2 mg chlorpheni-ramine maleate	325 mg aceta-minophen	B	safety of phenyl-propanolamine not established; Rx to OTC switch (first two ingredients)
Histosal Tablets (Ferndale)	20 mg phenyl-propanolamine hydrochloride	12.5 mg pyrilamine maleate	324 mg aceta-minophen + 30 mg caffeine	B	safety of phenyl-propanolamine not established; Rx to OTC switch (first two ingredients)

Cold and Cough Medicines: Product Ratings (contd)

Product and Distributor	Decongestant	COMBINATION PRODUCTS Antihistamine	Pain-Fever Reliever/Other	Rating*	Comment
Allerest Sinus Pain Formula Tablets (Fisons)	30 mg pseudoephedrine hydrochloride	2 mg chlorpheniramine maleate	500 mg acetaminophen	A	Rx to OTC switch (first two ingredients)
Allergy-Sinus Comtrex (Bristol-Myers Squibb)				A	Rx to OTC switch (first two ingredients)
Sine-Off Maximum Strength Allergy/Sinus Caplets (SmithKline-Beecham)				A	Rx to OTC switch (first two ingredients)
Codamil Tablets, Capsules (Central)	30 mg pseudoephedrine hydrochloride	2 mg chlorpheniramine maleate	325 mg acetaminophen	A	Rx to OTC switch (first two ingredients)
Sinarest Tablets (Fisons)				A	Rx to OTC switch (first two ingredients)

Product and Distributor	Cough Suppressor	Decongestant	Antihistamine	Pain-Fever Reliever	Rating*	Comment
Children's Tylenol Cold Tablets (McNeil-CPC)		7.5 mg pseudoephedrine hydrochloride	0.5 mg chlorpheniramine maleate	80 mg acetaminophen	A	children's dosage; Rx to OTC switch (first two ingredients)
Liquids						
Children's Tylenol Cold Liquid (McNeil-CPC)		15 mg pseudoephedrine	1 mg chlorpheniramine maleate	160 mg acetaminophen	A	children's dosage; amounts per teaspoonful; Rx to OTC switch (first two ingredients)
Benadryl Cold Liquid (Parke-Davis)		10 mg pseudoephedrine hydrochloride	8.3 mg diphenhydramine hydrochloride	167 mg acetaminophen	A	dosage per teaspoonful; Rx to OTC switch (first two ingredients)

COUGH-SUPPRESSORS

Product and Distributor	Cough Suppressor	Decongestant	Antihistamine	Pain-Fever Reliever	Rating*	Comment
Tablets and Capsules						
Comtrex Capsules or Tablets (Bristol-Myers)	10 mg dextromethorphan hydrobromide	30 mg phenylpropanolamine hydrochloride	2 mg chlorpheniramine maleate	325 mg acetaminophen	B	phenylpropanolamine not proved safe; Rx to OTC switch (phenylpropanolamine, chlorpheniramine)

*Author's interpretation of FDA critera. Based on contents, not claims.

Cold and Cough Medicines: Product Ratings (contd)

COMBINATION PRODUCTS

Product and Distributor	Cough Suppressor	Decongestant	Antihistamine	Pain-Fever Reliever	Rating*	Comment
Contac Severe Cold & Flu Hot Medicine Powder (SmithKline-Beecham)	20 mg dextromethorphan hydrobromide	60 mg pseudoephedrine hydrochloride	4 mg chlorpheniramine maleate	650 mg acetaminophen	A	R to OTC switch (pseudoephedrine, chlorpheniramine)
Contac Severe Cold Formula Caplets (SmithKline-Beecham)	15 mg dextromethorphan hydrobromide	12.5 mg phenylpropanolamine hydrochloride	2 mg chlorpheniramine maleate	500 mg acetaminophen	B	phenylpropanolamine not proved safe; R to OTC switch (phenylpropanolamine, chlorpheniramine)
Multisymptom Tylenol Cold Medication Tablets and Caplets (McNeil CPC)	15 mg dextromethorphan hydrobromide	30 mg pseudoephedrine hydrochloride	2 mg chlorpheniramine maleate	325 mg acetaminophen	A	R to OTC switch (pseudoephedrine, chlorpheniramine)
NyQuil LiquiCaps (Richardson-Vicks)	15 mg dextromethorphan hydrobromide	30 mg pseudoephedrine hydrochloride	25 mg diphenhydramine hydrochloride	250 mg acetaminophen	A	R to OTC switch (pseudoephedrine, diphenhydramine)

Product and Distributor	Cough Suppressor	Decongestant	Antihistamine	Rating*	Comment
Tylenol No Drowsiness Cold Caplets (McNeil-CPC)	15 mg dextromethorphan hydrobromide	30 mg pseudoephedrine hydrochloride	325 mg acetaminophen	A	℞ to OTC switch (pseudoephedrine)
Liquids					
Actifed with Codeine Cough Syrup (Burroughs Wellcome)	10 mg codeine phosphate	30 mg pseudoephedrine hydrochloride	1.25 mg triprolidine hydrochloride	A	℞ to OTC switch (pseudoephedrine, triprolidine)
Bromanyl Syrup (generic)	10 mg codeine phosphate		12.5 mg bromodiphenhydramine	C	antihistamine not approved in OTC review
Bromodiphenhydramine Hydrochloride with Codeine Liquid (generic)	10 mg codeine phosphate			C	see previous comment
Effective Strength Cough Formula Liquid (Barre-National)	15 mg dextromethorphan hydrobromide		2 mg chlorpheniramine maleate	B	one teaspoonful is too little chlorpheniramine; two teaspoonfuls is too much dextromethorphan; ℞ to OTC switch (chlorpheniramine)
Phenergan with Codeine Syrup (Wyeth-Ayerst)	10 mg codeine phosphate		6.25 mg promethazine hydrochloride	B	promethazine not proved safe

*Author's interpretation of FDA criteria. Based on contents, not claims.

Cold and Cough Medicines: Product Ratings (contd)

COMBINATION PRODUCTS

Product and Distributor	Cough Suppressor	Decongestant	Antihistamine	Rating*	Comment
Prometh with Codeine Syrup (generic)				B	see previous comment
Ryna-C Liquid (Wallace)	10 mg codeine phosphate	30 mg pseudoephedrine hydrochloride	2 mg chlorpheniramine maleate	A	2 tsp provide correct adult dosage; Rx to OTC switch (pseudoephedrine, chlorpheniramine)
Triacin-C Cough Syrup (several makers)	10 mg codeine phosphate	30 mg pseudoephedrine hydrochloride	1.25 mg triprolidine hydrochloride	A	Rx to OTC switch (pseudoephedrine, triprolidine)
Tricodene Forte Liquid (Pfeiffer)	10 mg dextromethorphan hydrobromide	12.5 mg phenyl-propanolamine hydrochloride	2 mg chlorpheniramine maleate	B	phenylpropanolamine not proved safe; Rx to OTC switch (phenylpropanolamine, chlorpheniramine)

EXPECTORANTS + OTHER INGREDIENTS

Product and Distributor	Expectorant	Cough Supressor	Decongestant	Rating*	Comment
Tablets and Capsules					

Product					Comment
Congestac Caplets (Menley & James)	400 mg guaifenesin	60 mg pseudoephedrine hydrochloride		A	Rx to OTC switch (pseudoephedrine)
Glycofed Tablets (Pal-Pak)	100 mg guaifenesin	30 mg pseudoephedrine hydrochloride		A	Rx to OTC switch (pseudoephedrine)
DayCare Caplets (Richardson-Vicks)	100 mg guaifenesin	30 mg pseudoephedrine hydrochloride	10 mg dextromethorphan hydrobromide	A	Rx to OTC switch (pseudoephedrine)
Dimacol Caplets (Robins)				A	see previous comment

Liquids

Product					Comment
Cheralin Expectorant Liquid (Lannett)	88 mg potassium guaiacolsulfonate + 88 mg ammonium chloride + 1 mg antimony potassium tartrate			C	too many expectorant active ingredients; disapproved expectorant ingredients
Fedahist Expectorant Syrup (several makers)	200 mg guaifenesin	30 mg pseudoephedrine hydrochloride		A	Rx to OTC switch (pseudoephedrine)
Robitussin-PE Liquid (Robins)	100 mg guaifenesin	30 mg pseudoephedrine hydrochloride		A	Rx to OTC switch (pseudoephedrine)
Conex Syrup (Forest)	100 mg guaifenesin	12.5 mg phenylpropanolamine hydrochloride		B	phenylpropanolamine not proved safe
Triaminic Expectorant (Sandoz)				B	

Cold and Cough Medicines: Product Ratings (contd)

COMBINATION PRODUCTS

Product and Distributor	Expectorant	Decongestant	Cough Supressor	Rating*	Comment
Fedahist Expectorant Pediatric Drops (several makers)	40 mg guaifenesin per drop	7.5 mg pseudoephedrine hydrochloride per drop		A	children's dosage; R to OTC switch (pseudoephedrine)
Naldecon EX Children's Syrup (Apothecon)	100 mg guaifenesin per tsp	6.25 mg phenyl-propanolamine hydrochloride per tsp		B	phenylpropanolamine hydrochloride not proved safe; R to OTC switch (phenyl-propanolamine)
Cheracol Syrup (Roberts)	100 mg guaifenesin		10 mg codeine phos-phate	A	
Guiatuss AC Syrup (generic)				A	
Robitussin A-C Syrup (Robins)				A	
Iopen-C Liquid (several makers)	30 mg iodinated glyc-erol		10 mg codeine phos-phate	C	disapproved expectorant
Iotuss Liquid (Muro)				C	
Terpin Hydrate and Codeine Elixir (generic)	85 mg terpin hydrate		10 mg codeine	C	terpin hydrate not approved as OTC expectorant

Product	Ingredient		Antitussive/Codeine	Category	Comments
Calcidrine Syrup (Abbott)	152 mg calcium iodide anhydrous		8.4 mg codeine	C	calcium iodide anhydrous not approved as OTC drug
Nucofed Pediatric Expectorant Syrup (SmithKline Beecham)	100 mg guaifenesin	30 mg pseudoephedrine hydrochloride	10 mg codeine phosphate	A	Rx to OTC switch (pseudoephedrine)
Pediacof Syrup (Sanofi Winthrop)	75 mg potassium iodide	2.5 mg phenylephrine hydrochloride	5 mg codeine phosphate	C	also includes antihistamines; expectorant not approved as OTC drug; combination is not approved
Cheracol D Cough Liquid (Roberts)	100 mg guaifenesin		10 mg dextromethorphan hydrobromide	A	
Guaituss-DM Liquid (several makers)	100 mg guaifenesin		10 mg dextromethorphan hydrobromide	A	
Contac Cough Formula Liquid (SmithKline Beecham)	67 mg guaifenesin		10 mg dextromethorphan hydrobromide	A	
Benylin Expectorant Liquid (Parke-Davis)	100 mg guaifenesin		5 mg dextromethorphan hydrobromide	A	
Terpin Hydrate with Dextromethorphan Hydrobromide Liquid (generic)	85 mg terpin hydrate		10 mg dextromethorphan hydrobromide	C	terpin hydrate not approved as OTC expectorant

*Author's interpretation of FDA criteria. Based on contents, not claims.

Cold and Cough Medicines: Product Ratings (contd)

COMBINATION PRODUCTS

Product and Distributor	Expectorant	Decongestant	Cough Supressor	Rating*	Comment
Vicks Children's Cough Syrup (Richardson-Vicks)	50 mg guaifenesin	3.5 mg dextromethorphan hydrobromide		A	dosage for children
Vicks Pediatric Formula 44e (Richardson-Vicks)	33.3 mg guaifenesin	3.3 mg dextromethorphan hydrobromide		A	dosage for children
Dihistine Expectorant Liquid (several makers)	100 mg guaifenesin	30 mg pseudoephedrine hydrochloride	10 mg codeine phosphate	A	Rx to OTC switch (pseudoephedrine)
Isoclor Expectorant Liquid (Fisons)				A	
Novahistine Expectorant Liquid (Marion Merrell Dow)				A	
Ryna-CX Liquid (Wallace)				A	
Novahistine DMX Liquid (Marion Merrell Dow)	100 mg guaifenesin	30 mg pseudoephedrine hydrochloride	10 mg dextromethorphan hydrobromide	A	Rx to OTC switch (pseudoephedrine)
Ru-Tuss Expectorant Liquid (Boots)				A	

EXPECTORANT + DECONGESTANT + COUGH SUPRESSOR + OTHER INGREDIENTS

Product and Distributor	Expectorant	Decongestant	Cough Supressor	Other Ingredients	Rating*	Comment
Contac Cough & Chest Cold Liquid (SmithKline Beecham)	50 mg guaifenesin	15 mg pseudoephedrine hydrochloride	5 mg dextromethorphan hydrobromide	125 mg acetaminophen	A	℞ to OTC switch (pseudoephedrine)
Cough Formula Comtrex Liquid (Bristol-Myers)	50 mg guaifenesin	15 mg pseudoephedrine hydrochloride	7.5 mg dextromethorphan hydrobromide	125 mg acetaminophen	A	℞ to OTC switch (pseudoephedrine)
DayCare Liquid (Richardson-Vicks)	33.3 mg guaifenesin	10 mg pseudoephedrine hydrochloride	3.3 mg dextromethorphan hydrobromide	108.3 mg acetaminophen	A	℞ to OTC switch (pseudoephedrine)
Father John's Medicine Plus Liquid (Oakhurst)	30 mg guaifenesin + 83.3 mg ammonium chloride	2.5 mg phenylephrine hydrochloride	7.5 mg dextromethorphan hydrobromide	1 mg chlorpheniramine maleate	C	too many expectorant ingredients; ammonium chloride not approved; ℞ to OTC switch (chlorpheniramine)
Quelidrine Cough Syrup (Abbott)	40 mg ammonium chloride + 0.005 ml ipecac fluid extract	5 mg phenylephrine hydrochloride + 5 mg ephedrine hydrochloride	10 mg dextromethorphan hydrobromide	2 mg chlorpheniramine maleate (antihistamine)	C	both expectorants disapproved; ℞ to OTC switch (chlorpheniramine)

*Author's interpretation of FDA criteria. Based on contents, not claims.

Cold-Sore Balms

A cold sore is an itchy, burning, blistery, and crusty eruption that appears on a corner of the mouth or the edge of the nose. It comes too often and then goes away too slowly. Such sores are caused by a virus, and are provoked to appear by sunlight and perhaps other environmental insults. They tend to recur and cannot be wholly prevented. Cold sores also are called *fever blisters* and *sun blisters*. Although they cannot be cured, cold sores can be effectively treated to relieve the pain and irritation.

Reviewers noted that one self-treatment method that does not use drugs has been reported to curb cold sores at their incipient stage. Another preventive measure recently has been reported in the medical literature (*See* Prevention of Cold Sores, further on.)

COLD-SORE BALMS is based on the report on External Analgesic Drug Products by the FDA's Advisory Review Panel on OTC Topical Analgesic, Antirheumatic, Otic, Burn and Sunburn Prevention and Treatment Drug Products; and on the report "Orally Administered Drug Products for the Treatment of Fever Blister" by the FDA's Advisory Review Panel on OTC Miscellaneous Internal Drug Products. Additionally, it is based on these more recent FDA documents: Proposed Rulemaking for Skin Protectants and for External Analgesic Drug Products for Fever Blister and Cold Sore Treatment Drugs; and the Tentative Final Monograph on Orally Administered Drug Products for Treatment of Fever Blisters.

Hurtful Herpes

The virus that causes cold sores is called *herpes simplex* type 1; the sores are sometimes called *herpes labialis*. The Latin word *labialis* means "lips," which is where they usually occur. The sores particularly seem to favor the corners of the mouth. The herpes simplex type 1 virus is spread by mouth-to-mouth and other physical contact.

The herpes simplex type 2 virus causes sores on the genitals that are called *herpes genitalis*. This venereal disease is spread mainly by sexual contact and has become one of the commonest but most difficult to treat. No cure is known. The discussion in this Unit relates solely to the type 1 virus, which causes *herpes labialis*; persons with *herpes genitalis* should consult a doctor for symptomatic relief.

Most people suffer minor herpes infections early in life, and are partially immunized by them. Protective substances called *antibodies* combat the infection—but they seem unable to wholly eliminate the virus from the body. It remains, in a dormant and perhaps incomplete form, inside nerve cells near the lips (or at other locations). It rejuvenates and provokes new cold sores when the body's defenses are temporarily under stress or weakened by fever, chilling, sunburn, windburn, menstruation, upset stomach, gastrointestinal distress, emotional pressures, or pure and simple excitement.

The new eruption—called *recurrent herpes*—usually begins with a mild burning or itching; the skin may feel unusually firm because fluid is collecting within. A red pimple then appears, enlarges, and fills up with clear-colored fluid. Several of these blisters may coalesce to form a single, large "water blister," which then may rupture. The fluid it contains is filled with the virus. Care should be taken not to spread it to other parts of your own body or to somebody else's (as, for example, by kissing).

After several days, the overlying skin layers slough off, scabs form, and the sore finally heals. If healing has not occurred within 7 to 10 days, experts recommend a visit to a doctor: The problem may not be a cold sore, and additional medical care may be needed.

Virologists say 150 million Americans have latent herpes and suffer 100 million recurrences yearly, so there is much interest in the causes of and in the ways to prevent these recurrences. New data on both questions have come to light in a research paper published recently in *The Lancet* (Dec. 7, 1991, pp. 1419-22): Scientists at the National Institutes of Health (NIH) and the University of California, Los Angeles School of Medicine, started with the assumption that sunlight is an important stimulus for cold sore-recurrences. They recruited sufferers of persistent cold sores and exposed their lips to strong pulses of ultraviolet B (UVB) light, like that from the sun. On one occasion, these subjects protected their lips with a sunscreen containing 2.8 percent glyceryl aminobenzoate and 3.3 percent padimate O, which absorb UVB light, and 5.6 percent oxybenzone, which absorbs ultraviolet A (UVA) light (*Total Eclipse AB*, Eclipse Laboratories). It had a sun protection factor (SPF) of 15. (*See* SUNSCREENS for a description of UV light and the ingredients that block it.) On another occasion, the subjects used a sunscreen that did not contain the active, UV light-absorbing ingredients. Neither subjects nor researchers knew which preparation was being used for which UV light exposure until afterward.

When the subjects were using the unprotective dummy sunscreen, 27 out of 38 of them (71 percent) developed cold sores within a few days. But when they used the real and protective sunscreen, only one subject developed a cold sore. These findings thus are strong evidence that cold sores can be and are prompted to erupt by the sun's UV light. They show, even more strongly, that a UVB sunscreen can prevent these recurrences—at least under experimental conditions.

Cold Sores versus Canker Sores

Many people confuse cold sores with canker sores. The two must be differentiated because they are entirely different diseases. Cold sores can be self-diagnosed and self-treated with nonprescription medicines, whereas canker sores (which may be called *aphthous stomatitis* or *aphthous ulcers*) may need to be examined by a dentist or a doctor, who can decide their cause and recommend an appropriate treatment. The cause of canker sores is unknown. Viruses are among the suspects.

Unlike cold sores, which mainly occur on the *outside* of the lips, canker sores arise *inside* the mouth—particularly on the inner lining of the lips or the cheeks or on the tongue, soft palate, or other mucosal surfaces. Canker sores are small, whitish, depressed areas, with red borders. Like cold sores, they can be quite painful.

Canker sores are a recurrent disease. They usually appear for the first time in late childhood or during the teen-age years, though both youngsters and oldsters sometimes are suddenly afflicted with them. They tend to recur when the mucosa has been scratched by a toothbrush bristle or injured in some other way, or as part of an allergic reaction or a hormonal change (such as menstruation). Emotional stress can provoke canker sores. If left untreated, they may require 10 to 14 days to heal.

Many topical remedies have been used to treat canker sores. They include dyes, resins such as myrrh, colloidal substances such as aloe, astringents and substances that act on protein (such as alum), and antibacterials, for example, hydrogen peroxide. (*See* Sore Mouth in MEDICAMENTS FOR SORE GUMS, MOUTHS, AND THROATS.)

Prevention of Cold Sores

One method for preventing recurrent cold sores has been reported in the medical literature: Treating the emerging sore with ice, for periods of 45 to 120 minutes. This treatment will work only if the ice is applied the *same* day the budding new sore first makes itself felt. The ice should be held gently against the sore until the area becomes uncomfortable, and then removed briefly before it is applied again. When this treatment is successful—and advocates say it often is—the cold sore vanishes by the following morning.

Another preemptive method, obviously, would be to use a sunscreen like the one described previously above. Note, however, that the FDA has not yet evaluated the use of sunscreens for this purpose.

Topical Drugs for Cold Sores

Drugs applied directly to the cold sore are the ones most commonly and successfully used for relief of the itching, burning, and pain. But some drugs are also promoted for internal use to relieve cold sores. (*See* further on under Internal Drugs for Cold Sores.)

The report on external cold-sore remedies is brief, and evaluators did not assess all the active ingredients in preparations used for treatment. Budgetary constraints in the early 1980s led the FDA to disband the Miscellaneous External Drugs Panel before it could finish its work. Therefore, an ingredient-by-ingredient assessment of the contents of topical cold-sore remedies was left for the FDA to perform at a later date. The FDA documents, however, are somewhat contradictory and confusing at this stage; the information that follows is very preliminary.

Cold sores (fever blisters) can be self-treated with two principal types of nonprescription drugs: skin protectants that cover, shield, and soften the sore, and itch-pain relievers that can be sprayed, dabbed, or spread onto the sore to relieve the discomfort it causes.

Claims

Accurate for skin protectants:

- "Relieves dryness and softens cold sores and fever blisters"
- "Softens crusts (scabs) associated with cold sores and fever blisters"

Accurate for external pain relievers:

- "For the temporary relief of pain and itching associated with cold sores"
- "...relief of itching associated with fever blisters and cold sores"

Skin Protectants

Some skin-protectant ingredients soften scabs by absorbing and holding body fluid next to the skin. Others, called *demulcents*, soothe the skin. Still others are skin softeners, or *emollients*.

Dampening or softening a cold sore keeps it from drying out and cracking, which can add to pain and discomfort and can allow bacteria to get in under the skin, causing secondary infections. Skin protectants prevent this dryness, and also provide a physical barrier against environmental irritants. The skin protectants useful for cold sores, listed as follows, are described briefly in the Unit UNGUENTS AND POWDERS FOR THE SKIN.

APPROVED SKIN-PROTECTANT ACTIVE INGREDIENTS

- ALLANTOIN *(0.5 TO 2 PERCENT): See* p. 972.
- COCOA BUTTER *(50 TO 100 PERCENT): See* p. 973.
- DIMETHICONE *(1 TO 30 PERCENT): See* p. 974.
- GLYCERIN *(20 TO 45 PERCENT): See* p. 974.
- PETROLATUM *(30 TO 100 PERCENT): See* p. 975.
- SHARK LIVER OIL *(3 PERCENT): See* p. 975.

CONDITIONALLY APPROVED SKIN-PROTECTANT ACTIVE INGREDIENTS

None.

DISAPPROVED SKIN-PROTECTANT ACTIVE INGREDIENTS

- BISMUTH SUBNITRATE: *See* p. 977.
- BORIC ACID: *See* p. 977.
- PYRIDOXINE HYDROCHLORIDE: The value of this drug, if any, is very unclear, the FDA says. For now its verdict is: not safe or effective.

Pain Relievers Applied to the Skin

The ingredients listed here are intended to relieve itching and pain. Most of them are described in ITCH AND PAIN REMEDIES APPLIED TO THE SKIN (*See* pp. 557-565.) The remainder are described here briefly.

APPROVED PAIN-RELIEVING ACTIVE INGREDIENTS

- BENZOCAINE: This is the active ingredient in many currently marketed cold-sore balms. The approved concentration is 5 to 20 percent.
- BENZYL ALCOHOL (10 TO 33 PERCENT)
- BUTAMBEN PICRATE (1 PERCENT)
- CAMPHOR (0.1 TO 2.5 PERCENT)
- CAMPHORATED METACRESOL (CAMPHOR 3 TO 10.8 PERCENT), METACRESOL 1 TO 3.6 PERCENT)
- THE COMBINATION OF CAMPHOR (3 TO 10.8 PERCENT) + PHENOL (4.7 PERCENT) IN LIGHT MINERAL OIL
- DIBUCAINE (0.25 TO 1 PERCENT)
- DIBUCAINE HYDROCHLORIDE (0.25 TO 1 PERCENT)
- DIMETHISOQUIN HYDROCHLORIDE (0.3 TO 0.5 PERCENT)
- DYCLONINE HYDROCHLORIDE (0.5 TO 1 PERCENT)
- JUNIPER TAR (1 TO 5 PERCENT)
- LIDOCAINE (0.5 TO 4 PERCENT)
- LIDOCAINE HYDROCHLORIDE (0.5 TO 4 PERCENT)
- PEPPERMINT OIL (MENTHOL) (0.1 TO 1 PERCENT)
- PHENOL (0.5 TO 1.5 PERCENT)

- *PHENOLATE SODIUM (0.5 TO 1.5 PERCENT)*
- *PRAMOXINE HYDROCHLORIDE (0.5 TO 1 PERCENT)*
- *RESORCINOL (0.5 TO 3 PERCENT)*
- *TETRACAINE (1 TO 2 PERCENT)*
- *TETRACAINE HYDROCHLORIDE (1 TO 2 PERCENT)*

CONDITIONALLY APPROVED PAIN-RELIEVING ACTIVE INGREDIENTS

- *GLYCOL SALICYLATE:* The FDA thus far has little to say about this ingredient. It finds it safe. But its efficacy remains to be demonstrated. (*See also* p. 565)
- *TROLAMINE SALICYLATE: See* p. 566.

DISAPPROVED PAIN-RELIEVING ACTIVE INGREDIENTS
None.

Other Active Ingredients

Several other ingredients, including alcohol and benzalthonium chloride, which both are antiseptics, are formulated into cold sore products. The FDA simply has not yet decided how to deal with these ingredients. So little can be said with certitude about them.

APPROVED MISCELLANEOUS ACTIVE INGREDIENTS
None.

CONDITIONALLY APPROVED MISCELLANEOUS ACTIVE INGREDIENTS

- *BISMUTH SODIUM TARTRATE:* Evidence is wanting that this compound is safe and effective, the FDA says.
- *PECTIN:* This ingredient has not been shown to be safe or effective for

fever blisters.

• *TANNIC ACID:* This is a tanning agent used to cure leather. Technically, it is an astringent. It is believed to pull foreign proteins out of burns, sores, and wounds while providing them with a protective cover. However, bacterial infections can fester under the crust. Tannic acid also is a liver toxin. Because of these effects, it has been ruled "not safe and effective" for most uses in skin disorders. However, it has been formulated into widely used cold-sore balms, and since these products are applied only to tiny areas of skin, it may be safe. Based on past usage and recent studies, it may also be effective. The FDA grants it tentative approval: not proved safe or effective.

• *ZINC SULFATE:* This is an astringent. (*See* pp. 897-899.) The FDA finds it safe but says its effectiveness for relieving cold sores remains to be proved.

Combination Products

Products marketed for cold-sore relief tend to contain two or more active ingredients. The FDA plans to approve for this purpose combinations of two safe and effective itch-pain relievers of two different chemical classes (-*amine* and -*caine* drugs—*See* ITCH AND PAIN REMEDIES APPLIED TO THE SKIN). Allowable amounts of camphor and phenol may be combined with other itch-pain relievers. Safe and effective amounts of benzyl alcohol, juniper tar, phenol, phenolate sodium, or resorcinol can safely and effectively be combined with camphor, and menthol can be combined with any single skin protectant or combination of skin protectants. Combinations of a safe and effective itch-pain reliever and one or more of the safe and effective skin protectants described in this Unit also are likely to be approved, and are considered for now to be safe and effective.

The FDA is not yet convinced there is merit in combining an itch-pain reliever and a sunscreen to both treat *and* prevent fever blisters. It lists benzocaine + phenol + alcohol as not proved safe and effective. The initial decision for pectin + bismuth sodium tartrate is the same. The combination of aqua ammonia + spirits of ammonia + phenol + camphor is disapproved.

As indicated before, the FDA's rule-making on cold sore balms still is in a rough and preliminary stage. For this reason, the ratings for specific products in the table Cold-Sore Balms: Product Ratings are quite tentative. Most of the products contain benzocaine, which is safe and effective at concentrations of 5 to 20 percent, with one or more skin-protectant ingredients.

Internal Drugs for Cold Sores

Several drugs that are taken internally have been claimed by manufacturers to relieve cold sores. They were evaluated by the Miscellaneous Internal Drugs Panel, which found some of the product claims misleading or unsupported by scientific data. The Panel specifically disapproves several claims.

 Claims

Disapproved
- "For the relief of discomfort of sun blisters"
- "Useful for fever blisters of herpetic origin"
- "Arrests the symptoms associated with cold sores and sun blisters on the lips"

The FDA plans to ban all of these products before the end of 1992.

APPROVED ACTIVE INGREDIENTS TAKEN INTERNALLY
None.

CONDITIONALLY APPROVED ACTIVE INGREDIENTS TAKEN INTERNALLY
None.

DISAPPROVED ACTIVE INGREDIENTS TAKEN INTERNALLY

The FDA has banned, as not safe and effective, three oral-drug ingredients. In the following discussion, two of these substances are considered together.

- *LACTOBACILLUS ACIDOPHILUS AND LACTOBACILLUS BULGARICUS:* These are bacteria, obtained from milk or from special cultures of yogurt, that are dried with milk sugar and then marketed. Some commercial preparations contain *L. acidophilus* alone; at least one contains a mixture of *L. acidophilus* and *L. bulgaricus*. These bacteria are also sold as antidiarrheal drugs, and the Panel concurs with other reviewers that these drugs are safe in dosages of up to 4 grams daily.

Almost a dozen studies have been conducted on the use of *Lactobacilli* against cold sores; the majority show promising results. But none meet the FDA's scientific standards.

How *Lactobacilli* might help relieve cold sores has not been explained. One hypothesis is that in some way the bacteria impart a herpes-virus resistance factor to saliva.

Although evaluators held out some hope that the two bacterial preparations *may* effectively treat cold sores, they say that more definitive test results are needed. Until this is accomplished, *L. acidophilus* and *L. bulgaricus*—alone or together—are judged to be safe but not effective against *herpes simplex*, type 1 virus, and cold sores.

- *LYSINE (LYSINE MONOHYDROCHLORIDE):* An essential amino acid, which is a constituent of protein, this substance is present in many of the foods we eat. Supplements are given for nutritional and medicinal reasons, and reviewers judge lysine safe in dosages of up to 3 grams a day.

Several clinical studies were reported in which cold-sore patients who were given lysine supplements showed faster healing and had far fewer recurrences than did untreated patients. Scientifically controlled studies were then undertaken. Disappointingly, the first such study showed that lysine had no effect on the appearance of the sores, the rate of healing, or the intervals between recurrences. A second study showed that lysine failed to hasten healing once a cold sore appeared. However, significantly fewer participants suffered new cold sores while on the lysine than did those participants taking dummy control preparation. The Panel concluded that lysine may be beneficial in some patients but, pending more conclusive studies, it listed the ingredient as safe but not proved effective as a cold-sore medication. No data has as yet emerged to prove it effective.

Safety and Effectiveness: Active Ingredients in Over-the-Counter Cold-Sore Remedies Applied to the Skin

Active Ingredient	Function	Assessment
allantoin (0.5 to 2%)	skin protectant	safe and effective
benzocaine (5 to 20%)	itch-pain reliever	safe and effective
benzyl alcohol (10 to 33%)	itch-pain reliever	safe and effective
bismuth sodium tartrate	function unclear	not proved safe or effective
bismuth subnitrate	skin protectant	not safe or effective
boric acid	skin protectant	not safe or effective
butamben picrate (1%)	itch-pain reliever	safe and effective
camphor (0.1 to 3%)	itch-pain reliever	safe and effective
camphor (2.5 to 10.8%) + phenol (4.7%)	itch-pain relievers	safe and effective
camphorated metacresol (camphor 3 to 10%, metacresol 1 to 3.6%)	itch-pain relievers	safe and effective
cocoa butter (50 to 100%)	skin protectant	safe and effective
dibucaine (0.25 to 1%)	itch-pain reliever	safe and effective
dibucaine hydrochloride (0.25 to 1%)	itch-pain reliever	safe and effective
dimethicone (1 to 30%)	skin protectant	safe and effective

dimethisoquin hydrochloride (0.3 to 0.5%)	itch-pain reliever	safe and effective
dyclonine hydrochloride (0.5 to 1%)	itch-pain reliever	safe and effective
glycerin (20 to 45%)	skin protectant	safe and effective
glycol salicylate	itch-pain reliever	safe, but not proved effective
juniper tar (1 to 5%)	itch-pain reliever	safe and effective
lidocaine (0.5 to 4%)	itch-pain reliever	safe and effective
lidocaine hydrochloride (0.5 to 4%)	itch-pain reliever	safe and effective
pectin	function unclear	not proved safe or effective
peppermint oil (menthol) (0.1 to 1%)	itch-pain reliever	safe and effective
petrolatum (30 to 100%)	skin protectant	safe and effective
phenol (0.5 to 1.5%)	itch-pain reliever	safe and effective
phenolate sodium (0.5 to 1.5%)	itch-pain reliever	safe and effective
pramoxine hydrochloride (0.5 to 1%)	itch-pain reliever	safe and effective
pyridoxine hydrochloride	skin protectant	not safe or effective
resorcinol (0.5 to 3%)	itch-pain reliever	safe and effective
shark liver oil (3%)	skin protectant	safe and effective
tannic acid	function unclear	not proved safe or effective

Safety and Effectiveness: Active Ingredients in
Over-the-Counter Cold-Sore Remedies Applied to the Skin (contd)

Active Ingredient	Function	Assessment
tetracaine (1 to 2%)	itch-pain reliever	safe and effective
tetracaine hydrochloride (1 to 2%)	itch-pain reliever	safe and effective
trolamine salicylate	itch-pain reliever	safe, but not proved effective
zinc sulfate	itch-pain reliever (astringent)	not proved safe or effective

Safety and Effectiveness: Active Ingredients in Over-the-Counter Cold-Sore Remedies Taken Orally

Active Ingredient	Assessment
Lactobacillus acidophilus	not safe and effective
Lactobacillus bulgaricus	not safe and effective
lysine (lysine monohydrochloride)	not safe and effective

Cold Sore Balms: Product Ratings

SINGLE-INGREDIENT PRODUCTS

Product and Distributor	Dosage of Active Ingredients	Rating *	Comment
benzalkonium chloride			
HVS 1 + 2 (Chemi-Tech)	**solution:** benzalkonium chloride in special base	C	not safe or effective for cold sores
tannic acid			
Zilactin Medicated (Zilactin)	**gel:** 7%	B	not proved safe or effective

For other, safe and effective single-ingredient products, such as petrolatum, *See* UNGUENTS AND POWDERS TO PROTECT THE SKIN pp. 981-983; for other safe and effective single-ingredient itch and pain relievers, *see* ITCH AND PAIN REMEDIES APPLIED TO THE SKIN, pp. 571-575.

COMBINATION PRODUCTS

Most of the combination products below are formulated in ointments, gels, or special liquids that will adhere to and protect the cold sore and surrounding skin, as well as medicate it.

Product and Distributor	Dosage of Active Ingredients	Rating *	Comment
Anbesol (Whitehall)	**gel:** 6.3% benzocaine + 0.5% phenol + alcohol	B	not proved safe and effective
Blistex Lip (Blistex)	**ointment:** 0.5% camphor + 0.5% phenol + 1% allantoin	A	

Product	Ingredients		Comments
Campho-Phenique Cold Sore Gel (Sterling)	**gel:** 10.8% camphor + 4.7% phenol in mineral oil	A	
Herpecin-L (Campbell Labs)	**lip balm:** pyridoxine hydrochloride + allantoin + padimate O	C	pyridoxine not safe and effective; combination with sunscreens not approved
Lip Medex (Blistex)	**ointment:** 1% camphor + 0.54% phenol + petrolatum and other skin protectants	A	
Orabase-O (Colgate-Hoyt)	**gel:** 20% benzocaine + mineral oil	A	
Pfeiffer's Cold Sore (Pfeiffer)	**lotion:** 7% gum benzoin + camphor + menthol + thymol + eucalyptus	C	eucalyptus not approved for this use; thymol not approved for this use either
Tanac (Commerce)	**liquid:** 10% benzocaine + 0.12% benzalkonium chloride + 6% tannic acid	C	not an approved combination; tannic acid not proved safe or effective
	stick: 7.5% benzocaine + 6% tannic acid + 0.12% tannic acid	C	
Total Eclipse AB (Eclipse Laboratories)	**liquid:** 2.8% glyceryl-aminobenzoate + 3.3% padimate O + 5.6% oxybenzone	C	this sunscreen combination (*see* SUNSCREENS) is not approved by FDA as safe and effective for cold sores; but the study described on p. 212, suggests that it is safe and effective

---

*Author's interpretation of FDA criteria. Based on contents, not claims.

Cold-Sore Relievers Taken Internally: Product Ratings

Product and Distributor	Dosage of Active Ingredients	Rating *	Comment
lactobacilli			
Bacia (Fisons)	**capsules:** at least 500 million viable *Lactobacillus acidophilus* organisms + carboxymethylcellulose	C	not safe and effective; banned for this use by FDA as of 12/92
Lactinex (HW & D)	**granules and tablets:** viable mixed culture of *Lactobacillus acidophilus* + L. bulgaricus	C	not safe and effective; banned for this use by FDA as of 12/92
Lysine Enisyl (Person & Covey)	**tablets:** 312 mg; 500 mg; 1000 mg	C	not safe and effective; banned for this use by FDA as of 12/92
L-Lysine (generic)		C	not safe and effective; banned for this use by FDA as of 12/92

*Author's interpretation of FDA criteria. Based on contents, not claims.

Contraceptives

Many women want to buy and use birth-control products freely, without seeing a doctor to get a prescription for oral contraceptives or to be fitted with a diaphragm or an intrauterine device (IUD). This Unit focuses on *vaginal contraceptives*, which women buy without prescription.

Rubbers, or *condoms*, are also sold over-the-counter. But since condoms contain no active chemical ingredients, technically they are not drugs—and so were not evaluated in the OTC Drug Review. However, some condoms are now coated at the factory with a thin layer of one of the spermicides described in this Unit. This spermicidal coating provides added protection against pregnancy in case the condom breaks or leaks.

The use of condoms has increased since the advent of acquired immune deficiency syndrome (AIDS). Some evidence suggests that nonprescription spermicides will stop the AIDS virus (HIV). But recent data indicates this is not so. No woman should rely on an over-the-counter spermicide for protection from AIDS. A condom provides

---

CONTRACEPTIVES is based on the report on vaginal contraceptives by the FDA's Advisory Review Panel on OTC Contraceptives and Other Vaginal Drug Products.

much better protection against AIDS than does a spermicidal cream or jelly.

How They Work

Vaginal contraceptives work in two ways to prevent pregnancy: They destroy sperm cells, and they block the entry of the sperm into the uterus. These contraceptives contain a spermicide (a sperm-killing drug) that quickly kills or immobilizes sperm cells by blocking their ability to break down and use the sugar *fructose*. This sugar, which is present in semen, provides the energy that sperm need to swim to and impregnate the ovum (egg)—the ultimate act of conception. "Since the activity of sperm depends on the metabolism of fructose," the Panel said, "the blocking of this process effectively destroys [their] capacity... to survive." A sperm cell dies within seconds after it encounters an effective spermicide.

The vaginal contraceptives' second line of defense is the cream or other substance with which the spermicide is formulated. This material forms the bulk of the product. It not only holds the spermicide in place during sexual intercourse but it also covers the *cervical os*, the narrow opening from the vagina into the uterus. It thereby creates a barrier that blocks the path of the sperm through the uterus to the fallopian tubes, where fertilization occurs.

 Claims for Vaginal Contraceptives

Accurate
- "Intended for the prevention of pregnancy"

False or Misleading
- "[10-hour] vaginal jelly"
- "Medically approved" or "medically tested"
- "Most frequently prescribed by physicians"
- "Remarkable birth-control invention"
- "Outstanding sperm effect in tests comparing it to other products"
- "Instantly lethal to male sperm"

Determinants of Efficacy

For women who want to follow the Panel's guidance, the range of options is extremely narrow: The reviewers approved only two currently marketed compounds, nonoxynol 9 and octoxynol 9, which they say are essentially identical. They are the spermicidal active ingredients in most vaginal contraceptives sold in the United States. These compounds are judged to be safe as well as effective, because they have been tested more carefully than other spermicides, and because major side effects rarely if ever have been reported as a result of their use. (*See* the Safety and Effectiveness table at the end of this Unit; it also lists the alternate chemical names for these ingredients.)

Vaginal contraceptives that contain nonoxynol 9 or octoxynol 9 may not all be equally effective, however. Products are formulated in different ways—as creams, jellies, aerosol foams, and semi-solid vaginal suppositories—that must be inserted into the vagina and used according to different sets of directions. For example, suppositories, which once were in vogue, require several minutes to melt, whereas foams may be used just before intercourse. These differences can affect the comparative effectiveness of the products.

The configuration of the vagina influences correct placement of a spermicidal contraceptive, as does a woman's awareness of how much should be used and where it should be placed. The vagina, 3 to 4 inches long, is not an open, hollow cavity, as is sometimes imagined. Until stretched during sexual activity, the lower third of its length is star-shaped. The middle third is shaped like the letter H. The upper third creates a crescent-shaped space around the cervix, which protrudes into the vagina.

A vaginal contraceptive product that is not inserted high enough into the vagina or is spread too thinly over the vaginal walls may not provide an adequate sperm-killing barrier at the critical entrance to the cervix. On the other hand, a suppository inserted high into the back of the vagina, immediately before intercourse, may not have time to melt and spread to cover the opening in the cervix. Moreover, some women dislike touching their vaginas, which makes it difficult for them to insert a vaginal contraceptive correctly.

Since *how* these contraceptives are inserted is such an important factor, it is difficult to say that any one is more effective than the others are. The evaluators did find "fragmentary evidence" that aerosol foams are better than other preparations, because they make correct placement of the spermicide easier. As for suppositories, the reviewers expressed concern over the lack of evidence on the proper placement, the melting time, and the duration of effectiveness of these semi-solid products, which have been promoted as being less messy than foams. The Federal Trade Commission, which regulates advertising, also was concerned about vaginal-suppository contraceptives and the claims made for them. The Commission told manufacturers they must stop saying and suggesting in their advertisements that suppositories are as effective as oral contraceptives and IUDs. Instead, they must say that the suppositories are comparable in effectiveness to vaginal foams, creams, and jellies. Also, advertisements must state that a waiting period of 10 to 15 minutes is required between the time the suppository is inserted and intercourse begins.

Two new delivery systems were introduced for spermicidal contraceptives in the 1980s. One is the spermicide-coated condom mentioned before. The second is the contraceptive sponge, which a woman inserts into her vagina before sexual intercourse; she should leave it in place for at least six hours thereafter. It is effective for 24 hours. Besides blocking conception, the sponge may have other, protective properties. In a study among prostitutes in Bangkok, Thailand, an organization called Family Health International found that use of a nonoxynol 9-impregnated sponge significantly reduced chlamydial infections and also reduced gonorrhea infections (*Journal of the American Medical Association*, vol. 257, pp. 2308-2312, 1987). But the women who used the sponge had a significantly *higher* rate of yeast infections (*Candida albicans*). (*See* 'YEAST' KILLERS FOR FEMININE ITCHING.)

The sponge has a relatively large dose of nonoxynol 9—one gram per sponge—and vaginal or penile irritation may occur.

A major factor influencing the effectiveness of these contraceptives is the care a woman takes in using the product. Studies have shown that vaginal contraceptives are among the least effective contraceptive methods. Between 2 and 36 of every 100 fertile women who use vaginal contraceptives become pregnant each year, according to *drug facts and comparisons* (1992).

These statistics indicate that there may be a far higher failure rate than was reported in manufacturers' studies, described further on, which the Panel used in judging nonoxynol 9 and octoxynol 9 to be effective. As experts explain it, the lower pregnancy rates *can* be achieved in well-motivated women who are carefully instructed on the products' use and who are reinforced in their decision to use the products correctly. For example, the high failure rates reported in some field trials using foam have been attributed to using too little, failing to shake the foam container vigorously enough, failing to recognize that the foam bottle is empty, failing to have the foam bottle available—or failing to interrupt love-making to use it.

Vaginal contraceptives are significantly *less* effective in preventing pregnancy than are oral contraceptives and other medically provided contraceptive methods.

Douching and Contraception

Many women believe douching after sexual intercourse is an effective contraceptive method. *It is not!*

As the American Pharmaceutical Association publication *Handbook of Nonprescription Drugs*, 9th ed. (1990), explains, douching is not at all reliable because sperm cells from semen enter the uterus too quickly to be washed away by water or other douching solutions. Sperm cells may reach the cervical opening within 30 seconds after ejaculation and may enter the cervix and uterus within 90 to 180 seconds. They can be in the fallopian tubes, where conception occurs, within five minutes. "Postcoital douching has no effect in removing sperm from the upper reproductive tract," the *Handbook* says, "and might, in fact, force sperm higher in the tract." The FDA agrees, stressing with capital letters:

"[Douching] does not prevent pregnancy."

Some women douche after intercourse whether or not they are protected by a contraceptive. This may be a costly mistake for women who use spermicides, for if they douche too soon they may wash the contraceptive material out while live sperm remain in the vagina. Experts recommend waiting at least 6 hours before douching.

Special Needs for Vaginal Contraceptives

Some women use vaginal contraceptives on a regular basis. Family-planning experts, manufacturers, and the Panel suggest several specific situations in which these products may be particularly useful:

- when teenagers who have sex infrequently do not wish to burden their bodies with hormonal oral contraceptives or an IUD

- when older women who have sex infrequently wish to avoid the risk of heart and artery disease and other complications that they face if they use oral contraceptives. (This is of special concern if they also are cigarette smokers.)

- for unprotected cycles when a woman is going onto or off the oral contraceptives, or in any cycle when she forgets to take one or two of the pills

- for added protection during highly fertile, mid-cycle days for couples who usually rely on condoms

- for use with a diaphragm if the spermicidal product prescribed with it runs out. (The same spermicidal active ingredients are present in *all* vaginal contraceptives.)

Combination Products

A vaginal contraceptive containing a single active ingredient is safer than a product containing two or more such ingredients, according to the evaluators. No products submitted for review contained two approved spermicidal ingredients. So there are no approved combination vaginal contraceptive products.

One combination contains methoxypolyoxyethyleneglycol 550 laurate and nonoxynol 9. This formula was judged safe but not proved effective, since the relative contribution of the two ingredients has not been established. All other combinations were rejected as unsafe or ineffective.

APPROVED CONTRACEPTIVE ACTIVE INGREDIENTS

The two approved surface-acting compounds are closely related chemically.

- **NONOXYNOL 9:** This is the active ingredient in the large majority of foams, creams, suppositories, and other over-the-counter vaginal contraceptives. It is the compound upon which the industry is essentially based at this time, and a variety of tests indicate that this substance is safe as well as effective. It has been fed in large doses to rats and dogs, applied to rabbits' sensitive skins and eyes, and inserted in large doses into dogs' vaginas. No significant adverse effects have been found. From these findings, as well as from wide clinical experience with human use, reviewers judged the compound to be safe.

The effectiveness of nonoxynol 9 has been established in a variety of test-tube studies involving precisely measured doses of human semen, and in a variety of more sophisticated experiments in which first the contraceptive and then human semen were introduced into women's vaginas. Samples were collected afterwards and assessed to see how many of the sperm cells survived. When an effective dose of nonoxynol 9 is used, most or all sperm cells are immobilized or dead after 20 seconds.

The results have been less spectacular in real-life trials. Reviewers summarized the results of six clinical experiments covering 425 women who used a nonoxynol cream preparation for a combined total of 4071 months. The pregnancy rate was 2.1 percent per year in women who used the product correctly, and 3.5 percent per year in women who used it incorrectly or irregularly. In other studies involving 1000 women who used nonoxynol 9 foam products for a combined total of 4634 months, the pregnancy rate was as low as 2.2 percent per year with correct use, and as high as 5.4 percent when use was incorrect or not regular.

Although these pregnancy rates appear low, they also suggest that each group of 100 women who used nonoxynol 9 products correctly throughout their fertile years could anticipate 50 unwanted pregnancies among themselves. And 100 women who used the products incorrectly or irregularly could expect as many as 100 unintended pregnancies during their fertile years. Moreover, the consensus of expert reports in the medical literature shows *much* higher pregnancy rates than the studies cited by the Panel. However, the panelists concluded that nonoxynol 9 is safe and effective as a vaginal contraceptive. Specific dosages depend on the way that the product is formulated, as do the instructions for use.

• *Octoxynol 9:* This substance is almost identical to nonoxynol 9 (*see* directly preceding); the Panel says the slight molecular variation between them has no significant effect on the biological or chemical properties of the compound. The failure rates are also quite comparable. Conclusion: Octoxynol 9 is safe and effective as a spermicide.

CONDITIONALLY APPROVED CONTRACEPTIVE ACTIVE INGREDIENTS

Two individual spermicides were evaluated as conditionally approved, as was one combination of nonoxynol 9 plus a second spermicidal surface-acting substance. In all three cases, the spermicide's effectiveness, not its safety, is in question.

• *DODECAETHYLENEGLYCOL MONOLAURATE:* This surface-acting substance is less well studied than nonoxynol 9. Evaluators based their decision that it is safe on two studies of rabbits and one study of women. In the latter, 50 women used a 5 percent concentration of this active ingredient in a jelly base. They applied it vaginally each night for 10 to 21 days. Neither the women nor the doctors who examined them found any problems during this brief period, so the Panel concluded that dodecaethyleneglycol monolaurate is safe.

Data on the effectiveness of this substance were even sparser. One study claiming to show that it blocks the cervical opening for up to 10 hours was conducted on a single human subject. No evidence was submitted showing the drug's sperm-killing ability in test tubes. Nor were there after-intercourse studies on the viability of sperm cells subjected to the substance in either animal or human vaginas. Therefore reviewers decided that, while safe, dodecaethyleneglycol's effectiveness remains to be proved.

• *LAURETH 10S:* Studies in dogs and rabbits showed no significant adverse changes in the animals or in their offspring. In one human study, a 2 percent concentration of laureth 10S in a jelly formulation produced no adverse effects in 10 women who put it into their vaginas daily for three weeks.

No evidence was presented on this substance's sperm-killing ability in the test tube or on its effectiveness in after-intercourse tests in animals, let alone in women. The verdict: Laureth 10S is safe but its effectiveness is yet to be shown.

• *METHOXYPOLYOXYETHYLENEGLYCOL 550 LAURATE + NONOXYNOL 9, COMBINED:* While nonoxynol 9 is both safe and effective (*see* earlier description), no scientific data were submitted on methoxypolyoxyethyleneglycol 550, so the evaluators could not assess its safety or efficacy or the contribution it may make to the combination product. The effectiveness of this ingredient and that of the combination product both remains to be established.

DISAPPROVED CONTRACEPTIVE ACTIVE INGREDIENTS

• PHENYLMERCURIC ACETATE (PMA): Weak concentrations of this mercury compound kill sperm, although they are no more effective, and may be less effective, than are commonly used concentrations of nonoxynol 9. The major problem with PMA is that mercury is readily absorbed from the vagina into the bloodstream, which carries it throughout a woman's body. It enters her breasts and may contaminate her milk if she is nursing. If, unknown to herself, she is pregnant at the time she uses a PMA vaginal contraceptive product, some of the mercury can pass through the placental barrier into the embryo or fetus—to which the mercury may be quite toxic.

Only a few cases have been reported of very severe *prenatal* (before-birth) mercury poisoning of children, and their mothers had taken the chemical through food or drinking water, *not* PMA contraceptives. In these tragic cases the babies' nervous systems functioned so poorly that they became grossly crippled. No documentation is available to show that infants born of mothers who used PMA vaginal contraceptives have been damaged as a result. But the evaluators believe that direct proof would be difficult, if not impossible, to obtain. Subtle changes that might show up only years later—for example, behavioral problems in school—would be particularly difficult to pin to the use of a mercury product. Yet animal studies suggest that such effects might occur.

Although the reviewers advise caution in using animal-study results to predict reactions in humans, they maintain that "the special susceptibility of the fetus and child to chemical pollutants such as mercury and the seriousness of mercury poisoning are generally recognized." So mercury compounds in "vaginal contraceptive preparations are potentially hazardous to the fetus and breast-fed infant."

Thus, the Panel decided that these products are unsafe and should be removed from the market.

• PHENYLMERCURIC NITRATE: The risks of PMA, described in the preceding paragraphs, extend to phenylmercuric nitrate and *all other mercuric compounds* that might be used in vaginal contraceptive products. The Panel said they are all unsafe.

Safety and Effectiveness: Spermicides in Over-the-Counter Vaginal Contraceptives

Active Ingredient	Chemical Name*	Assessment
dodecaethylene glycol monolaurate	polyethylene glycol 600 monolaurate	safe but not proved effective
laureth 10S		safe but not proved effective
methoxypolyoxyethylene glycol 550 laurate + nonoxynol 9		safe but not proved effective
nonoxynol 9	nonylphenoxypolyethoxyethanol, nonylphenoxy polyoxyethylene ethanol, polyoxyethylenenonylphenol	safe and effective
octoxynol 9	p-diisobutylphenenoxypolyeth oxyethanol, polyethylene glycol of mono-iso-octyl phenyl ether	safe and effective
phenylmercuric acetate (PMA)		not safe
phenylmercuric nitrate		not safe

* The shortened names are easier and commonly used, but package labels may list the longer chemical names, which are included here for consumers' guidance.

Contraceptives: Product Ratings

Product and Distributor	Dosage of Active Ingredients	Rating *	Comment
nonoxynol 9			
Conceptrol Birth Control (Ortho)	vaginal cream: 5%	A	
Delfen Contraceptive (Ortho)	vaginal foam: 12.5%	A	
Emko (Schering-Plough)	vaginal foam: 8%	A	
Encare (Thompson Medical)	vaginal suppositories: 2.27%	A	
Excita Extra (Schmid)	lubricated condom: 5.6%	A	
Gynol II Contraceptive (Ortho)	vaginal jelly: 2%	A	for use with vaginal diaphragm
Intercept Contraceptive Inserts (Ortho)	vaginal suppositories: 100 mg	A	
Koromex (Schmid)	vaginal jelly: 3%	A	
Ramses Extra (Schid)	lubricated condom: 5.6%	A	
Today (VLI)	sponge: 1 gram	A	
octoxynol 9			
Koromex (Schmid)	vaginal cream: 3%	A	for use with vaginal diaphragm

Contraceptives: Product Ratings (contd)

Product and Distributor	Dosage of Active Ingredients	Rating *	Comment
Ortho-Gynol Contraceptive (Ortho)	vaginal jelly: 1%	A	for use with vaginal diaphragm

*Author's interpretation of Panel criteria. Based on contents, not claims.

Corn and Callus Removers

Few pains are as intense as that of a toe-top O-corn, a hard, thick overgrowth of skin encircling a softer center. A bewildering selection of treatment preparations, including adherent films, creams and salves, and medicated pads, disks, and corn plasters, are sold to relieve O-corns and other painful or annoying corns and calluses.

But the choice of which drug to use is easy: Only salicylic acid is safe and effective. This acid is a *keratolytic agent*—a drug that eats away the bonds between the cells of the hard, outer portion of skin, causing it to peel.

 Claims

Accurate
- "For the removal of corns and calluses"
- "Relieves pain by removing corns and calluses"

CORN AND CALLUS REMOVERS is based on the report "Corn and Callus Remover Drug Products for OTC Human Use" by the FDA's Advisory Review Panel on OTC Miscellaneous External Drug Products, and the FDA's Tentative Final and Final Monographs on these products.

WARNINGS:
Do not use if you are a diabetic or have poor blood circulation.

Do not use on irritated skin or on any area that is infected or reddened.

If discomfort persists, see your doctor or podiatrist.

What Pressure Sores Are

Corns and calluses are caused by an overgrowth of the skin's horny outer layer as a reaction to long-standing friction or pressure. A *callus* is hard, thickened skin that has no central core. It usually arises on the sole of the foot. Calluses tend to be yellow in color, with normal skin-ridge patterns continuing across their surface. By contrast, *corns* usually have a definite central area or core, and they are commoner on the toes than on the soles of the feet.

Corns may be hard or soft or, like the O-corn, both hard and soft. They usually arise just over a toe bone, so there is pressure both from above and from below. *Hard corns* are raised, yellowish-gray sore sports, which are widest on the skin surface and taper inward to a point like an upside-down volcano that presses—painfully!—on underlying nerve endings. *Soft corns* are whitish skin thickenings in the toewebs. They tend to stay soft and sore because they are constantly moistened by sweat. *Seed corns* are tiny ingrowths in callused areas on the soles of the feet; they are rarely painful.

Corns that are red or blue—because they are filled with blood—are called *neurovascular corns*. They do not respond well to self-treatment.

A third major type of pressure sore on the feet is the *bunion*. A bunion is a swelling along the outside rear surface of the big toe. It forces the big toe and other toes out of line; the pressure causes secondary corns. A bunion may well require podiatric or medical care.

Treatment

Calluses and corns can often be removed with nonprescription medications. Those that fail to respond can be treated by a podiatrist, a physician, or an orthopedic surgeon who specializes in foot problems.

If you treat a callus or a corn with an over-the-counter medication, try at the same time to eliminate the rubbing or pressure that caused it—usually poorly fitting shoes or hosiery. If you do not, the condition is likely to recur. Remember, too, that a callus serves a protective function, so it should not be quickly or abruptly removed, particularly if it is not painful. It makes more sense to correct the underlying problem first. The outgrowth or ingrowth may then slowly recede without further treatment.

WARNING:

 Persons who have diabetes or poor circulation should not take care of their own calluses or corns but rather should let a foot doctor do it. Diabetics are highly vulnerable to infection; professional foot care helps prevent this development.

Forms of Treatment

The paucity of active ingredients to relieve corns and calluses is perhaps balanced by the variety of dosage forms in which they are made:

- A *collodion* is a solution of nitrocellulose in a solvent that dries quickly when applied and leaves a thin, cohesive film containing the active drug in contact with the skin. Some other, collodion-like preparations are also used to keep the active ingredient in touch with the callus or the corn.

- A *foot salve* is an ointment used on the feet.

- A *medicated plaster* is a topical medication in a skin-contact adhesive that is backed by a piece of fabric, plastic, or other material. It can be purchased in an appropriate size to cover a corn or a callus.

The Panel said collodions and plaster, disk, and pad dosage forms all are advantageous in treating calluses and corns because they adhere to and keep the medication in contact with the skin. They also hold in moisture, an advantage because the active ingredient, salicylic acid, works only in the presence of water. (This explains why it may be helpful to soak the foot in water for 15 to 30 minutes. Then dry it lightly before applying salicylic acid preparations.)

Combination Products

Evaluators could find no products containing two or more active ingredients that they felt could be approved as safe and effective. So none are approved for this purpose.

Skin-Peelers for the Feet

APPROVED SKIN-PEELING ACTIVE INGREDIENT

• SALICYLIC ACID (IN COLLODIONS AND MEDICATED PLASTERS): Salicylic acid is the only active ingredient legally present in corn and callus products. It is found in nature in wintergreen leaves and sweet-birch bark. Of course, salicylic acid is also manufactured synthetically (in huge amounts) because it is the parent compound for aspirin and several other pain-relieving drugs. However, salicylic acid does *not* act on corns and calluses as a pain reliever. Rather, it slowly eats away the unwanted skin.

Salicylic Acid for the Treatment of Corns and Calluses

Vehicles (Bases)	Approved Dosages
ointments and other non-adherent preparations	not recommended
in disks, plasters, and pads	12-40%
in collodions	12-17.6%

Too little salicylic acid is absorbed through the skin from a corn plaster to cause aspirin-poisoning. But it can easily dissolve normal skin as well as the thick skin of calluses and corns. So care must be taken to apply the drug *only* to overgrown skin areas.

With regard to safety, in two large studies of foot-clinic patients in the mid-1970s, investigators found that salicylic acid products caused few, if any, side effects and none that required a doctor's care. Reviewers accepted these findings and the absence of reported injury as evidence that salicylic acid is safe for nonprescription foot use.

Effectiveness was demonstrated to the evaluators' satisfaction in several scientifically controlled tests. In one study, 40 percent salicylic acid in medicated disks removed 73 percent of corns after five treatments over 11 days. This compares with 4 percent complete removal when the same disk was applied without the active drug. The treatment was less effective against calluses: After 11 days, only 15 percent of calluses were wholly gone. But then, the nommedicated disks did not remove *any* participant's callus within that time period.

In a more recent study, investigators used a variety of concentrations of salicylic acid (12, 20, 30 and 40 percent) to treat soft corns. All were effective. There was little difference in efficacy between the concentrations. Hence, you might wish to start with a relatively low concentration of this medication.

Based on these findings and other studies, evaluators say that salicylic acid is safe and effective for treating hard corns and calluses in concentrations of 12 to 40 percent in medicated plasters and in concentration of 12 to 17.6 percent in collodion or collodion-like vehicles. If a corn or a callus shows no improvement after 14 days, see a doctor.

CONDITIONALLY APPROVED SKIN-PEELING ACTIVE INGREDIENTS

None.

DISAPPROVED SKIN-PEELING ACTIVE INGREDIENTS

None.

Foot Salves: Preliminary Notes

A variety of salves, creams, lotions, and powders are sold over-the-counter to relieve tired and sore feet and prevent and cure minor foot ailments. Some serve as bases for other more active drugs. The Panel was planning to write a report on these foot preparations, but it was disbanded before it could do so. The FDA has not yet followed up on these ingredients and products.

Very preliminary judgments were, however, contained in the reviewers' rough-draft report on these drugs:

amyl salicylate	not effective
belladonna alkaloids	not effective
benzoic acid	not effective
calcium acetate	not proved safe or effective
camphor gum	not effective
chloroxylenol (PCMX)	not effective
dichlorophenyl trichloroethane	not effective
glyceryl monostearate	not effective
iodized botanical oil	not effective
lard	not effective
magnesium sulfate	not effective
methyl isobutyl ketone	not effective
oil of thyme	not effective
peppermint oil	not effective
pine-needle oil	not effective
potassium iodide	not effective
propylene glycol	not proved effective
salicin	not effective
sassafras oil	not effective
sodium bicarbonate	not effective
sodium chloride	not proved effective
sodium lauryl sulfate	not effective
sodium sesquicarbonate	not effective
sodium sulfate	not effective
tragacanth mucilage	not effective
witch hazel	not effective
zinc sulfate	not effective

Safety and Effectiveness: Active Ingredients in Over-the-Counter Products Sold for Removing Corns and Calluses

Active Ingredient	Assessment
salicylic acid in collodions and medicated disks, pads, and plasters	safe and effective

Corn and Callus Removers: Product Ratings

SINGLE-INGREDIENT PRODUCTS

Product and Distributor	Dosage of Active Ingredients	Rating *	Comment
salicylic acid			
Compound W (Whitehall)	collodion liquid or gel: 17%	A	
Dr. Scholl's Timed Release Medicated Disks (Schering-Plough)	medicated disks: 40%	A	only for corns
Freezone Solution (Whitehall)	flexible collodion: 13.6%	A	
Maximum Strength Wart-Off (Pfizer)	flexible collodion: 17%	A	
Mediplast (Beiersdorf)	plaster: 40%	A	

*Author's interpretation of FDA criteria. Based on contents, not claims.

Cradle-Cap Removers

In the first weeks of life, babies often develop a scaly scalp inflammation called *cradle cap*. It may be a residual accumulation of the fatty substance that covers the baby before birth or it may be an infantile form of seborrheic dermatitis. (*See* DANDRUFF AND SEBORRHEIC-SCALE SHAMPOOS AND OTHER TREATMENTS.) However, cradle cap usually goes away within a month and does not return. Occasionally it occurs later in infancy and sometimes spreads to other parts of the body.

Cradle cap is not dangerous. But its unsightliness disturbs many new parents. It may thicken because parents are afraid to wash their babies' scalps, even gently, for fear of pressing on the *fontanels*, the soft spots where the skull has not yet closed. A parent who has this concern should discuss it with a pediatrician and ask whether to use soap and water or a nonprescription preparation or some other method to remove the cradle cap and prevent its return.

CRADLE-CAP REMOVERS is based on the report "Dandruff, Seborrheic Dermatitis, Psoriasis Control Drug Products" by the FDA's Advisory Review Panel on OTC Miscellaneous External Drug Products and on the FDA's Tentative Final and Final Monographs on these products.

Drugs for Controlling Cradle Cap

Several drugs have been used to treat cradle cap. None at present meets the FDA's criteria for safety and effectiveness.

APPROVED ACTIVE INGREDIENTS

None.

CONDITIONALLY APPROVED ACTIVE INGREDIENTS

None.

DISAPPROVED ACTIVE INGREDIENTS

None.

Unclassified Active Ingredient

One ingredient, white petrolatum, listed by the present Panel as *inactive*, has been approved as generally safe and effective by another Panel (the FDA's Advisory Review Panel on OTC Topical Analgesic, Antirheumatic, Otic, Burn and Sunburn Prevention and Treatment Drug Products).

• PETROLATUM, WHITE: This petroleum derivative is widely used on babies to *prevent* diaper rash and to soften, lubricate, and cover dry skin. It is safe and effective for use as often as necessary. White petrolatum's specific value in dissolving cradle cap and in preventing it from forming again has not been directly assessed by any of the reviewing groups. But in one study white petrolatum was used to prevent cradle cap. Only 6 of 50 babies whose scalps were treated with this protectant developed cradle cap.

Safety and Effectiveness:
Ingredient in Over-the-Counter Cradle-Cap Treatments

Ingredient	Panel Assessment
petrolatum, white	safe and effective*

*Assessed only nonspecifically as a lubricant, a skin softener, and a protectant by the Advisory Review Panel on OTC Topical Analagesic, Antirheumatic, Otic, Burn and Sunburn Prevention and Treatment Drug Products.

Cradle-Cap Removers: Product Ratings

Product and Distributor	Dosage of Active Ingredients	Rating*	Comment
white petrolatum			
Vaseline (Chesebrough-Pond's)	ointment	A	

*Author's interpretation of FDA criteria. Based on contents, not claims.

Dandruff and Seborrheic-Scale Shampoos and Other Treatments

Dry, white flakes of dandruff falling from your hair certainly are unsightly. So, too, are the greasier flakes and scales that persistently appear on the scalp, eyebrows, and other hairy areas and body folds of people who suffer from the scalp and skin conditions called *seborrheic dermatitis*. Dandruff is mostly a nuisance. Seborrheic dermatitis is a disease.

Neither condition can be wholly cured. But several nonprescription drugs will safely and effectively control them.

"I haven't seen a patient for whom there is no help," says FDA dermatologist C. Carnot Evans, M.D. "Some cases are more difficult than others. But we have such an array of products, that we can almost always offer some relief!"

The shampoos, rinses, and other products covered in this Unit are *medicated*, meaning that they are medicinally active against dandruff and seborrheic scale. Of course, ordinary shampoos will wash

DANDRUFF AND SEBORRHEIC-SCALE SHAMPOOS AND OTHER TREATMENTS is based on the report "Dandruff, Seborrheic Dermatitis, Psoriasis Control Drug Products" by the FDA's Advisory Review Panel on OTC Miscellaneous External Drug Products; and FDA's Tentative Final and Final Monographs on these products, and other documents in the OTC Drug Review.

away dandruff, and if the problem is not too severe, then regular use of plain and unmedicated shampoos may suffice.

 Claims

Accurate
- "Controls the itching and scalp-flaking of dandruff"
- "For relief of the itching, irritation, and skin-flaking of seborrheic dermatitis of the skin and/or scalp"
- "Anti-dandruff…"

WARNING:

 These products should be kept out of the eyes or rinsed out quickly if they get in. If the condition fails to improve or worsens when self-treated, consult your family doctor or a dermatologist.

Fast Skin Turnover Forms Flakes

The flakes, or *scales*, as they are properly called, that characterize dandruff and seborrheic dermatitis principally consist of dead skin shed from the skin's outer layer. This outer layer, called the *epidermis*, and the inner layer, called the *dermis*, are cushioned on an underlying bed of fatty subcutaneous tissue.

Epidermal cells are formed constantly near the border with the dermis. These cells work their way up and out as they mature, changing their shapes, their traits, and their functions as they go. The normal life cycle for epidermal cells is 25 to 30 days. As they approach the surface, they harden and die.

The essential defect in both dandruff and seborrheic dermatitis appears to be the same: Epidermal skin is being re-created much more rapidly, and so must be shed much more rapidly, than is normal. In dandruff, the turnover rate is about 14 days, about twice the normal rate. In seborrheic dermatitis it may be even faster. Why these speed-ups occur is not known, although researchers have made a number of guesses. The result, though, is clearly visible on victims' heads and shoulders.

The flakes the two conditions produce can be relieved by many of the same drugs. But they can be controlled more effectively when people are aware of which disorder they have. The Flake Traits table can help you determine that.

Flake Traits

Factors	Common Dandruff	Seborrheic Dermatitis
site	scalp only	scalp, face, and body (especially in hairy areas and body folds)
redness (inflammation)	no	yes
appearance of flakes	dry, white to grayish	greasy, yellowish-brown
itching	sometimes	usually
irritants	winter weather	stress and illness

One long-standing explanation for dandruff is that it is caused by a yeast-like fungus, *Pityrosporum ovale*, which resides in the scalp. But virtually everyone has this fungus in his or her hair, and not everyone has dandruff. So many experts doubt that this organism causes dandruff. (But: *See* below.)

A long-standing theory put forth to explain seborrheic dermatitis is that excessive *sebum*, a fatty substance secreted onto the skin's surface by glands, provides a coating of oil that makes it easier for bacteria and yeast to grow. These microorganisms then produce irritating substances that damage the skin and cause it to turn over more quickly, producing scales. But it has not been proved that seborrheic dermatitis and *seborrhea*—the increased production of sebum—always go together. (The names chosen by the Panel to describe these conditions are confusing. *Seborrheic dermatitis* should mean a skin condition caused by or associated with excess sebum production: in other words, *seborrhea*. Yet the evaluators claim that seborrheic dermatitis can occur *without* seborrhea, which makes little sense. It is best not to take these terms too literally; the names used for skin conditions are frequently confusing and imprecise.)

Until we have a better understanding of their causes, dandruff and seborrheic dermatitis must be treated symptomatically.

Drugs Used

Classifications

The drugs used specifically to treat dandruff and seborrheic dermatitis fall into 5 different classes:

- *CYTOSTATIC AGENTS:* provide the most direct treatment approach. They slow the growth rate (-*static*) of skin cells (*cyto-*) so that the turnover time for the epidermis is longer. This means that production of dead cells—dandruff and seborrheic scales—is slowed.

- *KERATOLYTICS:* cause the flaking outer layer of the epidermis to peel away. The Panel believes these drugs dissolve the "cement" that holds the cells together. Keratolytics do not prevent scale formation, as cytostatic agents do, but loosen existing scales so that they are easier to wash away.

- *TAR PREPARATIONS:* are widely used to treat dandruff and seborrheic dermatitis, although no one knows for sure *how* they are helpful. They may impede cell growth and multiplication, or they may penetrate the skin and loosen the scales.

- *ANTIMICROBIALS (ANTISEPTICS):* kill bacteria and other microorganisms that were once thought to cause dandruff. Many experts doubt that they do, however, and it is noteworthy that in the Panel's judgment no antimicrobial agent has been proved effective in relieving dandruff or seborrheic dermatitis. *However:* The FDA has approved an antifungal cream, *ketoconazole*, as a prescription (℞) treatment for dandruff; it is believed to act against *P. Ovale.* So the notion that antimicrobials can relieve dandruff remains viable.

- *HYDROCORTISONE PREPARATIONS:* relieve inflammation, and so they alleviate the redness and itchiness of seborrheic dermatitis. They are of unproved safety and effectiveness against ordinary dandruff, and the FDA has granted only conditional approval for their sale and use for this purpose.

Four of the five drugs that are safe and effective for treating dandruff are also safe and effective for treating seborrheic dermatitis. The exception is sulfur preparations, which should not be used for the latter condition. (*See* further on.)

Combination Products

In the past, many shampoos and groomers that were used to treat dandruff and seborrheic dermatitis contained several active ingredients. Evaluators took an extremely dim view of these preparations, noting that very few studies have been conducted to justify their use. Only one combination of two different anti-dandruff drugs is approved as safe and effective: sulfur (2 to 50 percent) + salicylic acid (1.8 to 3 percent).

Anti-Flake Medications

The Panel assessed more than two dozen active ingredients formulated into products to treat ordinary dandruff and the greasier variety that is symptomatic of seborrheic dermatitis. FDA has made only a few later changes in these judgments.

APPROVED ANTI-SCALE ACTIVE INGREDIENTS

The FDA endorses six different active ingredients as safe and effective for the control of scales. They represent four of the five types of ingredients found in these products: cytostatic agents, hydrocortisone preparations, keratolytic agents, and tar preparations.

• COAL-TAR SHAMPOOS: These messy, black-brown, syrupy substances, extracted from soft coal, have long been mainstays of the skin doctor's trade. In fact, tars of various kinds have been used medicinally for thousands of years and, with sulfur, are the oldest drugs that have won approval from the contemporary medical scientists on the OTC Review Panels.

Coal tar contains, more or less, 2 to 8 percent light oils (principally benzene, toluene, and xylene); 8 to 10 percent middle oils (principally phenols, cresols, and naphthalene); and 8 to 10 percent heavy oils (naphthalene and derivatives), along with 16 to 20 percent anthracene oil and about 50 percent pitch.

Applications for Approved Over-the-Counter Anti-scale Drugs

Approved Ingredient	To Control Scalp Dandruff	To Control Seborrheic Dermatitis of Scalp	To Control Seborrheic Dermatitis of Body
coal-tar preparations	yes	yes	yes
hydrocortisone preparations (to relieve itching)	no	yes	yes
pyrithione zinc	yes	yes	no
salicylic acid	yes	yes	yes
selenium sulfide	yes	yes	yes
sulfur preparations	yes	no	no

Shampoos that contain coal tar may have a disagreeable odor. They can stain hair, skin, and clothing. But they have proved to be remarkably safe when applied to the scalp once or twice weekly and then rinsed off.

Coal-tar shampoos are helpful for both dandruff and seborrheic dermatitis of the scalp, although it is not clear how they work. The tar may take oxygen from the skin cells, slowing their reproduction, or it may penetrate the skin and somehow destroy scales. Alternatively, some tar constituents may react with sulfur-and-hydrogen elements (sulfhydryl groups) in the skin, much as sunlight does, to slow epidermal skin growth and lessen flaking.

Besides its apparent ability to act directly on dandruff flakes, coal tar narrows capillary blood vessels in the skin, kills bacteria, stops itching, and has an astringent effect on the scalp. Thus it would be a highly popular drug if it were not messy and smelly and if it did not sometimes stain the skin, hair, and clothing.

Despite long use and wide medical acceptance, coal tar has not been studied well in carefully controlled tests. Moreover, the tests that have been done have not all been encouraging. In one, a 5 percent coal-tar shampoo did not produce significantly better results after 8-weeks' use than did a dummy shampoo without the tar. However, in another study on patients suffering ordinary dandruff or dandruff associated with seborrheic dermatitis, a 5 percent coal-tar extract shampoo reduced flake counts by one-third to one-half after 4 weeks, compared with only a one-tenth to one-quarter reduction in users of the look-alike, non-medicated shampoo. From the latter study and others, reviewers concluded that coal-tar products are safe and effective for use in shampoos.

The approved dosage for coal tar shampoos, hair groomers, and other tar-containing scalp treatments is 0.5 to 5% coal tar or its equivalent in other tar formulations. Products intended for brief use, such as shampoos, should be used at least twice weekly or as directed by a doctor. Products formulated to stay on the skin or scalp, such as hairgrooms and lotions, can be applied up to four times daily or as directed by a doctor.

WARNINGS:

 Use caution in exposing skin to sunlight after applying a coal tar. It may increase your tendency to sunburn for up to 24 hours.

Do not use for prolonged periods without consulting a doctor.

• *COAL TAR GELS, LOTIONS, OINTMENTS, AND SOAP:* These coal tar formulations are used for treating seborrheic dermatitis in body areas other than the scalp. In the past, consumers have disliked the products because they tended to be messy and smelly and stained clothing and bed clothes. A major improvement, skin experts say, has been the development of a "tar gel," a colloid emulsion of coal tar that is medicinally effective, convenient and easy to apply to the skin, and cosmetically *much* more appealing than earlier products.

Coal-tar preparations have a long-established value in relieving the itching, scaling, and inflammation of seborrheic dermatitis. But questions were raised about whether their frequent and continuing use may increase the risk of skin cancer. Two studies of patients treated for long periods with these products have largely, but not totally, dispelled this safety issue, in the FDA's view. Verdict: Coal-tar preparations are safe and effective for treating seborrheic dermatitis. The approved dosage is 0.5 to 5 percent coal tar, to be applied 1 to 4 times daily or as directed by a doctor.

WARNINGS:

 Use caution in exposing skin to sunlight after applying this product. It may increase your tendency to sunburn for up to 24 hours after use.

Do not use in or around the rectum or in the genital area or groin except on the advice of a doctor.

Do not use for prolonged periods without consulting a doctor.

• *HYDROCORTISONE PREPARATIONS (HYDROCORTISONE, HYDROCORTISONE ACETATE) FOR SEBORRHEIC DERMATITIS:* These drugs belong to a class of potent chemicals called *corticosteroids*. They are available without prescription in relatively weak concentrations of up to 1 percent. Even at these strengths, however, they are safe and effective for relieving mild to moderate rashes and other manifestations of seborrheic dermatitis, as well as the other unsightly and irritating symptoms this condition provokes. (*See* ITCH AND PAIN REMEDIES APPLIED TO THE SKIN for a fuller discussion of these drugs).

• *PYRITHIONE ZINC:* This drug is a cytostatic agent, which means that it controls ordinary dandruff and seborrheic scaling by slowing cell growth and turnover in the epidermis. It is strikingly different from coal tar, described previously. Unlike the tar, which is a traditional remedy, pyrithione zinc is a new drug. It was first synthesized in 1950 and later was chosen as an anti-dandruff active ingredient through a sophisticated screening test of some 1300 drugs.

Pyrithione zinc has been demonstrated to be safe in a variety of tests in animals and on humans. It is nonirritating and nonallergenic. Since it also is insoluble in water, it is not absorbed through the skin.

A residue of about 1 percent of the applied dose remains on the skin after rinsing. This residue is believed to account for much of the drug's beneficial effect. More than 30 well-controlled studies have been conducted on this ingredient, with excellent results in treating the scaling of dandruff and the effects of seborrheic dermatitis. The drug continues to be effective after many months of repeated use. It is significantly better than most—if not all—of the single-ingredient and combinations drugs that have been tested against it.

Pyrithione zinc is safe and effective. Approved dosages are 0.3 to 2 percent pyrithione zinc in shampoos and 0.1 to 0.25 percent pyrithione zinc in hair groomers and other products that are intended to be applied to and left on the scalp or the skin.

• *SALICYLIC ACID:* A skin-peeling (keratolytic) drug, salicylic acid is effective against both ordinary dandruff and seborrheic scaling of the scalp and the skin of the body.

This drug is the parent compound of ordinary aspirin. Once obtained from wintergreen leaves and sweet-birch bark, it is now manufactured synthetically.

Long-term use on the skin can be dangerous, because salicylic acid increases skin's water absorption, and eventually softens and weakens the skin, causing it to peel. However, when used twice weekly and then rinsed off, salicylic acid is safe, as too little is absorbed into the skin to cause injury.

This ingredient appears to benefit sufferers of dandruff and seborrheic dermatitis by dissolving and removing scales. While widely used, it is less well tested than pyrithione zinc. (*See* previously). Evaluators could find only two controlled studies in which salicylic acid was assessed alone rather than in combination with other ingredients. In both studies, 2 percent salicylic acid was more effective than a dummy medication in clearing up dandruff flakes.

Conclusion: Salicylic acid is safe and effective in treating ordinary dandruff and scaling caused by seborrheic dermatitis. The approved dosage is 1.8 to 3 percent salicylic acid applied twice weekly or more often in a medicated shampoo, or up to 4 times daily applied to the scalp or the skin in a hairgroomer, lotion, or other formulation.

- **SELENIUM SULFIDE:** This compound is a growth inhibitor (cytostatic agent) that is safe and effective against ordinary dandruff and seborrheic dermatitis.

Selenium sulfide is bright orange in color and is insoluble in water. This is a saving virtue: While selenium itself is dangerous—it is a potent poison if taken internally—the sulfide salt makes it safe because it is not absorbed through unbroken skin. Quite clearly, however, selenium sulfide should not be used if you have open scalp wounds or rashes. The substance also is irritating to the eyes and should be rinsed out quickly if some of the shampoo drips in accidentally.

A few individuals who use selenium sulfide will experience a rebound effect; that is, scalp oiliness may increase. They should switch to a different type of medicated shampoo.

Because selenium inhibits growth of *P. ovale*, which is found in the hair and on the scalp, it has been thought to relieve dandruff in this way. More likely, a breakdown product of the selenium sulfide blocks enzyme systems required for the growth of skin tissue. This slows the turnover process in the epidermis (outer layer of skin) and so limits dandruff. Whatever the mechanism, reviewers added, there is no doubt that the drug reduces cell turnover, whether on normal scalps or on itchy, scaly ones.

Several large and carefully conducted comparative studies show that the 1 percent selenium sulfide available over-the-counter is as effective against ordinary dandruff as a 2.5 percent formulation of this product that is only available by prescription. Conclusion: safe and effective.

The approved dosage is 1 percent selenium sulfide twice weekly or oftener in a shampoo or a rinse, or up to 4 times daily in a hairgroomer, ointment, or other preparation designed to be left on the skin.

- **SULFUR PREPARATIONS:** These scale-removing (keratolytic) compounds are safe and effective against ordinary dandruff but *not* against the scales produced by seborrheic dermatitis.

Sulfur is an ancient skin remedy, and it continues to be widely used by dermatologists for treating acne and other skin conditions. The most common forms are *precipitated sulfur* (milk of sulfur), which is a smooth, fine, yellowish-white powder that lacks sulfur's characteristic smell, and *colloidal sulfur*, which is composed of minute particles of the element suspended in gelatin, egg albumin, or a similar vehicle (base).

In low concentrations, sulfur is not very toxic, although continuing use can produce a reddening and a thickening of the skin. Concentrations over 10 percent can be deadly. Basing its judgment largely on sulfur's long use and wide acceptance, the Panel concludes that this elemental medication is safe for use in dandruff shampoos and other products in the recommended concentrations and dosages.

Few reliable studies have been conducted on the dandruff-combating effectiveness of sulfur as a single ingredient. The findings that are available suggest that it is effective, but they are not wholly conclusive in sulfur's favor. Nonetheless, the FDA says that 2 to 5 percent sulfur shampoos and lotions are safe and effective in controlling ordinary dandruff. Use sulfur twice weekly or more often, or as directed by a doctor, as a shampoo or rinse, or 1 to 4 times daily in a cream, lotion, or other form that is applied to the scalp.

CONDITIONALLY APPROVED ANTI-SCALE ACTIVE INGREDIENT

The value of hydrocortisone preparations has not yet been determined.

• HYDROCORTISONE PREPARATIONS (HYDROCORTISONE, HYDROCORTISONE ACETATE) FOR DANDRUFF: Neither the safety nor the effectiveness of hydrocortisone in treating dandruff has been established to the FDA's satisfaction. They are safe and effective for treating seborrheic dermatitis. (*See* Hydrocortisone Preparations under Approved Active Anti-Scale Ingredients.)

DISAPPROVED ANTI-SCALE ACTIVE INGREDIENTS

None.

When Greater Relief Is Needed

A 2.5 percent selenium sulfide suspension, which can be used as a shampoo, is available by prescription. An FDA expert says it is very effective. Steroid lotions also are available with a prescription (℞) to relieve inflammation and itching. The antifungal agent ketoconazole has been approved as safe and effective as a prescription cream for treating dandruff.

Safety and Effectiveness: Combination Products Sold Over-the-Counter to Treat Dandruff and Seborrheic Dermatitis

Safe and Effective

sulfur (2-5%) + salicylic acid (1.8-3%) (for dandruff only)

Safety and Effectiveness: Active Ingredients in
Over-the-Counter Dandruff and Seborrheic Dermatitis Shampoos and Other Treatments

Active Ingredient	Type	Assessment	Effective Against Dandruff	Effective Against Seborrheic Dermatitis
coal tar	tar	safe and effective	yes	yes
hydrocortisone preparations: hydrocortisone and hydrocortisone acetate	corticosteroid	safe and effective for seborrheic dermatitis; not proved safe for dandruff	maybe	yes
pyrithione zinc	cytostatic	safe and effective	yes	yes
salicylic acid	keratolytic	safe and effective	yes	yes
selenium sulfide 1%	cytostatic	safe and effective	yes	yes
sulfur preparations	keratolytic	safe and effective	yes	no

Dandruff and Seborrheic-Scale Shampoos and Hair Dressings: Product Ratings

SINGLE-INGREDIENT SHAMPOOS

Product and Distributor	Dosage of Active Ingredients	Rating for Dandruff*	Rating for Seborrhea of Scalp*	Comment
coal tar				
DHS Tar (Person & Covey)	0.5% coal tar (USP)	A	A	
Neutrogena T/Gel (Neutrogena)	2% coal tar extract	A	A	
Pentrax Tar (GenDerm)	4.3% coal tar	A	A	
Tegrin Medicated (Block)	5% coal tar	A	A	
Tegrin Medicated Extra Conditioning (Block)	7% coal tar solution	C	C	product information does not indicate coal tar concentration
povidone-iodine				
Betadine (Purdue Frederick)	7.5%	C	C	disapproved
pyrithione zinc				
Danex (Herbert)	1%	A	A	
Zincon (Lederle)	2%	A	A	
DHS Zinc (Person & Covey)	2%	A	A	

Head & Shoulders (Procter & Gamble)		A	A	
salicylic acid				
P & S (Baker-Cummins)	2%	A	A	
X-Seb (Baker-Cummins)	4%	C	C	exceeds approved dosage, 3%
selenium sulfide				
Selenium sulfide (generic)	1%	A	A	
Selsun Blue (Ross)	1%	A	A	

COMBINATION SHAMPOOS

Product and Distributor	Dosage of Active Ingredients	Rating for Dandruff*	Rating for Seborrhea of Scalp*	Comment
Denorex Extra Strength (Whitehall)	12.5% coal tar solution + 1.5% menthol	C	C	menthol not approved
Denorex Medicated (Whitehall)	9% coal tar solution + 1.5% menthol	C	C	menthol not approved
Fostex Medicated Cleansing (Westwood Squibb)	2% sulfur + 2% salicylic acid	A	C	not approved for seborrhea
Maximum Strength Meted (GenDerm)	5% sulfur + 3% salicylic acid	A	C	not approved for seborrhea

Dandruff and Seborrheic Shampoos and Hair Dressings: Product Ratings (contd)

Product and Distributor	Dosage of Active Ingredients	Rating for Dandruff*	Rating for Seborrhea of Scalp*	Comment
Sebaquin (Summers)	3% iodoquinol	C	C	ingredient not submitted to or assessed in OTC Review
Sebulex (Westwood Squibb)	2% sulfur + 2% salicylic acid	A	C	not approved for seborrhea

MEDICATED HAIR DRESSINGS

Product and Distributor	Dosage of Active Ingredients	Rating for Dandruff*	Rating for Seborrhea of Scalp*	Comment
P & S (Baker-Cummins)	liquid: less than 1% phenol	C	C	phenol disapproved
Sebucare (Westwood Squibb)	lotion: 1.8% salicylic acid	A	A	

SEBORRHEIC DERMATITIS RELIEVERS FOR THE SKIN

Product and Distributor	Dosage of Active Ingredients	Rating for Seborrhea*	Comment
coal tar preparations			

AquaTar (Allergan)	**gel:** 2.5% coal tar	A
Balnetar (Westwood)	**liquid:** 2.5% coal tar	A
Estar (Westwood)	**gel:** 2.5%	A
Medotar (Medco Labs)	**ointment:** 1% coal tar	A
Neutrogena T/Derm (Neutrogena)	**oil:** 5% coal tar	A

hydrocortisone preparations

See pp. 571-572, hydrocortisone product ratings in ITCH AND PAIN REMEDIES APPLIED TO THE SKIN

pyrithione zinc

ZNP Bar (Steifel)	**bar soap:** 2%	A

salicylic acid

Panscol (Baker Cummins)	**lotion, ointment:** 3%	A	
Calicylic Creme (Gordon)	**cream:** 10%	C	too strong

selenium sulfide

selenium sulfide (generic)	**lotion:** 1%	A
Selsun Blue (Ross)		A

---

*Author's interpretation of FDA criteria. Based on contents, not claims.

Deodorants for Incontinence and Ostomies

Most body-odor problems can be overcome by adequate personal hygiene, by the use of cosmetics, or by the use of antiperspirants, mouthwashes, or other products. But some people face unfortunate situations in which their bodies produce strong, foul odors.

They include persons who are incontinent of urine or feces, which means they do not have control over their bladders or bowels, or who have an opening from the intestinal tract to the outside of their bodies. These openings (enterostomies) are created surgically, usually in the treatment of cancer, ulcerative colitis, or some other serious disease. Well over a million Americans are ostomates, and their ranks are increased by tens of thousands each year. A *colostomy* is an opening from the large intestine (colon) to the outside of the body. An *ileostomy* is an opening from the small intestine (ileum) to the outside of the body.

Fecal incontinence and *urinary incontinence*—soiling and wet-

---

DEODORANTS FOR INCONTINENCE AND OSTOMIES is based on the report "Deodorant/Drug Products for Internal Use" by the FDA's Advisory Review Panel on OTC Miscellaneous Internal Drug Products and on the FDA's Tentative Final and Final Monographs on these products.

ting—are messy and distressing handicaps for many older Americans, as well as for younger people who suffer them because they are physically or mentally disabled. The incontinence adds to their disability and makes it impossible for many of these people to continue living at home. The group homes and institutions where they must live may become terribly malodorous, to the intense discomfort of family members, staff people, and the incontinent individuals themselves. Remedies to reduce this noisome nuisance are thus sorely needed.

Some people, too, have superficial sores or injuries that do not heal readily and therefore smell bad. Others feel they are unable to control extremely bad smells emanating from the armpits, crotch, mouth, or feet.

These problems often respond to special hygienic measures suggested by a doctor or a rehabilitation counselor. They may also be relieved through the use of deodorant drugs that are taken internally. Two drugs are safe and effective in relieving colostomy and ileostomy odors. One of them, *chlorophyllin copper complex*, also effectively controls the smell of fecal incontinence. But it has not been proved effective against the odor of urinary incontinence or other foul body odors.

 ### Claims for Deodorants

Accurate

• "An aid to reduce odor from a colostomy or ileostomy"

For chlorophyllin copper complex:

• "An aid to reduce fecal odor due to incontinence"

APPROVED DEODORANT ACTIVE INGREDIENTS

• BISMUTH SUBGALLATE: This drug has been used successfully for three decades to control -*ostomy* odors and has the endorsement of the United Ostomy Association — the patients who live with this handicap.

The FDA has accepted the long history of the use of this ingredient with few complications as evidence for its safety and effectiveness. It has accepted this less-than-scientific evidence in lieu of the standard, objective studies, because a reduction in disagreeable smell is, after all, a subjective judgment, both for the patient and for the investigator who is trying to assess the odor-reducing drug. Additionally, one double-blind study in ileostomy patients, and one uncontrolled study in patients with ileostomies or colostomies added to the FDA's conviction that bismuth subgallate is safe and effective. Both showed significant benefit from the drug. The approved dosage is 200 to 400 mg four times daily for adults and children over 12; for younger children, consult a doctor.

- *CHLOROPHYLLIN COPPER COMPLEX:* This ingredient is derived from plant leaves; chlorophyll is the green, waxy pigment that converts sunlight into food energy for plant (and thus eventually animal) growth and development.

Long use has confirmed chlorophyllin copper complex's safety, although it may turn the stool green and can cause mild diarrhea and cramping. Several studies in patients with what FDA candidly calls "offensive odors" confirmed the preparation's value for *-ostomies* and fecal incontinence but not for urinary incontinence and malodorous open sores. "Odor was satisfactorily eliminated in all cases involving colostomy and ileostomy," the agency says.

In another study, patients with urinary or fecal incontinence or both who produced "strong odor" were "virtually odorless" by the seventh day of treatment with chlorophyllin copper. The data summarized by the FDA in its Final Monograph on these drugs indicates that the chlorophyllin-copper complex is effective against odors of both urinary and fecal incontinence. However, in analyzing the data, the agency concluded that the evidence is valid only for fecal incontinence, not for problems from urination. This conclusion is based in part on a double-blind test, in which urine samples from incontinent patients were taken into an odor-free room and sniffed by researchers. These researchers did not know whether a particular specimen came from a patient who had been given the chlorophyllin copper complex or from one who had been given dummy medication instead. The intensity of the odor in each sample was measured on a scale that included "maximum," "severe," and "terrible" odors. The drug did not significantly improve the odor of the patients' urine compared with the odor of urine from patients taking the dummy drug.

Based on these findings, the FDA approved chlorophyllin copper complex for the amelioration of *-ostomy* odors and fecal incontinence as safe and effective. The dosage for adults and children over 12 years is 100 or 200 mg per day and up to 300 mg per day if needed. For children under 12 years of age, ask the doctor.

CONDITIONALLY APPROVED DEODORANT ACTIVE INGREDIENTS

None.

DISAPPROVED DEODORANT ACTIVE INGREDIENTS

None.

When Greater Relief Is Needed

The manufacturer of a chlorophyllin copper complex product asked the FDA to approve significantly higher daily dosages of up to 800 mg daily. The agency declined to do so. If the approved dosages of these products do not significantly relieve your problem, it may be worth asking your doctor if a trial at a higher dosage might be warranted.

Safety and Effectiveness: Active Ingredients in Over-the-Counter Deodorants for Ostomies and Incontinence

Active Ingredient	Assessment
bismuth subgallate	safe and effective
chlorophyllin, water-soluble (potassium sodium copper chlorophyllin)	safe and effective*

---

* Effective against odors of fecal incontinence but not against those of urinary incontinence.

Deodorants for Ostomies and Incontinence: Product Ratings

Product and Distributor	Dosage of Active Ingredients	Rating *	Comment
bismuth subgallate			
Devrom (Parthenon)	tablets, chewable: 200 mg	A	
chlorophyllin copper complex			
Chloresium (Rystan)	tablets: 14 mg	A	

*Author's interpretation of FDA criteria. Based on content, not claims.

Diaper-Rash Relievers

Every baby suffers red, sore diaper rash from time to time. Older persons who become incontinent suffer many of the same symptoms and require similar treatment.

Diaper rash has many causes including urine and feces, both of which irritate tender skin. Microorganisms in these body wastes also contribute to the problem. Bacteria metabolize urine to produce ammonia, which can be highly irritating. The yeast *Candida albicans*, which is often present in a baby's stool, may multiply rapidly and produce a bright-red, very irritating rash with sharply delineated edges.

Ambient heat and body heat trapped by plastic diaper backings or rubber pants produce angry-looking red marks and itching, stinging, bumpy eruptions where tender wet skin rubs against clothing. This condition—called *prickly heat* or *miliaria*—occurs when the sweat glands become blocked by water or wastes and rupture into the adjacent skin.

The soaps, bleaches, and detergents used to launder reusable

DIAPER-RASH RELIEVERS is based on the unadopted draft report "OTC Diaper-Rash Drug Products" by the FDA's Advisory Review Panel on OTC Miscellaneous External Drug Products, and, more importantly, on FDA's four Tentative Final Monographs on skin protectants, anti-microbial agents, anti-fungal agents, and itch-pain relievers that are used in these products.

cloth diapers can also cause or contribute to diaper rash and prickly heat. So does chafing in the baby's skin folds. A red and inflamed diaper area may also be a signal that the baby is allergic to milk or some other food. Diaper rash thus can signal an underlying medical problem.

If simple preventive measures and treatment with over-the-counter medicated lotions and powders do not clear the condition in a couple of days, a pediatrician's help should be sought.

Simple Remedies

An ordinary, mild diaper rash—in which the skin is reddened (erythematous) but not broken—can often be relieved by frequent diaper changes and simple cleansing with water. Switching to a different kind of diaper may help, too. The Panel suggests changing from plastic-backed disposable diapers to all-cloth washable ones, which allow more air to reach the skin surface. Switching the other way, from cloth to disposable paper diapers, also may help, since disposable diapers, unlike cloth ones, have a highly absorbent inner layer that quickly draws moisture off the skin. What is more, disposable diapers are always free of fecal bacteria because they have not previously been used or laundered with other diapers. Another suggestion is to leave the diaper off while the baby is napping, so the skin is exposed to air.

Types of Medications

Diaper rash products contain ingredients from several categories of drugs. There are five classes of drugs formulated into diapering preparations for the relief of diaper rash and prickly heat:

- *Skin protectants* are supposed to act to sooth mild rashes.
- *Wound healers* are alleged to speed up the healing process.
- *Antifungals* are supposed to act specifically to cure rashes caused by the yeast *C. albicans*.
- *Antimicrobials* inhibit or kill bacteria and other microorganisms that cause irritation, inflammation, and infections.
- *Itch-pain relievers* act on nerve endings and inflamed tissues to temporarily reduce itching and painful sensations.

The ingredients that you may find listed on a tube, jar, or squeeze bottle of a diaper rash-relief product are sorted out, by drug type, in the table Safety and Effectiveness: Active Ingredients in Over-the-Counter Diaper Rash Relievers, beginning on p. 292.

A strong warning has been issued by the FDA with regard to *phenol*, which can damage babies' skin and which is also absorbed through the skin into the interior of the body. A baby's liver may not be able to break down and detoxify phenol, which means that it will accumulate in the body. Phenol is a dangerous nerve poison. Covering phenol with a diaper further increases the hazard by increasing the amount of the substance that is absorbed through the skin. The FDA's warning says flatly:

 "Do not use phenol for diaper rash."

Skin Protectants

If the baby's skin is only mildly irritated, *skin protectants* may relieve the rash. These substances tend to be physically soothing and chemically inactive, so they are safe for regular use. Many people apply them to the baby's skin routinely to prevent diaper rash whenever they change diapers.

Skin protectants that FDA has approved for use on infants' skin are listed in the table Safe and Effective Skin Protectants for Treating and Preventing Diaper Rash.

Safe and Effective Skin Protectants for Treating and Preventing Diaper Rash

Active Ingredient	Approved Concentrations (%)
allantoin	0.5-2
calamine	1-25
cod-liver oil	5-13.6 (only in combination products)
dimethicone	1-30
kaolin	4-20
lanolin	15.5 (only in combination products)
mineral oil	50-100

Safe and Effective Skin Protectants for
Treating and Preventing Diaper Rash (contd)

Active Ingredient	Approved Concentrations (%)
petrolatum preparations (petrolatum, white petrolatum)	20-100
talc	45-100
topical starch (corn starch)	10-98
zinc oxide	1-25, and up to 40 in ointments

Skin protectants include absorbents, which remove urine from the skin, or adsorbents, which bind, hold, and neutralize urine and other irritating and toxic substances such as amonia. Some of these ingredients form a physical barrier that protects the skin against urine. Skin protectants also soothe and soften the skin, and some lubricate it to prevent chafing. *Note that the only ingredients currently approved by FDA as safe and effective for the prevention and treatment of diaper rash are these skin protectants.*

Most of these ingredients were assessed, in general terms, by the FDA's Advisory Review Panel on Miscellaneous External Drug Products. The FDA assessments lean heavily on these findings. The Panel's assessments are summarized in the Unit UNGUENTS AND POWDERS FOR THE SKIN, and unless otherwise noted, the cross references for specific ingredients, below, are to that Unit in this Guide. For ingredients assessed initially by FDA rather than by the Panel, a summary of the agency's rationale will be found further on.

Ammonia Fighter

One drug, *methionone*, is sold over-the-counter in capsules for *internal* use for neutralizing the ammonia in urine. It thus may alleviate diaper rash in infants and also comparable rashes in adults who have urinary incontinence. Methionone appears to have escaped evaluation in the OTC Drug Review thus far. The trade name is *Uranap* (Vortech).

Claims for Skin Protectants

Accurate
- "Helps treat and prevent diaper rash"
- "Protects chafed skin due to diaper rash"
- "...helps seal out wetness"

Directions

Change wet and soiled diapers promptly, cleanse the diaper areas, and allow to dry. Apply ointment, cream, or powder liberally as often as necessary with each diaper change, especially at bedtime or any time when exposure to wet diapers may be prolonged. Note: Some skin protectants should not be applied to skin that has already broken into a rash. *See* Active Ingredients, further on.

APPROVED SKIN-PROTECTANT ACTIVE INGREDIENTS

There are now 13 safe and effective skin protectants for preventing and treating diaper rash:

- **ALLANTOIN:** Allantoin is a compound for which few, if any, adverse reactions have ever been reported in the medical literature. It appears to be non-toxic, non-allergenic, and non-irritating when applied to the skin. It has the ability to protect even very young and tender bottoms against the moisture and irritation of diaper rash. Allantoin also is a skin softener.

    In one series of controlled experiments, with an emulsion that contained allantoin, silicones, and the now-banned germicidal agent hexachlorophene, only 5 percent of several hundred babies developed diaper rash. In a control group of babies who were not so treated, the incidence of diaper rash was 3 times higher. In another part of this study, the skin of 34 out of 38 infants who already had diaper rash or a similar problem cleared up nicely after treatment with the emulsion. The investigators concluded that the allantoin-containing mixture was effective and relatively free from side effects. Allantoin is considered safe and effective for people of all ages when applied in a concentration of 0.5 to 2 percent, as often as needed.

- *CALAMINE (PREPARED CALAMINE AND CALAMINE LOTION):* A pinkish-colored anodyne, calamine protects the skin by absorbing moisture and chemical
irritants; it soothes, too. Calamine is 98 percent zinc oxide, which is
white. But it also contains about 0.5 percent—that is, one-half of 1
percent—of the iron compound ferrous oxide. This chemical's red
color imparts the pinkish cast, which is wholly "window dressing"
according to the experts. The iron contributes nothing to zinc oxide's
absorbent and protectant effect, which, like calamine's safety, is principally attested by consumer acceptance and long, trouble-free clinical
use. (*See* Zinc Oxide, further on.)

  The dosage, for all ages, is a 1 to 25 percent concentration of
calamine, applied as often as needed.

- *COD-LIVER OIL (IN COMBINATION PRODUCTS ONLY):* This smooth, slippery stuff—
from which most if not all of the cod fishes' fishy odor has been
removed—has been used in diapering preparations for over half a century, in combination products with other skin-protectant ingredients. It
softens the skin and protects it from urine and fecal material. Cod-liver
oil contains vitamins A and D, which are claimed to speed the healing
of diaper rashes. The FDA doubts this claim, as it doubts *all* "speedy
healing" claims, for want of convincing scientific evidence that healing
in fact is enhanced. Nevertheless, caught between these doubts and
manufacturers' insistence that these vitamins are helpful, the FDA has
temporarily taken itself off the hook by approving cod-liver oil as a safe
and effective skin protectant, at concentrations of 5 to 13.5 percent in
combination diaper care products, adding the proviso that the oil must
contain potentially-effective amounts of vitamins A and D — if, in fact,
as the makers claim, they *are* effective wound healers.

- *CORN STARCH: See* Topical Starch.

- *DIMETHICONE:* An inert, soothing, syrupy silicone, dimethicone is judged
to be remarkably free of toxicity. It is chemically similar to simethicone, which is taken internally to relieve symptoms of gas. (*See*
ANTI-GAS AGENTS.) Dimethicone clings to the skin and repels water.
It will effectively seal a wound against air, wind, and other drying or
frictional irritants. Because it can block the ammonia usually produced by bacterial decomposition of urine, this ingredient can be used
to treat and prevent diaper rash. Dimethicone also will seal and protect chapped skin and lips against further drying and chapping. It
should *not* be used on puncture wounds or infected wounds, however,
because some air must reach wound surfaces in order for them to
heal; without air they fester.

Dimethicone is safe and effective in a 1 to 30 percent concentration on the skins of people of all ages. It can be applied in generous amounts and as often as needed.

- **KAOLIN:** Also called *China clay, white bole, argilla,* and *porcelain clay,* kaolin is a powdery, earthy, clay-type material. Technically it is purified and hydrated aluminum silicate. It protects the skin through its ability to avidly absorb moisture and toxic substances dissolved in it.

    Kaolin has been used as an internal and external medication for hundreds of years. There are no reports of toxic reactions following its application to the skin. The substance absorbs perspiration and other moisture, and acts as a dusting powder to dry weepy skin conditions like eczema and the leaky blisters of poison ivy and poison oak. For people of all ages, kaolin is considered safe and effective in concentrations of 4 to 20 percent. It can be applied liberally, when needed.

- **LANOLIN (IN COMBINATION PRODUCTS ONLY):** This is an oily substance extracted from sheeps' wool. It long has been used in a diapering product, for the barrier it forms on the skin against urine and other irritants. Most studies of lanolin's safety and effectiveness as a skin protectant have been for problems other than diaper rash (for anal itching, for example). At high concentrations (50 percent) lanolin may be irritating. But in the lower concentrations used in diaper rash compounds irritation is rarely if ever a problem. Based on these considerations, FDA judges lanolin safe and effective as a skin protectant against diaper rash at a concentration of 15.5 percent, the amount present in the product it evaluated, in combination with one or more other active ingredients.

- **MINERAL OIL:** This syrupy substance is tasteless and odorless. It smooths, soothes, and softens the skin and provides a barrier against urine and feces. It has been widely studied as a skin protectant, but has not been studied specifically as a diaper rash reliever. Nevertheless, based on wide use on other body areas, and mineral oil's long use, without apparent problems, in diapering preparations, FDA rules it safe and effective in concentrations of 50 to 100 percent. (Lesser amounts of mineral oil are used as a vehicle for other drugs in some products. The FDA counts mineral oil as an *inactive ingredient*—one with no protective value—in concentrations that are under 50 percent.)

- **PETROLATUM PREPARATIONS: PETROLATUM AND WHITE PETROLATUM:** These petroleum derivatives can be used to soften, lubricate, and protect the skin. White petrolatum is chemically more refined than yellow or amber petrolatums, but their pharmaceutical properties are the same.

Petrolatum is the base (vehicle) for a variety of internal and external medications, and is regarded as extremely safe. For small, superficial burns, petrolatum by itself (or on a gauze dressing) will keep air out, prevent evaporation of moisture from the wound, and reduce pain. Petrolatum can also be used to relieve sunburn, chapping, and other forms of dry skin, and as an ammonia-blocking agent to prevent diaper rash. It should *not*, however, be used on puncture wounds, lacerated skin, or wounds that have become infected, since the lack of exposure to air retards healing and may cause the wound to form pus.

For persons of all ages, petrolatum preparations are safe and effective in 30 to 100 percent concentrations and can be applied as often as needed.

• *TALC:* This is the principal ingredient in many baby powders. It has been recommended for babies by the American Academy of Pediatrics because it clings to the skin, protecting it from irritation. Talc lubricates skin surfaces and so prevents chafing. It repels water and urine.

The FDA finds talc safe for use on unbroken skin, but says it should not be used on the open broken skin of severe rashes, where it can crust up and exacerbate the soreness. Parents also should take care that talc powder does not get into babies' faces where it could be inhaled and cause problems.

Talc is safe and effective as a skin protectant in concentrations of 45 to 100 percent.

• *WHITE PETROLEUM: See* Petrolatum preparations.

• *TOPICAL STARCH (CORN STARCH):* This is a powdery, kitchen-cabinet remedy—a food substance, really. Its protective power lies in its ability to absorb huge amounts of liquids when it is dusted on the skin. Topical starch absorbs 25 times more moisture than talc, which also is used for this purpose. Bacteria and their poisonous byproducts, as well as other noxious materials, can be absorbed and held away from the skin by topical starch and thus rendered harmless. Topical starch also smoothes and lubricates body surfaces that have been irritated by friction.

Topical starch feels bland to the skin. This helps explain why no adverse effects have as yet been attributed to dusting it on the body. For adults, children, and infants, the Panel says that a 10 to 98 percent topical starch preparation can safely and effectively be applied to irritated skin as often as needed.

• *ZINC OXIDE:* This fine, white powdery substance, sometimes known as *flowers of zinc* or *zinc white,* is the basic active ingredient in calamine preparations. Zinc oxide is used to cover the skin to protect it from dryness and other harmful environmental stimuli. It absorbs toxic substances and also serves as a lubricant. Zinc oxide is extremely safe, even when taken internally, and there have been no published reports of complications following its use on the skin. Its effectiveness is established by wide use and acceptance by consumers and doctors. It is the sole or principal ingredient in a wide variety of over-the-counter preparations.

Because of its cooling, slightly astringent, antiseptic, antibacterial, and protective actions, zinc oxide is considered particularly effective in treating diaper rash and prickly heat. It is also useful against eczema, impetigo, and many other itchy conditions. The approved concentration is up to 25 percent in powders and other formulations, and up to 40 percent in an ointment.

CONDITIONALLY APPROVED SKIN-PROTECTANT ACTIVE INGREDIENTS

The FDA lists a number of diapering-product skin-protectant ingredients that it says have not yet been proved safe and effective. They are:

- *ALDIOXA:* This is an aluminum salt of allantoin. (*See* Allantoin). The clinical studies on its use in treating rashes and other skin problems in infants simply have not convinced FDA that it is safe and effective.
- *ALUMINUM ACETATE:* A manufacturer claims that creams and ointments containing this ingredient act as a skin barrier and help restore the skin's natural acid-base balance. No supportive data were provided, and FDA, accordingly, says this ingredient is not proved safe and effective.
- *ALUMINUM HYDROXIDE:* This is a safe and effective skin protectant for adults. *See* p. 973. But there are no data on its efficacy or safety for treating diaper rash in infants. Verdict: not proved safe or effective.
- *COCOA BUTTER:* This protectant has not been tested or marketed in products labelled specifically for diaper rash. So there is no evidence on its safety or effectiveness, which is why it wins only conditional approval. *See* p. 973.
- *COLLOIDAL OATMEAL:* This substance is formulated as a bath additive, cleansing bar, or soak, after which, it leaves a thin starchy film on the skin that may resist urine and other diaper contents. But it also may

seal in wetness, which is undesired. The FDA was also unable to get a clear idea of the elemental constituents of colloidal oatmeal. For these reasons, and a couple of others, it said colloidal oatmeal is not proved safe and effective.

• *CYSTEINE HYDROCHLORIDE:* Inadequate data were sent by the manufacturer, FDA says. The result: not proved safe and effective.

• *DEXPANTHENOL:* Inadequate data. Verdict: not proved safe and effective.

• *GLYCERIN:* The FDA is worried about this soothing stuff, because it could hold urine against the skin, enhancing its damage. Over all, the relevant data in glycerin's favor were scant. So glycerin as yet is not proved safe or effective for preventing or treating diaper rash.

• *MICROPOROUS CELLULOSE:* This material is derived from corn cobs and other sources. It is very effective in absorbing water and other liquids. But no data were submitted to show specifically that it is safe or effective for preventing or treating infants' diaper rashes.

• *PERUVIAN BALSAM, PERUVIAN BALSAM OIL:* At low concentrations, this is an acceptable *fragrance*—an *inactive* ingredient—in diapering products. Manufacturers claim, however, that it is medicinally useful — an *active* ingredient — at higher concentrations, in the realm of 1.5 to 3 percent. These claims are not backed by adequate data. Conclusion: Not proved safe or effective.

• *SHARK-LIVER OIL: See* p. 975. The data submitted to FDA are inadequate to prove that this substance is a safe and effective skin protectant, the agency says. Shark-liver oil contains vitamins A and D, which manufacturers claim speeds wound healing; the FDA also doubts this claim. Verdict: not proved safe or effective.

• *SODIUM BICARBONATE (BICARBONATE OF SODIUM, BAKING SODA):* This common kitchen substance may be safe and effective for occasional use to relieve irritated skin, as the Panel reported. *See* pp. 975. But there is no data on its safety when used repeatedly in diapering — and FDA has some qualms about it. No specific data were available, either, on its effectiveness for preventing or treating diaper rash. Verdict: sodium bicarbonate is not proved safe or effective.

• *ZINC ACETATE: See* p. 976. There is no data on the safety or the effectiveness of this substance in preventing or treating diaper rash. The FDA's tentative judgment: not proved safe or effective.

• *ZINC CARBONATE:* This ingredient has not been marketed in diaper rash products, and there are no data to show it is safe and effective for this specific purpose. *See* p. 976.

DISAPPROVED SKIN-PROTECTANT ACTIVE INGREDIENTS

The FDA is worried about the hazards of some ingredients that are marketed in products sold for the prevention and treatment of diaper rash.

- **BISMUTH SUBNITRATE:** No satisfactory data were submitted to show it is safe. It can be poisonous if accidentally ingested by a baby. The nitrate can be converted to nitrite in the gut, which in turn can cause a variety of symptoms including cardiac arrest. Conclusion: not safe and not effective.
- **BORIC ACID:** Several panels have stated that boric acid is toxic and is not safe for use on the skin. The FDA concurs.
- **SULFUR:** This element is unsafe for repeated use on the skin; it can exacerbate rashes and other injuries. *See* p. 593. The FDA says: Not safe or effective.
- **TANNIC ACID:** Once widely used, this ingredient has lost the confidence of doctors and government regulators. *See* p. 595. It is not safe or effective, FDA says.

Wound Healers

Some manufacturers claim they have products that encourage, speed, or enhance wound-healing of rashes and other, more serious diaper zone eruptions, including blisters and open sores, that may follow. The FDA simply does not believe *any* claim for *any* wound-healing ingredient has ever been convincingly proved with scientific data. So it appears the FDA will not even permit a wound-healing classification of drugs in its final ruling on diapering products.

But FDA is also between a rock and a hard place: Many diaper care products have been promoted, for years, for their ability to heal rashes and other skin symptoms of exposure to urine and feces. To avoid further conflict, FDA indicates that it might let manufacturers keep their wound-healing ingredients—if not their claims for them—if in some other way they could justify the ingredients' presence in the products. Vitamins A and D, for example, for which wound-healing claims long have been made, are present in rich amounts in cod-liver oil and shark-liver oil, which also lubricate the skin and protect it from urine and other irritants. These vitamins may therefore continue to show up, in some form, in diapering preparations. Manufacturers meanwhile have time, before FDA's final ruling, to prove to the agency that these "wound healers" in fact do help heal wounds.

Some other putative wound-healers appear to lack a second, saving grace. Unless quickly proved safe and effective, they are likely to be banned.

APPROVED WOUND-HEALING ACTIVE INGREDIENTS
None.

CONDITIONALLY APPROVED WOUND-HEALING ACTIVE INGREDIENTS

The problem with "wound-healing" agents is the same—lack of convincing evidence that they are either safe or effective—and so they simply will be listed rather than described.

- CHOLECALCIFEROL (VITAMIN D)
- CYSTEINE HYDROCHLORIDE
- LIVE YEAST-CELL DERIVATIVE
- PROTEIN HYDROLYSATE (L-LEUCINE, L-ISOLEUCINE, L-METHIONONE, L-PHENYLALANINE, AND L-TYROSINE)
- RACEMETHIONONE
- VITAMIN A
- VITAMIN D

DISAPPROVED WOUND-HEALING ACTIVE INGREDIENTS
None.

Antifungals

The moist, warm, alkaline environment inside an unchanged diaper is conducive to the vigorous growth of various funguses; one of them, *C. albicans*, produces a bright red rash. The FDA does not think that parents can adequately diagnose and treat a baby's fungal infection; diagnosis may require sending a skin scraping to a medical laboratory to find out exactly which organism—it may be a fungus, but it also *might* be a bacteria—is causing the infection. The FDA plans to ban antifungal claims and ingredients in diaper-rash products.

APPROVED ANTIFUNGAL ACTIVE INGREDIENTS

None.

CONDITIONALLY APPROVED ANTIFUNGAL ACTIVE INGREDIENTS

None.

DISAPPROVED ANTIFUNGAL ACTIVE INGREDIENTS

- CALCIUM UNDECYLENIC ACID: This antifungal agent has been approved for use against jock itch and athlete's foot (*see* p. 589) but is reported to be ineffective against *C. albicans*; it was not recommended for children under 2 years of age. Some evidence has been submitted to show that calcium undecylenic acid relieves diaper rash. But FDA says it does not believe parents can safely and effectively diagnose and treat diaper rash fungal infections in their babies. The verdict for calcium undecylenic acid is: not safe and effective.
- SODIUM PROPIONATE: For the reasons just cited for calcium undecylenic acid, this ingredient is not safe and effective for use by parents in the treatment of infections that arise under diapers.

   Some other antifungal agents may still be marketed in diaper-rash products. The FDA summarily dismisses them as unsafe and ineffective for this purpose. They are:

- BENZETHONIUM CHLORIDE: *See* p. 590.
- BORIC ACID: *See* p. 590.
- CAMPHOR: *See* p. 594.
- CHLOROXYLENOL (PCMX): *See* p. 591.
- 8-HYDROXYQUINOLINE
- MENTHOL: *See* p. 594.
- PHENOL: *See* p. 592.
- RESORCINOL: *See* p. 594.
- SALICYLIC ACID: *See* p. 593.

Antimicrobials

Two schools of thought exist on whether antimicrobial drugs should be applied to babies' skins in diaper-rash products or in ordinary soaps to prevent or treat bacterial infections. One view, in a comment submitted to the FDA, implicitly favors the use of these compounds, suggesting that labels for them should say "Helps kill germs associated with diaper rash" or "Helps kill germs that may aggravate diaper rash."

The opposite view states that bacterial or fungal infections that may accompany diaper rash are sometimes-serious secondary events that require diagnosis and treatment by a pediatrician or family physician—if and when they occur. In this view, diaper-rash products are intended to protect the skin from irritation by urine and feces but *not* to treat secondary infections.

The FDA currently "agrees" with the second viewpoint. The agency's position is that

"A rash in the diaper area that does not clear up in a reasonable amount of time may indicate the presence of a secondary bacterial or fungal skin infection... These conditions should not be treated with OTC drugs, and... an infection in the diaper area or a diaper rash that has persisted a week or more should be taken to a physician for appropriate diagnosis and therapy."

Given this point of view, the agency did not look kindly on claims for antimicrobials used for diaper rash. However, it did not look unkindly on any of the compounds that were submitted to it for this purpose.

The agency reviewed the literature on the relationship between bacterial flora and diaper rash. The microorganism *Staphylococcus aureus* is found more often inside the diapers of babies with rashes than it is found inside the diapers of babies who do not have a rash. But it is not clear whether *S. aureus* is the cause of the rash—or a result of it. It also is not clear, the FDA said, whether it is wise or safe to change the bacterial flora that normally is present on any baby's skin by treating him or her with an antimicrobial drug.

"There does not appear to be a generally recognized theory at this time to support OTC treatment or prevention of ordinary, mild diaper rash with antimicrobial drug products," the FDA adds. Some antimicrobials, such as triclocarban and triclosan, may be absorbed through the skin. These substances normally are degraded and excreted through physiological mechanisms that may not be fully developed until infants are six months of age. If this is so, the FDA says, these compounds could build up in the body to dangerous levels in babies' bodies.

 ## Claims for Antimicrobials

Accurate
None.

False, Misleading, Unproved or Inappropriate
• "Treats infection"
• "Kills millions of diaper rash germs"
• "Kills bacteria that cause diaper rash and odor"
• "Medicated formula, inhibits the growth of bacteria"

APPROVED ANTIMICROBIAL ACTIVE INGREDIENTS
None.

CONDITIONALLY APPROVED ANTIMICROBIAL ACTIVE INGREDIENTS

• **BENZALKONIUM CHLORIDE:** This is a quaternary ammonium compound, or "quat." (*See* p. 422). When used briefly, in small amounts, the FDA says this substance is safe. But its safety when used repeatedly on large areas of skin, under diapers, has not been fully established. It is not known if babies become sensitized to it, and if so, it is also not clear how much is absorbed through the skin. To what degree benzalkonium chloride may irritate babies' skin is not known either. Safety studies to answer these questions are needed. The studies submitted to demonstrate the effectiveness of benzalkonium chloride in preventing and treating diaper rash are also flawed, the agency said. Verdict: The drug's safety and efficacy for use in diapering products need to be shown.

• **BENZETHONIUM CHLORIDE:** This "quat" is very similar to benzalkonium chloride, just described. (*See also* p. 422). Both the safety and the effectiveness of this compound as an antimicrobial ingredient in diapering products remain unresolved.

• *CALCIUM UNDECYLENATE:* This ingredient is rated safe and effective for treating jock itch in adults and older children (*see* p. 589), but it is not approved for infants.

Calcium undecylenate is a normal constituent of human sweat, so its safety, generally speaking, can be inferred, the FDA says. But whether baby powders containing up to 15 percent calcium undecylenate also are safe, under a diaper, cannot be directly inferred from the substance's natural role in sweat. Tests to establish its safety thus far are inconclusive. The studies submitted to establish the compound's effectiveness all are flawed or inadequate, the FDA says. So: Both the safety and effectiveness of calcium undecylenate as a diapering antimicrobial need to be proved.

• *CHLOROXYLENOL (PCMX):* This is a phenol-like compound that is widely used as an antiseptic. The FDA is suspicious of it and finds that the studies submitted thus far to establish its safety and its effectiveness under the pressure-cooker conditions inside wet diapers are inadequate. Some tests in animals (rats) suggest that chloroxylenol may be hazardous. Tentative verdict: not proved safe or effective.

• *METHYLBENZETHONIUM CHLORIDE:* This "quat" is very similar to benzethonium chloride, described previously. The studies that have been done to establish the safety and effectiveness of methylbenzethonium chloride are different from those done on the related quats. But the FDA's verdict, for now, is the same: not proved safe and not proved effective.

• *OXYQUINOLINE (8-HYDROXYQUINOLINE):* Several Panels have evaluated oxyquinolines, and none was very positive or very negative about it. The general verdict, which the FDA agrees with, is that their safety and effectiveness remain to be proved. Virtually no data were submitted to establish oxyquinoline's safety and efficacy in diapering products. For now, the FDA says: not proved safe or effective.

• *PROPIONATE:* A lot of old, irrelevant and unconvincing data were submitted to several Panels, and to the FDA, in support of this compound's safety and effectiveness as a nonprescription drug. Very little of this information spoke directly to its use in preventing and treating diaper rash. More information is needed, the FDA says. Its current assessment is that sodium propionate is not proved safe or effective.

• *TRICLOSAN:* This ingredient is formulated into soaps and other personal cleansing products. Tests have been conducted in which baby rhesus monkeys and human babies have been washed with it, and no harm appears to have resulted. But the FDA finds these tests unconvincing. The agency also is not persuaded that simply killing bacteria on babies' skin—which triclosan certainly will do—is either safe or useful. "The agency considers the benefit-to-risk ratio to be unacceptably small if there is any potential risk at all," the FDA says. The available data is inconclusive, the agency analysts add. Triclosan is not proved safe or effective.

DISAPPROVED ANTIMICROBIAL ACTIVE INGREDIENTS

* BORIC ACID: Several Panels list boric acid as unsafe for use on the skin. Based on these findings, the FDA labels it unsafe for use in diapering products.
* P-CHLOROMERCURIPHENOL: The one manufacturer who included this compound in a diaper-rash product has withdrawn it. This compound is both a *mercurial* and a *phenol*—and both are dangerous. The FDA's verdict on *p*-chloromercuriphenol: not safe.
* PHENOL: This drug can be absorbed through the skin, and it is toxic. (*See* PHENOL: SPECIAL NOTE.) The FDA warns that it is not safe to use any phenol preparation in treating diaper rash.
* RESORCINOL: This is a phenol-like drug that is safe when used in limited amounts in older people. It is not safe in infants and young children. Some deaths have been reported when resorcinol-containing products were used on infants' skins. The FDA's verdict: not safe.

Itch-Pain Relievers

Several currently marketed diaper rash products contain benzocaine or other drugs intended to relieve itching and pain from diaper rash. The FDA believes these ingredients should not be used for this purpose. Infants cannot clearly communicate with adults to tell them what kind of distress they are feeling—and where. So symptoms cannot be treated specifically. What is more, some drugs used to reduce itching and pain are, in and of themselves, irritants—and could complicate rather than relieve the baby's discomfort without the parent knowing that he or she is making matters worse.

If one of these drugs is applied under a warm and an eventually wet diaper, it may be more readily absorbed into the skin than might be the case if the same drug were applied on a dry, exposed skin surface. Some of these drugs can damage the skin and may also cause systemic damage.

Although manufacturers advertise and sell creams and ointments that contain these itch-pain relievers, they declined to submit information to FDA that might show—specifically—that the drugs are safe and effective for treating diaper rash. Based on all these reasons, FDA has tentatively decided to ban itch-pain relievers in over-the-counter diaper rash products.

APPROVED ITCH-PAIN RELIEVERS

None.

CONDITIONALLY APPROVED ITCH-PAIN RELIEVERS

None.

DISAPPROVED ITCH-PAIN RELIEVERS

The following disapproved ingredients all are described elsewhere in this Guide under different headings. Unless manufacturers or others quickly provide the FDA with data demonstrating that these ingredients are safe and effective, all will soon be banned from diapering products.

* BENZOCAINE
* CAMPHOR
* DIBUCAINE
* EUCALYPTOL
* HYDROCORTISONE ACETATE
* MENTHOL
* OIL OF CADE (JUNIPER TAR)
* OIL OF EUCALYPTUS
* PHENOL
* PRAMOXINE OXIDE
* RESORCINOL
* TETRACAINE

Combination Products

Many diaper rash products are combinations of two or more active ingredients. The FDA approves as safe and effective only combinations of two or more skin protectants, in the approved concentrations. (*See* the table Safety and Effectiveness: Combination Products Sold Over-The-Counter to Prevent and Relieve Diaper Rash.)

When Greater Relief Is Needed

A festering diaper rash can quickly develop into a pediatric emergency. There is little need to wait for an emergency. If a diaper rash does not quickly abate, take the baby to the pediatrician. That's why he—or she—is there!

Safety and Effectiveness: Combination Products Sold Over-the-Counter to Relieve Diaper Rash

Safe and Effective Combinations

> 2 or more approved skin protectants at approved concentrations

Conditionally Safe and Effective Combinations

> 1 skin protectant + 1 conditionally approved antimicrobial
> protein hydolysate + cysteine hydrochloride + racemethione

Unsafe or Ineffective Combinations

> 1 skin protectant + 1 antifungal
> 1 skin protectant + 1 itch-pain reliever
> all other combination products

Safety and Effectiveness: Active Ingredients In Over-the-Counter Diaper-Rash Medications

Active Ingredient	Purpose	Assessment
allantoin	skin protectant	safe and effective
aluminum acetate	skin protectant	not proved safe or effective
aldioxa (aluminum dehydroxy allantoinate)	skin protectant	not proved safe or effective
aluminum hydroxide	skin protectant	not proved safe or effective
benzalkonium chloride	antimicrobial	not proved safe and effective
benzethonium chloride, in bar soap	antimicrobial	not safe or effective
as skin antiseptic	antimicrobial	not proved safe or effective
benzocaine	itch-pain reliever	not safe or effective
bicarbonate of sodium (see sodium bicarbonate)		
bismuth subnitrate	skin protectant	not safe or effective
boric acid	skin protectant	not safe
calamine (calamine lotion, prepared calamine)	skin protectant	safe and effective
calcium undecylenate	antimicrobial	not proved safe or effective
camphor (0.1-2.5%)	itch-pain reliever	not safe or effective

chloroxylenol (PCMX) in bar soap	antimicrobial	not proved safe or effective
as skin antispetic	antimicrobial	not safe or effective
cod-liver oil	as skin protectant	safe and effective only in combination products
cod-liver oil	as wound healer	not proved effective
colloidal oatmeal	skin protectant	not proved safe or effective
cornstarch (see topical starch)		
cysteine hydrochloride	wound healer	not proved safe or effective
dexpanthenol	skin protectant	not proved safe or effective
dibucaine	itch-pain reliever	not safe or effective
dimethicone	skin protectant	safe and effective
glycerin	skin protectant	not proved safe or effective
8-hydroxyquinoline	antimicrobial	not safe or effective
kaolin	skin protectant	safe and effective
lanolin	skin protectant	safe and effective only in combination products
live yeast-cell derivative	wound healer	not proved safe or effective
menthol	itch-pain reliever	not safe or effective
methylbenzethonium chloride in bar soap	antimicrobial	not safe or effective

Safety and Effectiveness: Active Ingredients in Over-the-Counter Diaper-Rash Medications (contd)

Active Ingredient	Purpose	Assessment
as skin antiseptic	antimicrobial	not proved safe or effective
microporous cellulose	skin protectant	not proved safe or effective
mineral oil	skin protectant	safe and effective
oil of cade (juniper tar)	itch-pain reliever	not safe and effective
oil of eucalyptus (eucalyptol)	itch-pain reliever	not safe or effective
oxyquinoline (8-hydroxyquinoline)	antimicrobial	not proved safe or effective
p-chloromercuriphenol	antimicrobial	not safe or effective
peruvian balsam, peruvian balsam oil (1.5-3%)	skin protectant	safe, not proved effective
petrolatum	skin protectant	safe and effective
phenol	antimicrobial	not safe
pramoxine hydrochloride	itch-pain reliever	not safe or effective
protein hydrolysate (1- leucine, 1-isoleucine, 1-methionone, 1- phenylalanine, 1- tyrosine)	wound healer	not proved safe or effective
racemethionine	wound healer	not proved safe or effective
resorcinol (resorcin) 0.5 -3%	antimicrobial	not safe

shark-liver oil	skin protectant	safe and effective only in combination products
sodium bicarbonate	skin protectant	not proved safe or effective
sodium propionate	antimicrobial	not proved safe or effective
talc	skin protectant	safe and effective
tannic acid	skin protectant	not safe or effective
tetracaine	itch-pain reliever	not safe or effective
topical starch	skin protectant	safe and effective
topical starch	wound healer	not proved safe or effective
triclosan	antimicrobial	not proved safe or effective
vitamin A	wound healer	not proved safe or effective
vitamin D	wound healer	not proved safe or effective
zinc acetate	skin protectant	not proved safe or effective
zinc carbonate	skin protectant	not proved safe or effective
zinc oxide	skin protectant	safe and effective

Diaper Rash Relievers: Product Ratings

Product and Distributor	Dosage of Active Ingredients	Rating *	Comment
A and D (Schering-Plough)	**ointment:** fish liver oil [vitamin A & D]	A	
Caldesene (Fisons)	**ointment:** 54% white petrolatum + 15% zinc oxide	A	
Desitin (Pfizer)	**ointment:** 40% zinc oxide + cod-liver oil [vitamin A & D] + petrolatum + lanolin	A	
Diaparene (Lehn & Fink)	**powder:** 0.55% methylbenzethonium chloride + corn starch + magnesium carbonate	B	methylbenzethonium not proved safe or effective
Diaparene Peri-Anal Medicated (Lehn & Fink)	**ointment:** 0.1% methylbenzethonium chloride + zinc oxide + cod-liver oil [vitamin A & D] + mineral oil + white petrolatum + starch + lanolin	C	methylbenzethonium not proved safe or effective; too many skin protectants
Mexsana Medicated (Schering-Plough)	**powder:** triclosan + zinc oxide + kaolin + eucalyptus oil + camphor + cornstarch	C	triclosan not proved safe or effective; too many protectants

Panthoderm (Jones Medical)	cream: 2% dexpanthenol	B	not proved safe or effective
Vaseline Pure Petroleum Jelly (Chesebrough-Pond's)	ointment: white petrolatum	A	if simplest is best, then this is best

*Author's interpretation of FDA criteria. Based on contents, not claims.

Diarrhea Remedies

Diarrhea, often called "the runs" or "the trots," can be both embarrassing and physically incapacitating. Abdominal cramps, nausea, vomiting, and headache frequently compound the misery it brings.

A variety of illnesses, certain parasitic infestations, and unwisely ingested foods and beverages all can cause diarrhea. If the condition is severe—and it may be life-threatening, particularly for infants—or if it continues for longer than two days, the Panel recommends: *Consult a physician!*

The available over-the-counter products offer no more than symptomatic relief, and work best for the mildest kinds of diarrhea. Self-treatable cases, the Panel says, are those in which the victim is not feverish and is not passing bloody stools. Both of these symptoms require a doctor's attention. Mild and self-treatable diarrhea usually goes away by itself in a day or two. But meanwhile a nonprescription antidiarrheal drug may relieve some discomfort.

DIARRHEA REMEDIES is based on the report of the FDA's Advisory Review Panel on OTC Laxative, Antidiarrheal, Emetic, and Antiemetic Drug Products and on FDA's Tentative Final Monograph on OTC Antidiarrheal Drug Products.

Claims

Accurate
- "For the treatment of diarrhea"
- "Reduces the number of bowel movements in diarrhea"
- "Improves consistency of loose, watery bowel movements in diarrhea"

WARNING:

 Do not use for more than two days, or in the presence of fever, or for children under 3 years of age unless directed by a doctor.

Remedies Available

Given that virtually everyone suffers diarrhea at one time or another, there have been surprisingly few safe and effective nonprescription remedies to treat it. One such drug, polycarbophil, was called to the Panel's attention by the FDA; it has since been formulated into a number of nonprescription preparations. The FDA has also approved activated attapulgite as safe and effective. A third drug, loperamide hydrochloride (*Imodium A-D*; McNeil) is more powerful than the others. It long has been used as a prescription (℞) antidiarrheal. At the manufacturer's request, FDA approved loperamide as safe and effective for short-term self-treatment of acute diarrhea.

Replacing Lost Body Salts: Preliminary Notes

The gravest risk of severe diarrhea, particularly in children, is loss of body fluids and, worse, loss of electrolytes — salt substances that are required to maintain the body's fluid, chemical, and physiological balances. Depletion of one or the other of these body salts can be fatal in a surprisingly short time. *Infants and toddlers with diarrhea require medical attention.*

The Advisory Review Panel on OTC Miscellaneous Internal Drug Products was to have assessed several electrolyte replacements.

Specifically, these drugs included: calcium chloride, magnesium chloride, potassium chloride, sodium bicarbonate, sodium chloride (table salt), and sodium lactate. But the group was disbanded before this work could be done. The FDA or another supplemental Panel may complete this effort.

Medically sanctioned preparations are already available: For infants and young children, the World Health Organization endorses an oral hydration solution that is being widely distributed in Third World countries and is now becoming available without prescription in the United States, as *Pedialyte Solution* (Ross) and *Rehydralyte Solution* (Ross), among others. Alternatively, the Federal Centers for Disease Control (CDC), in Atlanta, suggest the do-it-yourself regimen (*see* the box below).

Meanwhile a new epidemic of the waterborne disease *cholera*— a severe kind of diarrhea—has spread from Asia to South America, and more recently Central America. Some cases have occurred in Americans traveling abroad in epidemic areas.

Home Treatment for Diarrhea

This is the regimen proposed by the Centers for Disease Control (CDC) in Atlanta.

Prepare 2 separate drinking glasses as follows:

Glass Number 1

orange, apple, or other fruit juice (rich in potassium)	8 oz
honey or corn syrup (contain glucose necessary for absorption of essential salts)	½ tsp
table salt (contains sodium and chloride)	1 pinch

Glass Number 2

water (carbonated or boiled if tap water is contaminated)	8 oz
baking soda (sodium bicarbonate)	½ tsp

Drink alternately from each glass. Repeat through the day. Supplement as desired with carbonated beverages, water, or tea. Avoid solid foods. It is important that infants continue breast-feeding and receive plain water as desired, while receiving these salt solutions. Older persons can take OTC antidiarrheal drugs along with these fluids.

Cholera, once often fatal, now can be successfully treated. The primary treatment is to replace the body fluids and electrolytes that are being lost be diarrhea and also by vomiting. The best way to do this, particularly in people who are severely dehydrated and ill, is with electrolyte solutions infused into a vein. This requires hospital care—which should be sought at once. An emergency alternative for people traveling in, or just returned from epidemic areas, is to drink copious amounts of electrolyte replacement fluids like the ones described above. The *Merck Manual*, 12th edition, recommends that solutions containing sugar, salt, potassium, and baking soda, or similar mixtures be given in amounts comparable to the fluid that is being lost. Warm the fluids to close to body temperature, the *Manual* says. Seek medical help.

A Word about Lomotil

One of the most popular antidiarrheal drugs, the world around, is diphenoxylate hydrochloride, which is most familiar under its trade name *Lomotil* (Searle); it also is sold under many other names, including *Lofene* (Lannett) and *Low-Quel* (Halsey). Diphenoxylate is an opiate-like narcotic, although a weak one, that can cause addictive symptoms if taken in large amounts. An overdose can be fatal. To frustrate narcotics abuse, this drug is formulated with a small amount of atropine, which causes dry skin, flushing, rapid heartbeat, and other unpleasant effects.

Diphenoxylate relaxes the colon, which reduces cramping pain. This slows the fecal stream so that more of the water can be reabsorbed before the residue is expelled. The drug thus can provide effective symptomatic relief of diarrhea.

In the United States, *Lomotil* and similar preparations are controlled substances but since they are considered to have only a limited potential for narcotic abuse, they may be obtainable without prescription. In many foreign countries, which is where American travelers may be most likely to want them, diphenoxylates are nonprescription drugs.

Some experts say these drugs may do "more harm than good" in treating traveler's diarrhea, because slowing the bowel's movement may hold back the bacteria that are causing the cramps and diarrhea. The symptoms thus may be "worsened" by taking the drug. The CDC therefore recommends that diphenoxylate be used "with caution" and for not more than two or three days. Also, this drug should not be used by persons with fever or with blood or mucus in their stools, and should not be given to children under 2 years of age except under a doctor's supervision.

Combination Products

The Panel judged most combination preparations as useless, because they contained too little of one or another drug to contribute significantly to the product's over all effectiveness. Tests are required to show that each ingredient makes a statistically significant contribution to the product's antidiarrheal effect. Pending submission of data showing the contribution of each ingredient to the product's effectiveness, the Panel granted only *conditional* approval to a half-dozen oral-dosage combinations. A decade later, the FDA had not granted full approval to any of them, or to any others. (*See* the table Safety and Effectiveness: Combination Products at the end of this Unit).

It would make sense, of course, to have combination products of antidiarrheal ingredients with safe and effective drugs that relieve nausea and vomiting. But no such combination has been found. To mix antidiarrheals with other kinds of active ingredients does *not* make sense unless such a mixture would meet the specific needs of an identifiable group of sick people. None has. So, for the time being all antidiarrheal combinations are disapproved.

Some substances that are active ingredients in other types of drugs are present in small amounts in antidiarrheals. They are intended to improve the products' taste or texture or are included for other pharmacological reasons. They cannot be identified as active ingredients, and claims cannot—or at least should not—be made for the antidiarrheals based on these added ingredients.

Antidiarrheal Drugs

The Panel and FDA judged 2 dozen ingredients in terms of their ability to inhibit or control diarrhea in a safe and effective way. Only a few weathered their critical scrutiny.

APPROVED ANTIDIARRHEAL ACTIVE INGREDIENTS

• ATTAPULGITE, ACTIVATED: Although formulated as both tablet and liquid preparations, attapulgite naturally is a solid, earthen stuff—a special clay (aluminum magnesium silicate), originally dug from a mother lode

that stretches south from Attapulgus, Georgia, to the Florida border.
Other sources have since been found.

Attapulgite's great virtue as an anti-diarrheal is its avid ability
to bind, hold, and hence, thicken water or watery liquids: It is 33
times more absorbent than kaolin (*see* further on) and *absorbs* 8 times
its weight in water. This stuff is inert and had been shown to be nontoxic to animals; the Panel and FDA had little doubt about its safety.
The drug's efficacy was established conclusively in a study in which
patients suffering from diarrhea were given either attapulgite or look-
alike tablets that contained a *placebo*, an inactive dummy drug. The
FDA summarizes the findings in this way:

"Results... indicated that... the active [drug] group had significantly fewer bowel movements, better stool consistency, and fewer
cramps than the subjects in the placebo group." In other studies, which
included 3000 children and 2000 adults, there were no serious complications, albeit 4 percent of adults suffered constipation as a presumably
welcome side effect of this antidiarrheal therapy. Verdict: safe and
effective. *See* the Dosages for Approved Diarrhea Remedies table.

Attapulgite's Other Role: Cleaning Up Behind Cats

Attapulgite is one of a very few safe and effective antidiarrheal drugs
for self-treatment in people. It perhaps has a larger role to play in
society, as a basic ingredient in cat box litter. In Quincy, Florida,
which is a center for cat litter production, the manager of one company was quoted as saying (*New York Times*, Aug. 12, 1984):

"Attapulgite's got probably one of the best absorbencies of any
mineral you're going to find... we use it about as fast as they can
bring it in. We use anywhere from 150 to 200 tons a day."

The United States has some fifty million cats, which eat over two
billion pounds of cat food per year. With attapulgite, the kitty litter industry appears to have a sure-fire winner.

Claims for Attapulgite

Based on the findings described here, the following special claim for attapulgite is accurate:

> • "Relieves cramps in diarrhea"

• *LOPERAMIDE:* This drug is considered significantly more effective than other nonprescription remedies for diarrhea. It has a record of two decades' use as a prescription (℞) drug, and continues to be marketed for prescription use as well as over-the-counter use.

   Loperamide's safety and prompt effectiveness in relieving diarrhea have been demonstrated in several scientifically controlled studies. The exact mode of action is unknown, but it appears to slow the contractile movements in the gut, and so slows down and firms up bowel movements. Less fecal matter is produced; stools become thicker and denser; less water and fewer electrolytes are lost in the fecal stream.

   Loperamide is a synthetic, opium-like drug, but it is not addictive. The American Medical Association reports in its *Drug Evaluations Annual* 1991 that "no significant adverse reactions or drug interactions have been reported."

   The FDA-approved indication is

   • "For the control and symptomatic relief of acute nonspecific diarrhea."

WARNING:

 Do not use for more than 2 days unless directed by a doctor.

   Loperamide is safe for adults and for children over 6 years of age, and is available in liquid and tablet form. *See* the table Dosages for Approved Diarrhea Remedies.

• *POLYCARBOPHIL AND CALCIUM POLYCARBOPHIL:* Polycarbophil is an indigestible synthetic resin with an astonishing capacity to hold fluids: It will absorb 60 times its weight in water. For this reason, it is effective as an antidiarrheal. Polycarbophil absorbs free fecal water, forming a gel. This partially dries out the intestine and allows the fecal matter to solidify into formed stools.

   Animal studies indicate that polycarbophil is safe, and clinical studies in human sufferers of acute and chronic diarrhea have demonstrated the ingredient's effectiveness. It is the only over-the-counter antidiarrheal approved for young children.

Calcium polycarbophil is essentially identical to polycarbophil, but the calcium salt dissolves in water, allowing the compound to be formulated as a liquid medication.

CONDITIONALLY APPROVED ANTIDIARRHEAL ACTIVE INGREDIENTS

• *BISMUTH SALTS: BISMUTH SUBNITRATE AND BISMUTH SUBSALICYLATE:* Products containing bismuth salts are claimed to coat and protect the digestive tract. But tests with animals, which were studied directly, and with people, who were studied with a special internal camera, failed to confirm such an action. Also, it seems clear that most people probably use bismuth compounds after they develop diarrhea and not before. So a protective coating against infectious agents or other toxic substances may not do them much good.

On the *plus* side, the evaluators reviewed some evidence that shows that large and frequent doses of bismuth subsalicylate will control diarrhea in visitors to foreign countries, and more evidence along this line was published after the Panel filed its report. One recent report shows that chewing high-dose bismuth subsalicylate tablets several times a day helps prevent traveler's diarrhea in U.S. visitors to Mexico. However, the FDA has looked at a manufacturer's studies on bismuth subsalicylate as a treatment for traveler's diarrhea, and wrote back to say the data are "insufficient" to demonstrate the effectiveness of the ingredient.

Bismuth subsalicylate is widely used and generally regarded as safe. But the safety of bismuth subnitrate has not been established. Its effectiveness remains to be proved for both of these compounds.

• *CALCIUM HYDROXIDE:* In solution this substance is commonly called *lime water*. It sometimes has a constipating effect when used as an antacid. While it is judged safe, its effectiveness as an antidiarrheal needs to be proved.

• *CHARCOAL, ACTIVATED:* Activated charcoal is obtained by distilling wood pulp, which is then treated to increase its ability to grab and hold onto nearby molecules of chemical substances. Each particle has an enormous surface area available for this purpose—for which reason activated charcoal is a valuable antidote for poisoning. It is considered safe, but no studies show that it is an effective antidiarrheal.

- **KAOLIN:** The virtue of this powdered aluminum clay is that it is quite inert, so it is judged safe. Proponents claim that it grabs and holds some poisons, bacteria, and viruses and may solidify (and thus slow) the flow of the fecal stream.

    In one study, in which monkeys were fed a diarrhea-inducing diet of oranges, carrots, cabbage, and prune juice, the kaolin firmed the animals' stools somewhat, but it did not decrease the number of stools. Evaluators accepted these results but questioned their relevance to diarrhea in humans. Kaolin's effectiveness remains unproved.

- **PECTIN:** Pectin is a plant extract that is used to make jellies jell. The Panel judges it safe when taken in modest amounts. It is not at all clear how the substance may contribute to the relief of diarrhea. In tests in which monkeys were fed diarrhea-inducing diets, pectin, like kaolin (*see* previously), firmed the animals' stools but did not diminish their number. When the diarrhea was induced by disease germs (like those of cholera) or by castor oil or other chemicals, pectin and kaolin both dried up the animals' stools and reduced the number of stools. But clear-cut evidence of pectin's effectiveness in relieving human diarrhea has yet to emerge.

DISAPPROVED ANTIDIARRHEAL INGREDIENTS

- **POTASSIUM CARBONATE:** This chemical was judged safe but not effective as an antidiarrheal because the Panel found it to be an *inactive*, not an active, ingredient.

- **RHUBARB FLUID EXTRACT:** Reviewers were not altogether clear whether it is Chinese rhubarb (*Rheum officinale*) or American rhubarb (*Rheum rhabarbarum*) that they were assessing. But in either case the reviewers gave this substance the verdict: not safe, not effective.

When Greater Relief is Needed

Persistent diarrhea can turn rapidly into a medical emergency, in adults as well as children. Care should be sought at a hospital emergency room if no private physician is available.

The benchmark for diarrhea therapies is *traveler's diarrhea* in tourists, students, or professional visitors (including doctors who study themselves) to such foreign countries as Mexico or Egypt. These are places where Americans run a high risk of this sickness, and where limited time and tight schedules magnify the loss of a day spent cooped up in a hotel room, close to a toilet and a bed.

The current champion among these regimens is the prescription antibiotic combination drug trimethoprim-sulfamethoxazole (*Bactrim*, Roche) alone or in combination with loperamide. A single high dose of *Bactrim* can kill the infectious agent and relieve traveler's diarrhea within an hour, gastroenterologist Charles D. Ericsson, M.D., and several colleagues reported in the *Journal of the American Medical Association* (Jan. 12, 1990). But the most effective regimen was Bactrim + loperamide. The treatment starts with 4 mg of loperamide, and continues with 800 mg and 320 mg respectively of trimetoprim-sulfamethoxazole if the loperamide fails to quell the symptoms quickly. The antibiotic is repeated twice daily for up to three days; the antidiarrheal (2 mg) is repeated after each loose stool. Diarrhea was relieved, on average, *within one hour* with this combination regimen in Dr. Ericsson's study.

Travelers planning to visit countries with poor water supplies and questionable hygienic practices for raw food and water should consider obtaining and carrying these two drugs with them, along with their doctors' instructions on how and when to take them.

Opium Available Over Some Counters

The narcotic drug opium and its refined product, *paregoric* (camphorated tincture of opium) are very effective diarrhea remedies. They are sold over-the-counter in some states and locations, although legally opium is not an OTC drug. Rather, it is a *controlled substance*—a narcotic that has a low potential for abuse. A little atropine is added to make the substance relatively unpleasant, giving the person who takes it a clammy, sweaty feeling, and thereby discouraging abuse.

Opium powder, tincture of opium, and paregoric are sold as antidiarrheals in a diminishing number of nonprescription products, in a slowly-diminishing number of states. By and large, it is the states and locales that allow OTC sales of codeine (another Schedule V narcotic) for coughs that allow opium to be sold for diarrhea. See p. 142 , for a list of states where opium anti-diarrheals may be available without a prescription. Note: Diphenoxylate hydrochloride, described on p. 313, is likely to be available without prescription in these same states.

Dosages for Approved Diarrhea Remedies

Age Group	Activated Attapulgite	Polycarbophil or Calcium Polycarbohil
Adults and children over 12 years	1200 mg after first loose bowel movement, and 1200 mg after each successive bowel movement, not to exceed 8400 mg in 24 hr	1 gram 4 times a day or 2 grams 3 times a day, not to exceed 6 grams in 24 hr
Children 7 to 12 years	600 mg after first loose bowel movement, and 600 mg after each successive bowel movement, not to exceed 4200 mg in 24 hr	0.5 to 1 gram 3 times a day, not to exceed 3 grams in 24 hr
Children 3 to 5 years	300 mg after first loose bowel movement, and 300 mg after each successive bowel movement, not to exceed 2100 mg in 24 hr	0.33 to 0.5 grams 3 times a day, not to exceed 1.5 grams in 24 hr
Children under 3	consult a doctor	consult a doctor

Age Group	loperamide
Adults and children over 12 years	4 mg after first loose bowel movement, and 2 mg after each successive bowel movement, not to exceed 8 mg in 24 hr
Children 9 to 11 years	2 mg after first loose bowel movement, and 1 mg after each successive bowel movement, not to exceed 6 mg in 24 hr
Children 6 to 8 years	2 mg after first loose bowel movement, and 1 mg after each successive bowel movement, not to exceed 4 mg in 24 hr
Children under 6 years	consult a physician

Safety and Effectiveness: Active Ingredients in Over-the-Counter Diarrhea Medications

Active Ingredient	Assessment
attapulgite, activated	safe and effective
bismuth subnitrate	not proved safe or effective
bismuth subsalicylate	safe but not proved effective
calcium polycarbophil	safe and effective
calcium hydroxide	safe but not proved effective
charcoal, activated	safe but not proved effective
kaolin	safe but not proved effective
loperamide	safe and effective
pectin	safe but not proved effective
polycarbophil	safe and effective
potassium carbonate	safe but not effective
rhubarb fluid extract	not safe or effective

Safety and Effectiveness: Combination Products Sold Over-the-Counter to Treat Diarrhea

Safe and Effective

Conditionally Safe and Effective

any combination of 2 or 3 approved ingredients in which 1 or more is present in less than the minimum dosage set by the Panel

any combination of 2 or 3 ingredients in which 1 or more is only conditionally approved

activated attapulgite + pectin

kaolin + pectin

kaolin + hydrated alumina powder

Unsafe or Ineffective

any combination containing an unsafe or an ineffective active ingredient

any combination in which an ingredient is present at a dosage above the maximum set by the Panel

Diarrhea Remedies: Product Ratings

Product and Distributor	Dosage of Active Ingredients	Rating *	Comment
attapulgite (activated)			
Children's Kaopectate (Upjohn)	chewable tablets: 300 mg liquid: 600 mg per tablespoon	A A	
Donnagel (Robins)	liquid: 600 mg per tablespoon chewable tablets: 600 mg	A A	
K-Pek (Rugby)	suspension: 600 mg per table-spoon	A	
Kaopectate Advanced Formula (Upjohn)	liquid concentrate: 600 mg per tablespoon	A	
Parepectolin (Rhone-Poulenc Rorer)		A	
Rheaban Maximum Strength (Pfizer)	tablets: 750 mg	A	
bismuth subgallate			
Devrom (Parthenon)	chewable tablets: 200 mg	C	not submitted to Over-the-Counter Drug Review

Diarrhea Remedies: Product Ratings (contd)

Product and Distributor	Dosage of Active Ingredients	Rating*	Comment
bismuth subsalicylate			
Pepto-Bismol (Procter & Gamble)	**liquid:** 262 mg per tablespoon **chewable tablets:** 262 mg	B B	not proved effective not proved effective
Pink Bismuth (generic)	**liquid:** 262 mg per tablespoonful	B	not proved effective
charcoal, activated			
Charcoal (Paddock)	**tablets:** 325 mg	B	not proved effective
Charcocaps (Requa)	**capsules:** 260 mg	B	not proved effective
loperamide hydrochloride			
Imodium A-D (McNeil-CPC)	**liquid:** 1 mg per tsp. **tablets:** 2 mg	A A	Rx to OTC switch Rx to OTC switch
Loperamide Hydrochloride (Perrigo)	**liquid:** 1 mg per tsp.	A	Rx to OTC switch
polycarbophil			
Mitrolan (A.H. Robins)	**chewable tablets:** 500 mg as cal-cium carbophil	A	
FiberCon (Lederle)		A	

NARCOTIC COMBINATION PRODUCTS[†]

Product and Distributor	Dosage of Active Ingredients	Rating[*]	Comment
Lomotil (Searle)	**tablets, liquid:** 2.5 mg per tablet or tsp. + 0.025 atropine sulfate	A	This FDA-approved drug is outside the OTC Review; it is a Schedule V narcotic that is available OTC in some states and locations, not others. The manufacturer notes on the package information for doctors: "This is *not* an innocuous drug…. dosage recommendations should be strictly adhered to especially in children…"
Diphenoxylate hydrochloride + atropine sulfate (generic)		A	
Parepectolin (Rhone-Poulenc Rorer)	**suspension:** 15 mg opium [3.7 ml paregoric] + 5.5 g kaolin + 162 mg pectin per 2 tablespoonsful	B	neither kaolin nor pectin proved effective
Kaopectolin with Paregoric (generic)		B	*see* previous comment

[*] Author's interpretation of FDA criteria. Based on contents, not claims.
[†] Not available in all states, or on open shelves. Ask your pharmacist for these products.

Diarrhea Remedies: Product Ratings (contd)

NON-NARCOTIC COMBINATION PRODUCTS

Product and Distributor	Dosage of Active Ingredients	Rating*	Comment
Kaolin with pectin (generic)	**suspension:** 5.85 g kaolin + 130 mg pectin per 2 tablespoonsful	B	neither ingredient proved effective
Kaopectolin (generic)		B	*see* previous comment

*Author's interpretation of FDA criteria. Based on contents, not claims.

Digestive Aids

This Unit exemplifies the slow, grinding pace of the Over-the-Counter Drug Review to purge drug stores of worthless, dubious and trivial products—to consumers' great advantage. When the Review began in the late 1960s, more than a hundred ingredients were sold in hundreds, perhaps thousands of products, whose manufacturers stridently claimed they relieved a wide range of digestive distress. Some of these ingredients had odd or exotic names like dog grass, horsetail, and golden seal. Others, such as belladonna were potentially hazardous. (They all are listed in the first edition of this reference work, The Essential Guide to Nonprescription Drugs, *Harper & Row, 1983, pp. 263-66).*

Through the work of the Panel and the follow-up study by FDA analysts and regulators, these drugs have been winnowed out. Some, particularly antacids, have been found to be safe and effective and are reviewed elsewhere in this guide (See ANTACIDS.) *But most have simply been discarded as worthless or unproved. The result: Only two active ingredients remain under consideration as possibly safe and effective*

DIGESTIVE AIDS is based on the report "Digestive Aid Drug Products for OTC Human Use" by the FDA's Advisory Review Panel on OTC Miscellaneous Internal Drug Products and on FDA's Tentative Final Order on these products.

Digestive Aids.

Consumers should, however, observe this caution: Many of these worthless ingredients—which cannot pass scientific scrutiny as drugs— are showing up in health food stores and other retail outlets (and in mail order catalogues), where they may be listed as "nutritional supplements" or under some other rubric. The labels on these ingredients (or products) don't say what their intended use is. So selling them may be legal. But these substances are no more worthwhile and certainly no less hazardous when purchased in this unregulated way than they would be if labeled "nonprescription drug." The only remedies that can be reliably taken to relieve digestive distress—or any other symptom—are those sold as OTC or prescription (R) "drugs" with FDA's approval.

Almost everybody suffers an occasional stomachache after eating. Some people suffer stomachaches quite frequently.

Influenced by advertisements, consumers may blame their problem on "gas" and reach for one of the popular over-the-counter drugs that is claimed to relieve "gas distress." While the discomfort certainly is real, the Panel says that "gas" is probably not its cause—and is almost certainly not the cause if the distress comes in the first half-hour after eating.

Swallowed air accounts for abut 70 percent of the gas in the gut. Everybody swallows air in and with food when they eat. Between meals, gum chewing and cigarette smoking can cause people to swallow air. Many people swallow air when they are anxious. Lesser amounts of gases—including hydrogen, carbon dioxide, and methane— are produced by bacterial breakdown of certain foods, most notably beans and onions, in the large intestine.

A lot of this gas is eliminated from the body by burping or belching. Some gas is absorbed into the bloodstream, and excreted from the lungs in exhalations when we breathe. Much is passed from the anus as *flatus*: One may relieve oneself of one-third to one-and-a-half liters of gas daily in this way!

Surprisingly, people who complain of "gas" may not have any more gas in their guts than others. In a provocative study, gastroenterologists at the Minneapolis Veterans Administration Hospital discovered that "gas-pain" victims had a normal volume of gas but experienced difficulty in moving it outward toward the anus. They also were more likely than normal persons to suffer movement of gas *upward*— that is, from the intestines back into the stomach. Because of these problems they suffered pain from a volume of gas that might not bother other people.

These and related findings convinced the Panel that so-called excessive gas is not the cause of distress immediately after eating and may not be the cause of intestinal distress either.

If not gas, then what is the cause of after-eating discomfort? The reviewers conceded that they do not know for sure. Perhaps distress after eating may result from eating too much. Intestinal distress may also reflect problems in the time it takes food to get through the intestines, the nature of the food eaten, or the behavior of the intestinal bacteria that share our dinners with us.

FDA Griped About 'Gripe Water'

Regulators at FDA take a dim view of a traditional English remedy for infants' upset stomachs. The products they are concerned about are Woodward's *Gripe Water* and gripe waters by other manufacturers.

Woodward's, of London, claims its product relieves "minor tummy upsets" in infants, as well as hiccups and the pain of teething. Gripe waters sometimes are used for *colic*, the much more intense and upsetting distress that many babies — and their parents — experience during the third to sixth month of life. The implicit assumption is that these problems are "gas" pains: Woodward's claims their product provides "the safe and gentle way of relieving baby's wind."

The FDA disagrees and has issued an order to prevent the importation of gripe waters into the United States, where it turns up from time to time in the upscale drugstores and pharmacies.

The Woodward's product contains, among other things, dill oil, dill water, sodium bicarbonate, and about 4 percent alcohol.

Sodium bicarbonate is an acceptable antacid — but only for adults. Dill oil and dill water do not even appear in FDA's master lists of "OTC Drug Review Ingredients." Alcohol does appear, of course, but it is not approved for use in infants, and how it might aid digestion is unclear.

A New York City pediatrician says the only way gripe water might work is by "getting babies a little tipsy." A few teaspoonfuls of gripe water, he and other experts add, is not likely to harm an infant. But given that the preparation contains abut the same alcohol content as beer, perhaps it would be more beneficial for the nanny or the parent to take it—rather than give it to the baby.

Types of Distress

To try to sort out the symptoms and appropriate treatment for what in a simpler age was called simply "upset stomach," "stomachache," or, in children, "a tummy ache," the Panel made the following distinctions:

• *Distress that appears after eating* (postprandial distress). Symptoms arise within a half-hour after a meal. They include feelings of abdominal bloating, distention, fullness, or pressure.

• *Intestinal distress* Symptoms arise from half an hour to several hours after eating. Because of the longer time interval, they may involve the small and large intestines as well as the stomach. They also may be felt lower in the abdomen (below the belly button) as well as in the stomach. Symptoms of intestinal distress also include bloating, distention, fullness, and pressure but may include abdominal pain and cramps or anal flatus (breaking wind).

Panel evaluators say that both forms of digestive distress are brief, self-correcting problems, unrelated to any known organic disease. Symptoms that result from swallowing an excess of air—technically called *aerophagia*—are not considered as belonging to either group. Also, digestive distress is different from stomach acidity, constipation, or diarrhea, which produce different symptoms and require different treatments. *See* the Symptom Key to Drugs for Gastrointestinal Problems.

The Panel's division of digestive complaints into two categories did not please drug manufacturers and others who complained that *bloating*, *fullness*, and *distention* occur both before and after the Panel's 30-minute time mark. These critics argued that consumers pay little attention to *when* these symptoms appear and are not skilled in deciding whether they arise above or below the belly button.

The critics asked that this distinction between *postprandial distress* and *intestinal distress*—which some observers, at least, found useful—be dropped. The FDA agreed to do so, relegating the Panel's effort at clarity to bureaucratic limbo. With this caveat, the Symptom Key to Drugs for Gastrointestinal Problems, on pp. 319-320, will help readers identify the source of gastrointestinal distress they may be enduring, and indicate which unit in this Guide describes the nonprescription drugs that may relieve their symptoms.

How Drugs *Might* Relieve Digestive Distress

Given the lack of knowledge about what really causes digestive distress, evaluators found it hard to define how nonprescription drugs—or any others—might effectively relieve it. Several possibilities are summarized here.

- The active ingredient lowers surface tension on stomach contents. This facilitates absorption of digestive juices, which in turn speeds up digestion and the passage of food contents out of the stomach and into the small intestine.

- The active ingredient speeds up stomach-emptying by changing the stomach's acidity or by some similar mechanism.

- The active ingredient works by increasing contractions of the stomach's smooth muscles, hastening stomach-emptying.

The experts remain unconvinced that any of these mechanisms accounts for the beneficial action of ingredients used to relieve distress after eating — if in fact they have any beneficial action. If you take a drug for after-meal distress, the Panel says you should wait until you feel the symptoms and *not* take the drug before eating, as a preventive measure. No evidence exists to show that any of these medications is effective when taken in advance of the symptoms.

The Panel says that if intestinal distress persists over days or weeks, you should see a doctor. These symptoms could signal the onset of an organic disease that requires medical care.

Combination Products

Reviewers could not find any individual active ingredients that they felt were safe and effective for treating immediate distress after eating or intestinal distress. So, naturally, it follows that no combination of ingredients is wholly approved either.

Symptom Key to Drugs for Gastrointestinal Problems

Symptoms	*Drug Group*	*See*
Acid indigestion, sour stomach, heartburn	antacids	Antacids

Symptom Key to Drugs for Gastrointestinal Problems (contd)

Symptoms	Drug Group	See
Gas pain	anti-gas agents	ANTI-GAS AGENTS
	digestive aids*	this Unit
Constipation	laxatives	LAXATIVES
Diarrhea	anti-diarrheals	DIARRHEA REMEDIES
Digestive distress	digestive aids*	this Unit
Overindulgence in food and drinks	no group name	HANGOVER AND OVERINDULGENCE RELIEVERS

* No approved drugs.

 Claims

Accurate (if a drug is proved safe and effective for this purpose, which none as yet has been)

• "Digestive aid"

• "For the relief of symptoms of gastrointestinal distress such as fullness, pressure, bloating or [a] stuffed feeling (commonly referred to as gas)"

• "For relief of pain and/or cramping which occur after eating"

APPROVED DIGESTIVE-AID ACTIVE INGREDIENTS

None.

CONDITIONALLY APPROVED DIGESTIVE-AID ACTIVE INGREDIENTS

The Panel decided that the following ingredients are, generally speaking, safe in the doses recommended for the relief of immediate after-meal distress. The problem is lack of proof that these drugs are really effective.

• CHARCOAL, ACTIVATED, AND CHARCOAL, WOOD: These preparations appear to be safe. But charcoal can bind and hold any number of commonly used medications, inactivating them, so its safety when used over long periods of time is not clear. Reviewers say therefore that charcoal can be regarded as safe only when taken in dosages of no more than 10 grams per day for up to 7 days. The full 10-gram daily dose should be divided into several smaller doses and taken at different times during the day. Also, persons taking other drugs should ask their doctors whether they can safely use nonprescription charcoal medications.

The binding and inactivating properties mentioned above are termed *adsorption*. Many noxious substances can be neutralized by adsorption, so there is justification for believing that the process may be effective in relieving bloating and other intestinal distress symptoms caused by substances in food. Further, because activated charcoal is one-third more effective in this regard than wood charcoal, the Panel recommends that the former be used for intestinal-distress products.

Nonetheless, until definitive proof of effectiveness is established, the evaluators granted these charcoals only conditional approval.

DISAPPROVED DIGESTIVE-AID ACTIVE INGREDIENTS
None.

When Greater Relief Is Needed

If eating more slowly, or eating less food at a sitting, does not relieve digestive distress, and if the other drugs available over-the-counter for gastrointestinal symptoms are similarly unavailable (*see* Symptom Key for Gastrointestinal Problems), then consider a visit to a gastroenterologist. Ask your family doctor for a referral or phone the university medical center nearest your home for a clinic appointment or a private consultation.

Safety and Effectiveness: Active Ingredients in
Over-the-Counter Products Used to Treat Digestive Distress

Active Ingredient	Panel's Assessment
charcoal, activated	safe, but not proved effective
charcoal, wood	safe, but not proved effective

Safety and Effectiveness: Combination Products Sold
Over-the-Counter to Relieve Digestive Distress

Safe and Effective
None

Conditionally Safe and Effective
acetaminophen + 1 conditionally approved aid for digestive distress

Unsafe or Ineffective
All others

Digestive Aids: Product Ratings

Product and Distributor	Dosage of Active Ingredients	Rating *	Comment
charcoal preparations			
Charcoal (Paddock)	tablets: 325 mg	B	not proved effective
Charcocaps (Requa)	capsules; activated: 260 mg	B	not proved effective
Charcoal Capsules (Rugby)	tablets: 260 mg	B	not proved effective

*Author's interpretation of FDA criteria. Based on contents, not claims.

Douches and Other Vaginal Drugs

Women douche for a variety of reasons, some of which make sense, a few of which do not. Douching may help a woman feel cleaner and fresher. It may relieve itching and minor vaginal irritation. But douching before love-making has not been proved to increase the likelihood of conceiving a boy, as some doctors say it may; and douching after making love certainly will not prevent pregnancy, as more than a few women have learned to their regret.

The Panel defined *vaginal douche* as a liquid preparation used to irrigate the vagina over an indeterminate period of time for one or more of these purposes

cleansing

soothing and refreshing

deodorizing

relieving minor vaginal irritations

reducing the number of pathogenic organisms

changing the vagina's acidity to encourage the growth of normal

DOUCHES AND OTHER VAGINAL DRUGS is based on the report of the FDA's Advisory Review Panel on OTC Contraceptives and Other Vaginal Drug Products.

      vaginal flora (microorganisms)
producing an astringent effect
lowering surface tension
dissolving vaginal discharge and debris

Douching products are sold as pre-mixed liquids, as concentrates, and as powders that must be diluted for use. They may be directed into the vagina from rubber or plastic douche bags, from single-use disposable containers, or from bulb syringes. Alternatively, they can be introduced into the vagina as suppositories that melt when heated to body temperature, releasing their active ingredients. A few vaginal self-treatment drugs are available as ointments or gels.

 Claims

Accurate

For products that contain safe and effective active ingredients for the relief of minor irritations:

- "For temporary relief of minor vaginal irritation and itching"
- "For relief of minor vaginal soreness"

For products that contain safe and effective active ingredients that lower surface and tension, produce a mucolytic or proteolytic effect, or both:

- "Removes vaginal discharge"
- "Removes vaginal secretions"
- "Mild detergent action"
- "Thins out vaginal mucus discharge"

False, Misleading, or Unproved

- "Intimately understood"
- "Contains only the mildest of ingredients"
- "Completely refreshes"
- "Complete feminine hygiene"
- "Intended for all women who want to enjoy extra confidence in meeting people"
- "Complete feminine daintiness"
- "Intimate cleanliness"
- "Gentle"
- "Safe"

- "Removes contraceptive jellies and creams"
- "Safe for delicate membranes"

References to "cleansing," "refreshing," "soothing," or "deodorizing" are *cosmetic* claims that need not be proved and are outside the scope of the OTC Drug Review.

WARNING:

 For products that contain safe and effective ingredients: If a minor irritation has not improved after one week of use, consult your doctor. If symptoms continue, or if redness, swelling, or pain develops, stop douching. Consult your physician if these symptoms persist.

Douches: Cosmetics or Drugs?

The FDA previously treated douches as *cosmetics*, requiring them to carry one of these notices:

- "For cleansing purposes only, after menstruation and after marital relations"
- "For cleansing purposes only. Do not use more than twice weekly unless directed by a physician"

More recently, the FDA and the Panel have decided—on the basis of revisions in the Federal Food, Drug, and Cosmetic Act—that douches may be cosmetics, or drugs, or both. Some reasons for douching (for example, cleansing, soothing and freshening, and deodorizing) are for the most part *cosmetic* reasons. Cosmetics are outside the OTC Review's jurisdiction. If, however, a douche contains medicinal amounts of any active drug ingredient, or if the label claims that it may prevent, mitigate, or otherwise be useful for treating any illness, injury, or disease condition, then it is a *drug*.

These distinctions are sometimes quite fine. Thus, insofar as a product kills bacteria or inhibits their growth, thereby reducing vaginal odor, it is a drug. But these distinctions also are important for consumers to bear in mind because cosmetic ingredients are not required to meet scientific standards for effectiveness. Drug ingredients are. So a buyer can have greater confidence in the effectiveness of a drug ingredient—particularly one that the evaluators have assessed as safe and effective—than in the effectiveness of a cosmetic ingredient for which no proofs are asked.

Douching and Contraception

Many women have become mothers because of their belief that douching after sexual intercourse is an effective contraceptive method. *It is not!* Sperm cells enter the uterus too quickly to be washed away by water or other douching solutions. In fact, they may reach the cervical opening within 30 seconds after ejaculation. Within 90 to 180 seconds, they are securely inside the cervix. As described in the American Pharmaceutical Association publication *Handbook of Nonprescription Drugs*, 9th Ed. (1990): "Post-coital douching has no effect in removing sperm from the upper reproductive tract, and might, in fact, force sperm higher in the tract." The Panel, which shares this judgment, recommends that all douching product labels state explicitly that the products are not intended to prevent pregnancy.

Some women douche after intercourse, whether or not they are protected by a contraceptive. This may be a mistake for women who use spermicides, for if they douche too soon they may wash the contraceptive out while viable sperm cells remain in the vagina. The Panel suggests: Wait at least 6 hours before douching.

Is It Wise to Douche?

The answer is: probably no. In the Panelists' opinion there is widespread overindulgence in douching, for which there is no clear-cut scientific support. They cite "tradition, ignorance, and commercial advertising" as major contributors to the persistence of this practice.

The other side of the coin is that there has seemed to be no good reason *not* to douche. So the reviewers also say that for the normal, healthy, nonpregnant woman who believes she derives some benefit from the practice, there is no medical reason not to. (Douching during pregnancy is discussed further on.)

However, in the decade since the Panel wrote its report—which is long overdue for updating by the FDA—disquieting news about douching has appeared in the medical literature:

- Douching appears to double the risk of *ectopic pregnancy*. This is a dangerous condition in which the embryo develops in a fallopian tube or in the abdomen rather than in the uterus, and must be removed surgically. Researchers reported in the *American Journal of Obstetrics and Gynecology* (vol. 153, no. 7) that among women who had experienced tubal pregnancies, 17 percent douched at least once a week. Among a control group of women who had not had ectopic pregnancies, only 8 percent douched weekly or oftener. Women who used commercial douches were at highest risk. Women who douched with water, or vinegar and water, had only minimal risk. Women who douched less frequently than once weekly had no increased risk of ectopic pregnancy in this study group of women in Salt Lake City, Utah, and Seattle, Washington.

- Women who douche weekly or oftener have a four-fold higher risk of cervical cancer than do women who douche less often or not at all. This finding, too, is in women from Utah, the majority of whom are Mormons. These findings were reported in the *American Journal of Epidemiology* (Feb. 15, 1991).

- *Pelvic inflammatory disease* (PID), which is caused by an infectious microorganism (*Chlamydia*), is commoner in women who douche than in those who do not. Researchers at the University of Washington, in Seattle, reported in the *Journal of the American Medical Association* (April 11, 1990) that women who douched once or twice a month were 1½ times more likely to have PID than were randomly selected women in the population at large. The risk was 3½ times higher for women who douched three or more times per month. Water and vinegar-and-water douching was less risky than the use of commercial douches in disposable bottles. "Long-term [adverse] effects on the vaginal environment of some commercial preparations, particularly those with antimicrobial [drug] activity, might be greater than that of water with vinegar," the researchers say.

Vaginal Hygiene

The vagina is naturally self-cleansing. It is a 3- to 4-inch-long tissue sheath lined on the inside by a unique and relatively thick mucous membrane that is highly responsive to cyclical changes in blood levels of the female sex hormones estrogen and progesterone. A thin superficial layer develops only at *menarche*, when a girl begins to menstruate. It is shed into the vagina itself each month under the influence of estrogen and then regrows. After menopause, this layer vanishes.

The vaginal mucosa is naturally bathed by a variety of secretions: mucus, water, proteins, and salt. Vaginal fluids also include sloughed-off superficial cells from the uterine cavity and vaginal walls, blood, microorganisms and the debris they produce, possibly seminal fluid, and debris from contraceptive and other drugs that have been introduced into the vagina or from tampons.

During menstruation, and throughout the month as well, vaginal secretions gravitate downward and outward. Douching may enhance this natural self-cleansing process.

The Vaginal Flora

The vagina is naturally inhabited by large numbers of microorganisms that together are called the *vaginal flora.* Major components are

cocci

coliforms

diphtheroids

facultative anaerobes

fungi (including *Candida albicans*)

lactobacilli (Döderlein's bacilli)

Micrococcacus

Trichomonas

The normal acidity of the vagina (pH 4.0), sustained by lactic acid secretions from the resident lactobacilli, is required for maintenance of the normal vaginal flora. It also helps protect against overgrowth by resident bacteria or other organisms from outside sources.

Under abnormal conditions, some microorganisms that normally are present in the vagina overgrow. This results in vaginal discharge, itching and irritation, and vaginal malodor—the symptoms of *vaginitis*. The symptoms may also be produced by microorganisms invading from the outside.

It may be impossible for a woman to decide for herself which kinds of organisms are causing vaginitis. This may make effective self-treatment difficult, since different microorganisms respond to treatment by different drugs. At the same time, many women come to recognize two of the commonest types of vaginitis: those caused by *Candida albicans* and related yeasts and those caused by the flagella *Trichomonas vaginalis*. Both "yeast" and "tric," as they have come to be called, produce intense itching, inflammation, and malodorous vaginal discharge, which in the case of yeast tends to be whitish in color. The Contraceptive and Vaginal Drug Panel believed that these infections should be diagnosed by a doctor who should then supervise their treatment. But the Antimicrobial II Panel said there is a place for self-treatment for yeast infections in the form of nonprescription drugs, and the FDA has concurred, with this proviso: The first time a woman experiences the intense—sometimes agonizing—itching of a yeast infection, she should seek medical help. If she subsequently suffers another attack that she recognizes as "yeast," she can treat herself, using one of the potent antifungal agents that the FDA recently switched to over-the-counter status for this purpose. (*See* 'YEAST' KILLERS FOR FEMININE ITCHING.) No over-the-counter drug is approved for the self-treatment of self-diagnosed trichomoniasis.

Changes in the vaginal flora will alter a woman's vaginal odor, and infectious microorganisms can produce unpleasant smells as well as itching and other symptoms. If douching successfully eliminates an unpleasant or unaccustomed odor, and clears up minor symptoms that accompany it, then a woman has no further cause for concern. But if these symptoms persist for several days, experts advise consulting a doctor.

Risks for Pregnant Women

Some douche ingredients are irritating or cause allergic reactions. A woman who notices redness, swelling, itching, or other symptoms after douching should stop using the product temporarily and consider changing to a different brand. A more insidious hazard, in the Panel's view, is systemic poisoning resulting from the absorption of douche ingredients across the vaginal wall and into the bloodstream.

Many factors influence vaginal absorption of drugs, including the type of drug and its base, the user's age, and the stage of her menstrual cycle. What *is* certain is that absorbed drugs can be directly injurious to the woman herself and may cross the placenta and damage her fetus if she is pregnant.

The evaluators have taken one step to reduce this risk: They have identified as "unsafe" a number of douche ingredients that are general poisons. A second step is up to women: Do not douche if you are pregnant, the Panel says, except with the approval of your physician!

The risk of drug absorption is not the only reason for pregnant women to avoid douching. Panel members who are obstetricians report from their own experiences with pregnant patients, as well as from reports in the medical literature, that the proliferation of blood vessels in the placenta and in the vaginal and uterine walls can set the stage for serious douching mishaps. The worst possible risk is the introduction of an air bubble into one of the uterine blood vessels. In one reported case, when the air reached the woman's brain, she died.

Douching solutions that enter the uterus can induce abortion. If they pass through the fallopian tubes, they may carry microorganisms into the abdominal cavity—seeding a severe, possibly life-threatening infection. While these are uncommon risks, experts urge that pregnant women douche only after consulting their doctors, if at all.

Combination Products

No combination douching products now marketed warranted the Panel's approval as safe and effective. Conditional approval was granted to 8 combinations that were submitted for its assessment. The balance were rejected as unsafe or ineffective. (*See* the Safety and Effectiveness: Combination Products table at the end of this Unit.)

Categories of Products

The Panel divided the active drug ingredients in douches into four groups:
- *Anti-irritants* relieve minor itching and irritation, principally by killing or inhibiting the causative microorganisms.
- *Acidifiers* are alleged to encourage normal flora (which dis-

courage infectious microorganisms) by enhancing the acidity of vaginal secretions. A few active ingredients have the opposite, or *alkalizing*, effect.

• *Astringents* pucker the vaginal mucosa and pull protein-type substances out of the vaginal secretions. This may *feel* good, but the Panel's report offers no explanation of how or why this is a medicinal benefit.

• *Detergents* lower surface tension on the walls of the vagina and soften, loosen, and help remove mucus and other secretions.

The active ingredients that actually or allegedly provide these benefits are described under their respective headings, which follow. Because some ingredients are said to provide two or more of these actions, they are assessed separately under each appropriate heading.

Anti-irritants

Perhaps the commonest medicinal claim made for douches is that they relieve minor vaginal itching, irritation, and soreness. Two dozen ingredients for which this claim is made were submitted for assessment, but only one ingredient was approved. Given the Panel's many unfavorable reports, some of the claims made for douche products seem particularly immodest.

 Claims for Anti-irritants

Accurate
• "For relief of minor vaginal irritation and itching"
• "For temporary relief of minor vaginal irritation and itching"
• "For relief of minor vaginal soreness"

Unproved, False, or Misleading
• "Complete feminine hygiene"
• "Reduces the number of pathogenic organisms"

WARNING:

 If minor irritation has not improved after one week, consult your doctor. If redness, swelling, or pain develops, stop douching. Consult your doctor if symptoms persist.

APPROVED ANTI-IRRITANT ACTIVE INGREDIENTS

• *POVIDONE-IODINE 0.15 TO 1.3 PERCENT:* This preparation puts iodine, which reliably kills germs, into a chemical complex with povidone, which holds the iodine, and releases it slowly onto the vaginal surface or other tissues that this complex may come in contact with. (*See* Povidone-Iodine in FIRST AID ANTISEPTICS.) A wide variety of studies have been performed in animals and on people to assess the safety of povidone-iodine. The Panel said it is safe, and FDA agrees.

Is it also effective? The evidence cited by the Panel to show that povidone-iodine relieves vaginal irritation and itching was skimpy at best. Nevertheless, its judgment is—safe and effective.

CONDITIONALLY APPROVED ANTI-IRRITANT ACTIVE INGREDIENTS

• *ALLANTOIN:* No report has ever appeared in the medical literature suggesting that this ingredient causes side effects, so the Panel grants that it is safe. But evaluators were given no data to show that allantoin relieves minor vaginal irritations. Conclusion: safe but not proved effective.

• *ALOE VERA, STABILIZED GEL:* This leaf substance from the aloe vera plant has been used medicinally since ancient times. The crude plant extract deteriorates within hours, but one manufacturer claims to have stabilized the active substance in a medicinal gel. Standard animal tests have demonstrated the basic safety of stabilized aloe vera, and in the one hundred reports submitted to the present Panel not one adverse effect was reported. Clearly the substance is safe.

Effectiveness is another matter. Tests in the laboratory demonstrated that aloe vera kills a number of microorganisms that cause vaginal itching and irritation. These include *C. albicans, Staphylococcus aureus, Streptococcus viridans,* and *T. vaginalis.* But clinical reports on the use of aloe vera in treating women were found wanting. So the Panel says its effectiveness remains to be proved, even though aloe vera is safe.

• **BENZALKONIUM CHLORIDE AND BENZETHONIUM CHLORIDE:** These compounds, assessed together, have long been used in douches and vaginal compounds. Practically no complaints have been received from women saying the products were ineffective or caused adverse reactions. But the Panel says the medical and scientific view of these drugs—once highly favorable—has now changed. There is concern that while they effectively kill microorganisms in the test tube, they may be far less serviceable in actual use. They are, for example, inactivated by many natural and manufactured substances including soaps, human tissue, proteins, and even the containers in which they are packaged. Also, some bacterial organisms resist these drugs and, in fact, may actually grow more rapidly in their presence, a risk evaluators believe must be assessed.

On top of the new questions that have arisen about the safety of benzalkonium chloride and benzethonium chloride, reviewers received no data that clearly show that these drugs really work in treating minor vaginal irritation. So the Panel concludes that both the safety and effectiveness of these ingredients must be proved if they are to be granted a better than conditional approval.

• **BENZOCAINE:** A highly effective anesthetic, benzocaine has an impressive safety record; because of this the present Panel rates benzocaine safe, despite a paucity of data on its use in the vagina. The effective concentration of benzocaine is generally recognized as being between 5 and 20 percent. The concentrations in vaginal suppositories assessed by the Panel are much lower (between 0.2 and 0.65 percent) and the experts doubt that they are strong enough to effectively relieve vaginal itching and irritation. So if manufacturers wish to continue to market such low doses of benzocaine, evaluators say, they must demonstrate through scientific studies that low doses of this anesthetic are in fact effective.

• **BORON COMPOUNDS: BORIC ACID, BOROGLYCERIN, SODIUM BORATE, SODIUM PERBORATE:** These compounds have been widely used medicinally, and they do kill some microorganisms. But they also have been discovered to be extremely potent poisons, so their use as drugs has fallen off rapidly in recent years. The Panel claims that "a serious question of safety exists" when these compounds are used in concentrations over 1 percent. In addition to their questionable safety no evidence was presented to show that boric acid and related compounds are effective in treating self-diagnosable, minor vaginal irritations. The Panel concluded that boric acid and related compounds are not proved safe or effective.

• *EDETATE DISODIUM AND EDETATE SODIUM:* The edetates hold (bind) mineral particles, including calcium and zinc. Theoretically this action prevents these essential "nutrients" from being eaten by microorganisms that are causing vaginal complaints.

Edetates are widely used in food processing and have been assumed to be safe. But the Panel notes that loss of zinc in the early stage of human embryonic development can lead to serious birth defects, so it questions the safety of the edetates and strongly warns pregnant women not to use them.

If the safety issue were clearly resolved, the evaluators believe these compounds might win a permanent place as safe and effective anti-irritants: They do appear to be effective against *T. vaginalis*, which causes trichomoniasis. But further studies are still needed to establish this effectiveness when the drugs are used in self-treatment. In sum, both the safety and effectiveness of edetate disodium and edetate sodium remain to be proved. However, these compounds may be recommended by a doctor for treating trichomoniasis once it has been determined that this organism is responsible for itching, irritation, or other vaginal symptoms. Treatment with edetate compounds should be under a doctor's supervision.

• *NONOXYNOL 9 AND OCTOXYNOL 9:* These two closely related compounds (*see* Approved Spermicides in CONTRACEPTIVES) are considered safe. The Panel reviewed studies that suggest that when one of these compounds is used in a douche, it will reduce the count of microorganisms responsible for vaginal irritation. Studies in culture dishes indicate that the flagella *T. vaginalis*—the cause of "tric"—are inhibited by the *-oxynol* drugs. The reviewers were impressed by this evidence, but not convinced. They call for testing to see if effectiveness can be clearly demonstrated. Verdict: safe but not proved effective.

• *OXYQUINOLINE CITRATE AND OXYQUINOLINE SULFATE:* These compounds were once used to treat gonorrhea and other infections. No adverse effects were reported. In recent years, however, it has been suggested that they might cause cancer and genetic damage. Until such questions are settled, their safety remains in doubt.

As to whether they really work, the Panel received no data to show that these drugs are effective in relieving minor vaginal irrita-

tion, despite their long use as antimicrobial agents. So both safety
and effectiveness must be proved.

• PHENOL AND PHENOLATE SODIUM (UNDER **1.5** PERCENT): Phenol is the antiseptic
ingredient that has that characteristic "medicinal" smell. Phenol also
is the active ingredient in phenolate sodium. In recent years, phenol
has been shown to be extremely toxic. The present Panel concurs
with the Antimicrobial I Panel that in concentrations above 1.5 percent it is too dangerous to use, but lower concentrations may be safe.
(*See* PHENOL: SPECIAL NOTE.) The reviewers believe phenol may
effectively relieve vaginal irritation, but studies to prove this have not
yet been done. At present, phenol at 1.5 percent concentration or less
is listed as not proved safe or effective.

• SODIUM BORATE: *See* Boron Compounds.

• SODIUM EDETATE: *See* Edetate Disodium and Edetate Sodium.

• SODIUM PERBORATE: *See* Boron Compounds.

DISAPPROVED ANTI-IRRITANT ACTIVE INGREDIENTS

• PHENOL AND THE PHENOL COMPOUNDS: Including phenolate sodium and sodium salicylic acid phenolate (over 1.5 percent phenol)

These compounds are hazardous because phenol is a potent
nerve poison. There is little doubt that it will be absorbed through the
vaginal wall and into the bloodstream when these compounds are
applied to the vagina in douches or other over-the-counter medications. Although, generally speaking, phenol is mildly effective as a
topical antimicrobial agent, the reviewers said that studies submitted
on its use as a vaginal drug were inadequate. Conclusion: Phenol and
its derivatives are unsafe and ineffective if used in concentrations
over 1.5 percent phenol in douches or other nonprescription vaginal
drug products.

• SODIUM SALICYLATE: The Panel says it is not aware of any data to show
that sodium salicylate is either safe or effective when used intravagi-
nally. In sum: not safe and not effective.

• SODIUM SALICYLIC ACID PHENOLATE: *See* Phenol and the Phenol Compounds.

Vaginal Acidifiers and Alkalizers

Vaginal secretions are somewhat acidic; they have a pH of about 4.0.
This acidity is maintained by bacteria, called lactobacilli, that secrete

lactic acid. Vaginal acidity helps prevent overgrowth of invasive, irritating, disease-producing bacteria, most of which cannot thrive in an acid milieu. The acidic nature of this region also appears to prevent these dangerous bacteria from migrating upward through the cervix, where they could cause infections in the uterus and the abdominal cavity.

Women have apparently long understood the hygienic value of maintaining vaginal acidity; how else can one explain the wide use of vinegar for douching! Other acids are included in commercial preparations. What remains unclear is whether douching adds enough acid for a long-enough period of time to stimulate the normal flora (microorganisms). Also unclear is whether this stimulation helps relieve vaginal symptoms. (For the use of lactobacilli to acidify the vagina and control yeast infections, *see* p. 1037 "Will Yogurt Stop Yeast?")

Claims for Acidifiers and Alkalizers

Accurate (If a manufacturer should prove it to be so)
• "Helps keep vagina in its normal acid state"

Unproved, False, or Misleading
• "Completely compatible with normal vaginal environment"

• "Formula like the natural environment in your own body"

• "Buffered to control a normal vaginal pH"

• "pH 3.5"

• "Alters vaginal pH"

The claim is made by some manufacturers that *reducing* the vaginal acidity by using an alkalizing or neutralizing agent will help restore the natural vaginal flora. Evaluators have the same doubts about this claim as they do about those made for acidifiers. Two of the conditionally approved ingredients, sodium bicarbonate and sodium carbonate, are alkalizers and are identified as such.

WARNING:

 If vaginal itching, redness, swelling, or pain develops, douching should be discontinued. If the symptoms persist, consult a physician.

APPROVED ACTIVE INGREDIENTS FOR CHANGING ACID-BASE BALANCE

None. The Panel evaluated a number of mild acids used for douching. It could not find any one of them that it could say, with confidence, is safe and effective.

CONDITIONALLY APPROVED ACTIVE INGREDIENTS FOR CHANGING ACID-BASE BALANCE

The Panel gave tentative assent to most of the acidifiers and alkalizers it considered. Its principal findings are summarized here.

- *ACETIC ACID:* Acetic acid is the acid in household vinegar, which has a venerable history of use for douching; it contains 4 to 6 percent acetic acid. The usual dose is 1½ teaspoonfuls of vinegar in a quart or a liter of water. Reviewers believe this dosage is safe. Vinegar may also be effective in encouraging the growth of normal vaginal flora, but studies that could clearly establish this remain to be done. Therefore the verdict is: safe but not proved effective.

- *BORIC ACID:* This acid, described as an anti-infective on p. 378, has not been shown to be either safe or effective in altering the acid-base balance in the vagina.

- *CITRIC ACID:* Like vinegar, this is a douche material with long years of use. With no reports of toxicity or irritation, evaluators judged citric acid safe. No hard data were present to prove that citric acid douches in fact change the vaginal acidity or have a beneficial effect on the vaginal flora. In short: As a douche ingredient citric acid is safe in the currently marketed concentrations of 0.1 to 0.5 percent, but proof of effectiveness is lacking.

- *LACTIC ACID AND THE COMBINATION OF LACTIC ACID + SODIUM LACTATE:* These ingredients have for a long time been used for douching, and they have the theoretical advantage that lactic acid is the principal *natural* acid in the vagina. Concentrated lactic acid can be quite corrosive, but the weak concentrations found in douches (0.4 to 1.3 percent) were judged safe. Sodium lactate is neutral and nontoxic, and no reports of serious toxic consequences exist despite a long history of use in douches.

  Although there is every reason to believe that lactic acid and lactic acid combined with sodium lactate will help maintain the normal, acidic atmosphere of the vagina, it has not been satisfactorily demonstrated that these chemicals remain there long enough to do very much good. So, pending studies that clarify this question, the Panel's assessment of lactic acid, alone or in combination with sodium lactate, is that it is safe but not proved effective.

• SODIUM BICARBONATE: A common household chemical better known as *baking soda*, sodium bicarbonate does not acidify the vagina. On the contrary, it alkalizes, or neutralizes, it—at least briefly. Although evaluators could find no evidence to substantiate sodium bicarbonate's safety when used in douching, the compound is so widely used in food and as a home remedy that the Panel accepts it as safe.

But the reviewers claim to have no idea how neutralizing the vaginal secretions might enhance the growth of normal bacterial flora. In fact, no studies submitted show that brief treatment with sodium bicarbonate has any lasting effect whatsoever. So while safe, the chemical's effectiveness remains strongly in doubt.

• SODIUM BORATE: *See* Boric acid.

• SODIUM CARBONATE: Like sodium bicarbonate, this compound has an alkalizing effect. It is quite corrosive at high concentrations. Even in the extreme dilutions in which it is formulated into douches its safety has not been well established. Neither is it clear to reviewers what, if any, effect its use has on the normal microorganisms of the vagina. Conclusion: Both safety and effectiveness need to be proved.

• SODIUM PERBORATE: *See* Boric acid.

• TARTARIC ACID: This weak acid is a byproduct of grape fermentation in the production of wine. At low concentrations, it is considered safe. But the Panel received no data from manufacturers to show that adding tartaric acid to a douche will enhance vaginal acidity or that this will encourage the growth of normal vaginal flora. While safe, tartaric acid is yet to be shown effective as a vaginal acidifier.

• VINEGAR: *See* Acetic acid.

DISAPPROVED ACTIVE INGREDIENTS FOR CHANGING ACID-BASE BALANCE

None.

Astringents

The Panel has virtually nothing to say about whether an astringent is pharmacologically useful—and, if so, how—in a douche or other vaginal preparation. Generally speaking, astringents create a puckery sensation when applied to the skin or mucous membranes. They also pull proteins—including cellular debris and microorganisms—out of solution and concentrate them. This may facilitate their removal from the body.

APPROVED ASTRINGENT ACTIVE INGREDIENTS

None.

CONDITIONALLY APPROVED ASTRINGENT ACTIVE INGREDIENTS

• *ALUM:* Alum is a widely used astringent that may consist of ammonium aluminum sulfate (*See* p. 895) or potassium aluminum sulfate, both of which are aluminum salts. Alum has a long medicinal history in the treatment of animals and humans, and while it is mildly toxic in high concentrations, the Panel says that the doses used in vaginal products (between 0.03 and 0.06 percent) appear to be safe. These doses, however, are far below the concentrations at which alum is usually regarded as being effectively astringent. So their effectiveness must be proved. Also, if alum is to be used at concentrations of 0.5 to 5 percent—doses generally recognized as effective—then its safety ought to be proved. At present no data are available to show that these concentrations are safe for intravaginal application. Here the Panel's verdict is twofold: Alum can be considered not proved safe *or* not proved effective, depending on the dosage.

• *BORON COMPOUNDS: BORIC ACID, BOROGYLCERIN, SODIUM BORATE, SODIUM PERBORATE:* These aforementioned compounds have not been shown to be either safe or effective astringents for use in the vagina.

• *ZINC SULFATE:* The dose of zinc sulfate currently used in douches, 0.02 percent, is low enough to be safe, but it is far below what are considered to be effective astringent levels. So if the currently used dose is maintained, it must be proved effective. And if the dose generally accepted as effective is used, it will have to be proved safe for use in the vagina. In short, depending on the concentration in which it is used, zinc sulfate is assessed as either not proved safe *or* not proved effective for use in the vagina.

DISAPPROVED ASTRINGENT ACTIVE INGREDIENTS

None.

Detergents

Many douche products contain ingredients that lower surface tension on the vaginal wall. This reduction facilitates the removal of vaginal secretions, discharge, and debris. Such preparations are said to have a cleansing or a *detergent* effect.

 Claims

Accurate
- "Removes vaginal discharge"
- "Removes vaginal secretions"
- "Mild detergent action"
- "Thins out vaginal mucus, discharge"

WARNING:

 If vaginal itching, redness, swelling, or pain develops, stop douching. Consult your physician if symptoms persist.

APPROVED DETERGENT ACTIVE INGREDIENTS

The four vaginal detergents considered safe were assessed in pairs by the Panel. They are treated this way in the discussion that follows.

- *DIOCTYL SODIUM SULFOSUCCINATE AND SODIUM LAURYL SULFATE:* Pharmacologically, these are similar compounds. They are generally recognized as wetting, solubilizing, mucus-removing agents. Although toxic in high doses, they are judged safe at the levels used in douches: 0.002 percent of dioctyl sodium sulfosuccinate; 0.01 to 0.02 percent of sodium lauryl sulfate.

The Panel cites no data to show that these ingredients are specifically useful. Nevertheless, on the basis of the compounds' recognized detergent properties and wide use in various drugs, they were judged effective as well as safe for vaginal application as long as the aforementioned dose levels are maintained.

These drugs are also safe and effective for the treatment of trichomoniasis when this condition has been diagnosed by a physician, who then supervises their use in treating the infection.

• NONOXYNOL 9 AND OCTOXYNOL 9 When used in spermicides these surface-acting compounds were found to be safe. The Panel's report does not mention any specific evidence of how well these compounds work to soften and loosen discharge and debris from the vagina. The vote for a rating of "effective" is based on how well they perform in other products used for wetting, solubilizing, and mucus removal.

The safe and effective dose for products that contain nonoxynol 9 is 0.0176 percent. The safe and effective dose of octoxynol 9 is 0.088 percent.

CONDITIONALLY APPROVED DETERGENT ACTIVE INGREDIENTS

The Panel was able to grant only conditional approval to several drugs that are alleged to help remove mucus and other debris from the vaginal wall. In most instances it is effectiveness rather than safety that remains in doubt.

• ALKYL ARYL SULFONATE Animal studies confirm that this substance, commercially used as an insecticide, is safe. But no studies were submitted to show that alkyl aryl sulfonate removes mucus from the vagina. The Panel has doubts about its effectiveness. The reviewers categorize the compound as safe, but stipulate that its effectiveness must be established through testing if this preparation is to remain on the market.

• BORON COMPOUNDS: BORIC ACID, BOROGYLCERIN, SODIUM BORATE, SODIUM PERBORATE: The potent toxin boron makes these substances doubtfully safe for vaginal use. No evidence was presented to show that boron derivatives actually work to soften, loosen, or remove mucus or other secretions and debris. The Panel's decision: not proved safe or effective.

- **PAPAIN:** This protein-dissolving enzyme from the papaya tree is the principal ingredient in meat tenderizers. Papain has seen long-term use for the treatment of open wounds. Since no adverse effects have been reported, the present Panel feels that papain is safe for use in the vagina, even though no *specific* toxicity studies were submitted. No data were submitted to show that this enzyme effectively removes secretions from the vaginal wall when used in a douche. Conclusion: safe but not proved effective.
- **SODIUM BICARBONATE:** The Panel lists this substance (household baking soda) as safe but not proved effective as a detergent-type drug for use in the vagina.

DISAPPROVED DETERGENT ACTIVE INGREDIENT

None.

INACTIVE INGREDIENTS

A variety of inactive ingredients are put into douches and other vaginal self-treatments for cosmetic or formulary purposes.

For the most part they are harmless, but the Panel expresses concern about the safety of two of them. Silica (fine) is abrasive and potentially dangerous to the soft tissues of the vagina. Camphor is readily absorbed through mucosal tissues and is highly toxic. (*See* CAMPHOR: SPECIAL NOTE.)

- *ALCOHOL*
- *AMERCHOL L 101*
- *AROMATIC OILS*
- *CAMPHOR*
- *CETYL ALCOHOL*
- *CHLOROTHYMOL*
- *EUCALYPTOL*
- *FRAGRANCE*
- *GLYCERIN*
- *ISOPROPYL MYRISTATE*
- *LACTOSE*
- *MENTHOL*
- *METHYLPARABEN*

- *METHYLSALICYLATE*
- *OIL OF EUCALYPTUS*
- *OIL OF PEPPERMINT*
- *POLYSORBATE 20*
- *POTASSIUM HYDROXIDE*
- *PROPYLENE GLYCOL*
- *PROPYLPARABEN*
- *PURIFIED WATER*
- *SILICA, FINE*
- *SODIUM CHLORIDE*
- *STEARIC ACID*
- *SODIUM SULFATE*
- *THYMOL*
- *TRAGACANTH*
- *WATER-SOLUBLE INGREDIENTS OF CHLOROPHYLL*

Vaginal Moisturizers May Relieve Dryness

Dryness in an organ that normally should remain moist distresses many women—some 25 million of them according to one manufacturer. The dryness causes irritation, itching, and other discomfort. It is painful and can frustrate sexual intercourse.

Lubricant products have long been sold for use immediately before sexual intercourse. But in recent years, some manufacturers have begun to produce long-acting vaginal moisturizer products that are claimed to sustain internal moisture in the vagina when applied as infrequently as three times a week. They are advertised as specifically useful for new mothers, menopausal women, and others who suffer from vaginal dryness.

These products were not assessed in the Over-the-Counter Drug Review. It is not clear which of their ingredients, if any, are considered to be active ingredients by the agency and which are not. One product contains the moisture-holding substance polycarbophil, which the FDA considers an active ingredient when it is used as a remedy for diarrhea. (*See* pp. 304-305.)

Safety and Effectiveness: Panel's Assessment of Active Ingredients in Over-the-Counter Douches and Other Vaginal Applications

Active Ingredient	As Anti-Irritant	As Acidifier or Alkalinizer	As Astringent	As Detergent
acetic acid (vinegar)		safe but not proved effective		
alkyl aryl sulfonate				safe but not proved effective
allantoin	safe but not proved effective			
aloe vera, stabilized gel	safe but not proved effective			
alum			safe but not proved effective	
ammonium aluminum sulfate (See alum)				
benzalkonium chloride	not proved safe or effective			
benzethonium chloride	not proved safe or effective			

Safety and Effectiveness: Panel's Assessment of Active Ingredients in Over-the-Counter Douches and Other Vaginal Applications (contd)

Active Ingredient	As Anti-irritant	As Acidifier or Alkalinizer	As Astringent	As Detergent
benzocaine	safe but not proved effective			
boric acid	not proved safe or effective	not proved safe or effective	not proved safe or effective	not proved safe or effective
boroglycerin	not proved safe or effective	not proved safe or effective	not proved safe or effective	not proved safe or effective
citric acid		safe but not proved effective		
dioctyl sodium sulfosuccinate				
edetate disodium	not proved safe or effective			safe and effective
edetate sodium	not proved safe or effective			
lactic acid		safe but not proved effective		safe but not proved effective

lactic acid + sodium lactate	safe but not proved effective	
nonoxynol 9	safe but not proved effective	safe and effective
octoxynol 9	safe but not proved effective	safe and effective
oxyquinoline citrate	not proved safe or effective	
oxyquinoline sulfate	not proved safe or effective	
papain		safe but not proved effective
phenol (under 1.5%)	not proved safe or effective	
phenol (over 1.5%)	not safe or effective	
phenolate sodium (under 1.5% phenol)	not proved safe or effective	
phenolate sodium (over 1.5% phenol)	not safe or effective	
potassium aluminum sulfate (See alum)		
povidone-iodine	safe and effective	

Safety and Effectiveness: Panel's Assessment of Active Ingredients in Over-the-Counter Douches and Other Vaginal Applications (contd)

Active Ingredient	As Anti-irritant	As Acidifier or Alkalinizer	As Astringent	As Detergent
sodium bicarbonate (alkalizer)		safe but proved effective		safe but not proved effective
sodium borate	not proved safe or effective	not proved safe or effective	not proved safe or effective	not proved safe or effective
sodium carbonate (alkalizer)		not proved safe or effective		
sodium lactate		safe but not proved effective		
sodium lauryl sulfate				safe and effective
sodium perborate	not proved safe or effective	not proved safe or effective	not proved safe or effective	not proved safe or effective
sodium salicylate	not safe or effective			
sodium salicylic acid phenolate	not safe or effective			
tartaric acid		safe but not proved effective		

	safe but not proved effective
vinegar (*See* acetic acid)	
zinc sulfate	

Safety and Effectiveness: Combination Products Sold Over-the-Counter for Douching and Other Vaginal Self-Treatment

---

Safe and Effective

Conditionally Safe and Effective

citric acid + papain
oxyquinoline sulfate + alkyl aryl sulfonate + edetate disodium
oxyquinoline citrate + boric acid + alum + zinc sulfate
nonoxynol 9 + edetate sodium
alum + zinc sulfate
benzalkonium chloride + edetate disodium
sodium borate + sodium lauryl sulfate
phenol + sodium phenolate
sodium lactate + lactic acid + octoxynol 9
sodium lauryl sulfate + sodium bicarbonate + sodium carbonate
sodium perborate + sodium borate + sodium lauryl sulfate
stabilized aloe vera gel + allantoin

Not Safe or Not Effective

phenol (greater than 1.5%) + sodium borate + sodium salicylate
sodium salicylic acid phenolate (phenol greater than 1.5%) + boroglycerin + benzocaine
sodium salicylic acid phenolate (phenol greater than 1.5%) + boroglycerin + benzocaine + povidone-iodine

Douches: Product Ratings

SINGLE-INGREDIENT PRODUCTS

Product and Distributor	Dosage of Active Ingredients	Rating *	Comment
acetic acid (vinegar)			
Massengill Disposable (SmithKline-Beecham)	liquid	B	not proved effective
Massengill Vinegar + Water Extra Mild (SmithKline-Beecham)		B	
Summer's Eve Disposable (Fleet)		B	
povidone-iodine			
Betadine Medicated Disposable Douche (Purdue Frederick)	solution: 0.3% when reconstituted	A	
Betadine Medicated Premixed Disposable Douche (Purdue Frederick)	solution: 0.3%	A	
Summer's Eve Medicated Disposable Douche (Fleet)	solution: 0.23% when reconstituted	A	

Douches: Product Ratings (contd)

Product and Distributor	Dosage of Active Ingredients	Rating *	Comment
sodium bicarbonate			
Massengill Baking Soda Freshness (SmithKline-Beecham)	**solution:** sodium bicarbonate in sanitized water	B	not proved effective

COMBINATION PRODUCTS

Product and Distributor	Dosage of Active Ingredients	Rating *	Comment
Massengill (Beecham Products)	**liquid concentrate:** lactic acid + sodium lactate + sodium bicarbonate + octoxynol 9	B	first two ingredients not proved effective
	powder: ammonium alum + phenol	C	not an approved combination; phenol not proved safe and effective
Trichotine (Reed & Carnrick)	**liquid:** sodium lauryl sulfate + sodium perborate	B	sodium perborate not proved safe or effective
Triva (Boyle)	**powder:** 2% oxyquinoline sulfate + 35% alkyl aryl sulfonate + 0.33% disodium edetate	B	not proved effective

*Author's interpretation of Panel criteria. Based on contents, not claims.

Ear-Care Aids

Ear disorders are difficult to self-diagnose; they usually require medical attention and prescription drugs. For these reasons the FDA has approved only one type of nonprescription self-treatment of the ear: agents that soften and loosen ear wax. Earache, drainage of fluid from the ear, itching, any hearing impairment, and ringing in the ears or other unusual sensations all require medical attention. (Specialists who provide this ear care are called *otologists* or *otolaryngologists*.)

One other condition, *swimmer's ear*, may be amenable to preventive and self-treatment measures. But the FDA is not convinced yet that the time-honored remedies for swimmer's ear in fact do what they are supposed to do. So these self-treatments still are only conditionally approved.

Heat is a popular remedy for earache. The Panel does not object to the hot-water bottle approach to this pain. But it recommended that if you have an earache, see a doctor.

EAR-CARE AIDS is based on the report "OTC Topical Otic Drugs" by the FDA's Advisory Review Panel on OTC Topical Analgesic, Antirheumatic, Otic, Burn, and Sunburn Prevention and Treatment Drug Products and the FDA's two Tentative Final Orders and Final Order on these drugs.

Earache

In the judgment of FDA medical experts and drug regulators, it is not safe for consumers to self-diagnose and then treat earache (external otitis) with nonprescription drugs. To underscore this belief, the agency has removed from the market all nonprescription ear drugs that contain pain-relieving active ingredients.

Ear Wax

Cerumen, the technical name for ear wax, is a yellowish-brown material composed of several substances secreted from glands in the outer part of the ear canal. Ear wax is water-repellent and it plays a role in protecting the ear from moisture, injury, and infection.

The protective action of ear wax may be lost as the result of overzealous cleansing or picking at an ear. "Cotton tips are for cleaning belly buttons, not ears!" an official of the American Academy of Otolaryngology/Head and Neck Surgery, representing the nation's ear doctors, has recently declared.

The ear canal is self-cleansing: When you chew food, the motion of the jaw muscles moves the wax in the ears, and sloughed-off cells and other debris are gently forced outward. Panel reviewers say that the best thing to do about ear wax is leave it alone. If something *must* be inserted to remove some of it, the object of choice is the tip of a finger. The evaluators frown on sticks and hairpins but reserve their greatest scorn for the cotton-tipped wood applicators. These devices push the wax inward rather than pull it outward and may even injure or puncture the eardrum.

Many people have misconceptions about ear wax. Experts explain that

- it does not cause deafness
- it does not cause the normal loss of hearing that occurs with age
- it does not imply poor hygiene
- it does not require daily removal

For most people, occasionally wiping off the outer ear with a washcloth is treatment enough for removal of excess ear wax. But a minority of individuals have a tendency—possibly inherited—to accumulate this wax, which from time to time must be removed by other means. These people may feel the buildup of wax as a sense of fullness in the ear. To relieve the condition, self-treatment with the one approved nonprescription ear-wax softening agent is judged to be safe and effective. This substance infiltrates, softens, and loosens the wax so that it can be gently flushed out with warm water. If the wax has become hard-packed, however, its removal should be left to a doctor.

 Claim

Accurate

- "For occasional use as an aid to soften, loosen and remove excessive ear wax"

WARNING:

 Do not use if you have ear drainage or discharge, ear pain, irritation, or rash in the ear or are dizzy; consult a doctor. Do not use if you have a perforation (hole) in the ear drum or after ear surgery unless directed by a doctor. Do not use for more than four days.

Drugs for Ear-Wax Removal

The softening agent approved for nonprescription use infiltrates, softens, and loosens the wax mechanically, so that it can be gently flushed out with warm water from an ear syringe. (An NIH specialist notes, however, that a jet of water from an ear syringe can injure the ear or cause an infection—particularly if the eardrum has been perforated.) *Cerumnolytic agents* are solvents that melt the wax. They are stronger than the approved softening agent, and they are *not safe* for nonprescription use.

If symptoms of fullness persist following self-removal of ear wax, or if the maneuver causes pain or dizziness, seek a doctor's help. You should not attempt to remove wax accumulations if you have an earache, an ear drainage, or a perforated eardrum. Also, wax softeners should not be used on children under 12 years except as specified by a doctor.

APPROVED EAR WAX-REMOVAL ACTIVE INGREDIENT

• CARBAMIDE PEROXIDE, IN GLYCERIN: The substance *carbamide peroxide*—which also is known as *urea hydrogen peroxide*—effervesces (bursts into bubbles) when brought in contact with body tissue in the ear. The hydrogen peroxide releases its oxygen component, which in turn loosens tissue debris and wax. The urea also acts to remove loose, dead bits of tissue.

FDA specifies that 6.5 percent by weight is the safe concentration of carbamide peroxide, dissolved in anhydrous glycerin. The mixture's safety and effectiveness in softening ear wax has been established by long clinical use; no acceptable studies confirm them.

Directions for use: Put 5 to 10 drops into the ear with a medicine dropper and keep it there by tilting the head. After 15 minutes, the medication and ear-wax debris can be removed with lukewarm water injected *very gently* from an ear syringe. This treatment can be performed once or twice a day, if necessary, for up to four days.

CONDITIONALLY APPROVED EAR WAX-REMOVAL ACTIVE INGREDIENTS

None.

DISAPPROVED EAR WAX-REMOVAL ACTIVE INGREDIENTS

None.

Swimmer's Ear

People who swim and dive often emerge from the ocean or a pool with water trapped in their outer ear canals. This water can break down the protective layer of ear wax that lines these canals (*see* above), leaving the skin wet and sodden, which encourages bacterial and fungal infections.

The afflicted ear(s) at first may feel full and blocked, then become swollen, runny, itchy, and painful. Hearing may be temporarily impaired. The ear is painful to the touch. This is *swimmer's ear* — and if you have these symptoms, seek help from a doctor. But: Early self-treatment may prevent this otic affliction.

Several products long have been sold to dry water-clogged ears and prevent swimmer's ear. For some reason, the Panel failed to formally assess their active ingredients. So the FDA took the task on itself.

 Claims

Accurate for swimmer's ear prevention
None.

Unproved for swimmer's ear prevention
- "Aids in the prevention of swimmer's ear (external otitis) by helping to dry moisture in the ear..."
- "Aids in the prevention of swimmer's ear by restoring the normal acidity of the ears"

Unproved for drying water-clogged ears
- "Helps dry water in the ears"
- "Helps relieve the discomfort of water-clogged ears by drying excess water"

APPROVED ACTIVE INGREDIENTS FOR PREVENTION OF SWIMMER'S EAR
None.

CONDITIONALLY APPROVED ACTIVE INGREDIENTS FOR PREVENTION OF SWIMMER'S EAR

The FDA lists these ingredients and combinations as safe, but not proved effective:

- ACETIC ACID 2 PERCENT, IN DISTILLED WATER OR PROPYLENE GLYCOL: This is the acid that is found in vinegar. At low concentrations of 5 percent or less, acetic acid is completely innocuous to human tissues; indeed, it is a natural chemical constituent of the human body.

Historically, the panel noted, vinegar was probably the first germ-killer (antibiotic) used by Ancient Man. A number of studies have confirmed that this acid effectively kills some funguses and a wide range of bacteria, including some that thrive in warm, moist ears and that are known to cause swimmer's ear. The theory is that the acid will kill these germs, restore the ear's normal, acidic balance, or both, and so discourage the growth of germs. However, only a few studies of acetic acid's actual use in swimmers' ears were sent to the agency, by one drug manufacturer. The FDA found these studies defective, and inadequate for a label claim for effectiveness against swimmer's ear. So the agency's tentative judgement is: safe but not proved effective.

How to Prevent Swimmer's Ear

America's ear doctors are less circumspect than FDA in endorsing a method to unstop water-clogged ears and prevent swimmer's ear. Here are instructions from the American Academy of Otolaryngology/Head and Neck Surgery:

1. Tilt head sideways, with the water-filled ear up.

2. Pull ear upward and backward.

3. Carefully squeeze into the ear a medicine-dropper full of a rubbing alcohol, such as isopropyl alcohol, or a half-and-half mix of rubbing alcohol and white vinegar from the kitchen. "Alcohol dries out the ear, and kills any bacteria or fungus," the Academy says.

4. Wiggle ear to move the solution all the way down into it.

5. Finally, re-tilt head so that the affected ear now is *down*, and let the fluids drain out. Gently tapping the opposite, upper side of the skull may help.

The ear doctors suggest that swimmers bothered by this minor affliction carry a medicine bottle of alcohol or alcohol-vinegar mix in their swim bags. Also possibly helpful: Put a little mineral oil or baby oil in each ear *before* swimming.

WARNING:

 Do not use these methods if you have a perfo-rated eardrum.

- *ANHYDROUS GLYCERIN 5 PERCENT, IN ISOPROPYL ALCOHOL 95 PERCENT:* The Glycerin is a syrupy stuff that tends to stay put when placed in the ear. *Anhydrous* means that the glycerin is made without water—and so tends to absorb it.

  Glycerin has been used medicinally since its discovery two centuries ago, and FDA is convinced it is safe. But the one study submitted to demonstrate its effectiveness in drying out water-clogged ears was somewhat defective: Water was squirted gently into children's ears, and then one ear of each child (the right one) was treated with anhydrous glycerin in isopropyl alcohol. Five minutes later, the doctor who conducted the study examined all ears and concluded that the anhydrous glycerin + alcohol had significantly dried out the right ears of 42 of his 49 subjects, compared with their water-filled-but-untreated left ears.

  The FDA faults this study because the same (right) ear was used for the drug in all cases, and the doctors who put the water and the glycerin alcohol preparations into the ears also scored the results — which therefore could have been biased in favor of the treatment. A better clinical study is needed, FDA said, to show the medication helped dry out water-clogged ears. Further, the agency added, the study did not prove that drying out wet ears prevents swimmer's ears: that remains to be proved. Conclusion: anhydrous glycerin + isopropyl alcohol is safe but not proved effective for either drying water-clogged ears or preventing swimmer's itch.

- *ISOPROPYL ALCOHOL:* Alcohol is a drying agent and also a germ-killer. (*See* p. 421, and *also see* box, p. 358.) Its role in a preparation for drying water-logged ears and preventing swimmer's ear needs to be defined, FDA says. Also, unless the glycerin or the alcohol is designated an *inactive ingredient*, their independent and relative contributions to these claims for ear-drying and the relief of swimmer's ear will need to be proved. The FDA has not yet formally rated isopropyl alcohol, alone or in combination with glycerin for the treatment of swimmer's ear.

DISAPPROVED ACTIVE INGREDIENTS FOR PREVENTION OF SWIMMER'S EAR

None.

When Further Relief Is Needed

An itchy, painful, runny ear that develops after swimming has passed the moment when self-treatment can be attempted. See a doctor at once—preferably an ear specialist (otologist or otolaryngologist)—for this condition, or any other earache.

Safety and Effectiveness: Active Ingredients in Over-the-Counter Ear-Care Products

Active Ingredient	Action	Assessment
acetic acid	swimmer's ear preventive	safe, not proved effective
anhydrous glycerin	ear-drying aid, swimmer's ear preventive	safe, not proved effective
carbamide peroxide (urea hydrogen peroxide), in glycerin	ear-wax softener	safe and effective
isopropyl alcohol	ear-drying aid, swimmer's ear preventive	not assessed
vinegar	swimmer's ear preventive	not assessed

Ear Care Aids: Product Ratings

Product and Distributor	Dosage of Active Ingredients	Rating *	Comment
Debrox (Marion Merrell Dow)	**ear drops:** 6.5% carbamide peroxide in glycerin	A	
Dri/Ear (Pfeiffer)	**ear drops:** 2.75% boric acid + isopropyl alcohol	?	neither ingredient has as yet been assessed by FDA for treating swimmer's ear.
E.R.O. (Scherer)	**ear drops:** 95% glycerin	B	not proved effective
Murine Ear Drops (Abbott)	**ear drops:** 6.5% carbamide peroxide in glycerin	A	

* Author's interpretation of FDA criteria. Based on contents, not claims.

Eye Drops and Ointments

The eye is one of the most sensitive organs that people self-treat with nonprescription drugs. Structurally, the eyes are well protected from disease and injurious objects. But they are also vulnerable and may easily sustain serious damage. A principal hazard of self-care with nonprescription eye drops and ointments is that self-diagnosis, which may be based on guesswork, can lead to incorrect self-treatment, which in turn can worsen the symptoms or condition. The Panel warns that the drugs described in this unit should not be used for more than 72 hours without a doctor's diagnosis and supervision. *Ophthalmologists* (medical doctors who care for eyes) are the specialists to consult when something is wrong with your eyes.

"There are very few disorders of the eye which are amenable to treatment with OTC ocular preparations," the Panel says. These drugs for the most part only "relieve symptoms." They "do not have any truly curative effect."

The safety of eye drugs is easier to test than most other drugs,

EYE DROPS AND OINTMENTS is based on the report of the FDA's Advisory Review Panel on OTC Ophthalmic Drug Products and on the FDA's Tentative Final and Final Monograph on these products.

because of a very responsive—but now quite controversial—method called the Draize test. Chemicals are put into the eyes of rabbits, which are held in stockades so they cannot remove the drugs by pawing at their eyes or by rubbing their eyes against their cages. Rabbits' eyes are considered to be more sensitive than people's, and irritation, inflammation, and other adverse changes caused by the material being tested are easy to detect. The problem, animal rights advocates say, is that the Draize test is cruel. Advocates of these tests reply that it is better to discover that a drug is harmful in rabbits' eyes than in those of people. Currently, the rabbits' eyes are winning out over people's eyes; the Draize test is falling into disuse.

Data on the effectiveness of nonprescription eye drugs, as with many other groups of over-the-counter drugs, is scantier than one might wish. Because of the limited number of well-controlled, well-executed studies, the Panel and the FDA have had to rely on some less-scientific data, such as long use, acceptance by doctors, and manufacturers' marketing data on user satisfaction.

Most of the drugs described in this unit, which are called *astringents*, *demulcents*, and *emollients* (defined later) can be used to treat dryness and minor discomfort and irritation in the eyes. A fourth class, *vasoconstrictors*, relieves the redness in eyes that have become mildly bloodshot owing to irritation.

Drug analysts at the FDA have not finally made up their minds on two other classes of drugs that are sold over-the-counter for eye care. But the Panel's and the FDA's preliminary assessments were negative. These two classes of drugs are Antiseptics and Anti-infectives. There are no approved ingredients or claims for drugs in either class.

 ## Claims

Accurate for Astringents, Demulcents, and Emollients
• "For the temporary relief of discomfort due to minor eye irritations"

Additional approved claims for demulcents and emollients appear in the following sections on these drugs.

Accurate for Vasoconstrictors
• "Relieves redness of the eye due to minor eye irritation"

WARNING:

 If you experience eye pain, changes in vision, continued redness or irritation of the eye, or if the condition worsens or persists for more than 72 hours, discontinue use of any nonprescription drug and consult a doctor.

It is wrong to suggest that cosmetic benefits result from use of these drugs. The FDA banned all references to eye appearance in labeling claims on the grounds that they promote continuing use of eye drugs; such extended use could be dangerous. No eye product is particularly suitable or helpful for people of any particular age or group.

Which Eye Conditions are Self-treatable?

The conservatism of the evaluators prompted them to define far more specifically than most other Panels the disorders it believes should—and should not—be self-treated. The FDA, still more conservatively, limited the self-treatment even more narrowly. The recommendations of the Panel and the FDA follow.

Self-Treatable Conditions

Tear insufficiency

This condition, sometimes called "dry eye," is caused by sun, wind, and chemical irritants and also by aging and several serious eye diseases. The over-the-counter drugs that relieve the symptoms of tear insufficiency are called *artificial tears.* They moisten the eye and supplement its protective tear-fluid (*See* EYES: ARTIFICIAL TEARS). Some contact-lens wearers use these products to maintain a moist, protective environment where the plastic lenses meet eye surfaces. However, this use falls outside the purview of the FDA's over-the-counter drug review and will not be considered in this Guide.

Corneal edema

This is a serious condition in which the cornea swells with fluid. It can cause excruciating pain and dim the vision. Corneal edema *can* be treated with nonprescription drugs *but only under a doctor's supervision.*

(This disease and its treatment are described more fully in the Unit EYES: CORNEAL EDEMA.)

Foreign bodies in the eye

When acid or some other chemical splashes into the eye, emergency care is required. Treatment is also needed (although perhaps less urgently) for pollen, dust, smog, and other solid, liquid, and gaseous pollutants that enter and irritate the eye. Eyewashes, lotions, and eye-irrigating solutions are available for diluting these substances and washing them out. (Their emergency and first-aid uses are described in the Unit EYEWASH.)

All chemical burns of the eye require medical attention after emergency measures have been taken. If you cannot remove a foreign body from an eye, you should see a doctor immediately.

Irritation and inflammation

If mild, these conditions can be self-treated. They principally affect the *cornea*, the transparent front part of the eyeball; the *sclera*, or the "whites" of the eyes; and the *conjunctiva*, the pinkish-white areas. These surfaces need to be slippery and moist. Normally moisture is provided by tear fluid.

When the conjunctiva are irritated (conjunctivitis), the eye responds by weeping copiously. If this tearing fails to remove the irritant, the eye tissue absorbs fluids and swells up, and blood vessels *dilate* (widen) and fill with blood, creating what is called "red eye" or, more commonly, "bloodshot eyes." When this occurs the eyes may itch, smart, burn, and continue to drip. If the pain is intense, a doctor's help should be sought—in a hospital emergency room if need be.

Red eye is not always caused by environmental pollutants. Eye drugs, even those prescribed by a doctor, can also cause it. So can trauma (for example, being hit on or near the eye) and allergic reactions, infections, and increased pressure inside the eyeball, which can occur with a serious underlying disease like glaucoma. Since there is often no way for a person to know what is causing the inflammation and irritation, self-treatment with over-the-counter drugs should not continue for more than three days. If the symptoms worsen in this time, consult a doctor at once. Persons who know they have glaucoma should *never* self-treat their eyes except under their doctors' supervision, because doing so may worsen an already serious condition or delay getting urgently needed prescription drugs or other treatment.

The Panel approves self-treatment for red eye that results when a foreign object has been successfully removed from the eye. It also approves self-treatment for inflammation and irritation caused by gases, smoke, and other air pollutants and by the water in chlorinated swimming pools. Reddening of the eyes is very often an allergic response. Cold compresses over the eye may bring relief, or the redness, itching, and tearing may be safely relieved by over-the-counter drugs. If self-treatment fails to relieve the irritation, inflammation, and swelling, seek a doctor's help.

Conditions Possibly Self-Treatable

Evaluators say several types of minor infections might suitably be self-treated with over-the-counter drugs—*if* safe and effective drugs were available for the purpose. But the Panel says no such products exist at present.

The FDA takes an even tougher stance than the Panel on self-treatment of eye infections. The FDA says that the symptoms of minor infections and of serious infections are often so similar that the ordinary lay person has no way of distinguishing between them. Therefore, the FDA has decided that the risks of self-treating minor infections outweigh the benefits. It has tentatively decided to announce, at the next stage of the OTC Drug Review of ophthalmalic products, that the use of nonprescription drugs to self-treat eye infections is unsafe, and that such products should be banned.

The minor infections that the Panel—but not the FDA—would allow to be self-treated are as follows.

Granulated eyelids

Redness, itching, burning, and crusting along the eyelid margins is called *blepharitis*: *blepharo-* means "eyelid"; *-itis* means "inflammation." The cause is likely to be a staph infection, or dandruff, or the two together. When staph is the principal cause, the scales that form on the lids tend to be small and dry; when dandruff is principally to blame, the scales are oily. Persons affected by the latter variety usually have scalp dandruff.

The treatment for granulated eyelids is control of head dandruff, removal of scales on the eyelid margin by using a cotton applicator, which you *can* do yourself, and treatment with an anti-infective ophthalmic ointment, which requires a doctor's prescription.

Pink eye

The Panel draws a not-altogether-clear distinction between red eye, which is mild conjunctivitis due to allergic response (and which is unquestionably self-treatable), and pink eye, which is a more serious conjunctivitis that may be allergic but may also be caused by bacterial or viral infections. One point *is* clear: With eye conditions, "pink" is *worse* than "red." The panelists were cautious, although not wholly opposed to attempts to self-treat the pink eye provided an individual sees a doctor if the eye does not clear up within three days.

Two signs of pink eye are redness and discharge. The main symptom is a feeling that sand is in the eye. Vision is not impaired and there is little pain. If the pink eye is bacterial in origin, the cause is likely to be pneumococcus, *Staphylococcus aureus*, homophilus bacteria, or hemolytic streptococci. The FDA recommends that *all* such eye infections be treated by a doctor.

Sty

This infectious condition, technically called *hordeolum*, is a staphylococcal abscess that develops in skin glands on the edge of the eyelid. A sty on the eye looks red and swollen and may be quite sore. Warm, moist compresses and anti-infective drugs—which now require a prescription—are the usual treatments. These infections tend to recur.

Conditions Not Self-Treatable

A number of eye problems definitely require medical assistance; they include:

Embedded foreign body

If an eyewash will not clear a foreign body from the eye, help must be sought from a doctor or other qualified health professional.

Uveitis

This is inflammation that affects the iris—the tissue that makes eyes blue, brown, or green—or related structures inside the eyeball. Uveitis is a serious disease and medical care is necessary.

Glaucoma

This disease is characterized by the increased pressure inside the eyeball, which often leads to blindness. The eyes may appear red, prompting attempts at self-treatment with nonprescription vasoconstrictors (preparations that constrict blood vessels). This is a mistake. Only a doctor can decide which drug is needed, and a vasoconstrictor is unlikely to be the drug of choice.

Flash burns

The ultraviolet rays emitted by welding torches can cause flash burns that redden the eye. These burns will heal, but medical attention is a must.

Tear-duct infections

In these rare infections the inner corner of the eye becomes swollen, sore, and red. Pus appears. It is essential that a doctor provide treatment.

Corneal ulcers

Besides being quite painful, these sores, which may be caused by microorganisms or other factors, endanger vision. Medical treatment is the only answer.

▬▬▬

Special Needs of Eye Medications

Treating the eye with drugs is harder than it may seem. For one thing, the drugs do not stay put: The normal turnover time for tear fluid in the eye is 16 percent per minute. This means that at the end of three minutes, almost half of a drug dose will have vanished down the tiny drainage holes in the corners of the eyes through which tears drain into the nostrils. Ointments applied under the lower lid may stay in place longer than liquid eye drops.

▬▬▬

Combination Products

This Panel, like others, took a dim view of combination products. Single-ingredient products are safer. But it approved a few combinations, particularly of two or three demulcents and the one approved astringent, or a vasoconstrictor, or both. Two or more emollient ingredients also may be combined.

The Panel dealt with what might appear to be a bewildering array of eye-drug ingredients. But for consumers who wish to restrict themselves to safe and effective single-ingredient products or combinations, the choice is narrower (and thus simpler) than it may seem.

There is only one safe and effective *ocular astringent*: zinc sulfate.

Reviewers approved four *ocular vasoconstrictors*, but only allow one vasoconstrictor per product.

The remainder of the approved ingredients, *demulcents* and *emollients*, are more useful for their physical properties (their ability to soothe and protect the eyes) than for their chemical activity, which is minimal at most.

Vasoconstrictors

Ocular vasoconstrictors constrict blood vessels in the eye. Those approved are all *sympathomimetic amines*. They mimic the natural action of the involuntary nervous system, acting by tightening smooth muscle, thus constricting or making blood vessels in the eye narrow. Bloodshot eyes are "whitened" in this way.

However, most of these preparations can provoke a rebound effect, in which the blood vessels dilate again and the eyes appear red again. If this happens, the treatment is to stop using the drug—*not* to use more of it, which unfortunately is what some people are tempted to do.

Vasoconstrictors may also dilate the pupil. This is a particular risk for persons who wear contact lenses or whose corneas may have been scratched by other objects. Pupillary dilation can even lead to glaucoma, a very serious eye condition.

However, in view of the low concentrations used in over-the-counter products, these risks are slight enough that the evaluators say vasoconstrictors are safe. But the FDA warns that persons with diagnosed glaucoma, which could be made worse by the use of vasoconstrictors, should not use them.

 ## Claims for Vasoconstrictors

Accurate

• "Relieves redness of the eye due to minor eye irritations"

Inappropriate
• For "tired eyes"

APPROVED VASOCONSTRICTOR ACTIVE INGREDIENTS

• **EPHEDRINE HYDROCHLORIDE:** This substance occurs naturally in the MaHuang plant, and the Chinese used it medicinally over 5000 years ago. Ephedrine was introduced into Western medicine in 1924 and now is usually produced synthetically. A 0.123 percent concentration of ephedrine has been used for years to treat minor eye irritation. It may be particularly valuable when the eyes are swollen by allergic reactions. The drug is safe and effective for adults and children. Correct dosage is 1 to 2 drops of a 0.123 percent concentration of ephedrine hydrochloride per eye, up to 4 times daily.

• **NAPHAZOLINE HYDROCHLORIDE:** In the low concentrations of 0.01 to 0.03 percent, for which it is approved in nonprescription eye products, this vasoconstrictor is safe and effective. At higher dosages, however, it can dilate the pupils.

Tests show that naphazoline hydrochloride will correct and may prevent the red eyes that some people suffer when they swim in chlorinated swimming pools. For adults and for children, the approved dosage is 1 to 2 drops per affected eye of a 0.01 to 0.03 percent concentration of naphazoline hydrochloride, up to 4 times each day.

• **PHENYLEPHRINE HYDROCHLORIDE:** This vasoconstrictor has been a standard ingredient in over-the-counter eye products for a long time. Studies in animals and in humans show that it effectively re-whitens eyes that have been reddened with irritating substances for experimental purposes. In several tests, for example, phenylephrine hydrochloride was compared with eye-soothing preparations that did not contain a vasoconstrictor. Subjects were humans whose eyes had been reddened by exposure to the irritating body chemical *histamine* or to chlorinated water like that found in swimming pools. In all tests, the phenylephrine hydrochloride, in a 0.12 percent solution, was more effective than the preparation that lacked it. So this drug is judged safe and effective in dosage of 1 to 2 drops of 0.08 to 0.2 percent phenylephrine hydrochloride, used no more than 4 times per day.

• **TETRAHYDROZOLINE HYDROCHLORIDE:** This drug has been shown to be effective in relieving conjunctivitis caused by allergies and by chemical and physical irritants. In one study of 348 patients, an investigator reported that 96 percent obtained relief from the drug. In another study of 808 patients, relief was obtained by 87 percent of the participants.

Tetrahydrozoline hydrochloride has the advantage that it rarely if ever dilates the pupil of a healthy eye. No cases of rebound conjunctivitis have been reported either. Thus, this ingredient is assessed as safe and effective. The approved dosage is 1 to 2 drops of a 0.01 to 0.05 percent solution of tetrahydrozoline hydrochloride in each affected eye, up to 4 times daily.

CONDITIONALLY APPROVED VASOCONSTRICTOR ACTIVE INGREDIENTS

None.

DISAPPROVED VASOCONSTRICTOR ACTIVE INGREDIENTS

None.

Astringents

An *astringent* is a substance that "pulls" particles out of a solution, holding and solidifying them. For the most part astringents do not enter body cells; they act on the outer layers of cells or between individual cells. These substances will draw the surface molecules of cells together, puckering the skin and mucosal surfaces. Only very weak astringent concentrations are found in nonprescription ophthalmic preparations. Reviewers believe they act mainly to clear mucin and perhaps other substances from the surface of the eye and do not otherwise act on the outer layers of the cornea or the conjunctiva (inner eyelid), which could be dangerous.

Manufacturers have made inflated claims for eye astringents, suggesting that they will cure hay fever and sty. Although astringents may *relieve* some symptoms of hay fever, such as itchiness and irritation, they will not *cure* it.

Claims for Astringents

Accurate
- for "the temporary relief of discomfort from minor eye irritations"

APPROVED ASTRINGENT ACTIVE INGREDIENT

- *ZINC SULFATE:* Some eye preparations contain zinc sulfate as their single active ingredient, but this astringent is usually combined with a vasoconstrictor and sometimes other ingredients as well. The safety of zinc sulfate is attested to by the sale of millions of bottles of these products over several decades, with only very few adverse effects having been reported. In a 20-day Draize test, rabbits' left eyes, treated with zinc sulfate, showed no greater irritation than did their right eyes, which were not treated.

    Evaluators conclude from the available evidence that zinc sulfate is both safe and effective. The dosage is 1 to 2 drops of a 0.25 percent solution in the affected eye, up to 4 times daily.

CONDITIONALLY APPROVED ASTRINGENT ACTIVE INGREDIENTS
None.

DISAPPROVED ASTRINGENT ACTIVE INGREDIENTS
None.

Demulcents

A *demulcent* is a substance that coats and protects mucous membrane surfaces. For the most part, these compounds are chemically inert and provide beneficial effects through their protective physical properties.

They help the tissues retain moisture and insulate them from sun, wind, and other environmental forces. They also slow the turnover of tear fluid, or serve to increase the water that is present on the eye surfaces. Demulcents are sometimes called *artificial tears*, and are also used as wetting agents for contact lenses.

This is the FDA's official definition of a demulcent:

"An agent, usually a water-soluble polymer, which is applied topically to the eye to protect and lubricate mucous membrane surfaces and relieve dryness and irritation."

 ## Claims for Demulcents

Accurate

- "For the temporary relief of burning and irritation due to dryness of the eye"

- "For the temporary relief of discomfort due to minor irritation of the eye or to exposure to wind or sun"

- "For use as a protectant against further irritation or to relieve dryness of the eye"

- "For use as a lubricant to prevent further irritation or to dryness of the eye"

APPROVED DEMULCENT ACTIVE INGREDIENTS

The Panel assessed the demulcent ingredients listed here. All of them were judged both safe and effective.

- *CELLULOSE DERIVATIVES:* carboxymethylcellulose sodium; hydroxyethyl cellulose; hydroxypropyl methylcellulose; methylcellulose
- *DEXTRAN 70*
- *GELATIN*
- *LIQUID POLYOLS:* glycerin; polyethylene glycol 300; polyethylene glycol 400; polysorbate 80; propylene glycol; polyvinyl alcohol
- *POVIDONE*

For a more detailed discussion of these compounds and their use in relieving tear insufficiency ("dry eye"), *see* EYES: ARTIFICIAL TEARS. Demulcents are also formulated into safe and effective combination products that contain a vasoconstrictor, an astringent, or both.

CONDITIONALLY APPROVED DEMULCENT ACTIVE INGREDIENTS

None.

DISAPPROVED DEMULCENT ACTIVE INGREDIENTS

None.

Emollients

The *emollients*, like the demulcents, are inert, bland, soothing substances, with the difference that they are oily and therefore less readily washed away by tear fluids. They soften the skin and hold in moisture, so they are useful for treating teary and irritated eyes. They also cover skin and mucosal surfaces, keeping out water-soluble irritants, air, and airborne bacteria. Emollients lubricate tissue (for example, the surfaces of the eyeball and the eyelids) and are also widely used as bases for other drugs for eye care.

This is FDA's long-labored-over and clear and succinct definition of an emollient:

"An agent, usually a fat or oil, which is applied locally to the eyelids to protect or soften tissues and to prevent drying and cracking."

Emollients are usually formulated as ointments. To apply them, you gently pull down the lower eyelid and apply a ¼-inch-long ribbon of the product to the inside of the lid.

 ## Claims for Emollients

Accurate

- "For the temporary relief of burning and irritation due to dryness of the eye"
- "For the temporary relief of discomfort due to minor irritation of the eye or to exposure to wind or sun"
- "For use as a protectant against further irritation or to relieve dryness of the eye"

• "For use as a lubricant to prevent further irritation or dry-ness of the eye"

APPROVED EMOLLIENT ACTIVE INGREDIENTS

The FDA approved 10 emollients, in two categories, as grouped here. All are safe and effective.

• LANOLIN PREPARATIONS: ANHYDROUS LANOLIN AND LANOLIN: These substances are obtained from sheep-skin secretions that are extracted from wool. Lanolin contains about 25 percent water; anhydrous lanolin is lanolin with the water removed. Lanolin is a yellowish semi-solid fat with little or no odor. A few people are allergic to it, but the reviewers believe that the small amounts in ophthalmic drugs are unlikely to cause allergic reactions. However, the more refined and purified *nonionic lanolin derivatives* are even less likely to cause an allergic reaction. One such product has been marketed for years and no serious adverse effects have been reported as the result of its use.

Vision may blur briefly when lanolin preparations are first put in the eyes; this is not harmful. In emollient products intended for use in the eye, lanolin is present in concentrations of 1 to 10 percent, in combination with white petrolatum, mineral oil, or another oily emollient.

Basing their assessment on wide usage and the protective and lubricating qualities of these preparations, FDA evaluators judged these lanolins to be safe and effective emollients and lubricants. The dosage for adults and children is a ¼-inch-long streak of ointment applied to the inside of the eyelid.

• OILY INGREDIENTS: LIGHT MINERAL OIL, MINERAL OIL, PARAFFIN, PETROLATUM, WHITE OINTMENT, WHITE PETROLATUM, WHITE WAX, YELLOW WAX: These are bland and essentially inert substances that are the bases—with or without lanolin—for virtually all ophthalmic ointments. All are derived from petrolatum except white wax, which is made by bees and has a honey-like odor. White wax and paraffin are harder than the other oily ingredients listed here and are used to increase the consistency of ointment products; they are not used alone as emollients.

Long use attests to the safety of these substances. An eye surgeon reported using ointments made with these substances on more than 20,000 surgical patients, with no ill effects as the result. The safe and effective dosage for these emollient preparations for adults and children is a ¼-inch-long streak applied to the inner side of the lower eyelid.

CONDITIONALLY APPROVED EMOLLIENT ACTIVE INGREDIENTS

None.

DISAPPROVED EMOLLIENT ACTIVE INGREDIENTS

None.

Anesthetics

An anesthetic relieves, and so can mask pain. The Advisory Panel and the FDA believe it is very dangerous to self-treat an eye with an anesthetic.

This self-care pain relief may dangerously delay a search for medical help for a rapidly deteriorating eye problem caused by a corneal abrasion, which is a wearing away of the eyeball's outer layer, or by a foreign body embedded in the eye, or some other serious eye condition. Worse, anesthetic agents used in eye drugs can themselves cause serious damage to the eye, even after a single application. So the judgment of whether, when, and how to use eye anesthetics must be made by a doctor.

APPROVED ANESTHETIC ACTIVE INGREDIENTS

None.

CONDITIONALLY APPROVED ANESTHETIC ACTIVE INGREDIENTS

None.

DISAPPROVED ANESTHETIC ACTIVE INGREDIENTS

The Panel and the FDA assessed two anesthetics and found both wanting.

- *ANTIPYRINE:* The 0.4-percent antipyrine solution that one manufacturer submitted to the OTC Review was found to have only slight anesthetic effect. So the drug is ineffective, as well as unsafe (for the reasons described above).
- *PIPEROCAINE HYDROCHLORIDE:* This drug is an effective ocular anesthetic in the 2-to 4-percent ointments that are sold by prescription (R). It may be effective at the lower dosages that have been sold without prescription. But because the use of this drug could allow a person to temporize, and not seek appropriate medical help, the FDA says: not safe.

Anti-Infectives

An anti-infective kills or limits the growth and multiplication of bacteria and other microorganisms. Self-treatment of an eye infection with nonprescription anti-infective drugs is controversial. The Panel said that minor infections on the external surfaces of the eye—that is, infections that are not on or in the eyeball—usually are not dangerous. They will heal by themselves rather quickly. So self-treatment could be recommended if safe and effective drugs were available for the purpose. But none of the anti-infectives in OTC products meets the test for safety and effectiveness. The infectious conditions that might be self-treatable, the Panel said, include sty, granulated eyelid, and pink eye, or conjunctivitis.

APPROVED ANTI-INFECTIVE ACTIVE INGREDIENTS

None.

CONDITIONALLY APPROVED ANTI-INFECTIVE ACTIVE INGREDIENTS

- *SILVER PROTEIN, MILD:* There is no doubt that silver can stop or slow bacterial growth. But there is considerable doubt about its effectiveness in nonprescription eye preparations that contain relatively small amounts of this substance. So, while the FDA currently considers it safe, it believes that the effectiveness of mild silver protein needs to be proven.

DISAPPROVED ANTI-INFECTIVE ACTIVE INGREDIENTS

• BORIC ACID: Eye drops and ointments containing this anti-infective have been widely used for decades. In low concentrations, of about 1 percent, boric acid may be valuable in adjusting a product's acidity to the needs of the eye. But its antimicrobial potency when put into the eye has not been proven.

   Without doubt, boric acid will kill bacteria. To be truly effective in this task, it must remain in contact with the bacteria for at least 24 hours. However, liquid ingredients put into the eye are diluted by tear fluid 10 times within a matter of minutes. Ointments may keep the boric acid in contact with the eye for a while longer. But even so, the Panel did not think that boric acid ointment is strong enough to adequately control bacterial growth. The FDA said: not effective.

• MERCURIC OXIDE, YELLOW: Reports from eye doctors indicate that some people delay seeking treatment for eye infections while they self-treat eye conditions with mercuric oxide, a drug that has been used in the eyes for more than a century. One manufacturer said he had sold more than a million units of a yellow mercuric oxide preparation, yet had received only a few minor complaints. Nevertheless, beyond concerns about its safety, FDA was not persuaded that the drug is effective in retarding bacterial growth. So its judgment is that yellow mercuric oxide is not safe and not effective.

When Greater Relief Is Needed

See an eye specialist (ophthalmologist) at once for any eye condition that affects your vision or is painful, worrisome, or distressing in any way. If you cannot schedule an emergency appointment with a private eye doctor, go to the emergency room of your nearby hospital; there will be an ophthalmologist in the hospital or on-call at all times.

Safety and Effectiveness: Combination Products Sold Over-the-Counter for the Care of the Eyes

Safe and Effective

Each ingredient must be approved, and must be present in an approved dosage, and the final marketed product must be shown to be safe and effective.

zinc sulfate (astringent) + vasoconstrictor

any 2 or 3 demulcents

2 or 3 demulcents + 1 vasoconstrictor

zinc sulfate + 1 vasoconstrictor + 1, 2, or 3 demulcents

2, 3, or more emollients

Safety and Effectiveness: Active Ingredients in Over-the-Counter Eye-Care Products

Active Ingredient	Drug Group*	Assessment
anhydrous lanolin (1-10%)	emollient	safe and effective
antipyrine	anesthetic	not safe and effective
boric acid	anti-infective	not effective
carboxymethylcellulose sodium (0.2-2.5%)	demulcent	safe and effective
dextran 70 (0.1%)	demulcent	safe and effective
ephedrine hydrochloride (0.123%)	vasoconstrictor	safe and effective
gelatin (0.01%)	demulcent	safe and effective
glycerin (0.2-1%)	demulcent	safe and effective
hydroxyethyl cellulose (0.2-2.5 %)	demulcent	safe and effective
hydroxypropyl methylcellulose (0.2-2.5%)	demulcent	safe and effective
lanolin (1-10%)	emollient	safe and effective
lanolin, anhydrous (1-10%)	emollient	safe and effective
mercuric oxide, yellow	anti-infective	not safe and effective
methylcellulose (0.2-2.5%)	demulcent	safe and effective

mineral oil (up to 50%)	emollient	safe and effective
mineral oil, light (up to 50%)	emollient	safe and effective
naphazoline hydrochloride (0.01-0.03%)	vasoconstrictor	safe and effective
paraffin (up to 5%)	emollient	safe and effective
petrolatum (up to 100%)	emollient	safe and effective
petrolatum, white (*See* white petrolatum)		
phenylephrine hydrochloride (0.08-0.2%)	vasoconstrictor	safe and effective
piperocaine hydrochloride	anesthetic	not safe
polyethylene glycol 300 (0.2-1%)	demulcent	safe and effective
polyethylene glycol 400 (0.2-1%)	demulcent	safe and effective
polysorbate 80 (0.2-1%)	demulcent	safe and effective
polyvinyl alcohol (0.1-4%)	demulcent	safe and effective
povidone (0.1-2%)	demulcent	safe and effective
propylene glycol (0.2-1%)	demulcent	safe and effective
silver protein, mild	anti-infective	safe, but not proved effective
tetrahydrozoline hydrochloride (0.01-0.05%)	vasoconstrictor	safe and effective

Safety and Effectiveness: Active Ingredients in Over-the-Counter Eye-Care Products (contd)

Active Ingredient	Drug Group*	Assessment
white ointment (up to 100%)	emollient	safe and effective
white petrolatum (up to 100%)	emollient	safe and effective
white wax (up to 5%)	emollient	safe and effective
yellow wax (up to 5%)	emollient	safe and effective
zinc sulfate (0.25%)	astringent	safe and effective

* These terms are explained in the text.

Eye Drops and Ointments: Product Ratings

SINGLE-PURPOSE PRODUCTS

Product and Distributor	Dosage of Active Ingredients	Rating*	Comment
boric acid			
Boric acid (generic)	ointment: 5%	B	not proved effective
Boric Acid (Lilly)	ointment: 5%	B	not proved effective
	ointment: 10%	B	not proved effective
mercuric oxide, yellow			
Stye (Commerce)	ointment: 1%	C	not safe or effective
Yellow mercuric oxide (generic)	ointment: 1% and 2%	C	not safe or effective
silver protein, mild			
Argyrol S.S. 10% (Iolab)	solution: 10%	B	not proved effective

VASOCONSTRICTORS

Product and Distributor	Dosage of Active Ingredients	Rating*	Comment
naphazoline hydrochloride			
Allerest Eye Drops (Pharmacraft)	solution: 0.012%	A	
Clear Eyes (Ross)		A	

Eye Drops and Ointments: Product Ratings (contd)

Product and Distributor	Dosage of Active Ingredients	Rating *	Comment
Naphcon (Alcon)		A	
VasoClear (Iolab)	solution: 0.02%	A	
Comfort Eye Drops (Sola/Barnes-Hind)	solution: 0.03%	A	
oxymetazalone hydrochloride			
OcuClear (Schering)	solution: 0.025%	A	℞ to OTC switch
phenylephrine hydrochloride			
AK Nefrin Ophthalmic (Akorn)	solution: 0.012%	A	
Isopto Frin (Alcon)		A	
tetrahydrozoline hydrochloride			
Murine Plus Eye Drops (Ross)	solution: 0.05%	A	
Soothe Eye Drops (Alcon)		A	
Tetrahydrozoline hydrochloride (generic)		A	
Visine Eye Drops (Leeming)		A	

DEMULCENTS

see pp. 394-395 Product Ratings in EYES: ARTIFICIAL TEARS

EMOLLIENTS

Product and Distributor	Dosage of Active Ingredients	Rating*	Comment
Duratears Naturale (Alcon)	**ointment:** white petrolatum + anhydrous lanolin + mineral oil	A	
Lacri-Lube S.O.P. Ointment (Allergan)	**ointment:** 55% white petrolatum + 42% mineral oil	A	

COMBINATION PRODUCTS

Product and Distributor	Dosage of Active Ingredients	Rating*	Comment
Clear Eyes (Ross)	**eye drops:** 0.012% naphazoline hydrochloride + 0.2% glycerin	A	
Clear Eyes ACR (Ross)	**eye drops:** 0.012% naphazoline hydrochloride + 0.2% glycerin + 0.25% zinc sulfate	A	
Collyrium with Tetradrozoline (Wyeth-Ayerest)	**eye drops:** 0.05% tetrahydrozoline hydrochloride + 1% glycerin	A	
Optised (generic)	**eye drops:** 0.12% phenylephrine hydrochloride + 0.25% zinc sulfate	A	

Eye Drops and Ointments: Product Ratings (contd)

Product and Distributor	Dosage of Active Ingredients	Rating*	Comment
Relief (Allergan)	**eye drops:** 0.12% phenyephrine hydrochloride + 0.1% antipyrine	C	antipyrine not safe
Visine A.C. (Pfizer)	**eye drops:** 0.05% tetrahydrozoline hydrochloride + 0.25% zinc sulfate	A	

*Author's interpretation of FDA criteria. Based on contents, not claims.

Eyes: Artificial Tears

Our eyes must remain moist. Dry eyes quickly become excruciatingly painful. Severe and permanent damage, including blindness, may follow.

Fortunately, effective over-the-counter drugs are available to relieve dryness, whether due to sun or wind exposure, illness, the effects of old age, or serious eye disease. These medications are called eye soothers (*ocular demulcents*), and the Panel that assessed them says they are one of the very few kinds of eye preparations that are safe and effective for people to use as self-treatment.

Most of these medications can absorb large amounts of water. Administered by dropper, they coat dry mucous membranes and other raw surfaces, protecting them from environmental irritants (including the air itself). The medications lubricate eye surfaces and hold in their natural moisture. Some ocular demulcents act by thickening and retaining the tear fluid in the eye. Most of these preparations are formulated as sterile-water solutions that have about the same saltiness and acidity as natural eye secretions. These drugs are popularly called "artificial tears."

EYES: ARTIFICIAL TEARS is based on the report of the FDA's Advisory Review Panel on OTC Ophthalmic Drug Products and the FDA's Tentative Final and Final Monographs on these products.

It recently has been demonstrated scientifically that dry eyes see a little less sharply and clearly than the same eyes do when adequately moist. This has prompted an editorialist in the *Lancet* (vol. 339, p. 1389, June 6, 1992) to suggest that individuals who suffer from this condition remember to use their artificial tears when driving, especially at night, when glare is a problem. Air travelers and crews, who are subjected to dry, air-conditioned air in plane cabins, also should remember to take artificial tears along, and use them, the editorialist says. Dry-eyed photographers and people who work on visual-display screens, such as word processors, also should use these products, if necessary, since they blink less frequently than is normal—which can exacerbate a dry-eye condition.

 Claims

Accurate

- "For the temporary relief of burning and irritation due to dryness of the eye"
- "For the temporary relief of discomfort due to minor irritations of the eye or to exposure to wind or sun"
- "For use as a protectant against further irritation to relieve dryness of the eye"
- "For use as a lubricant to prevent further irritation or relieve dryness of the eye"

WARNING:

 If you experience eye pain, changes in vision, continued redness or irritation of the eye, or if the condition worsens or persists for more than 72 hours, discontinue use of any nonprescription drug and consult a doctor.

Dry Eye

When exposure to sun, wind, chemicals, or other drying environmental influences produces what is technically called *tear insufficiency,* a person experiences dry eye. This may be felt as a burning sensation or as the feeling that a foreign body is caught in the eye. The eye itself may become red.

Dry eye is common in older people and causes them greater suffering during waking hours than at night, when closed lids retain the eyes' moisture. The flow of tears from the lacrimal glands may also be reduced by any of several diseases, including a condition called by the jaw-breaker medical term *keratoconjunctivitis sicca*. Scarring or damage to the tear-fluid system is one of this disorder's main causes.

Demulcents

Artificial-tear products consist principally of water. But their action goes beyond the replacement of tear-fluid—which would be of brief benefit at best since it is washed away so quickly. *Demulcents* (soothers) thicken and hold water and natural tear secretions so that they flow more slowly across and out of the eye. They may double the turnover time of tears. Demulcents also coat dry eye-surfaces, postponing evaporation of left-over moisture. By holding moisture in contact with the eye and lubricating dry surfaces, as tears normally do, the artificial tears reduce friction and irritation.

The demulcent active ingredients may constitute only 1 percent or so of the product. Panel reviewers say that such a product should also contain a preservative to prevent bacterial contamination, along with buffers that would approximate the acid and salt content of normal tears and tonicity ingredients to aid in maintaining normal physiological tone and tension.

Demulcents do not react with the eye tissue or with each other. For these reasons, reviewers approved combinations of 2 or 3 safe and effective demulcents, but no more. They also would permit demulcents to be combined with ocular astringents and vasoconstrictors (blood-vessel narrowers) to relieve irritation and slow the passage of the other ingredients from the eye (*See* Combination Products in EYE DROPS AND OINTMENTS.

The same artificial-tear products used by active people for temporary relief of dry eye—for example, after a day of hang-gliding, boat racing, or suntanning on the beach — are also used routinely by older people and others with chronic tear insufficiency. But the experts warn that self-treatment of a self-diagnosed dry-eye condition for more than 72 hours is potentially a very dangerous mistake. After 72 hours, consult a doctor.

For persons with severe dry-eye conditions, the moisture provided by nonprescription artificial tears may disappear too quickly to provide ongoing relief, and a prescription product may be needed.

APPROVED DEMULCENT ACTIVE INGREDIENTS

These substances appear to be among the safest and most effective of any assessed in the review of over-the-counter drugs; the FDA has evaluated 13 demulcent ingredients that it judged to be safe and effective. The following descriptions follow the reviewers' practice of evaluating some ingredients individually and others (cellulose derivatives and liquid polyols) in groups.

• CELLULOSE DERIVATIVES: CARBOXYMETHYLCELLULOSE SODIUM, HYDROXYETHYL CELLULOSE, HYDROXYPROPYL METHYLCELLULOSE, METHYLCELLULOSE: Cellulose derivatives have been used in the eye for 40 years; they are the bulk-providing ingredients in half of all prescription eye-drugs. Most studies on the safety and effectiveness of cellulose derivatives have been based on methylcellulose, one of the first of this group to be used in the eye. There is no reason to believe the others are less safe or less effective. Reviewers concluded that there are no known adverse reactions to the use of cellulose derivatives. The dry crusts of this material that may form on the eyelids are harmless and can be easily wiped off,

Cellulose derivatives have been shown to remain in the eye two to four minutes after use. One report says that a solution of 1 percent hydroxypropyl methylcellulose remained in the eye for an average of 6½ minutes—a remarkably long time.

Dosage for adults and children is 1 to 2 drops of an aqueous solution containing 0.2 to 2.5 percent of total cellulose derivatives.

• DEXTRAN 70: This substance is a grouping of sugary subunits produced by bacteria that grow on table sugar. This kind of long-chained molecular structure, made up of many similar or identical subunits, is called a *polymer*. One of the polymers' most useful traits is that they are chemically inert (inactive).

For a long time, dextran has been used as a volume expander for plasma used in blood transfusions. When dextran is applied to the skin, it can cause hives, swelling, and other intense allergic reactions. But when put into rabbits' eyes in the low concentrations used in artificial-tear preparations, no significant reactions occurred. In one of the few tests on human subjects, the only adverse reactions were brief periods of stinging and blurred vision. Though dextran has not been extensively studied as an eye drop, reviewers believe the approved dose—0.1 percent dextran 70—is safe and effective, though the substance must be combined with another approved polymer-like demulcent ingredient to reach an effective dosage level.

- **GELATIN:** A natural polymer (*See* the discussion of polymers under Dextran 70), gelatin is widely used in foods. It is colorless or faintly yellow, transparent, brittle, practically odorless, and has no taste of its own. Before cellulose derivatives became available gelatin was widely used in formulating ophthalmic (eye) drugs as a substitute for the natural, water-soluble proteins in tear fluid.

    The effectiveness of gelatin in artificial-tear products has not been studied, but the Panel nevertheless evaluates it as effective as well as safe in concentrations of 0.01 percent (one-hundredth of 1 percent) if it is combined with other polymeric demulcents.

    The safe dosage for adults and children is 1 to 2 drops of a 0.01 percent gelatin concentration in a water solution with another approved polymer-type demulcent.

- **GLYCERIN :** *See* Liquid Polyols.

- **HYDROXYETHYL CELLULOSE:** *See* Cellulose Derivatives.

- **HYDROXYPROPYL METHYLCELLULOSE:** *See* Cellulose Derivatives.

- **LIQUID POLYOLS: GLYCERIN, POLYETHYLENE GLYCOL 300, POLYETHYLENE GLYCOL 400, POLYSORBATE 80, AND PROPYLENE GLYCOL:** These substances are all gooey, clear, water-soluble fluids that tend to be bland, stable, and nontoxic. They are widely used as vehicles (bases) and solvents for other active drugs as well as in moisturizers and other cosmetics. Although their safety and effectiveness as eye-drug ingredients have not been well studied, their few side effects and their ability to "coat" tissue surfaces led evaluators to deem these ingredients effective and safe as demulcents and eye lubricants.

    For adults and children dosage is 1 to 2 drops of 0.2 to 1 percent concentration in water solution, applied as needed.

- **METHYLCELLULOSE:** *See* Cellulose Derivatives.

- **POLYETHYLENE GLYCOL 300 AND POLYETHYLENE GLYCOL 400:** *See* Liquid Polyols.

- **POLYSORBATE 80:** *See* Liquid Polyols.

- **PROPYLENE GLYCOL:** *See* Liquid Polyols.

- **POLYVINYL ALCOHOL:** This alcohol has been widely used as a base for prescription eye medications. It has been carefully tested. Serious side effects have not been found and minor ones have been uncommon, even though millions of product units of polyvinyl-alcohol eye preparations have been sold.

Polyvinyl alcohol is less syrupy than methylcellulose and other artificial tear substances, so evaluators guess that it acts by forming a protective film, which lubricates eye surfaces and holds in moisture. It is formulated into products that wearers of hard contact lenses use to reduce eye irritation.

The safe and effective dosage for children and adults is 1 to 2 drops of water solution containing 0.1 to 4 percent polyvinyl alcohol, administered as needed.

• *POVIDONE:* This substance is essentially inert, so it is widely used as an inactive ingredient in the manufacture of drugs. Although less well studied as an eye drug than polyvinyl alcohol (*see* directly preceding), a 1968 report from the National Academy of Sciences indicates that a 3 percent povidone product probably is safe and effective for use in soothing and lubricating dry eyes and for enhancing the comfort of contact lenses. The Panel and the FDA concur with this judgment of safety and effectiveness.

For adults and children, approved dosages are 1 to 2 drops of 0.1 to 2 percent povidone, used as needed.

Safety and Effectiveness: Active Ingredients in Over-the-Counter Eye Soothers (Demulcents)

Active Ingredient	Assessment
carboxymethylcellulose sodium	safe and effective
dextran 70	safe and effective
gelatin	safe and effective
glycerin	safe and effective
hydroxyethyl cellulose	safe and effective
hydroxypropyl methylcellulose	safe and effective
methylcellulose	safe and effective
polyethylene glycol 300	safe and effective
polyethylene glycol 400	safe and effective

Safety and Effectiveness: Active Ingredients in Over-the-Counter Eye Soothers (Demulcents) (contd)

Active Ingredient	Assessment
polysorbate 80	safe and effective
polyvinyl alcohol	safe and effective
povidone	safe and effective
propylene glycol	safe and effective

Artificial Tears: Product Ratings

Product and Distributor	Dosage of Active Ingredients	Rating*	Comment
Cellufresh (Allergan)	0.5% carboxymethylcellulose sodium	A	
Celluvisc (Allergan)	1% carboxymethylcellulose sodium	A	
Hypotears (Iolab)	1% polyvinyl alcohol	A	
Isopto Tears (Alcon)	1% hydroxypropyl methylcellulose	A	
Lacril (Allergan)	0.5% hydroxypropyl methylcellulose + gelatin	A	
Liquifilm Forte (Allergan)	3% polyvinyl alcohol	A	
Liquifilm Tears (Allergan)	1.4% polyvinyl alcohol	A	
Moisture Drops (Bausch & Lomb)	0.5% hydroxypropyl methylcellulose + 0.1% dextran	A	
Murine (Ross)	1.4% polyvinyl alcohol + 0.6% povidone	A	
Murocel (Bausch & Lomb)	1% methylcellulose + propylene glycol	A	

| Tears Naturale II (Alcon) | 0.1% dextran 70 + 0.3% hydroxypropyl methylcellulose | A |
| Tears Plus (Allergan) | 1.4% polyvinyl alcohol + povidone | A |

*Author's interpretation of FDA criteria. Based on contents, not claims.

Eyes: Corneal Edema

The cornea of the eye—the clear natural window through which we see—may become swollen because it has absorbed too much fluid. This condition is called *corneal edema*. Vision becomes blurred or foggy. Lights appear to be surrounded by halos. In some cases the eye may become quite irritated, and even excruciatingly painful, with the result that the sufferer cannot tolerate light.

Experts say that corneal edema can be at least partially corrected with sterile salt water available over-the-counter. But since the swelling is usually the symptom of a more serious underlying disorder that requires medical diagnosis and care, the panel stipulates that this sterile salt water be used only under a doctor's supervision.

 Claims

Accurate
- "For the temporary relief of corneal edema"

EYES: CORNEAL EDEMA is based on the report of the FDA's Advisory Review Panel on OTC Ophthalmic Drug Products and on the FDA's Tentative Final and Final Monographs on these products.

WARNINGS:

 Do not use except under the advice and supervision of a doctor. If you experience eye pain, changes in vision, continued redness, or irritation of the eye, or if the condition worsens or persists, consult a doctor.

Two to 5 percent salt solutions should *not* be used as an eyewash or to treat the eyes for problems other than corneal edema.

Corneal Edema: Causes and Treatment

A variety of problems can cause this condition. Contact lenses that fit badly or are not removed often enough to rest the eye can injure the cornea, causing it to absorb tear fluid and swell. Inflammatory reactions and infection can also produce this effect. Finally, the serious eye disease *glaucoma* can result in corneal edema, as can *iritis*, which is an inflammation of the colored part of the eye.

The sterile salt water (saline) solutions that can be safely used to treat this condition range from 2 to 5 percent salt. When put into the eye every 3 or 4 hours (as directed by a doctor) these solutions, called *ocular hypertonicity agents*, will draw water out of the cornea. This reduces the swelling. A demulcent (soother) to help hold the salt water is also allowed. (*See* the Unit EYES: ARTIFICIAL TEARS for a discussion of demulcents.)

APPROVED ACTIVE INGREDIENT (HYPERTONICITY AGENT)

• **SODIUM CHLORIDE:** Ordinary salt (in sterile water) is the one substance judged to be safe and effective in reducing corneal edema, providing the patient is under medical supervision. The safe and effective concentrations are from 2 to 5 percent.

These preparations, which are formulated as eye drops or as an ointment, may cause stinging, redness, and temporary discomfort in the eye. The reactions are not dangerous, but this mild discomfort should serve to prevent overdosing or use by persons who do not really need the medication.

Tests in rabbits and in humans indicate that such salt solutions will produce a 10 to 20 percent reduction in corneal swelling. The likelihood is that vision will sharpen and improve as a result.

The approved dosage for adults and children is 1 to 2 drops of a 2 to 5 percent concentration of salt water in each affected eye every 3 or 4 hours, as directed by a physician.

Safety and Effectiveness: Active Ingredient in Solutions Sold Over-the-Counter for Corneal Edema

Active Ingredient	Panel's Assessment
sterile salt water (2-5%)	safe and effective

Saltwater Preparations for Corneal Edema: Product Ratings

Product and Distributor	Dosage of Active Ingredients	Rating*	Comment
Adsorbonac Ophthalmic (Alcon)	**solution:** 2% sodium chloride + povidone	A	
	solution: 5% sodium chloride + povidone	A	
Muro-128 Ophthalmic (Bausch & Lomb)	**solution:** 2% sodium chloride + hydroxypropyl methylcellulose	A	
	solution: 5% sodium chloride + hydroxypropyl methylcellulose + propylene glycol	A	

*Author's interpretation of FDA criteria. Based on contents, not claims.

Eyewash

An eyewash is a sterile water solution that can be used to bathe the eye or to dilute and flush out irritating foreign matter. Dust, pollen, and air-borne pollutant gases and liquids—including smog and swimming-pool chlorine—that have dissolved in the eye's tear fluid can be removed with eyewash. Experts say that these washes, also called *eye lotions* and *eye-irrigating solutions,* should be present in sealed, sterile containers in first-aid and emergency kits in the home and workplace.

Eyewash products differ from all other over-the-counter prepara-tions in that the reviewing Panel insists they must not contain *any* active drug ingredients, that might worsen the irritation and pain. The FDA agrees: Only sterile water and inactive ingredients that approxi-mate ordinary tear-fluid's saltiness and acidity are allowed.

 Claims

Accurate

• "For flushing, or irrigating the eye to remove loose foreign

EYEWASH is based on the report of the FDA's Advisory Review Panel on OTC Ophthalmic Drug Products and the FDA's Tentative Final and Final Monographs on these products.

material, air pollutants, or chlorinated water"

- "For bathing the eye to help relieve burning and itching by removing loose foreign material, air pollutants (smog or pollen), or chlorinated water"

Emergency Treatment: Chemical Burns

When an acid or a caustic substance like lye (or any other potent chemical) splashes into the eye, definite steps must be taken at once to neutralize and remove the substance. The eye must be flushed out immediately, using large amounts of an eyewash or irrigating solution, or warm clean tap water, or both. The National Poison Center Network warns that a delay of only seconds may greatly increase the extent of injury. The Center offers these emergency instructions:

Forcibly hold eyelids open and immediately rinse eyes and face with gentle stream of warm running water from tap or pitcher for at least 15 minutes. Then take victim to the emergency department of a hospital or to an eye doctor (ophthalmologist).

The Panel concurs that in the absence of adequate amounts of prepackaged eyewash, copious flushing with water is a must followed by receiving medical care. The Panel adds this urgent warning:

WARNINGS:

 If you experience severe eye pain, headache, rapid change in vision (side or straight ahead), sudden appearance of floating spots, acute redness of the eyes, pain on exposure to light, or double vision, consult a physician at once.

If symptoms persist or worsen after use of (an eyewash), consult a physician.

The clear message in treating chemical burns—or any massive infiltration of alien material into the eye—is: Don't take chances. Don't wait. Give emergency care with eyewash or water. Get medical help.

Natural and Assisted Eye Irrigations

The tears are the eyes' first line of defense against noxious gases, liquids, and solid particles from the environment. They dilute and carry away these substances when they enter and irritate the sensitive whites of the eyes, the clear visual windows (the corneas), and the eyes' inner lids. Even very tiny foreign particles and liquid droplets can create a sand-in-the-eye sensation. Their presence can also redden the eye, cause it to swell, and produce uncontrollable blinking. Burning, smarting, stinging, and itching may be felt.

The irritant's presence quickly stimulates increased tear secretion as the eye attempts to cleanse itself. In a non-emergency situation, keeping the eye closed may facilitate this effort and help control pain. But an eyewash (to dilute and flush out the foreign matter) is the next step.

Some eyewash products come with a sterile eye cup. To use: Rinse the eye cup. Fill halfway up with the eyewash liquid and bending over it, press the eye cup tightly against the eye to avoid spillage. Tilt the head back, open the eyelids wide, and rotate the eyeball by tracking visual circles (i.e., as if following circles around the head). This helps ensure that all eye surfaces will be bathed by the fluid.

Eyewash products may also be packaged in a container that can be gently pressed to let a stream of the liquid go into the eye.

If these first-aid measures fail, a doctor's help should be sought. While the eye usually reacts sensitively to foreign bodies, it also may quickly accommodate them, so that the pain largely subsides. An embedded particle, however, can cause both physical and chemical damage; it must be removed by a doctor or other qualified health-care professional.

INGREDIENTS IN EYEWASHES

No active medicinal ingredients should be present in eyewash products. Thus none was approved, and any eyewash that includes an active ingredient would be disapproved as unsafe and misbranded. None of the active ingredients that are rated safe or effective in eye drops or ointments should be found in eyewashes. For a list of such substances *see* Eyewashes: Safety and Effectiveness table.

The principal *inactive* ingredient in all eyewashes is sterile water. Also included should be tiny amounts of one or more suitable preservatives (for example, benzalkonium chloride 0.01 percent); appropriate buffers, like weak concentrations of boric acid to establish an acidity to match that of normal tear-fluid; and compounds like sodium chloride (common table salt) to allow for a tearlike salinity (saltiness) of about 1 percent.

Eyewashes: Product Ratings

Product and Distributor	Dosage of Active Ingredients	Rating *	Comment
AK-Rinse (Akorn)	none[†]	A	
Blinx (Sola/Barnes-Hind)	none	A	
Collyrium Eye Lotion (Wyeth-Ayerst)	none	A	comes with eye cup
I Rinse (Americal)	none	A	
Lavoptik Eye Wash (Lavoptik)	none	A	comes with eye cup
Murine Regular (Ross)	none	A	
Ocu-Bath Eye Lotion (Commerce)	none	A	

* Author's interpretation of FDA criteria. Based on contents, not claims.
† No active drug ingredients should be found in eyewash products.

First-Aid Antibiotics

Antibiotics are germ products that fight other germs, or, as the Antimicrobial II Panel defines them: "chemical substances produced by a microorganism and having the capacity, in dilute solutions, to kill or inhibit the growth of other microorganisms." Although antibiotics originally were derived from living microorganisms—the well-known antibiotic called penicillin came from the bread mold *Penicillium notatum*, for example—now most are manufactured synthetically. Generally speaking, antibiotics are extremely powerful drugs.

Millions of tiny tubes of first-aid antibiotics have been sold over-the-counter in the last 40 years, and these antibiotics are also available to consumers in powders, creams, and sprays. But until recently, there was little scientific proof of their value in preventing infections in minor cuts, scrapes, and burns—which is the *only* approved use for them. Millions of tubes also were sold for the *treatment* of pre-existing infections. But the Panel and the FDA agreed that consumers cannot identify the bacterium or other microorganisms that

FIRST-AID ANTIBIOTICS is based on the report "Topical Antibiotic Products" by the FDA's Advisory Review Panel on OTC Antimicrobial Drug Products (Antimicrobial II Panel) and on the FDA's Tentative Final and Final Monographs on these products and several subsequent amendments.

are causing an infection and hence cannot rationally select a nonprescription antibiotic product to treat it. Hence, the sale of nonprescription antibiotic preparations to treat pre-existing infections has been banned. Consumers thus are encouraged to seek medical help for infections that do not drain and heal quickly when subjected to frequent hot water soaks—the standard self-care method.

However, in the mid 1980s, the FDA changed its mind about the value of nonprescription antibiotics in *preventing* infections. The change was based on two developments:

- The American Academy of Pediatrics published an extensive review of the medical literature on these drugs, and concluded—in an official position paper—that topical antibiotics may prevent infection after minor cuts, abrasions, and burns, and therefore may be appropriate as an "adjunct" to careful washing of the wound.

- A report was published on a 15-week study of 59 toddlers at a rural day-care center. The youngsters were examined daily, and half had their minor skin injuries and insect bites treated with an ointment containing the antibiotics neomycin sulfate, zinc bacitracin, and polymyxin B sulfate. The other children were treated with a drug-free ointment. Only 15 percent of the children treated with the active drugs suffered streptococcal (bacteria) skin infections, and none had a recurrence; only 1 needed treatment with an oral antibiotic. By contrast, 47 percent of the children who received the dummy medication suffered infections, and 5 had recurrences; 12 required oral antibiotic therapy. The topical antibiotic combination thus provided statistically significant advantage over the dummy medication.

Different antibiotics are effective against different species of bacteria. Since no one can anticipate in advance *which* types may infect a wound, it makes good sense to choose a combination product, like the one used on the day-care children, rather than a single-ingredient product. These combinations are listed below.

Choice of Treatments

The first-aider's first task, after calming the injured person, is to gently clean the wound, using cool, gently running water (or colder water if the injury is a burn). A mild soap also may be used for this cleansing if the wound is dirty, and if the soap does not increase the pain.

When the wound is clean, the first-aider now has three choices, as described in the Unit FIRST AID ANTISEPTICS. A small, clean wound, in which the skin repositions itself very closely to its normal alignment, may not require further treatment. But to kill germs that may have entered a relatively clean wound or may subsequently do so, a first-aid antiseptic or a first-aid antibiotic, such as the ones described in this Unit, may be used. For the most part, the antiseptic is the proper choice for larger, open skin wounds, but care should be taken to use nonirritating antiseptics for large, abraded areas of skin. Antibiotics may be the more appropriate choice for smaller injuries in body creases (such as on the finger or behind the knees), and on warm damp surfaces, or those injuries that are likely to come in contact with soil and other substances or fluids heavily contaminated with infectious microorganisms. Antibiotics should be used only on *small* areas of skin: those that can be covered with an adult's fingertip, for example. Use on wider areas, particularly in infants, can lead to absorption of the antibiotic through the damaged skin, resulting in a toxic reaction, such as (with neomycin) hearing loss.

It is unnecessary and probably unwise to treat a skin wound with both an antiseptic and an antibiotic. Choose one or the other, and stick with it. Wounds can be covered with a bandage or gauze dressing.

Combination Products

Some first-aid antibiotic products are combinations of two or three antibiotics. Different antibiotics kill or inhibit the growth of different groups of bacteria. Having two or more different antibiotics in a first-aid preparation can be advantageous, because each additional antibiotic extends the *spectrum*, or range, of bacteria that will be controlled.

The following are the approved single-ingredient and combination antibiotic products (most of them ointments) approved by FDA:

- *BACITRACIN*
- *BACITRACIN ZINC*
- *CHLORTETRACYCLINE HYDROCHLORIDE*
- *NEOMYCIN SULFATE*
- *TETRACYCLINE HYDROCHLORIDE*
- *BACITRACIN + NEOMYCIN SULFATE*

- *BACITRACIN + NEOMYCIN SULFATE + POLYMYXIN B SULFATE*
- *BACITRACIN + POLYMYXIN B SULFATE*
- *BACITRACIN ZINC + NEOMYCIN SULFATE*
- *BACITRACIN ZINC + NEOMYCIN SULFATE + POLYMYXIN B SULFATE*
- *NEOMYCIN SULFATE + POLYMYXIN B SULFATE*
- *OXYTETRACYCLINE HYDROCHLORIDE + POLYMYXIN B SULFATE*

In addition, to provide pain relief along with protection against germs, a single-ingredient or combination antibiotic may be combined with a -*caine* or -*amine* type of itch-pain reliever (topical anesthetic). *See* pp. 553 for more on these two types of pain relievers. These approved anesthetics are:

- *BENZOCAINE 5 TO 20 PERCENT*
- *BUTAMBEN PICRATE 1 PERCENT*
- *DIBUCAINE 0.25 TO 1 PERCENT*
- *DIBUCAINE HYDROCHLORIDE 0.25 TO 1 PERCENT*
- *DIMETHISOQUIN HYDROCHLORIDE 0.3 TO 0.5 PERCENT*
- *DYCLONINE HYDROCHLORIDE 0.5 TO 1 PERCENT*
- *LIDOCAINE 0.5 TO 4 PERCENT*
- *LIDOCAINE HYDROCHLORIDE 0.5 TO 4 PERCENT*
- *PRAMOXINE HYDROCHLORIDE 0.5 TO 1 PERCENT*
- *TETRACAINE 1 TO 2 PERCENT*
- *TETRACAINE HYDROCHLORIDE 1 TO 2 PERCENT*

 Claims

Accurate

- "First aid to help prevent infection in minor cuts, scrapes and burns"
- "… to decrease the risk of bacterial contamination…"
- "… to reduce the chance of skin infections…"

Directions

"Clean the affected area [and] apply a small amount of the ointment (an amount equal to the surface area of the tip of a finger)… 1 to 3 times daily. May be covered with a sterile bandage."

For powders: "…Apply a light dusting …"

For aerosols: "…spray a small amount …"

WARNINGS:

 Do not use in the eyes or apply over large areas of the body. In case of deep or puncture wounds, animal bites, or serious burns, consult a doctor.

Stop use and consult a doctor if the condition persists or gets worse. Do not use longer than one week unless directed by a doctor.

APPROVED ACTIVE INGREDIENTS

• *BACITRACIN:* This antibiotic, first isolated in 1943, is produced by a strain of bacteria called *Bacillus subtilis*. It kills gram-positive bacteria by blocking their ability to build cellular walls.

The drug usually is applied to small skin wounds in an ointment, which forms a protective physical cover over the wound. Bacitracin's established value, according to the Panel, is to reduce bacterial growth inside the ointment base itself and at the surface where the wound and ointment meet. Decision: safe and effective.

• *BACITRACIN ZINC:* Formulation of bacitracin as a zinc salt appears to enhance its antibacterial effect, the reviewers say. Bacitracin zinc is judged both safe and effective.

• *CHLORTETRACYCLINE HYDROCHLORIDE: See* Tetracyclines.

• *NEOMYCIN:* Neomycin is one of a class of potent antibiotics called *aminoglycosides*, which effectively kill bacteria by interfering with their ability to synthesize protein. When large amounts are used internally, these antibiotics can injure users' kidneys and damage hearing. However, they are unlikely to pose this hazard when small amounts are applied to skin wounds. The FDA says neomycin is safe and effective.

• *OXYTETRACYCLINE HYDROCHLORIDE: See* Tetracyclines.

• *POLYMYXIN B SULFATE:* This antibiotic is effective against only a few types of bacteria. But, since these organisms tend to be of the potentially dangerous *gram-negative* variety, polymyxin is a useful companion with bacitracin or other antibiotics that are more effective against *gram-positive* organisms. Polymyxin B sulfate is approved as safe and effective only in combination products with other approved antibiotics.

• *TETRACYCLINES:* Several tetracycline compounds will safely and effectively protect skin wounds against a wide range of bacteria; they include *chlortetracycline hydrochloride, oxytetracycline hydrochloride,* and *tetracycline hydrochloride.* These antibiotics interfere with the invading bacteria's ability to synthesize protein, thus inhibiting the growth and reproduction of these organisms.

Like all antibiotics, tetracyclines produce adverse effects in a small number of users. But the recommended dose—a dab of tetracycline ointment spread over the wound—is so small that these reactions are quite rare. So the tetracyclines are safe as well as effective.

CONDITIONALLY APPROVED ACTIVE INGREDIENTS
None.

DISAPPROVED ACTIVE INGREDIENTS
None.

Safety and Effectiveness: Active Ingredients in Over-the-Counter First-Aid Antibiotics

Antibiotic	Evaluation
bacitracin	safe and effective (active against gram-positive bacteria)
bacitracin zinc	safe and effective (against gram-positive bacteria)
neomycin	safe and effective (active against gram positive and some gram-negative bacteria)
polymyxin B sulfate	safe and effective (active primarily against gram-negative bacteria; approved only in combinations with other antibiotics that are active against gram-positive bacteria)

Safety and Effectiveness: Active Ingredients in Over-the-Counter First-Aid Antibiotics

Antibiotic	Evaluation
tetracyclines: chlortetracycline hydrochloride, oxytetracycline hydrochloride, and tetracycline hydrochloride	safe and effective (active against gram-positive and some gram-negative bacteria)

NOTE: The terms *gram-positive* and *gram-negative* are based on bacterial organisms' penchant for absorbing a dye, called *Gram's stain*, that colors them purple and so renders them clearly visible under a microscope. Organisms that absorb the dye are called *gram-positive*. *Gram-negative* bacteria absorb little or none of the dye and show up under the microscope with a faint pink color. Gram-negative organisms tend to be more dangerous than gram-positive ones. They also tend to be susceptible to different antibiotics, as indicated here.

First-Aid Antibiotics: Product Ratings

SINGLE-INGREDIENT PRODUCTS

Product and Distributor	Dosage of Active Ingredients	Rating *	Comment
bacitracin			
Bacitracin (generic)	**ointment:** 500 units per g	A	active against gram-positive bacteria
Baciguent (Upjohn)		A	active against gram-positive bacteria
chlortetracycline hydrochloride			
Aureomycin (Lederle)	**ointment:** 3%	A	active against gram-positive and some gram-negative bacteria
neomycin sulfate			
Myciguent (Upjohn)	**ointment; cream:** 3.5 mg per g	A	active against gram-positive and some gram-negative bacteria
Neomycin (generic)		A	active against gram-positive and some gram-negative bacteria
tetracycline hydrochloride			
Achromycin (Lederle)	**ointment:** 3%	A	active against gram-positive and some gram-negative bacteria

First-Aid Antibiotics: Product Ratings (contd)

COMBINATION PRODUCTS

Product and Distributor	Dosage of Active Ingredients	Rating *	Comment
Bactine First Aid Antibiotic Plus Anesthetic (Miles)	**ointment:** 5000 units polymyxin B sulfate + 3.5 mg neomycin base (as sulfate) + 400 units bacitracin + 10 mg diperodon hydrochloride per g	A	diperodon is a pain reliever
Campho-Phenique Antibiotic Plus Pain Reliever Ointment (Sterling Health)	**ointment:** 5000 units polymyxin B sulfate + 3.5 mg neomycin base (as sulfate) + 500 units bacitracin + 40 mg of lidocaine per g	A	lidocaine is a pain reliever
Medi-Quick (Mentholatum)	**ointment:** 5000 units polymyxin B sulfate + 3.5 mg neomycin base (as sulfate) + 400 units bacitracin per g	A	polymyxin adds protection against gram-negative bacteria
Neosporin (Burroughs Wellcome)	**ointment:** 5000 units polymyxin B sulfate + 3.5 mg neomycin base (as sulfate) + 400 units bacitracin per g	A	polymyxin adds protection against gram-negative bacteria

First Aid Antiseptics

Spectrocin Plus (Numark)	**ointment:** 5000 units polymyxin B sulfate + 3.5 mg neomycin base (as sulfate) + 400 units bacitracin + 5 mg lidocaine per g	A	lidocaine is a pain reliever

---

*Author's interpretation of FDA criteria. Based on contents, not claims.

First-Aid Antiseptics

An antiseptic is a drug that kills bacteria and other microorganisms on the skin or other body surfaces or retards their growth and spread. People use antiseptics mainly to prevent these infections, but also because of the sense of cleanliness they confer.

Antiseptics are formulated as swab-on liquids, sprays, powders, and moist paper-wipes, as well as in other ways. They are commonly used to wipe babies' bottoms and to remove germs after contact with human or animal wastes or with other disagreeable and presumably germ-laden substances. Their most important use, however, is in first aid—to cleanse and de-germ the skin around splinters, cuts, scratches, and other superficial wounds.

First-aid antiseptics are specifically defined by the FDA as a "germicide," or inhibitor of germs' growth that is applied to the skin "to help prevent infection in minor cuts, scrapes, and burns."

FIRST-AID ANTISEPTICS is based on the report of the FDA's Advisory Review Panel on OTC Antimicrobial Drug Products for Repeated Daily Human Use (Antimicrobial I Panel); the FDA's first two Tentative Final Monographs on OTC Antimicrobial Products; and two reports by the FDA's Advisory Review Panel on OTC Miscellaneous External Drug Products: "Alcohol Drug Products for Topical Antimicrobial OTC Use" and "Mercury-Containing Drug Products for Topical Antimicrobial OTC Human Use."

Though they may contain identical chemicals, there is a distinction between *antiseptics* and *disinfectants*. An antiseptic is intended to cleanse and de-germ the skin and other body surfaces. A disinfectant is used to clean and de-germ inanimate objects—from surgical instruments to toilet seats to hospital floors.

 Claims

Accurate

- "First aid to help prevent infection in minor cuts, scrapes and burns"
- "...decreases the risk of bacterial contamination ..."
- "...reduce[s] the chance of skin infection..."

WARNINGS:

 For external use only. Do not use in the eyes or apply over large areas of the body. In the case of deep puncture wounds, animal bites, or serious burns, consult a doctor.

Stop use and consult a doctor if the condition persists or gets worse. Do not use longer than one week unless directed by a doctor.

What To Do

The abundant variety of first-aid treatment products should not blind first-aiders to the simplicity or the priorities of their task. When you or someone else suddenly has been injured, the first priority is to try to sustain—or regain—some semblance of composure and calm.

The injured *person*, and then the extent of his or her injury, should be assessed. If the injury victim is unconscious, is bleeding severely, is pale and sweaty (which may mean *shock*), or appears to have a broken bone or other major injury, then standard first-aid measures should immediately come into play. Stay calm. Call out for medical help if someone is there to hear and respond. Put the injured person flat on his or her back. Use your fingers to clear any foreign matter that may be in the mouth or windpipe. Tilt the person's head back (unless the neck appears to be injured). This opens the airway to the lungs.

If the individual is not breathing, start mouth-to-mouth resuscitation. Check to see if the person's heart is beating by pressing fingers against the carotid artery in the neck, just behind the Adam's apple. If no pulse can be felt, the heart is not beating. Quickly raise the legs and/or lower the head. Give *CPR*—cardiopulmonary resuscitation—by pressing rhythmically down and releasing the chest, alternating this with continued mouth-to-mouth resuscitation to restore both heartbeat and breathing. Staunch blood flow if the victim is bleeding heavily. Obtain emergency medical aid. (These directions are taken from the *American Medical Association Handbook of First Aid and Emergency Care* [New York: Random House, 1990]. It pays to own and study a first aid handbook like this one; mouth-to-mouth and CPR techniques are taught by medical, paramedical and emergency services experts in most communities.)

If the injury is relatively minor (a skinned knee, a cut finger, or a first-degree burn from touching the stove, for example), you can probably treat it satisfactorily yourself. The first task, particularly with children, is to calm and reassure the injured person. If the problem is a skin wound—which is what this Unit is mostly about—the overlying clothing should be removed, and the injury examined and cleaned. Use cool, gently running water to cleanse the wound; but use colder water longer for burns (*see* p. 969).

Some first-aiders say mild soap should be used for wound cleansing, particularly if soil, dirt, or grit is stuck to the injured skin. Other first aiders worry about washing a skin wound with soap for fear its alkalinity will exacerbate the injury and pain. Use your judgment. If soap increases the pain, ease off on its use.

Some antiseptic preparations, particularly alcohol, are excellent wound cleansers. But alcohol is quite irritating to injured skin, so you would not use it for a wide, raw injury (a skinned knee for example) or for a burn. (For more on when to use alcohol, see Alcohol, further on.)

Once the injured area is clean, and the bleeding, if any, has been slowed (cold water will do this by shrinking the tiny blood vessels in and under the skin), you have basically three choices: (1) Pat the wound dry with a clean cloth or paper towel and leave it untreated, or (2) Treat it with a first aid antiseptic—one of the products described in this Unit, or (3) Treat it with a first-aid antibiotic. (*See* FIRST-AID ANTIBIOTICS.) Judgment is required to decide among these options. A clean, bloodless cut may need no further treatment if the skin around it is mostly intact and in its normal position. On the other hand, an elbow scraped on the playground probably could use treatment to kill microorganisms that may have gotten into the wound, and, perhaps, to keep other microorganisms from entering.

The *first-aid antiseptics* described here are germ-killing chemical agents. *First-aid antibiotics*, another option, contains special, potent germ-killing substances called *antibiotics* (defined on p. 404) that help to prevent infections. Many first-aid antibiotic products are formulated as ointments, with petrolatum as their vehicle (base)—although the Antimicrobial II Panel says that antibiotics in solution or cream bases are more effective.

'Drugs' and 'Cosmetics' Defined

The line between a "drug" and a "cosmetic" may seem vanishingly thin, since some ingredients, such as antimicrobials, can be found in *both* kinds of products. But these compounds are regulated far more rigorously when they are active ingredients in drugs.

The difference between the two classes of products depends in part on the type of chemical that is involved—and, obviously, to be *both* a drug and a cosmetic ingredient, it must be quite safe. Also, the difference depends in part on the claims made for it on the label and in promotional material. This is how the Food Drug & Cosmetic Act, the law under which the FDA regulates these compounds, defines the two classes:

A "drug" is an article "intended for use in the diagnosis, cure, mitigation, treatment or prevention of disease," or a substance "intended to affect the structure or any function of the body."

A "cosmetic," on the other hand, is an article "intended to be rubbed, poured, sprinkled, or sprayed on, introduced into, or otherwise applied to the human body or any part thereof for cleansing, beautifying, promoting attractiveness, or altering the appearance ..."

Both drugs and cosmetics must be safe to use, but only drugs must be proved effective. The Over-the-Counter Drug Review is intended, precisely, to ensure consumers that when it is finished, *all* such products that they buy will be certified safe and effective by the FDA.

Must a first-aider use *both* an antiseptic and an antibiotic? Probably not: One or the other is likely to suffice. The antiseptic, which will dry on the skin, or which can be covered with a bandage, may be the better choice for *superficial* injuries on wide, open skin areas. The ointment-based antibiotic, however, may be better for smaller, deeper cuts and puncture wounds, particularly those in body creases and other areas where it is difficult to protect the wound site from dirt and infection.

The final issue is pain relief. Many injuries will stop hurting by themselves within a half hour or so. However, other injuries, such as burns, may continue to hurt. Many antiseptic and antibiotic preparations are formulated as sprays or creams that also contain topical pain relievers; or the pain reliever can be applied separately. For a summary of these ingredients, *see* ITCH AND PAIN REMEDIES APPLIED TO THE SKIN.

Alcohols

Some of the most effective antiseptics are alcohols. They kill bacteria on contact, within seconds. They are, however, less effective against viruses and even less effective against funguses.

Besides killing "germs," alcohols are solvents and astringents. They loosen, dissolve, and remove grease and oil, protein-type matter, and other dirt and debris from the skin. And they evaporate quickly. The mild burning sensation felt when alcohol is rubbed on the skin offers a relaxing counterirritant effect for persons suffering from aches and pains.

Alcohols are colorless and do not stain clothing or the skin. This means that alcohol, unlike Mercurochrome or other dark-staining antiseptics, does not mask skin-color changes, particularly the inflammatory redness that may signal a developing infection. Another benefit of plain alcohol is it is likely to be far less expensive than other, less effective antiseptic products.

On the deficit side, alcohols may irritate underlying tissues. They therefore should not be used on deep or wide wounds or on puncture wounds, and they should not be used to irrigate deeply embedded splinters before an attempt is made to remove the splinters. Deep wounds require medical care. Mucosal tissue, such as the lips, is more sensitive to alcohol than regular skin and so should not be treated with strong alcohols. Because it is irritating, alcohol should not be used for treating burns.

Mercurials

The heavy liquid metal *mercury* and its salts have been used medicinally for thousands of years. But unlike alcohols, the use of mercurials as drugs, particularly as skin antiseptics, is waning.

A major difficulty with mercury is that it is readily absorbed through broken or unbroken skin, from the gastrointestinal tract when swallowed, and from the respiratory tract when inhaled as mercury vapor. Mercury is highly toxic. Once absorbed it can cause major damage, even death. Small amounts applied to minor skin wounds probably do not pose a serious or lethal hazard. But they can produce an itchy contact dermatitis and may provoke an allergic reaction.

However, the principal complaint against mercury as an antiseptic is not its lack of safety but its lack of effectiveness. Although Mercurochrome, Merthiolate (also called thimerosal), and related compounds were the standard applications for minor cuts and scratches a generation ago, they have since fallen into disuse. The reason is that experiments conducted in the 1940s showed that mecurials do stop bacteria from growing—but they often fail to kill them. The organisms revive and multiply anew once the mercury compound is removed, diluted, or neutralized.

The most striking discovery about mercury was that the human serum—the clear liquid portion of the blood—inactivates mercurial antiseptics. When Merthiolate is suspended in human serum, it requires 14,000 times more of the antiseptic to inactivate a test dose of infectious bacteria (*Salmonella typhosa*) than is needed when the antiseptic is suspended in salt water. Since mercurials used on the skin are likely to come into contact with serum, pus, and other body fluids, their effect on the bacteria they are supposed to kill may be nil.

For these reasons, the Panel declared that all topical mercurials are ineffective as antiseptics and that some are dangerous as well. Therefore, all medical claims for them are misleading and examples of misbranding. If the Panel's view prevails, all mercurial antiseptics will be removed from the nonprescription drug-marketplace in the United States before long.

Assessing Drugs and Claims

Alcohol and mercurial antiseptics were assessed by the FDA's Advisory Panel on Miscellaneous External Drugs. Many other antiseptics described in this unit were evaluated by the Antimicrobial I Panel.

Several that got lost in the shuffle have since been initially assessed by the FDA.

Combination Products

A first-aid antiseptic active ingredient may be combined with an external pain reliever or with a skin protectant. (*See* ITCH AND PAIN REMEDIES APPLIED TO THE SKIN for pain relievers, and UNGUENTS AND POWDERS TO PROTECT THE SKIN for skin protectants.) Several specific combinations and complexes of ingredients also are safe and effective, as described in this section, and listed in the table Safety and Effectiveness: Active Ingredients in First Aid Antiseptics.

APPROVED ANTISEPTIC ACTIVE INGREDIENTS

A number of ingredients are rated as safe and effective:

Single Ingredients

* *BENZALKONIUM CHLORIDE (0.1 TO 0.13 PERCENT):* *See* Quaternary Ammonium Compounds.
* *BENZETHONIUM CHLORIDE (0.1 TO 0.2 PERCENT):* *See* Quaternary Ammonium Compounds.
* *ETHYL ALCOHOL (48 TO 95 PERCENT BY VOLUME):* This is the oldest and best-known alcohol. It is the alcohol in liquor and wine, and has been used for centuries for its nutritional, intoxicant, and medicinal properties. When sold in drugstores for medicinal use it contains additives that make it unpalatable. Ethyl alcohol may also be called *absolute alcohol*, *alcohol*, *denatured alcohol*, or *ethanol*. Its technical name, in FDA parlance, now seems to be simply *alcohol*. But this is confusing, since several other types of alcohol also are approved for various medical uses.

  The long and universal use of ethyl alcohol in beverages attests to its relative lack of toxicity when taken in small quantities. As to external applications, it is not safe to use ethyl alcohol on large, open wounds, both because it is irritating and because it kills white blood cells. However, evaluators say it is safe to use for small wounds:

allergic reactions and other side effects are extremely rare.

Ethyl alcohol starts killing bacteria within seconds. Dipping your hands into it for one minute kills more bacteria than scrubbing them in water for six minutes. Ethyl alcohol also will kill or inactivate many common viruses, including flu virus and some herpes viruses. It is less effective against funguses, so it is not used to treat conditions like athlete's foot.

Daily or routine use of alcohol as an antiseptic is unwise. It kills the normal bacteria on skin surfaces so effectively that it may make the skin susceptible to the growth of other, disease-causing, bacteria.

Ethyl alcohol works best in the presence of water. So the Panel stipulates that these preparations contain at least 5 percent water by volume. The safe and effective concentrations of ethyl alcohol are 48 to 95 percent by volume.

• HEXYLRESORCINOL (0.1 PERCENT): Hexylresorcinol is a relatively old drug, used to clean wounds, that the *Handbook of Nonprescription Drugs* (9th edition) lists as safer but less toxic than phenol (*see* below) as an antiseptic for inhibiting bacterial growth. The Panel and the FDA, with few words, evaluate it as safe and effective.

• HYDROGEN PEROXIDE (3 PERCENT): This tried and true drug has been listed as a topical anti-infective for years in the *United States Pharmacopeia* (*U.S.P.*). A manufacturer submitted fresh data demonstrating that it inhibited the growth of a wide variety of bacteria and stopped all growth of *Staphylococcus aureus* within 10 minutes. FDA said: safe and effective.

• IODINES (IODINE TINCTURE 2 PERCENT, AND IODINE SOLUTION 2 PERCENT): This stinging, elemental antiseptic, dissolved in either alcohol or water, has been a standard household first-aid antiseptic for more than 130 years. Neither the Panel nor the FDA had any doubts about its effectiveness, but both worried that iodine might irritate the skin and thus retard wound healing. A number of studies then were conducted in which small wounds were induced on shaved patches of animals' skins; wounds treated with iodine were compared with wounds that were not treated with this antiseptic. No significant skin damage was detected in the iodine-treated animals, so the FDA changed its ruling on iodine preparations to safe and effective.

• ISOPROPYL ALCOHOL (50 TO 91.3 PERCENT BY VOLUME): Obtained principally from petroleum, isopropyl alcohol (also called *isopropanol)* is unfit to drink. It is more toxic than ethyl alcohol (*see* Ethyl acohol) and if accidentally swallowed, medical care should be sought at once. The vapors of isopropyl alcohol are poisonous enough that it should be used as an alcohol rub only in a well-ventilated room. Nevertheless, there is little if any risk in using isopropyl alcohol as an antiseptic, so the Panel lists it as safe.

When swabbed on the skin, isopropyl alcohol begins killing *Staphylococcus aureus*, *Escherichia coli*, and other bacteria within seconds. It works more slowly and less effectively against viruses and does even more poorly against funguses (for which other antiseptics are needed).

This alcohol works better in the presence of water, which should be present in no less than approximately 9 percent. At concentrations of 50 to 91.3 percent, isopropyl alcohol is assessed as both safe and effective.

- **METHYLBENZETHONIUM CHLORIDE (0.13 TO 0.5 PERCENT):** *See* Quaternary Ammonium Compounds.
- **PHENOL (0.5 TO 1.5 PERCENT):** This classic drug, the one with the "medicinal" smell, relieves itching and pain. *See* p. 811. Based on a review of the medical literature, the FDA upgraded it from the Panel's "safe but not proved effective" to an approved rating: safe and effective.
- **QUATERNARY AMMONIUM COMPOUNDS:** These "quats," as they are called, include benzalkonium chloride, benzethonium chloride, and the very closely related methylbenzethonium chloride. They are old, very strong antiseptic ingredients. The FDA reviewed a wide range of old and new studies on them, including some that showed that, contrary to the Panel's fears, quats are not inordinately irritating to the skin. Based on this review, the FDA re-listed all three compounds as safe and effective.

Combinations

Thus far, only one combination, which contains several antiseptic ingredients, has been approved as safe and effective:

- **EUCALYPTOL 0.091 PERCENT + MENTHOL 0.042 PERCENT + METHYL SALICYLATE 0.055 PERCENT + THYMOL 0.063 PERCENT + ALCOHOL 26.9 PERCENT:** None of these ingredients, singly, is safe and effective as a first-aid antiseptic. What is more, this combination violates several proposed rules for these products. Nevertheless, a manufacturer submitted data on a mouthwash product of this formulation, that showed that it is a more potent germ-killer than any of the individual ingredients—and that it is quite effective in this antiseptic capacity. Based on this, and considerably more data, the FDA placed the specific product formulation in the "safe and effective" category.

First aid antiseptics may be combined with safe and effective itch-and-pain relievers (*see* p. 567).

Complexes

Three chemical complexes of antiseptic ingredients are approved as safe and effective:

• CAMPHOR 10.8 PERCENT + PHENOL 4.7 PERCENT IN LIGHT MINERAL OIL: This preparation is described on p. 127.

• CAMPHORATED METACRESOL (3 TO 10.8 PERCENT CAMPHOR + 1 TO 3.6 METACRESOL, IN A 3 TO 1 RATIO): Products containing this ratio of camphor and metacresol have a long history of problem-free use. In submitting a large volume of new and old data on this complex of two active ingredients, a manufacturer declared the ingredients are widely applied, professionally, by doctors and nurses. Metacresol, the FDA agreed, is less toxic than phenol, to which it is similar—and which has been approved as safe in combinations with camphor. A little reluctantly, it would seem from its printed decision, FDA approved camphorated metacresol as safe and effective. (*See* p. 128.)

WARNING:

 Do not put a bandage over a wound treated with camphorated metacresol because it may irritate and burn the skin, and because bandaging may increase the amount of the drug that is absorbed internally.

• POVIDONE-IODINE COMPLEX (5 TO 10 PERCENT IODINE): The povidone holds the iodine, and slowly releases it onto the skin. This extends the preparation's effectiveness, and allows higher initial concentrations of iodine to be used than would be possible with iodine alone. An enormous literature has been developed to demonstrate the safety and efficacy of povidone-iodine. Unlike some of the other approved first aid antiseptics, this one is particularly effective in stopping fungal infections. Since fungal infections tend to develop in warm, damp areas of skin, povidone iodine may be particularly effective for treating them. Verdict: safe and effective.

CONDITIONALLY APPROVED ANTISEPTIC ACTIVE INGREDIENTS

Single Ingredients

- *BENZYL ALCOHOL:* This aromatic alcohol is not harmful to the skin. But it is not a very potent antiseptic, either. It is safe but its effectiveness must be proved.
- *CALOMEL (MERCUROUS CHLORIDE):* This mercurial is safe. But it has not been shown to be very effective.
- *CHLOROBUTANOL:* This is a fairly toxic alcohol, although in low concentrations (under 5 percent) it is not likely to be harmful. It kills bacteria only slowly. Tentative verdict: safe but not proved effective.
- *CHLOROXYLENOL:* This preparation is widely used in hospitals and doctors' offices as an antiseptic. It is safe, FDA says. But the finished product contains a number of other ingredients besides chloroxylenol. FDA wants to see proof that the active ingredient, alone, is effective before ruling that in fact it is. Current status: safe but not proved effective.
- *MERBROMIN:* This is the antiseptic that is better known as Mercurochrome. It effectively dyes the skin red. But it does little else—least of all kill germs with dispatch. A half-century ago, one investigator discovered that Mercurochrome's antiseptic power may have come from the alcohol, or acetone, in which it is formulated. While no harm comes of painting the skin with Mercurochrome, no help does either, according to the Panel. The verdict is: safe but not proved effective.
- *MERCUFENOL CHLORIDE (ORTHO-HYDROXYPHENYLMERCURIC CHLORIDE, ORTHO-CHLOROMERCURIPHENOL):* The FDA says these compounds are safe. But it has yet to see clear evidence that they are effective. So it says: safe but not proved effective.
- *PHENYLMERCURIC NITRATE:* While this compound has been found less toxic to human skin cells than some other commonly used mercurial antiseptics, there is no evidence that it effectively combats microorganisms in the low concentrations in which it is formulated into nonprescription products. The Panel's judgment therefore is that it is safe but not proved effective.
- *SECONDARY AMYLTRICRESOLS:* This category slipped past the Panel. The FDA wants clear evidence that these preparations are safe and effective.

- *TICLOCARBAN:* This antiseptic is most frequently used in antimicrobial bar soaps. *See* p. 454. But FDA remains unconvinced, based on the data submitted, that it is effective as a spray-on or a liquid antiseptic. Judgment for now: safe but not proved effective.
- *TRICLOSAN:* This compound, like triclocarban, is more likely to be found in an antimicrobial bar soap than in a first-aid antiseptic. It has a long regulatory history, and some of the safety tests, now being redone, were performed in a laboratory whose work FDA no longer accepts because of "numerous problems" there. Pending re-review of the massive data base, the FDA labels triclosan safe but not proved effective as a first-aid antiseptic.

Combinations and/or Complexes

- *IODINE COMPLEX (AMMONIUM ETHER SULFATE + POLYOXYETHYLENE SORBITAN MONOLAURATE):* The FDA has little to say about this formulation other than that it will need more data before declaring the formulation safe and effective. This particular iodine complex is conditionally approved for now.
- *IODINE COMPLEX (PHOSPHATE ESTER OF ALKYARYLOXY POLYOXYETHYLENE GLYCOL):* Not proved safe or effective as a first-aid antiseptic.
- *MERCUFENOL CHLORIDE + SECONDARY AMYLTRICRESOLS:* It is safe, FDA says, But its effectiveness is not established.
- *NONYLPHENOXYPOLY (ETHYLENOXY) ETHANOLIODINE:* Not proved safe or effective for use as a first-aid antiseptic.
- *POLOXAMER IODINE COMPLEX:* Proof of safety and efficacy are wanting for this complex, too.
- *TRIPLE DYE:* Proof still is lacking that this preparation is safe or effective.
- *UNDECOYLIUM CHLORIDE IODINE COMPLEX:* This formulation is not currently marketed over-the-counter in the United States. The FDA must be persuaded, by data, that the formulation is safe and effective as a first-aid antiseptic.

DISAPPROVED ANTISEPTIC ACTIVE INGREDIENTS

Single Ingredients

- *AMMONIATED MERCURY:* This is a toxic form of mercury that has been used to treat psoriasis, ringworm, and other skin conditions. The incidence of mercury poisoning is high. Therefore, the Panel concludes that ammoniated mercury is not safe, and like other mercurials, it is not effective as an antiseptic.

• *CLOFLUCARBAN:* Not safe or effective for use on the skin.

• *FLUOROSALAN:* Not safe for use on the skin.

• *MERCURIC CHLORIDE (MERCURY CHLORIDE):* The reviewers found no data on this compound's use as an antiseptic, so they summarily disapproved it.

• *MERCURIC OXIDE, YELLOW:* Not safe or effective.

• *MERCURIC SALICYLATE:* Little data is available on this mercurial antiseptic. It is not safe and not effective unless proved otherwise.

• *MERCURIC SULFIDE, RED:* Little data is available on this mercurial, so FDA obligingly placed it in the category *not safe and effective.*

• *MERCURY:* No data is available on the use of mercury as an antiseptic. It is hazardous, however, because it is absorbed through the skin and can cause internal poisoning. Not safe. Not effective.

• *MERCURY OLEATE:* This mercurial, similarly, is categorized not safe and not effective.

• *MERCURY SULFIDE:* Little data available. Not safe and not effective.

• *NITROMERSOL:* Little or no information available. So Panel and agency concur: Not safe. Not effective.

• *PARA-CHLOROMERCURIPHENOL:* Like other mercurials, this one is summarily dismissed by Panel and agency: Not safe and not effective.

• *THIMEROSAL (MERTHIOLATE):* This mercurial antiseptic once was widely used for first aid. It has since been found to be very damaging to human skin cells. It also is highly allergenic: In one survey, 1 of every 6 military recruits was found to be allergic to the drug. Apart from the question of safety, Merthiolate has also been found to slow bacterial growth but not kill the bacteria. So the Panel calls the drug neither safe nor effective.

• *TRIBROMSALAN:* This ingredient is judged not safe for use as an antiseptic.

• *VITROMERSOL:* As one more mercury compound about which evaluators could find no data, vitromersol was summarily disapproved as not safe and not effective.

• *ZYLOXIN:* This is a mercurial. No data on its value as an antiseptic were found, and it was summarily dismissed as not safe and not effective.

When Greater Relief Is Needed

Wide, deep, dirty, or scary wounds should be shown to a doctor. If your private physician is not immediately available, go at once to the Emergency Room of your community hospital.

Safety and Effectiveness: Active Ingredients in Over-the-Counter First-Aid Antiseptics

Active Ingredient	*Assessment*
amyltricresols, secondary	not proved safe and effective
benzalkonium chloride 0.1-0.13%	safe and effective
benzethonium chloride 0.1-0.2%	safe and effective
benzyl alcohol	safe but not proved effective
calomel	not proved safe and effective
chlorobutanol	safe but not proved effective
chloroxylenol (PCMX)	safe but not proved effective
cloflucarban	not safe or effective
ethyl alcohol (48-95%)	safe and effective
ethyl alcohol (under 48%)	safe but not effective
fluorosalan	not safe and effective
hexylresorcinol 0.1%	safe and effective
hydrogen peroxide 3%	safe and effective
iodine, topical solution 2%	safe and effective
iodine, tincture of (2%)	safe and effective
isopropyl alcohol (50-91.3%)	safe and effective

Safety and Effectiveness: Active Ingredients in Over-the-Counter First-Aid Antiseptics (contd)

Active Ingredient	Assessment
isopropyl alcohol (under 50%)	not effective
merbromin *see* Mercurochrome	
mercufenol chloride	not proved safe and effective
mercuric chloride (mercury chloride)	not safe or effective
mercuric oxide, yellow	not safe and effective
mercuric salicylate	not safe and effective
mercuric sulfide, red	not safe and effective
Mercurochrome	safe but not proved effective
mercury	not safe and effective
mercury, ammoniated	not safe or effective
mercury oleate	summarily disapproved
methylbenzethonium chloride 0.1-0.5%	safe and effective
nitromersol	not safe and effective
orthochloromercuriphenol *see* Mercufenol chloride	
orthohydroxyphenylmercuric chloride *see* Mercufenol chloride	
para-chloromercuriphenol	not safe and effective
phenol (0.5-1.5% in aqueous or alcoholic solution)	safe and effective
phenol (greater than 1.5% in aqueous or alcoholic solution)	not safe
phenylmercuric nitrate	safe but not proved effective
thimerosal	not safe or effective
tincture of iodine 2%	safe and effective
tribromsalan	not safe

Safety and Effectiveness: Active Ingredients in Over-the-Counter First-Aid Antiseptics (contd)

Active Ingredient	Assessment
triclocarban	safe but not proved effective
triclosan	safe but not proved effective
vitromersal	not safe or effective
zyloxin	not safe or effective

Safety and Effectiveness: Combination and Complex Products Sold Over-the-Counter as First Aid Antiseptics

Safe and Effective

camphorated metacresol (camphor 3 to 10.8% + 1 to 3.6% metacresol) in a 3:1 ratio

camphorated phenol (camphor 10.8% + phenol 4.7% in light mineral oil)

eucalyptol 0.091% + menthol 0.042% + methyl salicylate 0.055% + thymol 0.063% in 26.9% alcohol

povidone-iodine complex 5 to 10%

Conditionally Safe and Effective

iodine complex (ammonium ether sulfate + polyoxyethylene sorbitan monolaurate)

iodine complex (phosphate ester of alkylaryloxy [get correct sp.] polyoxyethylene glycol)

mercunfenol chloride + secondary amyltricresols

nonylphenoxypoly (ethyleneoxy) ethanoliodine

poloxamer-iodine complex

triple dye

undecoylium chloride iodine complex

Unsafe or Ineffective

None

First-Aid Antiseptics: Product Ratings

SINGLE-INGREDIENT PRODUCTS

Product and Distributor	Dosage of Active Ingredients	Rating*	Comment
benzalkonium chloride			
Benza (Century)	solution: 1:750	A	
Zephiran (Sanofi Winthrop)	tincture: 1:750 tincture spray: 1:750	A	
ethyl alcohol (48% to 95%)			
Alcare (Calgon Vestal)	foam: 62%	A	
Ethyl alcohol (generic)	liquid: 48% to 95%	A	
hexylresorcinol			
S.T. 37 (Menley & James)	solution: 0.1%	A	
hydrogen peroxide			
Hydrogen peroxide (generic)	solution: 3%	A	
iodine			
Iodine topical solution (generic)	solution: 2% iodine + 2.4% sodium iodide in purified water	A	

Tincture of iodine (generic)	swabs: 2% iodine + 2.4% sodium iodide + 47% alcohol	A	
isopropyl alcohol (50% to 91.3%)			
Alcohol Swab (Becton Dickinson)	swab: 70%	A	
Isopropyl alcohol (generic)	**liquid:** 70%	A	
mercurochrome (25% mercury + 20% bromine)			
Mercurochrome (generic)	**liquid:** 2%	B	not proved effective (after all these years!)
povidone-iodine			
Betadine (Purdue-Frederick)	**antiseptic gauze pads:** 10% available iodine **solution:** 10% available iodine **spray:** 5% available iodine	A	
Operand (Redi-Products)	**solution:** 10% available iodine; also: ointment, spray, swabsticks	A	
Polydine (Century)	**solution:** 10% available iodine	A	
Povidone-Iodine (generic)	**liquid, ointment, solution:** 10% available iodine	A	

First-Aid Antiseptics: Product Ratings (contd)

Product and Distributor	Dosage of Active Ingredients	Rating*	Comment
thimerosal			
Mersol (Century)	**solution:** 1:1000 **tincture:** 1:1000 + 50% alcohol	C C	not safe or effective not safe or effective
Thimerosal (generic)	**solution:** 1:1000 **tincture:** 1:1000 + 50% alcohol	C C	not safe or effective not safe or effective
triclosan			
SeptiSoft (Calgon Vestal)	**solution:** 0.25%	B	not proved effective

COMBINATION PRODUCTS

Product and Distributor	Dosage of Active Ingredients	Rating*	Comment
Campho-Phenique (Winthrop)	**liquid:** phenol 4.7% + camphor 10.8% in mineral oil	A	
Listerine Antiseptic (Warner-Lambert)	**liquid:** 0.06% thymol + 0.09% eucalyptol + 0.09% methyl salicylate + 0.04% menthol	A	

ANTISEPTIC/ANESTHETIC COMBINATION PRODUCTS

Product and Distributor	Dosage	Antiseptic	Anesthetic	Rating*	Comment

Product	Form			Rating*	
Aerocaine (Aeroceuticals)	spray	0.5% benzethonium chloride	13.6% benzocaine	A	
Anbesol (Whitehall)	liquid, gel	0.5%, phenol + 70% alcohol	6.3% benzocaine	A	
Bactine Antiseptic Anesthetic (Miles)	liquid, aerosal spray	0.13% benzalkonium chloride	2.5% lidocaine	A	
Maximum Strength Anbesol (Whitehall)	liquid, gel	0.5% phenol + 60% alcohol	20% benzocaine	A	
Medi-Quick (Mentholatum)	spray	0.13% benzalkonium chloride	2% lidocaine	A	
Unguentine Plus (Mentholatum)	cream	2% chloroxylenol + 0.5% phenol	2% lidocaine	B	chloroxylenol not proved effective

*Author's interpretation of FDA criteria. Based on contents, not claims.

Fluoride Toothpastes and Rinses for Cavity Prevention

Treating the teeth with tiny amounts of sodium fluoride—or other fluorine compounds—will significantly decrease the number of cavities that develop. The easiest, cheapest, and most effective form of fluoride supplementation is fluoridation of each community's drinking water. Just over half of all Americans—53 percent of them in 1989, according to government figures—are protected in this way. See Map, p. 445. One national health objective for the year 2000 is to extend optimal fluoridation to 75 percent of Americans served by community water systems.

The FDA Dental Panel said that fluoride dental products can further reduce the number of dental cavities that develop in people who live in places where water is fluoridated. But these over-the-counter preparations may be particularly valuable for the many Americans who live in towns and cities without adequate natural or supplemental fluoridation.

The toothpastes, powders, rinses, and gels sold to prevent cavi-

FLUORIDE TOOTHPASTES AND RINSES FOR CAVITY PREVENTION is based on the report "Anticaries Drug Products for OTC Human Use" by the FDA's Review Panel on OTC Dentifrice and Dental-Care Drug Products, and on the FDA's two Tentative Final Monographs on these products.

ties are categorized as drugs, and regulated by the government as such, because they prevent dental disease. The technical word for cavities is *caries*.

 Claims

Accurate
- "Aids in the prevention of dental cavities"
- "Aids in the prevention of dental caries (decay)"

False or Misleading
- "For a healthier mouth with less decay"
- "Raising your natural resistance to tooth decay"
- "Reduces mouth acidity"

Why Teeth Decay

It is *acid* that erodes tooth enamel, causing cavities. This acid is produced by bacteria that are a part of the sticky, smelly, gel-like film called *dental plaque* (or *bacterial plaque*) that builds up on the surfaces of teeth. It sticks stubbornly and gradually hardens into a resistant coating called *tarter* that cannot be adequately brushed away; professional cleaning by a dentist may be the only way to remove it. (*See* TEETH: ANTI-PLAQUE PRODUCTS).

Cavities start early. It has been estimated that by age two, half of all American children have at least one cavity. This early dental decay has been attributed to the propping of bottles of milk or juice in babies' mouths so they can suck themselves to sleep. This keeps sugars and the bacteria that feed on them in the mouth for longer-than-normal periods of time. At age six years, more than three-quarters of children have cavities, and by the time they leave school, only 2 percent of young Americans remain free of dental decay. The average 20-year-old American has 14 teeth that are decayed, have fillings, or are already missing.

The conventional wisdom in dentistry is that plaque and, by extension, cavities are caused by table sugar (sucrose) and other carbohydrates that nourish the acid-producing bacteria. So it is thought that eating less sugar and maintaining a more balanced diet can help control acid and cavities. But the Panel ruefully conceded that sugar consumption continues apace, despite widespread efforts to educate the public about its effects on dental health. *Chewing gum* also is high on the list of offending substances, as are cereals, desserts, soft drinks, and sweet, gooey foods that linger in the mouth and stick to the teeth. But children love them. Given children's cravings for sweets, which some scientific studies suggest may be wholly natural and normal, less-restrictive methods seem needed to prevent tooth decay.

Fluorides

How They Help

When infants and young children swallow fluoride, it is incorporated into the developing teeth, as hard, insoluble crystals. This substance, *fluorapatite,* replaces some of the natural outer-tooth enamel, and, to a lesser extent, it is incorporated into the deeper layers of the teeth. Later, after these teeth erupt into view, the fluoride-enriched enamel resists dissolution by acid.

Fluoride may do more than simply harden developing teeth, according to recent studies. Fluoride in the saliva, or in overlying dental plaque, may aid in the re-mineralization of the enamel by encouraging the deposition of calcium and phosphate. So older children and adults also may benefit from continuing use of fluoride products.

The metal tin also protects against acid; the word *stannous* on a dentifrice label means that the product contains tin. This metallic element also may help kill plaque-forming bacteria. (*See* MOUTHWASH FOR ORAL HYGIENE.) Stannous fluoride contains both protective elements—fluorine and tin.

Sources

Americans' principal source of fluoride is drinking water. This is so even if the water is not artificially fluoridated, because most if not all ground, river, and lake waters contain some natural fluoride. In places where the water contains about 1 part per million (1 ppm), which is considered to be the optimal amount, the prevalence of dental decay is about 60 percent lower than it is in low-fluoride areas. The-1 ppm level of fluoridation poses no risk to people who drink the water.

Of 132 million people who live in U.S. communities where the water contains 0.7 ppm or more fluoride particles, 9 million are drinking naturally fluoridated water, while 124 million use water that contains fluoride supplements. This supplementation usually is added in the amounts needed to bring the level up to 1 ppm. (These statistics come from the National Institute of Dental Research, in Bethesda, MD.)

Alternative sources of fluoride include professional applications by a dentist or a dental hygienist; periodic mouth rinsings with higher concentrations of fluoride (which is provided in some schools); and home treatment with fluoride toothpastes, treatment rinses, and treatment gels. Fluoridated water is helpful only until a child's adult teeth erupt, at about age 12 years. Fluoride toothpastes and similar products that are applied topically to the teeth provide additive benefit that continues through life.

Effectiveness

The complex data in the dental literature has been summarized as follows (*Journal of the American Medical Association*, Dec. 22-29, 1989, p. 3461):

- Community water fluoridation at 0.7 to 1.2 ppm used over a lifetime yields a 50 to 65 percent reduction in cavities (assuming no fluoride toothpastes, or other products are used)

- School water fluoridation at about four times the optimal level, consumed daily, starting at age 5 or 6 years, in communities where the water is fluoride-deficient yields a 40 percent reduction in cavities

- Fluoride drops or tablets taken at home, daily, to age 13 years, in communities where the water is fluoride-deficient yield a 50 to 65 percent reduction in cavities

- Fluoride tablets taken 1 mg per day, in school, from preschool to 8th grade in communities where the water is fluoride-deficient, yield a 25 to 40 percent reduction in cavities

- Fluoride mouth rinses, used through the school years, with 0.05 percent sodium fluoride daily or 0.2 percent sodium fluoride weekly yield a 30 to 40 percent reduction in cavities

- Fluoride toothpastes, used twice daily for life, with 0.76 percent or 1.2 percent monofluorophosphate, or 0.24 percent sodium fluoride, yield a 20 to 40 percent reduction in cavities

• Fluoride application by a dentist, once yearly, with 2 percent sodium fluoride + 8 percent stannous fluoride, or with acidulated phosphate fluoride (1.2 percent fluoride) yields a 30 to 40 percent reduction in cavities

Encouragingly, these findings indicate that the simplest and cheapest method—which is supplementing the water supply when it is fluoride-deficient—is the most effective way to prevent cavities.

Water fluoridation long has been fought by a concerned—some might say *paranoid*—segment of the population. These people say fluoride is poisonous and may cause cancer, and they may hint, darkly, that it is put into the water supply as part of a deadly plot.

None of these fears has ever proved out. People who live in areas where the water is naturally fluoridated, sometimes to levels well in excess of the 1-ppm goal of supplementation, do not have any more cancers than people in other communities do. In the 1980s, one laboratory study indicated that fluoride might induce a rare kind of cancer in rats. This possibility was studied exhaustively by the U.S. Public Health Service's National Toxicology Program. Early in 1991, the Public Health Service reported that its year-long investigation "has found no evidence establishing an association between fluoride and cancer in humans."

Dosage Forms

Fluoride is available in over-the-counter products in dentrifices and treatment mouth rinses and also may be available in treatment gels. Some of these products indicate the *type* of fluoride supplement but not the dosage. The Panel recommended that the dosage be listed. But the FDA says that manufacturers are not required to do so. Nevertheless, the spirit, if not the letter of the Food, Drug & Cosmetic Act, and of the Over-the-Counter Drug Review, is that consumers should know the names and the *amounts* of the active ingredients in the products they buy and use.

Most fluoride toothpaste is made by large companies, and the concentrations of the supplement are well known to dental experts and the government. Nevertheless, there are now, or soon may be two dosages of acidulated phosphate fluoride treatment rinses, 0.01 percent and 0.02

percent, the first to be used twice daily, the second only once. Consumers may need to differentiate these products from each other. It would seem wise, therefore, if these treatment rinses, and by extension *all* fluoride supplements, were labeled to show the dosage in a standard dose (say, an ounce of a rinse or a one-inch toothpaste ribbon).

Dentifrices

A dentifrice is a toothpaste, powder, or other substance that is used with a toothbrush. The first fluoride toothpaste, which contained stannous fluoride, was introduced in the United States in 1955. The main technical obstacle that needed to be overcome was to find an abrasive (a cleansing and polishing substance) that did not inactivate the fluoride. The first such abrasive, calcium pyrophosphate, was described in the dental literature in 1954; there have been others since then.

The American Dental Association (ADA) has classified several fluoride toothpastes as "accepted," and allows manufacturers to use its ADA Seal of Acceptance on their products along with an endorsement that says the product "has been shown to be an effective decay-preventive dentrifice that can be of significant value when used in a conscientiously applied program of oral hygiene and regular professional care."

Treatment Rinses

Fluoridated treatment rinses are newer and less widely investigated than dentifrices. Nevertheless, more than 20 extensive studies noted by the Panel indicate that use of these products can significantly reduce cavities. Some rinses have ADA endorsement. Treatment rinses should be spat out after rinsing. However, if you live in an area where the water has fewer than 7-ppm fluorine, your dentist may advise you to allow children ages 3 to 14 years to rinse with a treatment rinse and then *swallow* the material so that it can be usefully absorbed into unerupted teeth and bones. If you live in such an area, ask your dentist what to do.

Treatment Gels

The few studies on fluoride gels that had been published when the evaluators wrote their report provided what they called "reasonable documentation" of their effectiveness. The reviewers stipulated, however, that these gels should be used *in addition* to a dentifrice rather than as a substitute for it. Treatment gel formulations are not intended to be used as toothpastes.

Risk Factors

At concentrations far above those attained in dental-health programs, fluoride can be quite toxic. As noted above, the best cavity-preventing dose in drinking water is 1 ppm. When drinking water contains 2 to 10 ppm of fluoride, it may discolor children's teeth. At far higher concentrations (20 to 80 ppm in drinking water) fluoride may severely affect the bones. They become too dense and too fragile, and the joints may no longer work properly.

Many dental researchers have studied the question of whether fluoridated water or fluoride dental products will lead to toxic changes. The Panel believed, on the basis of available evidence, that they will not. One investigator found, for example, that in an average brushing no more than 0.25 mg of fluoride would be swallowed, and probably a lot less. Reviewers think that this is considerably below any toxic range.

To forestall the remote possibility that a child would eat the contents of a tube of fluoride toothpaste or drink a bottle of a treatment rinse, the Panel recommended—and the FDA agreed—that dentifrice packages contain no more than 260-mg total fluoride and that treatment rinse and gel packages contain no more than 120 mg.

The risk of fluoride-caused tooth discoloration is greatest in childhood years, when adult teeth are still developing under the gums. Therefore experts recommend that fluoride treatment rinses and gels be labeled for use only by adults and children over six years old, and that fluoride dentifrices be labeled for use by adults and children only when over the age of two years. Children under 12 years should be supervised by their parents or another adult when using these products.

Anticavity Preparations

APPROVED ACTIVE INGREDIENTS

All approved cavity-preventing ingredients are fluorides. For most of them there now are two or more approved dosage forms. The FDA says that enhanced protection against cavities can be obtained if children use both a fluoride toothpaste and a fluoride treatment rinse. One wonders if that is not too much of a good thing!

Concentrations of Approved Ingredients

Active Ingredient	Approved Concentrations in Dentifrice	Approved Concentrations in Treatment Rinse
acidulated phosphate fluoride		0.01 or 0.02%
sodium fluoride	0.22%	0.02 or 0.05%*
sodium monofluorophosphate	0.76%	
stannous fluoride †	0.4%	0.1%

* or in concentrate, with direction to dilute to those dosages.

†In treatment gel, 0.4% is the approved concentration when diluted from concentrate.

• *ACIDULATED PHOSPHATE FLUORIDE (TREATMENT RINSE):* In the amount of fluoride it delivers and in its safety, this preparation is comparable to the better-studied sodium fluoride rinses (*See* further on). Several studies that have been conducted with acidulated phosphate fluoride rinse show no harmful local or systemic effects. This rinse appears to be more effective for people who live in areas without fluoridated drinking water than it is for residents of communities that have fluoridated water. People who rinse with acidulated phosphate fluoride preparations may anticipate about a 30 to 40 percent reduction in cavities as a reward for their effort.

The approved daily dosage for adults and children over six years of age is one 1-minute swishing through the teeth with a rinse containing 2 tablespoons of 0.02 percent acidulated phosphate fluoride. For weaker treatment rinses containing 0.01 percent acidulated phosphate fluoride, two treatments daily are recommended.

• *SODIUM FLUORIDE (DENTIFRICE):* This fluoride has been broadly studied, and the test results led evaluators to conclude that it is safe and effective as a cavity-preventive dentifrice ingredient. In six 16 to 36-month clinical trials, 0.22 percent sodium fluoride with a 40 percent high-beta-phase calcium pyrophosphate abrasive system was tested against similar toothpastes without the fluoride. Results showed a statistically significant reduction in dental decay for the fluoride preparation.

These fluoride preparations also appear to be safe. A 150-pound man would have to eat the contents of 20 to 40 full tubes of sodium fluoride toothpaste to ingest a lethal dose. Lesser amounts conceivably could cause tooth discoloration in young children who regularly swallowed large amounts of the toothpaste and also consumed large amounts of naturally or artificially fluoridated water. Evaluators noted, however, that in the 15 years since these toothpastes first were widely marketed, there was no documented rise in the incidence of such discoloration.

The safe and effective dose for children over 2 years old and adults is one or more tooth-brushings daily with a 0.22 percent sodium fluoride dentifrice that contains a suitable abrasive system.

• *SODIUM FLUORIDE (TREATMENT RINSE):* Daily rinsing with a 0.05 percent solution of sodium fluoride has been shown to reduce the number of cavities that develop in children's teeth by 25 to 50 percent.

One early study showed that one of these rinses irritated the gums. But follow-up studies did not confirm this finding. As with sodium fluoride dentifrices (*see* immediately preceding), many containers of rinse would have to be consumed to cause lethal poisoning. Reviewers agree with the ADA that a 0.05 percent sodium fluoride rinse—swished through the teeth for a minute, once daily—is a safe and effective way to prevent cavities.

• SODIUM MONOFLUOROPHOSPHATE (DENTIFRICE): This compound may be less toxic in a single dose than sodium fluoride (*see* immediately preceding) simply because the fluoride particles are released from it more slowly. But over the long haul the two compounds are comparable in safety.

A number of studies, using toothpastes with a variety of abrasives, show that sodium monofluorophosphate effectively reduces the number of new cavities that will develop over a 2- to 3-year period by 20 to 30 percent. The safe and effective dosage for children over 2 years of age and adults is at least one brushing daily with a 0.76 percent sodium monofluorophosphate dentifrice that contains suitable abrasive ingredients.

• STANNOUS FLUORIDE (DENTIFRICE): This ingredient contains fluorine and tin, both of which act to harden teeth against acid and decay. The tin does not significantly increase the fluoride's toxic potential, but it may stain dental plaque and debris yellow. This, however, is a rare occurrence, and the stain can be removed.

Stannous fluoride has been widely tested in dentifrices containing several different abrasive mixes. Most, but not all, studies show that it reduces cavities by statistically significant numbers.

The safe and effective dosage for adults and children over 2 years of age is one or more thorough brushings daily with a 0.4 percent stannous fluoride toothpaste containing a suitable abrasive formulation.

• STANNOUS FLUORIDE (TREATMENT RINSE): This formulation is judged safe and effective, although the data on its effectiveness were less convincing to the Panel than was the case with other approved stannous fluoride and sodium fluoride formulations. Of the four long-term studies evaluated, two showed highly positive results; one failed to show consistently positive responses; and the last indicated that the rinse did not lower the occurrence of caries. By and large, reviewers suggest, stannous fluoride rinses are valuable for people who do not have fluoridated water, but perhaps less useful for people whose water is fluoridated.

The safety of stannous fluoride rinses does not differ significantly from that of stannous fluoride dentifrices. The occasional yellow staining that occurs in people who do not brush their teeth often enough can be removed by a dentist, and will not recur if the teeth are subsequently brushed well.

The rinse must be made up just before use because the active ingredient is chemically unstable when dissolved in water. The approved dosage for adults and children over 6 years old is one rinse per day of 10 ml (2 teaspoons) of a freshly prepared 0.1 percent rinse. It should be swished around between the teeth for one minute and then spit out.

• STANNOUS FLUORIDE (TREATMENT GEL): Evaluators found suitable documentation for the effectiveness of this preparation, in which the stannous fluoride is formulated in anhydrous (water-free) glycerin. In one ingenious study, teeth that were extracted after their owners had used a stannous fluoride gel over a period of time were found to be harder than teeth extracted from people who did not use the gel. Youngsters wearing braces on their teeth were far less likely to suffer calcium loss from the tooth enamel (which can happen with braces) if they regularly used a stannous fluoride gel.

Gel formulations of stannous fluoride do not significantly differ in safety from the dentifrice formulations described in this section. The evaluators say a 0.4 percent stannous fluoride gel is safe and effective for adults and children over 6 years of age when it is applied once daily to the teeth. But consumers should remember that gel formulations are not intended to be used as toothpastes. This ingredient may not yet be available over-the-counter.

CONDITIONALLY APPROVED ACTIVE INGREDIENTS
None.

DISAPPROVED ACTIVE INGREDIENTS
None.

When Greater Relief Is Needed

If a child develops frequent cavities in spite of good oral hygiene and the use of fluoride supplements, seek a dentist's help. He or she can prescribe stronger fluoridated supplements or mouthwash that will reduce plaque and so may forestall cavities. Another option: thin plastic occluded sealants, applied by a dentist to critical tooth surfaces, can significantly reduce and perhaps wholly prevent new cavities from developing.

Safety and Effectiveness: Active Ingredients in Over-the-Counter Cavity Preventives

Active Ingredient	*Assessment*
acidulated phosphate fluoride	safe and effective
sodium fluoride	safe and effective
sodium monofluorophosphate (dentifrice)	safe and effective
stannous fluoride	safe and effective

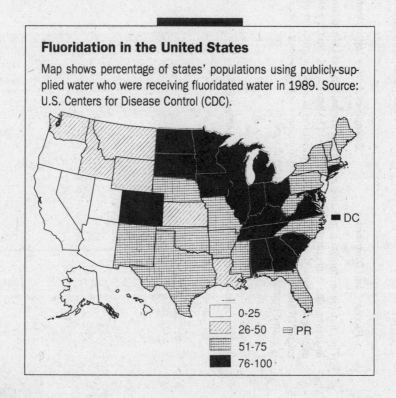

Fluoridation in the United States

Map shows percentage of states' populations using publicly-supplied water who were receiving fluoridated water in 1989. Source: U.S. Centers for Disease Control (CDC).

DC

0-25
26-50   PR
51-75
76-100

Fluoride: Product Ratings

Product and Distributor	Dosage of Active Ingredients	Rating *	Comment

The fluoride toothpastes, gels and rinses that are sold in the United States all apparently contain safe and effective ingredients, in appropriate concentrations, according to FDA standards. So they all would be rated "A" here. Many of these products, however, do not show the concentration of the fluoride active ingredient on the label. For this reason, any such product would be rated "B" here. Consumers are entitled to know—and may have a legal right to know—the concentration of dosage of medically active ingredients in nonprescription drugs.

*Author's interpretation of FDA criteria. Based on contents, not claims.

Germ-Killing Soaps

Millions of people routinely wash and bathe using expensive bar soaps that contain potent chemical ingredients that kill microbes (germs) or inhibit their growth on the skin. These soaps are promoted and used to prevent body odor, particularly underarm odor; for general cleanliness; and to a lesser extent to forestall skin infections.

An *antimicrobial* is an agent that kills or inhibits the growth and reproduction of microorganisms. A germ-killing soap contains one or more of these ingredients.

Do They Work?

Germ-killing soaps do kill germs and so apparently are able to help control underarm odor and other body odors. However, despite the huge sales of these soaps, there is little data on the number of microorganisms they kill. Soap and drug industry experts and research scientists were unable to provide evidence that directly shows the percentage

GERM-KILLING SOAPS is based on the report of the FDA's Advisory Review Panel on OTC Antimicrobial Drug Products Used for Repeated Daily Use (Antimicrobial I Panel), the initial Tentative Final Order on OTC Topical Antimicrobial Products, and related documents.

of underarm bacteria that must be killed to reduce body odor or the concentration of antimicrobial agents in soaps that are required to produce this effect.

The best the experts could do was to estimate, on the basis of tests, that about a 70 percent reduction in bacteria is required to control armpit and other body odors. While it remains to be proved, some germ-killing soaps may in fact reduce underarm bacterial counts by 70 percent or even up to 90 percent. But a second major question—one of safety—has arisen, and remains unanswered today: Is it wise or healthy to use such potent germ killers on a day-to-day basis for many years?

One concern, which was strongly expressed by the Panel in its report, is that some of these chemicals are absorbed into the body through the skin, even when the skin is not broken. They may accumulate in the liver and other organs—with dangerous consequences.

The other main worry is that most antimicrobial substances very effectively kill microorganisms in the class called *gram-positive bacteria*, which normally inhabit the skin. But they are far less effective against the class called *gram-negative bacteria*. (*See* p. 450.) The Panel's hypothesis, which it says is supported by several scientific studies, is that these soaps may kill relatively harmless gram-positive bacteria only to make room for and encourage the growth of gram-negative flora that can cause serious infection. A microbiologist at the National Institutes of Health said, however, that there is no evidence that this compensatory overgrowth of other organisms occurs on the skin. The Panel urged FDA to classify and regulate all germ-killing soaps and other products that contain these ingredients as *drugs*—not as cosmetics—so that the more stringent drug safety and effectiveness standards would be applied to them.

The Panel concluded that none of the antimicrobial agents used in these soaps is safe and effective. Only a conditional approval was granted to these antimicrobials, including the substances cloflucarban, triclocarban, and triclosan. They have been, and continue to be, widely used in germ-killing soaps.

A New Look

The Panel's adverse judgments provoked a flood of protest and the submission of new scientific research and data—much of it from major soap manufacturers, including Procter & Gamble and Colgate-Palmolive, and from drug companies such as Upjohn and CIBA-

GEIGY, that make the germ-killing substances. The manufacturers claimed their new data confirm the safety and effectiveness of triclocarban and other antimicrobial ingredients.

The FDA agreed in 1979 that much significant new data was available that needed to be assessed. It therefore reopened the administrative record. In effect the agency rolled back the OTC review process on these and other antimicrobial products to an earlier stage, so that new evidence could be submitted and evaluated. Final decisions on the safety and effectiveness of germ-killing soaps still are pending. The doubts originally raised by the Panel, and for the most part seconded by the FDA, remain unresolved.

Safety of Hexachlorophene and Other Antimicrobials

The development of potent antimicrobial chemicals for medical use before and during World War II led to the introduction of these substances into consumer products. One of the most effective and widely used antimicrobials was hexachlorophene. By 1972—the year that the review process and the Antimicrobial Panel were established—hexachlorophene was being formulated into 1500 over-the-counter cleansers and into other products. But that same year it became clear that hexachlorophene was a toxic substance. Significant amounts of the agent were found to be absorbed through the skin into the blood. In one study, concentrations ranging from 0.02 to 0.14 micrograms of hexachlorophene per milliliter (mcg/ml) of blood were found. The level rose to 0.38 mcg/ml in one volunteer who bathed in the substance.

Hexachlorophene was shown to cause systemic toxicity. The greatest danger was to newborn babies. Meanwhile, however, this substance had become widely used for bathing newborn babies to prevent infections. Some infants were washed with it two or more times daily.

Hexachlorophene was found to dig Swiss-cheese-like holes in babies' brain tissue after it was absorbed through the skin and carried to the brain in the bloodstream. In France, in the summer of 1972, 36 babies died after they were powdered with a baby powder that was accidentally contaminated at the manufacturer with up to 6.3 percent hexachlorophene. Some 168 other babies who were poisoned, but did not die, were still being studied a decade later to see if they had suffered permanent brain damage from their exposure to hexachlorophene.

Babies, it has been found, have difficulty eliminating hexachlorophene from their bodies. Older persons probably are better able to excrete it and so are less at risk. Nevertheless, the margin between a safe and effective hexachlorophene dose on the one hand and a dangerously poisonous dose on the other clearly is far too narrow. So, as its first substantive act in the OTC Drug Review, the FDA banned hexachlorophene from over-the-counter sales in the United States, in September of 1972.

The dismaying history of hexachlorophene no doubt prompted the Antimicrobial I Panel to look very critically at other germ-killing substances formulated into products designed for prolonged daily use—particularly bar soaps. The Panel proposed new testing guidelines to assess the safety of ingredients, and formulated a set of assumptions—strongly contested by the soap industry—about how much of these chemicals would be absorbed into the body in a bath or a shower.

The Panel calculated that 7 grams (roughly one-quarter of an ounce) of soap is used by an adult in bathing. A bar soap containing a 3 percent concentration of an antimicrobial thus would expose the user to 210 mg of the agent per bath. If it is assumed that all of the antimicrobial sticks to the skin, and that 3 percent of it is quickly absorbed through the skin to wind up in the bloodstream, a 150-pound man or woman would then be carrying about 1.26 micrograms of the agent per 1 milliliter of blood. In the case of hexachlorophene, this is a potentially toxic dose.

Effectiveness of Germ-Killing Soaps

In Reducing Odor

The unresolved questions of the safety of germ-killing soaps are matched by the paucity of convincing scientific data on their effectiveness. While the Panel and the FDA concur that these chemicals do reduce bacterial flora on the skin, this effect has never been directly correlated with reduction in body odor. The FDA will now require that claims related to deodorant effectiveness be based on demonstrated ability to reduce microbes or inhibit the growth of those microbes responsible for odor production.

In Preventing Infection

Besides cleanliness and control of body odor, the other benefit claimed for germ-killing ingredients in soaps is the prevention of skin infections. Several tests have been conducted, including studies at West Point and Annapolis. At West Point, cadets who showered with a germ-killing bar soap containing tribromsalan, triclocarban, and cloflucarban had 44 percent fewer boils but had more fingernail infections (paronychia) than did cadets who used ordinary bar soap. But a soap containing triclocarban and hexachlorophene did not lower the incidence of boils in naval cadets at Annapolis. A Panel consultant called these results equivocal, and it was decided that they were insufficient to support the conclusion that these soaps are effective in preventing infection. Also, if the products do indeed *increase* the potential for gram-negative or gram-positive streptococcal infections, any "deodorant benefit would probably be considerably outweighed by the potential hazard . . . when alternative methods of odor control are available."

 Claims

Accurate
- "Antimicrobial soap" or "antibacterial soap" (Elsewhere on the label manufacturers can say "reduces odor" or "deodorant soap.")

False or Misleading
Because no antimicrobial ingredient can truly ensure germ-free skin (and such a goal may not be desirable anyway) the FDA says that the claim "ensures bacterially clean skin" should *not* be made.

WARNING:
 Do not use on infants under 6 months of age.

Combination Products

Two chemically similar antimicrobial ingredients, triclocarban and cloflucarban, have been combined in some antimicrobial bar soaps. The FDA gives only *conditional* approval to this combination, pending proof that the two individual ingredients are safe and effective and do not become more toxic when mixed in a soap.

Germ-Killing Agents

APPROVED GERM-KILLING ACTIVE INGREDIENTS

None.

CONDITIONALLY APPROVED GERM-KILLING ACTIVE INGREDIENTS

- **CHLOROXYLENOL (PCMX):** Very little data on this substance—which also is designated parachlormetaxylenol, or PCMX—were submitted for evaluation. Even the additional material sent later to FDA leaves important safety and effectiveness questions unresolved. Chloroxylenol, like hexachlorophene, is a phenol derivative. Thus it should be very active against bacteria. But the evidence, in fact, is conflicting and inadequate. One report, published half a century ago, indicates that the substance is not very effective against bacteria on the skin. A more recent but inconclusive study shows that choroxylenol reduces microbial flora by 70 percent after 10 days' use. More studies are definitely needed.
- **CLOFLUCARBAN:** There are no *known* hazards associated with use of this germ-killer, which is often combined with triclocarban in antimicrobial bar soaps. But data to confirm its safety are wanting, and it is conditionally approved only in concentrations up to 1.5 percent.

  Cloflucarban, when ingested, is only about one-fiftieth as toxic as hexachlorophene. It also may be absorbed less readily through the skin. But data on blood levels following one or more baths and information about absorption into the body still are lacking.
- **PHENOL (UNDER 1.5 PERCENT AQUEOUS/ALCOHOLIC):** It is phenol—better known as carbolic acid—that lent the medicinal odor to some of the popular soap products that for many years were used to control body odor. While phenol is an effective germ killer, it is also highly toxic to the skin. Once absorbed through the skin, phenol can damage internal organs. (*See* PHENOL: SPECIAL NOTE.) Since safer antiseptics are

available, the Panel says that phenol—as sodium phenolate or secondary amyltricresols—is now far less commonly used.

The FDA evaluates phenol in hand soaps as safe but not proved effective at concentrations under 1.5 percent in water or alcoholic solutions. Phenol also is allowed in very low concentrations, of up to 0.5 percent, as an inactive ingredient, to give the product a medicinal smell—which some might consider deceptive.

WARNING:

 Phenol should never be used on diapers or on babies' skin, since an infant may be unable to excrete it once absorbed.

• *TRICLOCARBAN:* The effectiveness of triclocarban in killing microbial organisms has been demonstrated. But a clear correlation between reduced microbial counts and reduced body odor has not been demonstrated, so the FDA declined to certify triclorcarban as effective.

"The available evidence does not indicate that the use of triclocarban in bar soaps presents any known hazard to the general public," the FDA declared in 1978. "Based on blood-level data, [it] does not appear to be as toxic as hexachlorophene [which has been banned from OTC products]."

Studies conducted according to the Panel's guidelines show that a person who showers once or twice daily with a triclocarban soap will absorb roughly 500 to 1000 times *less* than the minimal toxic dose—a wide safety margin. However, because the enzyme pathways that rid the body of triclocarban develop only slowly after birth, this substance should not be used on babies under 6 months of age.

The possibility that triclocarban causes cancer has not been disproved. So the FDA grants only conditional approval in terms both of safety and effectiveness, and it limits the amount of triclocarban—alone, or in conjunction with cloflucarban—to 1.5 percent of the soap product in which it is formulated.

• *TRICLOSAN:* Although this is an effective antimicrobial, it has not been demonstrated that it kills the germs that cause body odor. So triclosan's effectiveness for this purpose in soaps remains to be proved.

About 12 percent of the triclosan deposited on the skin during a shower is absorbed into the skin: the highest amount for any antimicrobial now used in hand soaps. Most people excrete this chemical very rapidly. But some individuals are what the FDA calls "slow metabolizers" of triclosan. Their safety is of concern, because if triclosan is retained, it may damage their livers.

There is another cause for concern: Triclosan is used in a variety of consumer products. It is formulated into cosmetics, infant clothing, and diaper rinses. But the wisdom of this wide use has been questioned. Because the hazards of using triclosan have not been clearly established, it is one of the substances being re-evaluated. The FDA has lingering doubts about triclosan's effectiveness, apparently because it is not effectively against *Pseudomonas*, which is one of the most dangerous gram-negative bacteria.

DISAPPROVED GERM-KILLING ACTIVE INGREDIENTS

• **PHENOL (OVER 1.5 PERCENT AQUEOUS/ALCOHOLIC):** The Panel found phenol (carbolic acid) unsafe in concentrations greater than 1.5 percent. Although studies referred principally to formulations other than soap, phenol can be formulated as bar soap and evaluators wanted to rule out its use in these high concentrations to avoid risk of serious hazards such as severe skin burns, gangrene, and other forms of tissue damage.

Safety and Effectiveness:
Active Ingredients in Antimicrobial Soaps

Active Ingredient	Assessment
chloroxylenol (PCMX)	not proved safe or effective
cloflucarban	not proved safe or effective
phenol (under 1.5% or less in aqueous/alcoholic)	safe, not proved effective
phenol (over 1.5% aqueous/alcoholic)	not safe
triclocarban	not proved safe or effective
triclosan	not proved safe or effective

Germ-Killing Soaps: Product Ratings

Product and Distributor	Dosage of Active Ingredients	Rating *	Comment
Liquid Dial (Dial)	liquid soap: triclosan	C	not proved safe or effective; concentration not given on label
Liquid Safeguard (Procter & Gamble)	liquid soap: triclosan	C	not proved safe or effective; concentration not given on label
Safeguard (Procter & Gamble)	bar soap: triclocarban	C	not proved safe or effective; dosage (concentration) of this ingredient not given on label
Septi-Soft (Calgon Vestal)	solution: triclosan 0.25%	B	not proved safe or effective
Softsoap Antibacterial (Colgate)	liquid soap: chloroxylenol	C	not proved safe or effective; concentration not given on label
Zest (Procter & Gamble)	bar soap: triclocarban	B	not proved safe or effective

*Author's interpretation of FDA criteria. Based on contents, not claims.

Hair-Growth Stimulants and Baldness Preventives

The vanity-driven market for products that will retard baldness and stimulate hair growth on bald scalps has been in tumult in recent years. There are these developments:

- The FDA has banned all nonprescription baldness prevention drugs, saying that careful study in the OTC Drug Review has failed to find any one of them that scientifically can be shown to safely and effectively prevent hair loss or grow new hair.

- Small manufacturers and consumers of these hair-growth products have damned this decision—and some manufacturers have vowed to keep their products on the market by selling them as food supplements, without drug labels— which nevertheless, FDA says is illegal. At the time of the FDA's ban, some $200 to $300 million worth of these products were sold annually in the United States.

HAIR-GROWTH STIMULANTS AND BALDNESS PREVENTIVES is based on the report "Hair-Grower and Hair-Loss-Prevention Drugs" by the FDA's Advisory Review Panel on OTC Miscellaneous External Drug Products and the FDA's Tentative Final and Final Monographs on these products.

- The FDA has licensed one—and only one—prescription (℞) drug, minoxidil (*Rogaine*, Upjohn) as safe and effective for stimulating hair growth. The FDA first approved minoxidil, after two decades of research and development, for the typical "pattern baldness" that occurs in many men. Early in 1992, Upjohn launched a promotional campaign for minoxidil as a treatment for the more patchy and diffuse baldness that afflicts some women. But minoxidil is not a "magic bullet." Upjohn investigators found that only a minority of men who used minoxidil (39 percent) have "at least a moderate amount of new hair growth." Successful users must continue applying the drug—which costs about $2 a day. When they stop, the new hair falls out.

- Hair growth and baldness has become a major, new research area for basic and medical scientists. They are developing a new understanding of the biological factors that turn hair growth on—and off. The hope is that this new understanding will lead to better baldness preventives and remedies.

"If we're going to understand hair growth," Yale dermatologist Kurt S. Stenn, M.D., told the *New York Times* (February 5, 1991), "we're going to do it through solid, methodical science... It's not going to come out in splashy, commercialized miracle cures!"

Under ordinary circumstances, when the FDA rules that a class of drugs, like hair growers and baldness preventives, is at least temporarily *kaput*, it would be dropped from this Guide. The agency's ban on hair growers and hair-loss preventives became effective on July 7, 1990. But because of the strong consumer interest in these products, and because manufacturers of banned nonprescription products have vowed to evade and defy the FDA's ban, this unit is retained here, so that readers will have a sense of what drugs have been dismissed by the agency, which now regards them, legally, as "not generally recognized as safe and effective" and also so readers will have some sense of the many shortcomings in the data produced by manufacturers and by some satisfied consumers to support the claims they make for these products.

To cite just one example of manufacturers' defiance of the FDA ruling, an official for Angio-Medical Products, Corp. of New York City, told *Newsday* (July 12, 1989, p. 43) that it would continue to sell its *Zomexin*, which the newspaper describes as "a derivative of pig intestines." The FDA's ban "doesn't affect us, because we don't make drug claims," the official explained. Theirs, he said, was a *cosmetic* claim: "A drug claim says it grows hair. A cosmetic claim says it looks like you have more hair."

Some advocates of formerly legal nonprescription hair growth preparations either are cynical—or dumb. Asked repeatedly to provide scientific data that could lead FDA to approve their products, some submitted laudatory articles from popular magazines instead. Others sent brochures or other material touting the products—but neglected to inform the FDA what the products were made of. The agency clearly had no choice but to reject such submissions.

Why Hair Grows and Then Stops Growing

The commonest type of baldness in men is the receding hairline. The frontal V of the balding scalp progresses relentlessly backward until it reaches a second balding area at the crown of the head. Only a horse-shoe-shaped remnant of hair is then left, along the side and the back of the head. This is called *male pattern baldness*. It is a hair trait that is inherited from your forebears—as are hair color, hair texture, and the curl or straightness of your hair.

Women do not suffer this severe baldness. Their hair may thin naturally as they grow older, but it usually does not wholly vanish. Hair loss over much of the scalp may occur as an aftermath of child-birth, fever, crash dieting, iron deficiency, exposure to X-rays (radi-ographs), and hormonal imbalances like hypothyroidism and hyperthy-roidism. It also can be caused by drugs, particularly the potent ones used to treat cancer. Smaller and sometimes very unsightly patches of baldness can be caused by fungus infections or by syphilis and other diseases. The hair may regrow normally in these forms of baldness if the hair follicle, where each hair sprouts from the scalp, has not been seriously damaged. Because sudden, excessive hair loss or an unusual pattern of baldness may signal an underlying illness, persons who expe-rience either symptom should consult a doctor.

Under normal circumstances each hair grows for four to six years, and then enters a three-week transitional stage in which growth slows, the follicle withers, and the hair is shed. Then there is a three-month dormant period, after which the cycle repeats as the follicle becomes active again and produces a new hair. Under normal circumstances, about 85 percent of the hair on a human scalp is in the growth phase.

A hair grows only in one direction: lengthwise, from the root outward. Above the root, a hair shaft is dead tissue, like a fingernail. It cannot grow longer or thicker no matter how industriously it is cared for or treated with drugs. Cosmetic substances that cling to the shaft can, of course, make it look and feel thicker.

Many products promoted to prevent baldness claim to strengthen and conserve the hair. Persons tempted to believe these claims may do well to bear in mind the Panel's unequivocal finding that "nothing done to the hair shaft once it emerges from the surface of the scalp will influence the hair growth. Anything that would influence regeneration of the hair would have to work on the hair root.... To demonstrate that an ingredient is a hair restorer, it must be proven that the substance gets into the hair root and causes stimulation of hair growth."

To provide this proof a manufacturer, a university, or an independent researcher would have to demonstrate the following results—none of which has been shown to date (except for the prescription drug minoxidil):

• an increase in the growth rate of the hair
• an increase in the diameter of the hair shaft
• a lengthening of the hair-growth phase
• an increase in the weight of treated hair

Hormones and Hair Growth

One factor that unquestionably does influence hair growth is the level of sex hormones that are circulating in the bloodstream and present in the body. Unfortunately, hormones have not been shown conclusively to affect hair growth when they are applied directly to the scalp or skin.

Hormones change the growth rate, thickness, and color of the hair on various body surfaces. At puberty, for example, *vellus*—which most people call "peach fuzz"—appears on a boy's chin. Under the influence of the male sex hormone testosterone, this changes to become thick, long, pigmented beard hairs. Around 20 or 30 years later, the changes that produce male pattern baldness essentially reverse this process. The scalp-hair follicles do not simply stop producing hairs; rather, the thick, long, pigmented hair on the scalp is replaced by thin, soft, vellus hairs. The hair-growth phases also become shorter, so that the hairs that are produced are shorter, too.

The Sebum Theory

Oiliness of the scalp is a condition that *can* be controlled by using shampoos and other drug and cosmetic products. Much of this natural oil, called *sebum*, is produced by glands in the skin called *sebaceous glands*.

One theory states that male baldness may be caused by sebum. If this is true, then so-called sebum hair-loss might be prevented by quickly removing these oily substances from the scalp.

The manufacturer of a hair-preserving regimen submitted studies published thirty years ago. These reports indicate that when human sebum was applied to rats' skins, their hair fell out. No recent studies and no studies in humans were presented to support this observation or the sebum-hair-loss theory itself, which evaluators say doctors do not accept. On the contrary, a study cited in medical textbooks shows that sebum secretions are essentially the same on men with bald scalps, on the hairy parts of balding men's scalps, and on the scalps of men with no signs of baldness. The Panel's conclusion: "Balding men did not have abnormally oily scalps, and [there was] no quantitative chemical difference" between the sebum of balding and non-balding men.

APPROVED ACTIVE INGREDIENTS IN BALDNESS PREPARATIONS

None.

CONDITIONALLY APPROVED ACTIVE INGREDIENTS IN BALDNESS PREPARATIONS

None.

DISAPPROVED ACTIVE INGREDIENTS IN BALDNESS PREPARATIONS

Not surprisingly, in view of the aforementioned information, the Panel discounted the effectiveness of all the active ingredients it assessed. It dismissed five of the ingredients rather summarily but discussed the female hormone *estradiol* (a form of estrogen) at length.

Similarly, combination products were also dismissed because all single-entity active ingredients are ineffective.

• ASCORBIC ACID (VITAMIN C): The manufacturer who submitted a product that contains this substance did not submit, and the Panel could not find, any evidence to show that—by itself or in combination with other ingredients—that ascorbic acid has any influence on hair growth. The Panel's verdict: not effective. The FDA's verdict: Not safe either.

• BENZOIC ACID: The findings and the verdict duplicate those for ascorbic acid. (*See* Ascorbic acid.)

Does the FDA Infringe on Consumers' Freedom?

The FDA received many letters from consumers—some of them quite anguished—objecting to the then-forthcoming ban on hair-growth products.

"Some of the comments expressed concern that the ban will interrupt ongoing hair grower treatment programs which consumers are satisfied with," FDA reports. "The comments urged that, because hair growth ingredients are not harmful, consumers should be allowed to decide whether they want to use [them]."

The agency noted that it is required by federal law to protect and promote public health by ensuring that drugs are not only safe, but effective. It cited the following agency statement (in a case where it banned a quack remedy for cancer) as its rationale for policing both the safety *and* the effectiveness of drugs:

"In passing the 1962 Amendments to the Food, Drug & Cosmetics Act—the Amendments that require that a drug be proved effective before it may be marketed—Congress indicated its conclusions that the absolute freedom to choose an ineffective drug was properly surrendered in exchange for the freedom from the danger to each person's health and well-being from the sale and use of worthless drugs.... To the extent that any freedom has been surrendered by the passage of the legislation... that surrender was a rational decision which has resulted in the achievement of greater freedom from the dangers to health and welfare represented by such [worthless] drugs."

• *ESTRADIOL:* This substance is a form of the female hormone estrogen. When very potent estradiol compounds are applied to the forehead of normal men, they reduce the production of oil, or sebum. But attempts to inhibit sebum production with estradiol skin creams have been unsuccessful.

Estrogens are readily absorbed through the skin. So there is concern about their use by men, since persistent exposure can cause feminizing changes. For example, male factory workers who handle estrogen develop abnormally large breasts.

To forestall this side effect, estrogenic baldness remedies—like estrogen skin creams that women use for other purposes—are labeled with instructions not to exceed a measured quantity of estrogen. This amount equals 666 International Units (IU) of the hormone per day. Evaluators believe this is a safe amount, and they note that in the 30 years that estradiol skin creams have been marketed, only a tiny handful of adverse reactions have been attributed to their use.

The major question, then, is whether estradiol assists hair growth and helps prevent baldness. Since the sebum-hair-loss theory has been scientifically discredited, reviewers had strong doubts about estradiol's effectiveness. The Panel reviewed four studies submitted and decided that three were "too subjective to be convincing, because they consisted only of favorable testimonials by dermatologists, as well as [by] men and women with hair loss.... No descriptions, photographs, or quantitative data on the hair loss of individual patients were given." While evaluators felt the fourth study was well planned, they believed it to be so badly conducted that no significance could be attached to the results.

These studies were based on the manufacturers' recommended regimen: application of a de-acidizing scalp conditioner, a scalp cleanser, a shampoo, the hair-growth stimulator, and an antiseptic dressing. The reviewers concluded that while the ingredients in this regimen are safe, neither all of them together nor estradiol alone is effective in preventing hair loss due to sebum or in stimulating hair regrowth.

In an effort to forestall the FDA's ban on estradiol, one manufacturer submitted several new studies to the agency in 1988, in which shampooing and conditioning regimens, with and without estradiol, were compared. The FDA says "there was a slight indication in the study that estradiol, with the cleansing agents, could be more helpful" than the cleansing agents alone. But a more astute and convincing scientific study than the ones provided would be needed to show this result. Wanting such proof, the FDA's decision, for now, is that estradiol is unsafe and ineffective for preventing baldness or stimulating hair to regrow.

* LANOLIN: Despite a manufacturer's submission of a product containing this substance, reviewers were not able to locate any evidence that lanolin (alone or in combination) affects hair growth. The verdict: safe but not effective. An FDA summary of the Panel's findings, puzzlingly, lists lanolin as unsafe as well as ineffective for hair growth.

* TETRACAINE HYDROCHLORIDE: The manufacturer who submitted a product that contains this ingredient said that it improves circulation, relieves scalp itching, and aids in the development of the hair follicle. But no evidence was submitted, or found, which shows that tetracaine hydrochloride has any effect on hair growth. The Panel concluded that the chemical is safe but not effective. The FDA added, not effective.

* WHEAT-GERM OIL: This substance—purported to be a source of vitamin E and of thiamine—was included in a baldness remedy submitted for review. But the maker furnished no data to show that wheat-germ oil (alone or in combination with other ingredients) has any effect on hair growth, nor could the Panel find any such evidence. Conclusion: topically applied wheat-germ oil is not safe or effective in restoring hair or preventing baldness.

OTHER DISAPPROVED INGREDIENTS IN BALDNESS PREPARATIONS

In the years between 1980, when the Panel's report was published in the *Federal Register*, and 1989, when FDA announced it would ban all nonprescription hair-growth and baldness-prevention drugs as not safe and effective, the agency considered petitions from manufacturers, doctors, consumers, and others for a number of putative remedies. It turned them all down, based on the evidence it was provided. These ingredients are listed in the table Safety and Effectiveness: Active Ingredients in Over-the-Counter Baldness Remedies.

The Panel and the FDA also made a list of *inactive* ingredients, including shampoos and conditioners, that may be found in hair growth regimens. These ingredients may help clean and groom the hair, but they have absolutely no proven medicinal value in preventing hair loss or making hair grow:

ammonium lauryl sulfate
benzethonium chloride
coconut oil
isopropyl alcohol
methyl ethyl ketone
mineral oil

polyethylene glycol 400
polysorbate 80
sodium hydroxide
sulfonated vegetable oil
vegetable/olive oil

When Greater Relief Is Needed

A man or a woman who is deeply concerned about hair loss should see a dermatologist, specifically one who specializes in hair-loss therapy. Minoxidil is one option. Transplants of hair from hairy to balding areas of the crown is another. The transplants can be satisfactorily effective for some people—though they are costly and can be uncomfortable as well.

At some point science merges into art, and dermatology melds into cosmetology, so that treatments that may or may not "grow hair" nevertheless may make it "*look* like you have more hair." If the price is right, this may be treatment enough for some who suffer painfully the loss of their hair.

Safety and Effectiveness: Banned Active Ingredients in Over-the-Counter Baldness Remedies

Active Ingredient	Assessment
amino acids	not safe and effective
aminobenzoic acid	not safe and effective
ascorbic acid (vitamin C)	not safe and effective
benzoic acid	not safe and effective
biotin and all other B vitamins	not safe and effective
dexpanthenol	not safe and effective
jojoba oil	not safe and effective
lanolin	not safe and effective
nucleic acids	not safe and effective
polysorbate 20	not safe and effective

Safety and Effectiveness: Banned Active Ingredients in Over-the-Counter Baldness Remedies (contd)

Active Ingredient	Assessment
polysorbate 60	not safe and effective
sulfanilamide	not safe and effective
sulfur 1% in carbon or a fraction of paraffinic hydrocarbons	not safe and effective
tetracaine hydrochloride	not safe and effective
urea	not safe and effective
wheat-germ oil	not safe and effective

Hair-Growth Stimulant and Baldness Preventives: Product Ratings

The FDA's judgement is that no over-the-counter drug product can safely and effectively stimulate hair growth or prevent baldness. So all products sold for this purpose must be rated "X"—not safe, not effective—and banned.

Hangover and Overindulgence Relievers

Almost every adult has had the experience of eating or drinking too much—and then feeling awful. Can anything be done, one despairingly wonders, to calm the stomach and steady the head?

Fortunately, help may be close at hand at a drugstore or a grocery, if not in the medicine chest. Reviewers who evaluated several familiar products that are sold to relieve these conditions say these preparations can provide significant relief.

What Kinds of Relief Are Needed?

The over-the-counter drugs assessed by the Panel are intended for the relief of symptoms of occasional overindulgence or intoxication; they may bring little comfort to chronic alcoholics or inveterate gluttons. As the Panel sees it, two somewhat different conditions may require

---

HANGOVER AND OVERINDULGENCE RELIEVERS is based on the report "OTC Orally Administered Drug Products for Relief of Symptoms Associated with Overindulgence in Alcohol and Food" by the FDA's Advisory Review Panel on OTC Miscellaneous Internal Drug Products, the FDA's Tentative Final Monograph on these products, and related documents in the OTC Drug Review.

treatment. *Upset stomach* due to overindulgence in food and alcohol results when one eats and drinks too much, together. The key symptoms are heartburn, a sense of fullness, and nausea. *Hangover* results when one simply drinks too much—perhaps even *far* too much—alcohol. The symptoms may include nausea, heartburn, thirst, tremor, unsteadiness, fatigue, aches and pains, headache, and feelings of dullness, depression, or irritability.

With this distinction in mind, the Panel divided the products and ingredients it assessed into three groups:

- ingredients and drugs intended to relieve overindulgence in food and alcohol
- ingredients and drugs intended to relieve hangover
- ingredients intended to minimize alcoholic inebriation

Upset Stomach Due to Overindulgence

The Panel decided that the symptoms of overindulgence experienced by people who eat *and* drink too much are distinct and identifiable. These symptoms are different from hangover alone (which results from alcohol overindulgence) or from overeating alone.

The evaluators' recognition of these symptoms was based mostly on unpublished studies supplied by drug manufacturers, in which persons who were encouraged to overindulge in rich food and drink were then asked to describe their ill feelings. The following symptoms were listed by these human guinea pigs: fullness, heartburn or a burning sensation, passing of gas, stomachache, headache, belching, rumbling stomach, thirsty or dry mouth, sluggishness, taste repeat, nausea, and bitter or acid aftertaste. In all the studies, most participants complained of heartburn, fullness, nausea, or a combination of these complaints. This led reviewers to identify these complaints as the principal symptoms of overindulgence. According to the Panel, the alcohol is more responsible for these symptoms than the food.

The Panel approached products used to treat upset stomach due to overindulgence with a certain degree of skepticism. One reason is that evaluators could not think of any single active ingredient that will safely and effectively relieve either nausea or fullness, two of the three main symptoms of overindulgence. The third key symptom, heartburn, can be relieved with a number of safe and effective antacid active ingredients.

Combination Products

A fair number of persons with upset stomachs due to overindulgence also suffer headaches and other minor aches and pains. So the experts approve of combining a safe and effective pain reliever—either aspirin or acetaminophen—with safe and effective active ingredients that quell upset stomach. The experts do not sanction combinations that include two different aspirin-like drugs (salicylates). The Panel also approves of one safe and effective stimulant—caffeine—in overindulgence preparations.

One preparation that is marketed for upset stomach due to overindulgence contains aspirin + citric acid + sodium bicarbonate. When this product is immersed in water, a chemical reaction occurs: The ingredients are converted into sodium acetylsalicylate (a pain reliever) + sodium citrate (an antacid) + bubbles of carbon dioxide gas. There is some residue of sodium bicarbonate, which also acts as an antacid. Another widely marketed combination product used to relieve overindulgence is acetaminophen + citric acid + caffeine.

 Claims for Overindulgence Relievers

Accurate
- "For the relief of upset stomach due to overindulgence in food and drink"
- "For the relief of upset stomach associated with nausea, heartburn and fullness due to overindulgence in food and drink"

Unproved
- "Fast relief"
- "Speedy relief"

Drugs for Upset Stomach Due to Overindulgence

The Panel and the FDA categorize two ingredients in upset-stomach calmers. They are discussed in the following section.

APPROVED OVERINDULGENCE-RELIEVING ACTIVE INGREDIENTS

• BISMUTH SUBSALICYLATE: This bismuth compound has been found safe as a medication to counteract diarrhea at higher dosages than are recommended for the treatment of upset stomach due to overindulgence in food and drink. So the Panel and FDA judge it safe.

The effectiveness of bismuth subsalicylate against upset stomach due to overindulgence was tested in three excellently constructed and well-controlled tests. Participants were randomly assigned either to a treatment group or a dummy-medication group; neither the participants nor the investigators knew which people were receiving the bismuth subsalicylate and which the dummy preparation until after the test was over. In one of these tests 132 normal, healthy, non-alcoholic men and women were wined and dined in a dinner-party setting, where they were offered unlimited amounts of champagne, wine, and cordials to drink. Not surprisingly, 91 of them developed gastrointestinal distress during the course of the evening—and they required drug treatment. Roughly half took the bismuth subsalicylate preparation and half the look-alike dummy medication.

When the results were tabulated, it turned out that 9 out of 10 overindulgers who had dosed themselves with bismuth subsalicylate experienced good-to-excellent relief from their distress—in particular, relief from nausea, fullness, and heartburn. But among overindulgers who took the dummy preparation, only a little more than half experienced good-to-excellent relief. These are significant findings in favor of bismuth's ability to combat both the over all overindulgence syndrome and its three principal symptoms.

Evidence from the two other studies assessed by the Panel was less convincing, but the general results led reviewers to judge bismuth subsalicylate effective for relieving overindulgers' upset stomach. Appropriate doses are 0.525 grams to be taken no more often than every 30 to 60 minutes, for a total dose of 4.2 grams (or 8 doses) per day.

WARNING:

 If taken with other salicylates, and ringing in the ears occurs, discontinue use.

If you are taking medication for anticoagulation (thinning of the blood), or have diabetes, gout, or arthritis, consult a physician before taking this product.

• *CITRIC ACID (SODIUM CITRATE IN SOLUTION):* As an overindulgence reliever, citric acid is very often formulated in tablets or granules, along with sodium bicarbonate—which is an *adjuvant*, or helper ingredient—and a pain-relieving active ingredient. It *effervesces*, or fizzes, when put into water. In the resulting reaction, the citric acid is converted to sodium citrate.

Citric acid has been approved as safe and effective as an antacid. (*See* ANTACIDS.)

Only one scientifically controlled study was submitted to support the claim that citric acid specifically relieves upset stomach associated with overindulgence in rich and spicy foods that are washed down with alcoholic beverages. A statistically significant benefit was recorded only on "the morning after," not during the night.

Although the data on citric acid's effectiveness are less convincing than those for bismuth subsalicylate (*see* previous discussion), on the basis of this one study, the Panel decided that citric acid is safe and effective in providing general relief of upset stomach due to overindulgence. The safe and effective dosage should not exceed approximately 16 grams of sodium citrate for persons under 60 years of age (half that amount for older persons).

WARNING:

 If you are on a sodium-restricted diet, do not take this product except under the supervision of a physician.

Hangover Relievers

The Panel defined *hangover* as the "noxious feelings encountered several hours after the occasional ingestion of large amounts of alcohol." The most common symptoms are nausea, heartburn, thirst, tremor, loss of balance, fatigue, aches and pains, and irritable, dull, or depressed feelings.

Sufferers have long used three kinds of drugs to relieve these symptoms: pain relievers like aspirin for the headache, antacids for the gastric distress, and caffeine (a stimulant) for the dullness and fatigue.

Reviewers decided these three types of drugs are logical choices, so they approved combinations that include safe and effective doses of all three. In essence, the Panel reversed the usual policy of the over-the-counter drug review; that is, it actually recommended that hangover remedies be formulated as combination products rather than as single-entity drugs.

The safe and effective pain relievers are acetaminophen and aspirin. In one preparation, aspirin is mixed with citric acid and sodium bicarbonate in such a way that when the product is put into water before it is swallowed, a chemical reaction occurs. The ingredients are converted into sodium acetylsalicylate (a pain reliever) + sodium citrate (an antacid) + bubbles of carbon dioxide gas + a residue of sodium bicarbonate.

The safe and effective stimulant is caffeine. The safe and effective antacids are aluminum hydroxide, aluminum hydroxide gel, citric acid (sodium citrate), magnesium carbonate, and magnesium trisilicate.

The FDA has proposed one significant change in these combination products: The removal of either the caffeine or the antacid. Antacids reduce stomach acidity, the agency points out. But caffeine is known to *enhance* stomach acidity. So they work at cross purposes. The agency therefore plans to ban all combination hangover remedies that contain both an antacid and caffeine.

 Claims for Hangover Relievers

Accurate

• "For the relief of hangover"

For products that contain aspirin or acetaminophen:

• "For the temporary relief of minor aches and pains associated with a hangover"

For products that contain caffeine:

• "Helps restore mental alertness or wakefulness when [one is] experiencing fatigue or drowsiness associated with a hangover"

Combination Products

Unlike virtually all other categories of nonprescription drugs, this one—for hangover and overindulgence relievers—contains *only* combination products. The category appears to specifically accommodate—with FDA's approval—a handful of venerable hangover remedies.

Consumers should choose combination hangover remedies that contain only the ingredients they need to relieve their symptoms. For example, if you are nauseated but have no headache or other aches and pains, then you probably do not require a pain reliever. If you have only a headache, on the other hand, a couple of acetaminophen or aspirin tablets should suffice.

Based on its decision that an antacid should not be combined with a caffeine, and studies on the safety and effectiveness of the individual active ingredients in nonprescription hangover relievers, FDA classifies them as follows:

APPROVED HANGOVER-RELIEF COMBINATIONS

acetaminophen + caffeine

aspirin + caffeine

aspirin + citric acid + sodium bicarbonate (which produce sodium acetylsalicylate + sodium citrate + carbon dioxide gas + sodium when they are mixed with water)

acetaminophen + citric acid + sodium bicarbonate (which produce acetaminophen + sodium citrate + carbon dioxide gas + sodium when they are mixed with water)

aspirin + an antacid

acetaminophen + an antacid

CONDITIONALLY APPROVED HANGOVER-RELIEF COMBINATIONS

None.

DISAPPROVED HANGOVER-RELIEF COMBINATIONS

Any combination that includes an antacid + caffeine.

Drugs to Relieve Hangover

Several types of ingredients are formulated into hangover relief products. They are described in the following sections.

APPROVED HANGOVER-RELIEVING ACTIVE INGREDIENTS

- **PAIN RELIEVERS:** Acetaminophen, aspirin, and sodium salicylate in solution are safe and effective. The approved dosage is 325 to 650 mg every 4 hours. *See* pp. 759-801.
- **STIMULANTS:** The approved (safe and effective) stimulant is caffeine. It should be taken in doses of 100 to 200 mg. (*See* STIMULANTS.)
- **ANTACIDS:** Safe and effective antacids commonly found in hangover relievers are aluminum hydroxide, aluminum hydroxide gel, citric acid (sodium citrate), magnesium carbonate, and magnesium trisilicate. (*See* ANTACIDS.)

CONDITIONALLY APPROVED HANGOVER-RELIEVING ACTIVE INGREDIENTS

None.

DISAPPROVED HANGOVER-RELIEVING ACTIVE INGREDIENTS

None.

Hangover Minimizers

The best way to minimize hangovers is to drink in moderation. Preparations are marketed with claims for minimizing hangover symptoms. The one active ingredient sold for this purpose is activated charcoal, which is claimed to prevent or minimize the symptoms of hangover.

Claims for Hangover Minimizers

Unproved

- "To minimize the symptoms of a hangover caused by alcoholic beverages"
- "Helps minimize the symptoms of a hangover ..."

APPROVED HANGOVER-MINIMIZING ACTIVE INGREDIENTS

None.

CONDITIONALLY APPROVED HANGOVER-MINIMIZING ACTIVE INGREDIENT

• CHARCOAL, ACTIVATED: This material has a honeycomb structure that allows it to hold and neutralize large amounts of chemical substances. For this reason, it is widely used as an antidote to accidental poisoning, and the Panel judges it safe for use at the lower doses that are recommended for minimizing hangover.

The claim that activated charcoal helps circumvent hangovers is based on the theory that it is the impurities in alcohol—not the alcohol itself—that are largely responsible for the unpleasant aftereffects of drinking. According to this theory, vodka, which is largely free of impurities, causes fewer symptoms than an equivalent amount of bourbon, which contains many of them. The problem is that while impurities have been shown to play some role in drunkenness, other studies indicate, fairly conclusively, that it is the *amount* of alcohol consumed—whether as vodka or whiskey—that largely determines drunkenness. Not surprisingly, therefore, another test showed that bourbon produces no worse hangovers than vodka. No direct evidence is available from studies in humans to show that activated charcoal will neutralize impurities or minimize hangover. Therefore, the FDA judges activated charcoal safe but not proved effective when taken for this purpose.

DISAPPROVED HANGOVER-MINIMIZING ACTIVE INGREDIENTS

None.

Safety and Effectiveness: Active Ingredients in Over-the-Counter Remedies to Relieve Upset Stomach Due to Overindulgence in Food and Drink

Active Ingredient	Assessment
acetaminophen	safe and effective
aspirin	safe and effective
bismuth subsalicylate	safe and effective
citric acid (sodium citrate)	safe and effective

Safety and Effectiveness: Active Ingredients in Over-the-Counter Remedies for Relieving or Minimizing Hangover

Active Ingredient	Function	Panel's Assessment
acetaminophen	pain reliever	safe and effective
aspirin	pain reliever	safe and effective
aluminum hydroxide	antacid	safe and effective
aluminum hydroxide gel	antacid	safe and effective
caffeine	stimulant	safe and effective
charcoal, activated	minimizer	safe but not effective
citric acid (sodium citrate)	antacid	safe and effective
magnesium carbonate	antacid	safe and effective
magnesium trisilicate	antacid	safe and effective

Hangover and Overindulgence Remedies: Product Ratings

OVERINDULGENCE RELIEF PRODUCTS

Product and Distributor	Dosage of Active Ingredients	Rating *	Comment
Alka-Seltzer with Aspirin (Miles)	**effervescent tablets:** 325 mg aspirin + 1.9 g sodium bicarbonate + 1 g citric acid	A	
Extra Strength Alka-Seltzer (Miles)	same as above, but with 500 mg aspirin	A	
Bromo Seltzer (Warner-Lambert)	**effervescent granules:** 325 mg acetaminophen + 2.781 g sodium bicarbonate + 2.224 g citric acid per capful measure	A	
Pepto-Bismol (Procter & Gamble)	**liquid:** 262 mg bismuth subsalicylate per tablespoonful	A	
	tablets, chewable: 262 mg bismuth subsalicylate	A	

HANGOVER RELIEF PRODUCTS

Product and Distributor	Dosage of Active Ingredients	Rating *	Comment

Product and Distributor	Dosage of Active Ingredients	Rating*	Comment
Alka-Seltzer Advanced Formula (Miles)	effervescent tablets: 465 mg sodium bicarbonate + 280 mg calcium carbonate + 325 acetaminophen + 900 mg citric acid + 300 mg potassium bicarbonate	B	neither the calcium nor the potassium antacid is listed by FDA as approved for this use
Alka-Seltzer Antacid and Pain Reliever (Miles)	effervescent tablets: 325 mg aspirin + 1.9 g sodium bicarbonate + 1 g citric acid	A	
Alka-Seltzer Antacid and Pain Reliever Extra Strength (Miles)	same as above, but with 500 mg aspirin	A	
Bisodol (Whitehall)	powder: 716 mg sodium bicarbonate + 528 mg magnesium carbonate per teaspoonful	A	
BromoSeltzer (Warner-Lambert)	effervescent granules: 325 mg acetaminophen + 2.781 g sodium bicarbonate + 2.224 g citric acid per capful measure	A	

PRODUCTS TO PREVENT DRUNKENNESS OR MINIMIZE HANGOVER

Product and Distributor	Dosage of Active Ingredients	Rating*	Comment
Charcocaps (Requa)	capsules: 260 mg activated charcoal	B	not proved effective

*Author's interpretation of FDA criteria. Based on contents, not claims.

Hemorrhoid Medications and Other Anorectal Applications

*The U.S. government has spent over $50 billion to study
the backside of the moon, but not one red cent to study the
backsides of its citizens.*

—Leon Banov, M.D.

Few self-treatable conditions are as anguishing—physically and emotionally—as hemorrhoids. Reviewers who assessed the ointments and
suppositories used to relieve hemorrhoids point to these factors that
enhance this distress:

- The *anorectum*, or anorectal region, like the nearby genital
area, is richly endowed with sensory nerve receptors—and
so it hurts or itches quite badly when disturbed.

- Among body regions, the anorectum is a "social outcast."
Many people, doctors included, are shy about discussing it.

HEMORRHOID MEDICATIONS AND OTHER ANORECTAL APPLICATIONS is based on the report by the
FDA's Advisory Review Panel on OTC Hemorrhoidal Drug Products and the FDA's Tentative
Final and Final Orders on these products.

This may start with early childhood—when youngsters are encouraged to use euphemisms like "bottom," "fanny," or "behind." Code names are often taught both for defecation itself as well as for the place where this is done : the "rest room," "tinkle room," or "potty."

- A more frank and forthright acceptance of bowel functions would be beneficial. People could more easily and straight-forwardly ask for and receive medical help for anorectal disorders and thus might be spared much suffering.

The Anatomy of the Anorectum

Since it is difficult to see one's anus, reviewers offered this brief anatomical tour: Starting from outside, the *perianal area* is defined as the 3-inch-wide circle of skin immediately surrounding the anal opening. This skin is moist and is more vulnerable than most to pressure, frictional injury, and infection. The perianal area contains very sensitive pain-receiving nerve endings, which also transmit itching sensations.

The *anus* is the external opening through which bowel movements pass. The tight, inch-long passage above it is the *anal canal*. It normally stays tightly closed against leakage and seepage except when the bowels are moving or gas is being passed. Two sets of muscles open and close the canal. One, which surrounds part of the upper portion of the canal, is the *internal anal sphincter*; it is an involuntary muscle—that is, it functions outside our conscious control. Surrounding the lower portion of the canal is a muscular structure called the *external anal sphincter*, which one "pushes open" to defecate.

The anal canal is lined with skin and is studded with sensory nerve fibers that convey pain and itching. At its upper end is a demarcation, the *anorectal line*, where the skin gives way to mucosal surface. There the tight anal canal widens into a 5-inch-long hollow column, the *rectum,* where feces collect before defecation. Unlike anal skin, the rectal mucosa does *not* have superficial pain and itch receptors. But its underlying tissues do harbor pressure-sensitive nerves that tell us when to go to the toilet. These nerves also enable us to feel the difference between solid matter and *flatus* (gas). The anal canal and lower rectum are served by three major sets of blood vessels: the inferior (lower), middle, and superior (upper) hemorrhoidal arteries and veins. When affected by swelling, they may be a source of considerable discomfort and, sometimes, more serious disorders.

Disorders

Hemorrhoids

The anorectal disease of greatest concern to consumers is hemorrhoids, which sometimes are called *piles*. A hemorrhoid is a swollen or symptom-producing conglomeration of blood vessels, supportive tissues, and overlying mucous membrane or skin. It usually develops along the anal canal or in the lower end of the rectum. Blood may be discharged from the hemorrhoidal blood vessels. But bleeding is by no means the only symptom: Hemorrhoids typically cause burning, itching, inflammation, and swelling.

External hemorrhoids, which are those that arise below the anorectal line, constitute a substantial share of the problems for which consumers seek relief with over-the-counter hemorrhoidal medications. Internal hemorrhoids, which are less common, arise above the anorectal line. When an internal hemorrhoid extends down into the anal canal, or even out through the anus, it is said to be *prolapsed*.

The sluggish blood-flow through the hemorrhoidal vessels is believed to be a major contributing cause of hemorrhoids. The blood pools up and balloons out the veins and surrounding tissues. Humankind's upright stance may contribute to the problem. Blood in the human hemorrhoidal veins must be pumped upward, against gravity, to return to the heart. In most four-legged animals, on the contrary, the rectum is *higher* than the heart. Thus gravity carries the blood back, so it does not collect in vein-stretching pools.

Straining during defecation is another cause of piles because it compresses the hemorrhoidal veins; blood pressure builds up within the veins, dilating their walls. The increased pressure that pregnancy exerts on the pelvis commonly causes hemorrhoids. Another contributing factor may be the accumulation of fecal matter in small crypts (pockets) near the top of the anal canal. An increased intake of roughage may help clean out these pockets.

Perianal abscess

This condition can be defined as an infection and collection of pus due to bacterial penetration of underlying tissue.

Anal fissure

A painful crack or sore in the skin of the anal canal is referred to as an anal fissure.

Anal itchiness

Sufferers experience a persistent and often intense itching in the peri-anal area. Poor hygiene is a common cause of this complaint, which also may result from the consumption of peppery foods. In children, sudden attacks of intense itching at night often signal pinworm infections. (*See* WORM KILLERS FOR PINWORM INFESTATION.) If the child's anal itching does not vanish quickly, seek a doctor's help.

A warm sitz bath may resolve the itching in adults. Alternatively, OTC drugs that contain local anesthetics may bring relief. Hydrocortisone preparations also may be particularly helpful.

Poor anal hygiene can cause or contribute to anal itching. A number of cleaning aids, including medicated and non-medicated wipes and tissues are sold over-the-counter to relieve this distress.

Polyps

Polyps are benign tumors that arise in, or from just beneath, the mucous membrane of the rectum.

Anorectal cancer

Bleeding and a constant urge to defecate may result from a malignant tumor.

Treatment

Uncomplicated hemorrhoids and other minor, noncancerous anorectal disorders can be treated successfully with nonprescription drugs. But if the symptoms do not clear up completely within a week, they require medical attention. Bleeding from the anus, mucus discharge, seepage of fecal matter, and protrusion of a hemorrhoid or of rectal tissue outside the anal canal all are potentially serious medical problems. In these instances, a doctor should *always* be consulted.

Types of Drugs

- A *vasoconstrictor* temporarily shrinks swollen hemor-rhoidal blood vessels. An *astringent* concentrates and holds (binds) proteins—which may be bacteria, fecal matter, or festering body products—and keeps them away from the skin; it may also produce a bracing sensation. A *skin-peeling agent (keratolytic)* removes dead outer skin. *Local anesthetics* deaden pain; *protectants* provide a protective coating over irritated tissues, and *itch-pain relievers (antipruritics, analgesics, and anesthetics)* provide relief by temporarily damping down the receptivity of nerve endings in the skin.

For a synopsis of the hemorrhoid drug ingredients and the symptoms they relieve, *see* the table Drugs to Relieve Anorectal Symptoms.

Dosage Forms

Consumers use anorectal drug products to medicate two essentially different types of tissues: the perianal area and the rectum. These areas respond to drugs in different ways, and different methods are used to treat them. Drugs applied to the perianal area and anal canal are being used *externally*. Drugs slid or pushed through the anal canal into the rectum are being applied *intrarectally*.

Three different delivery systems are used in anorectal products: ointments, suppositories, and foams.

• OINTMENTS: Ointments are semi-solid preparations that may soften but will not melt into a liquid when they are subjected to normal body temperature of about 98.6° F. Panel reviewers included creams, gels, jellies, and pastes in their evaluation of anorectal ointments. These substances can be smeared on exposed surfaces and also can be forced upward into the anal canal with the fingertip.

When ointments are used intrarectally, they can be inserted through a tubular applicator that is sometimes called a *pile pipe*. This is slid past the anal sphincter muscle so that the medication is expelled from the tip and deposited within the rectum. The pile pipe should be flexible and should be well lubricated—perhaps with some of the ointment—so that it enters easily and does not injure the anal canal or the rectal mucosa. Even when they are applying an ointment intrarectally, many people prefer using their fingers—which the Panel says is even safer.

Dosages of anorectal products are hard to standardize. However, the evaluators concluded that the average suppository weighs 2 grams, about one-fourteenth of an ounce. Studies have shown that patients tend to apply about the same quantity of an anorectal ointment product

Drugs to Relieve Anorectal Symptoms

Symptom or sign	EXPECTATIONS FOR RELIEF						
	Local Anesthetics (which block nerve impulses)	Vasoconstrictors	Protectants	Astringents	Itch-pain relievers (which blunt sensory receptors in skin)	Skin-peeling Agents	Corticosteroids*
itching	yes	yes	yes	yes	yes	yes	yes
discomfort	yes	maybe	yes	yes	yes	yes	yes
irritation	yes	maybe	yes	yes	yes	yes	yes
burning	yes	no	yes	yes	yes	no	yes
swelling	no	yes	no	no	no	no	yes
pain	yes	maybe	no	no	yes	no	no
inflammation	no	no	maybe	no	no	no	yes
protrusion	should not be self-treated with over-the-counter products						
seepage	should not be self-treated with over-the-counter products						
bleeding	should not be self-treated with over-the-counter products						

*Source: *drug facts and comparisons*, Jan. 1992, p. 538, for 1% hydrocortisone preparations.

each time they use it. This amount is enough to provide an effective and protective layer over the anus and perianal area. So the Panel accepts 2 grams—which is the weight of 2 paper clips—as more or less the standard dose for an anorectal product.

• *SUPPOSITORIES:* Soft, usually slippery, solid formulations, suppositories are oval or bullet-shaped to slide easily through the anal canal and into the rectum. (Reviewers say an hour-glass shape would allow the suppository to stay in place longer.) Unlike an ointment, when a suppository is inserted into the rectum, little if any of the drug adheres to the anal canal. Suppositories are composed of materials that melt readily at normal body temperature.

This kind of medical treatment has been used at least since Biblical times. It continues to be popular, although current reviewers believe the benefit may be more in the mind than in the anorectum and the relief experienced may be dangerously deceptive; that is, you may feel a disorder is being *cured* rather than simply relieved, which could make you delay seeking appropriate medical attention.

Traditionally, suppositories are made of soap, tallow, candle wax, and, more recently, cocoa butter, hard fat, or glycerin. These substances also relieve constipation and help people move their bowels. The protectant substances in contemporary over-the-counter suppositories may lubricate the anal canal so that stools pass without tearing or irritating the tissue, but consumers are cautioned that the amount of lubricant may not be sufficient to act as a laxative. The principal use of suppositories as nonprescription anorectal medication is for local treatment of the lower rectum and anal canal, particularly for sufferers of internal hemorrhoids.

A normally functioning sphincter will keep much or all of an anal medication from seeping downward onto itch- and pain-sensitive anal surfaces. Also, caustic fluids normally present higher up in the rectum may quickly break down the active ingredients of these drugs. For these reasons, it may help people who do use suppositories to stand up straight after inserting one. This way the medicine will have a better chance of settling downward into the anal canal.

• *FOAMS:* Use of foams is new. This method was developed to overcome the shortcomings of suppositories in medicating the anorectum. Active drugs are incorporated into a foam that can be propelled into the anal canal under pressure.

Choice of Ingredients

The consumer with hemorrhoids or a troublesome itch may be daunted by the discovery that several different types of drugs are formulated into a variety of combination products that all promise symptomatic relief. The reviewers' sifting and sorting of these drugs—as summarized in the table Drugs to Relieve Anorectal Symptoms—should simplify the task of selection. This table allows you to pick the type of drug—local anesthetic, vasoconstrictor, and so on—most likely to relieve your principal symptoms.

'Witch Hazel' Still Fragrant With New Name

The flowers, bark, and leaves of the common, colorful American witch hazel shrub provided tonics and remedies to Native Americans. Today, natural witch hazel is one of a diminishing number of plant products that meet FDA standards for safety and effectiveness.

But the FDA, following other pharmacological authorities, has changed this bracing medication's name to *hamamelis water* to match the plant's Greek botanical name: *hama* means "together" and *mela* means "fruit." These plants are unusual because they bear their blossoms and fruits together, at the very same time of year, usually in autumn or winter. Witch hazels are thus also unique in being one of the very few types of plants that bloom—often for weeks at a time—in the dead of winter. (Most commercial witch hazel is grown in Connecticut.)

Flowers of the common, native witch-hazel shrub, *H. virginiana*, are ribbon-like clusters of yellow, orange, or red petals; the adjacent seed capsules, from the previous year's blossoms, will eject two black seeds a foot or so into the air when they burst.

Some experts have suggested that witch hazel's astringency is due at least in part to the alcohol in which the refined plant material may be dissolved. But traditionalists hold that the *astringent* and ultimately cooling and relaxing effect resides in the natural juices of this native plant, and at least one study by a manufacturer tends to confirm this view.

Then, in order to choose ingredients that have been approved as safe and effective, you should consult the Safety and Effectiveness table at the end of this Unit. This chart shows, for example, that a dozen protectant ingredients—which provide the bulk of most anorectal products—are safe and effective both for external application to the perianal area and for intrarectal administration in a suppository or with a pile pipe.

Only three other drugs from one other group, *vasoconstrictors*, are safe and effective for intrarectal use. So, a person's choice for safe and effective intrarectal drugs is, in fact, extremely limited.

The range is slightly wider for the consumer interested in choosing a safe and effective preparation for external use. When symptoms require this kind of medication, there are safe and effective agents in five other classes—local anesthetics, itch-pain relievers, astringents, skin-peeling agents (keratolytics), and corticosteroids—to consider.

Safety for Women and Children

Only very small amounts of drugs are absorbed into the bloodstream when they are applied externally to the perianal area. Therefore, evaluators say women can safely use all approved active ingredients in anorectal preparations. Safe and effective protectant ingredients that have no other pharmacological effect may also be used intrarectally. However, pregnant and nursing women should not use suppositories or intrarectally applied ointments and foams that contain other types of active ingredients.

Hemorrhoids and anorectal complaints are rare in children. When they do occur, the child should be taken to a doctor. The Panel stipulates that nonprofessional diagnosis and treatment of anorectal problems should not be attempted for children under 12 years of age. Exceptions can be made in the case of astringents (calamine, hamamelis water NF XI [better known as witch hazel] and zinc oxide) and approved protectants that can be used to relieve itching, burning, irritation, discomfort, and pain.

Combination Products

Most over-the-counter anorectal products contain a combination of active ingredients to treat two or more concurrent symptoms. Evaluators believe that two ingredients from two different drug groups are usually enough. But as many as four of the bland protectant ingredients may be combined if, together, they make up 50 percent or more of a finished product. Reviewers prefer single-ingredient products and believe a consumer should use a combination product only when he or she suffers all the symptoms found on the label.

 Claims

Accurate
- "For the temporary relief of the discomfort associated with hemorrhoids and other anorectal disorders"
- "Helps relieve anorectal itching"
- "Gives temporary relief of itching of piles (hemorrhoids)"

Drug Groupings

The active ingredients in anorectal products have been divided into several groups. To find which group a specific active ingredient belongs in, consult the list that follows. Each group is then described, and a table showing the safety and effectiveness of all ingredients in each group appears at the end of this unit.

Categorization of Anorectal Drugs

Active Ingredient	Pharmacologic Group
alcloxa	skin-peeling agent
aluminum hydroxide gel	protectant
benzocaine	local anesthetic
benzyl alcohol	local anesthetic
calamine (prepared calamine)	protectant and astringent
camphor	itch-pain reliever
cocoa butter (cacao butter)	protectant

Categorization of Anorectal Drugs (contd)

Active Ingredient	Pharmacologic Group
cod-liver oil	protectant
dibucaine	local anesthetic
dibucaine hydrochloride	local anesthetic
dyclonine hydrochloride	local anesthetic
ephedrine sulfate	vasoconstrictor
epinephrine	vasoconstrictor
epinephrine hydrochloride	vasoconstrictor
glycerin, aqueous solution	protectant
hamamelis water NF XI (witch-hazel)	astringent
hard fat	protectant
hydrocortisone	corticosteroid
hydrocortisone acetate	corticosteroid
juniper tar (oil of cade)	itch-pain reliever
kaolin	protectant
lanolin	protectant
lidocaine	local anesthetic
live yeast-cell derivative	wound healer
menthol	itch-pain reliever
mineral oil	protectant
petrolatum	protectant
phenylephrine hydrochloride	vasoconstrictor
pramoxine hydrochloride	local anesthetic
resorcinol	skin-peeling agent
shark-liver oil	protectant
tetracaine	local anesthetic
tetracaine hydrochloride	local anesthetic

Categorization of Anorectal Drugs (contd)

Active Ingredient	Pharmacologic Group
topical starch	protectant
witch hazel (See hamamelis water)	
white petrolatum	protectant
zinc oxide	protectant and astringent

Local Anesthetics

The symptoms that may be relieved by local anesthetics—which are also called *topical anesthetics*—include pain, burning, itching, irritation, and discomfort. They are the most important drugs for treating hemorrhoids and other anorectal disorders because they offer relief for a wider variety of symptoms than those of any other group. These drugs temporarily block the transmission of sensory nerve impulses from the skin receptors in the skin.

The experts disagreed about whether suppositories and other products intended for intrarectal use should contain anesthetics. The majority of the Panel said there is insufficient evidence to show that anesthetics are safe or effective when used intrarectally because drugs may be absorbed into the bloodstream from the rectal mucosa almost as rapidly as if they were injected directly into a vein. Moreover, when they are absorbed from the lower rectum, drugs may immediately enter the general circulation without passing through and being broken down by the liver. This is of concern because some local anesthetics with names ending in the suffix *-caine* can cause serious—even lethal— damage to the heart and nervous system if absorbed into the body in large amounts. The *-caine*-type anesthetic benzocaine is, however, free of this risk. There is another danger in putting anesthetics into the rectum: They may mask the feelings of fullness by which the body normally tells you to defecate.

Effectiveness also is at issue. The majority of the Panel said there are no known pain-receiving nerve endings on rectal surfaces; for example, cutting or burning the rectal mucosa during surgical treatments is not painful. This view is supported by two studies that show that test subjects could not differentiate between the pain-relieving effects of intrarectal products containing an anesthetic and look-alike dummy drugs.

Reviewers concluded that the usefulness of intrarectal anesthetics has yet to be established, so none were approved. The FDA has concurred in this judgment.

 Claims for Local Anesthetics

Accurate

• "For the temporary relief of itching, burning, and pain associated with hemorrhoids or other anorectal disorders"

• "For the temporary relief of the soreness of hemorrhoids [piles]"

APPROVED LOCAL ANESTHETIC ACTIVE INGREDIENTS

A number of ingredients were granted approval as local anesthetics for the treatment of hemorrhoids and other anorectal disorders. All are approved for external use only. Most of the anesthetics that follow are discussed in greater detail in the Unit ITCH AND PAIN REMEDIES APPLIED TO THE SKIN. Their application for anorectal problems is described here briefly.

• *BENZOCAINE:* While only a few studies have been done on the use of this anesthetic for anorectal distress, evaluators judged them adequate to establish its safety and effectiveness. In one study of 39 patients, for example, 20 percent benzocaine in an ointment relieved anorectal discomfort in all cases; lower concentrations resulted in a lower relief rate. So, 5 to 20 percent benzocaine is safe and effective when used up to 6 times in 24 hours. *See* p. 557.

• *DIBUCAINE PREPARATIONS (DIBUCAINE, DIBUCAINE HYDROCHLORIDE):* These pain relievers were evaluated by the Advisory Review Panel on Over-the-Counter Analgesic Drug Products and found to be safe and effective, in doses of 0.25 to 1 percent, for use on skin surfaces of the body. Based on this result, the FDA approved their use specifically for treating external hemorrhoids and other, minor anorectal distress. *See* p. 559.

• *DYCLONINE HYDROCHLORIDE:* This local anesthetic was approved by the FDA, in doses of 0.5 to 1 percent, based on the judgment that it is safe, generally speaking, for treating painful skin conditions. *See* p. 560.

- HYDROCORTISONE PREPARATIONS: HYDROCORTISONE, HYDROCORTISONE ACETATE: *See* p. 561.
- LIDOCAINE: This standard and effective pain-reliever was approved by the FDA for self-treatment of hemorrhoids on the basis of its earlier approval for treating itching and pain on a variety of skin surfaces of the body. *See* p. 562.
- PRAMOXINE HYDROCHLORIDE: This anesthetic active ingredient has been specifically tested in individuals with anorectal complaints. In one study of patients following hemorrhoid surgery, for example, 93 percent reported good-to-excellent pain relief. In another, 18 of 27 patients with hemorrhoids had improved enough after two weeks' treatment that they did not require surgery. The other nine reported some symptomatic relief. Patients with anal erosions also felt less pain when they used this drug. The approved dosage is a 2-gram dose of the 1 percent cream or jelly up to 5 times daily. *See* p. 563.
- TETRACAINE PREPARATIONS: TETRACAINE, TETRACAINE HYDROCHLORIDE: These local anesthetics were approved for external application to the perianal and anal surfaces on the basis of another panel's decision: They are safe and effective for treating pain and itching on skin surfaces at concentrations of 0.5 to 1 percent. *See* pp. 564-565.

WARNING:

 Do not use in large quantities, particularly on raw surfaces or blistered areas.

CONDITIONALLY APPROVED LOCAL ANESTHETIC ACTIVE INGREDIENTS

None.

DISAPPROVED LOCAL ANESTHETIC ACTIVE INGREDIENTS

None.

Vasoconstrictors

Vasoconstrictors temporarily tighten small blood vessels. Because hemorrhoids consist in large part of swollen blood vessels, vasoconstrictors can effectively relieve the discomfort of this swelling. Vasoconstrictors seem to offer relief from itching, although *how* is yet to be explained. Also, this itch relief is less than that offered by local anesthetics.

Squeezing an injured blood vessel, whether physically or chemically, is one way to make it stop bleeding. Vasoconstrictors may stop anorectal bleeding in this way. Evaluators warn, however, that blood coming from the anus may originate from a number of sites along the gastrointestinal tract. It could result from any one of several serious diseases—including ulcers and cancer—and so *never* should be self-treated. *If you are bleeding from the anus, see your doctor.*

The major risk of these drugs is that they may be readily absorbed through the hemorrhoidal vessels and carried to the heart, brain, and other central organs. They can raise blood pressure, cause irregular or arrhythmic heartbeats, and trigger restlessness, nervousness, sleeplessness, and tremor. Vasoconstrictors may overstimulate the thyroid, adrenal, prostate, and other endocrine glands. Prolonged use can lead to anxiety or even paranoia. Finally, vasoconstrictors can profoundly affect the actions of prescription drugs used to treat high blood pressure or mental illness. Reviewers specify that labels contain a warning.

WARNING:

 Do not use products containing vasoconstrictors if you have heart disease, high blood pressure, thyroid disease, diabetes, or difficulty in urination due to enlargement of the prostate gland, unless directed by a doctor. Do not use these products if you are taking a prescription drug for high blood pressure or depression without first consulting a doctor.

For similar reasons, consumers are warned not to use products containing vasoconstrictors for more than 7 days. In the nose, where they act as decongestants, and in other regions of the body, vasoconstrictors tend to be effective for only a few days. After that time there is a rebound effect in which the blood vessels relax again, and may become even more dilated than before.

Claims for Vasoconstrictors

Claims are made that vasoconstricting products "shrink" hemorrhoids. This may suggest permanent benefit, which these nonprescription medications cannot provide. So the word "shrink" must be coupled with the qualifier "temporarily."

Accurate
- "Temporarily reduces the swelling associated with irritated hemorrhoidal tissue and other anorectal disorders"
- "Temporarily shrinks hemorrhoidal tissue"

APPROVED VASOCONSTRICTIVE ACTIVE INGREDIENTS

Reviewers decided that four compounds provide safe and effective vasoconstrictive results when they are used to treat anorectal vascular swelling. Two were approved for both external use on the perianal area and intrarectal use in suppositories and ointment. Two were approved for external use only. However, anyone who plans to use these approved ingredients should note the Panel's warning for vasoconstrictors.

- **EPHEDRINE SULFATE, 0.1 TO 0.125 PERCENT (EXTERNAL AND INTRARECTAL USES):** This is a fine, white, odorless crystal or powder dissolved in water. It is readily absorbed from the rectal mucous membranes, for which reason dosage is restricted to amounts that have been shown to be safe when the drug is injected directly into a vein.

   At high doses, ephedrine can cause nervousness, insomnia, headache, heart palpitations, and other severe side effects, including anxiety and paranoid feelings. Even at therapeutic doses, death can occur in persons who are also taking certain drugs like phenothiazines (major tranquilizers) or MAO inhibitors. Ephedrine may also trigger cerebral hemorrhage or stroke.

   Persons who have heart trouble or thyroid disease, or who are taking digitalis, heart medicine, antidepressants, or other drugs that act on the nervous system should not use ephedrine except under a doctor's care.

   For people who do not have these problems, ephedrine sulfate used in the recommended doses is safe for self-treatment of anorectal swelling. However, most studies of effectiveness have been conducted on other body parts (like the nose). Moreover, while an ointment would be the most reasonable base for this drug, reviewers could find no studies of how it works against hemorrhoidal swelling when formulated this way. Nonetheless, because of ephedrine's recognized ability to temporarily constrict superficial vessels and reduce swelling, evaluators said it is effective as well as safe when used up to 4 times daily.

• *EPINEPHRINE, 0.005 TO 0.01 PERCENT (EXTERNAL USE ONLY):* This hormone preparation is pharmacologically quite similar to water-soluble epinephrine hydrochloride (*see* immediately below), even though it is not soluble in water. It is safe and effective for use up to 4 times daily.

• *EPINEPHRINE HYDROCHLORIDE, 0.005 TO 0.01 PERCENT (EXTERNAL USE ONLY):* This drug is a short-acting vasoconstrictor. Epinephrine hydrochloride is chemically unstable, so it degrades rapidly when stored in the medicine chest; it should not be kept long. Chemically, epinephrine hydrochloride is very similar to ephedrine, described previously. Thus it carries the same hazards. Note, too, the warning for vasoconstrictors on p. 492.

Although the effectiveness epinephrine hydrochloride has largely been established on sites other than the anus and the rectum, it is considered safe and effective for relief of anorectal swelling and itching when formulated as a 0.1 percent aqueous solution of which 100 to 200 micrograms of epinephrine hydrochloride are contained in each dosage unit. It may be used up to 4 times per day. This low dosage limit was set to avoid risk, even though it is unlikely that a toxic amount of the drug can be absorbed into the bloodstream when an ointment is applied externally.

• *PHENYLEPHRINE HYDROCHLORIDE, 0.25 PERCENT (EXTERNAL AND INTRARECTAL USES):* A potent vasoconstrictor, this drug is related chemically to the hormone epinephrine. But it is safer than epinephrine and the FDA says it is safe. It has little effect on the central nervous system or the rhythmical beats of the heart, although it does increase cardiac output in other ways. Phenylephrine hydrochloride also may be less likely than other vasoconstrictors to cause local irritation.

As with ephedrine and epinephrine, this substance should not be used by persons with hyperthyroidism, hypertension, or cardiovascular disease, or by persons taking MAO inhibitors or other potent psychiatric drugs except under a doctor's direction. Note the warning for vasoconstrictors on p. 492.

Phenylephrine hydrochloride is very efficient at constricting small blood vessels. Thus, the Panel accepted its effectiveness in relieving hemorrhoidal swelling, itching, and discomfort despite a lack of scientific data on application to the anorectum. Use up to 4 times daily.

CONDITIONALLY APPROVED VASOCONSTRICTIVE ACTIVE INGREDIENTS

None.

DISAPPROVED VASOCONSTRICTIVE ACTIVE INGREDIENTS

None.

Protectants

Most drugs act chemically on the body or on bacteria and other microorganisms. Protectants are different. They are for the most part bland, chemically inert, or inactive substances, which may be formulated as ointments, gels, lotions, creams, or powders. These preparations are intended to provide a physical barrier. That is, they coat and protect the skin or mucous surface where they are applied. In the anorectal area they can offer protection from rough, chemically irritating, bacteria-laden bowel movements. These protectants also prevent loss of moisture from anorectal surfaces, which is a major cause of irritation.

Protectants may absorb or bind and hold irritating substances, which keeps them away from exposed surfaces. Some of these ingredients also soften and lubricate skin tissue.

Few well-controlled scientific studies are available to prove the protectants' worth. Most of the ingredients approved here were judged on the basis of their wide use and few adverse reactions and, unless noted, are safe and effective at concentrations up to 50 percent (by weight) as single ingredients, or in combination products, as described in the following section.

Evaluators found little evidence that a combination of two, three, or four protectants is any more effective than one alone. Yet the Panel and the FDA have approved the use of up to four such substances provided, in most cases, that each ingredient constitutes 12.5 percent of the product by weight and that the protectant active ingredients constitute half of the product by weight. Since the standard dose of an anorectal product is about 2 grams, each application thus should provide about 1 gram of active substance. Protectants can be applied up to 6 times daily.

 Claims for Protectants

Accurate

For all protectants *except* aluminum hydroxide gel and kaolin:

- "Temporarily forms a protective coating over inflamed tissues to help prevent drying of tissues"
- "Temporarily protects irritated areas"
- "Temporarily relieves burning"
- "Provides temporary relief from skin irritations"
- "Temporarily provides a coating for relief of anorectal discomforts"
- "Temporarily protects inflamed, irritated anorectal surface from irritation and abrasions during bowel movement"
- "Temporarily protects inflamed perianal skin"

For aluminum hydroxide gel and kaolin:

- "For the temporary relief of itching associated with most anorectal conditions"

APPROVED PROTECTANT ACTIVE INGREDIENTS

The Panel and the FDA reached the safe-and-effective verdict for 14 protectant ingredients. With but one exception (glycerin), all were approved both for external application to the perianal area and for insertion into the rectum. Many of the ingredients discussed here are used as general skin protectants and are described for this use in UNGUENTS AND POWDERS FOR THE SKIN.

- *ALUMINUM HYDROXIDE GEL (EXTERNAL AND INTRARECTAL USES):* This white, powdery aluminum compound forms a gel when combined with water. Taken internally, it is widely used as an antacid, which attests its basic safety. (*See* ANTACIDS.) This substance, also called *gel of alumina*, has been marketed as a general skin protectant for almost a century.

Aluminum hydroxide gel appears to relieve most irritations of the anorectal surfaces—but not the irritation related to dry skin. In one study, an aluminum hydroxide gel thickened with kaolin relieved anal itching in 93 of 98 sufferers. This mixture may bind, hold, and neutralize fecal bacteria. It will not work if applied on top of petrolatum or other greasy substances.

Reviewers say that at a concentration of at least 50 percent of the dosage unit, aluminum hydroxide gel—by itself or with other protectants—is safe and effective when applied up to 6 times daily or after each bowel movement.

• CALAMINE (EXTERNAL AND INTRARECTAL USES): This pink mixture consists of at least 98 percent zinc oxide, which is white, and 0.5 percent ferrous oxide, which is red, and so gives the mixture its pinkish color. Its therapeutic effect is wholly due to the zinc oxide (*see* p. 500). Calamine absorbs moisture and chemical irritants and coats, covers, and protects the skin. The approved dosage is up to 25 percent calamine or a combination of calamine and zinc oxide, applied up to 6 times daily or after bowel movements.

• COCOA BUTTER (EXTERNAL AND INTRARECTAL USES): An oily, yellowish-white material, this chocolate-smelling extract of cacao beans has the property of remaining solid until it is warmed to within a few degrees of normal body temperature. Then it melts into a liquid without passing through any appreciable semi-soft stage. This quality makes cocoa butter an ideal basic substance for suppositories intended to lubricate the anal canal or soothe abraded and irritated anorectal tissue.

Although cocoa butter has never been studied scientifically as an anorectal drug ingredient, its long use in a variety of other drugs, and in cosmetics, suggests that it is safe and effective. Cocoa butter is judged to be safe and effective for anorectal use at concentrations of 50 percent or more by itself or with other protectants. It can be used up to 6 times daily or after bowel movements.

• COD-LIVER OIL (EXTERNAL AND INTRARECTAL USES): Although scientific studies of the use of this oil are few, the literature reveals no adverse effects when it is used as a skin-softener and protectant. It must be part of a combination product, and the product must provide 10,000 U.S.P. units of vitamins A and 400 U.S.P. units of cholecalciferol (vitamin D) in the recommended 24-hour dosage. Cod-liver oil was judged safe and effective when it constitutes at least 50 percent of the dosage unit. Such a product may be applied up to 6 times in 24 hours, or after each bowel movement.

• GLYCERIN, AQUEOUS SOLUTION (EXTERNAL USE ONLY): Sometimes called *glycerine* or *glycerol*, this clear, sweetish, syrupy stuff has been used to soothe the skin for some two centuries. Tests show glycerin to be safe when applied to rats' tails and the eyes, mucous membranes, and noses of dogs, cats, and rabbits. However, intrarectal application prompts rats, guinea pigs, and people to move their bowels.

When used by itself—that is, as anhydrous glycerin (without water)—this substance has a drying effect on the skin. But certain concentrations of glycerin in water will hold moisture in the skin and soften it. So glycerin is approved as safe and effective for external use in 10 to 45 percent aqueous solutions. It can be used up to 6 times daily or after each bowel movement. Glycerin is *not* approved for intrarectal application because of its laxative effect. (*See* p. 619.)

• HARD FAT (EXTERNAL AND INTRARECTAL USES): This is an opaque, which is to say *unclear* description for what apparently are a number of naturally derived fatty substances which also are called *witepsol*. They include *cocoa butter substitutes, hydrogenated coco-glycerides*, and *hydrogenated palm kernel glycerides*. Manufacturers submitted data that convinced the FDA that hard fat is safe and can reduce water loss through the skin significantly—by one-third to one-half.

Hard fat is solid at room temperature but melts in the body and so is a standard material for suppositories. But since it also soothes the skin, buffers it, and holds in moisture, the FDA agreed to classify it as an active ingredient. Hard fat is safe and effective when it constitutes 50 percent or more of an anorectal preparation or is part of a combination product that is 50 percent of the product weight. Products that contain it can be used up to 6 times daily.

• KAOLIN (EXTERNAL AND INTRARECTAL USES): Technically a purified and hydrated aluminum silicate, this substance is a powdery, earthy, clayish material. It can absorb large amounts of liquids and can bind, hold, and neutralize noxious substances, including fecal particles and bacteria. Although kaolin is useful for general skin disturbances, its safety in anorectal disorders has never been studied. But because it is inert, and because of its long history of successful use as a skin protectant, reviewers judged it safe. Kaolin is often combined with aluminum hydroxide (*see* above) in products sold to relieve itching due to moisture and irritation of the perianal area. It is ineffective when petrolatum or other greasy substances have been applied before it, so any of those preparations should first be washed away. The safe and effective dose for adults—for both external and intrarectal application—is at least 50 percent concentration per dosage unit, by itself or in combination with another appropriate protectant. It may be applied after bowel movements, but daily use should not exceed 6 times.

• LANOLIN (EXTERNAL AND INTRARECTAL USES): Mixed with water to produce what is called *hydrous wool fat*, lanolin is widely used as a cosmetic or medicinal skin softener (though its effectiveness for this purpose lacks scientific confirmation) and as a base for a variety of other kinds of products.

   Lanolin's safety as an anorectal medication has not been well studied. But evaluators concluded that its widespread use in so many preparations, over an extended period of time, suggests that it is effective as a skin-softening protectant. The approved dosage is: at least 50 percent by itself or in combination with other protectants. It can be used after bowel movements but should not be applied more often than 6 times a day.

• MINERAL OIL (EXTERNAL AND INTRARECTAL USES): This odorless, colorless, transparent oily liquid is refined from crude oil. It is relatively inert, does not turn rancid, and is widely used as a skin softener and as a base for creams and suppositories.

   Mineral oil is not absorbed through the skin, so it tends to remain where applied until accidentally or deliberately wiped off. It keeps out air, bacteria, and other irritating substances, holds moisture, and soothes and lubricates the skin. But the Panel could find no specific studies on the safety or effectiveness of mineral oil as an ingredient in anorectal products. Approval stems largely from its physical properties and its safe use on other parts of the body. The dosage should be at least a 50 percent concentration of mineral oil, by itself or with other protectants, and the preparation should be applied no more often than 6 times daily or after each bowel movement.

• PETROLATUM, WHITE PETROLATUM (EXTERNAL AND INTRARECTAL USES): Petrolatum usually is yellow, and the more purified form, white petrolatum, is whitish in color. Both forms are medicinally close to equivalent. They have been shown in tests to be the most effective ointment for protecting skin surfaces against water. Safety has been demonstrated through almost a century of wide use in pharmaceutical products and cosmetics. Although petrolatum has not been specifically studied as an anorectal medication, the Panel considers it effective as a physical barrier. It protects the anorectal area from irritants and may relieve their effects: burning, pain, or itch. The approved dosage is at least 50 percent concentration of petrolatum or white petrolatum in each dosage unit, by itself or in combination with other protectants. Apply liberally as often as needed.

• SHARK-LIVER OIL (EXTERNAL AND INTRARECTAL USES): This amber-to-brown-colored oily substance soothes and softens irritated skin. No data are available on the use of the oil for anorectal disorders, but experience with its application to other skin surfaces, as well as studies of cod-liver oil in diapering products, led evaluators to consider shark-liver oil safe and effective for softening and protecting anorectal surfaces and for relieving itching and irritation. This substance only can be used in combination with other protectants (usually, cod-liver oil), and the 24-hour dosage of the product must provide 10,000 U.S.P. units of vitamin A and 400 U.S.P. units of cholecalcitral (vitamin D). Like many of the other remedies described in this section, shark-liver oil products can be applied up to 6 times in 24 hours, or after every bowel movement.

• TOPICAL STARCH (EXTERNAL AND INTRARECTAL USES): Whether manufactured from corn or from rice, topical starch is an insoluble, chemically inactive substance that, weight for weight, can absorb huge amounts of moisture and noxious substances. It also smooths the skin and reduces friction. Its safety as a topical dusting powder is well established. Although starch is unstudied as an anorectal medication, the reviewers believe it is safe and effective in concentrations of 50 percent or greater per dosage unit—by itself or in combination with other protectants—when applied up to 6 times daily or after each bowel movement.

• ZINC OXIDE (EXTERNAL AND INTRARECTAL USES): Zinc oxide is applied in a paste or as a lotion to absorb excess moisture, or it may be sprinkled onto inflamed areas as a powder. It is the principal and the sole *active* ingredient in calamine. For anorectal application, the safe and effective dose is up to 25 percent concentration in a combination product (usually with calamine), that can be used up to 6 times daily or after defecating.

CONDITIONALLY APPROVED PROTECTANT ACTIVE INGREDIENTS

None.

DISAPPROVED PROTECTANT ACTIVE INGREDIENTS

None.

Astringents

The stingy, zesty feeling of witch-hazel lotions and similar astringents is easy to recall but hard to describe in sober, scientific words. An astringent puckers the proteinaceous outer membranes of skin and mucosal cells, shrinking them. An astringent can also absorb, concentrate, and hold loose proteinaceous substances on skin and mucosal surfaces—including fecal particles and bacteria—thereby reducing their irritancy. Astringents also have a drying effect.

An astringent will not significantly reduce hemorrhoidal swelling, but it may temporarily help relieve symptoms of burning, itching, discomfort, and irritation. Astringent-containing perianal pads and wipes are also useful for cleansing purposes and for relieving itching.

 Claims for Astringents

Accurate
- "Aids in protecting irritated anorectal areas"
- "For temporary relief of irritation and burning"

APPROVED ASTRINGENT ACTIVE INGREDIENTS

The Panel assessed astringents for both external use on the perianal region and intrarectal use as applied in suppositories and other intrarectal dosage forms.

- CALAMINE (EXTERNAL AND INTRARECTAL USES): This pinkish medication is at least 98 percent zinc oxide, dyed pink with a trace of red iron oxide.

The safety and effectiveness of calamine relate directly to that of zinc oxide (*see* further on). As an anorectal astringent, it is approved in dosages of 5 to 25 percent (based on the zinc oxide content) for external and intrarectal use when used up to 6 times in 24 hours, or after each bowel movement. It also is approved as a protectant, as described above on p. 497.

• HAMAMELIS WATER, NF XI (WITCH-HAZEL WATER) (EXTERNAL USE ONLY): This liquid is prepared by boiling crushed, dried twigs of the witch-hazel shrub (*Hamamelis virginiana*) for 24 hours. The residue is then distilled and mixed with 15 percent alcohol. It is clear and colorless, and has a pleasant fragrance. The Panel knows of no serious adverse reactions to witch hazel, although it may be allergenic.

The ingredient's astringency has been attributed to the minute amount of the original plant's volatile oil that is left in the final products. The Panel's guess was that the alcohol is the astringent, with the oil accounting only for the drug's appealing aroma. But a manufacturer claims to have proved that this is not so and that the witch hazel is medicinally active. A few studies have shown that witch-hazel water relieves itching, burning, and other discomforts when applied to the anorectal area. The substance is judged safe and effective in concentrations of 10 to 50 percent; it can be applied after each bowel movement or up to 6 times daily.

• ZINC OXIDE (EXTERNAL AND INTRARECTAL USES): This substance is widely used to treat skin disorders; it is the essential ingredient of calamine lotion. Zinc oxide's astringent properties are attributed to its ability to gather irritating proteins from the skin or mucosal surface and cover them with a protective film. The chemical appears to be more effective on injured than on unbroken skin. The safe and effective dosage is a 15 to 25 percent concentration of zinc oxide in a suitable base; it can be applied up to 6 times daily or after each bowel movement. It also is approved as a protectant, as described above on p. 500.

CONDITIONALLY APPROVED ASTRINGENT ACTIVE INGREDIENTS

None.

DISAPPROVED ASTRINGENT ACTIVE INGREDIENTS

None.

Itch-Pain Relievers

This category of drugs, originally called *counterirritants* in the OTC Drug Review, accommodates several old-time remedies that sting a little, cool a little, and soothe a little, and in these ways contribute a little to the relief of itching and pain. They do this by briefly reducing or blocking sensory receptors in the skin. These compounds probably are not appropriate for heavy-duty pain, for which the *Local Anesthetics,* described previously or a visit to the doctor would be the better choice.

These ingredients have been described at greater length in other Units and so will be covered only briefly here. They are for external use only, not for intrarectal use.

 Claims for Itch-Pain Relievers

Accurate
- "For the temporary relief of pain or burning"
- "Can help distract from pain"
- "May provide a cooling sensation"

APPROVED ITCH-PAIN RELIEVING ACTIVE INGREDIENTS

- CAMPHOR, *0.1 TO 3 PERCENT (EXTERNAL USE ONLY):* This substance produces both warming and cooling sensations. It has a pungent, aromatic taste and penetrating odor. After much debate among various Panels and the FDA, the agency decided that products containing camphor as a single ingredient in concentrations under 2.5 percent are safe; it approves a fractionally higher 3 percent limit for anorectal products. Few data were presented to bolster the claim that camphor relieves itching and pain in the anorectal area. Studies of its use elsewhere in the body indicate that it provides some relief. The FDA evaluators seem to be tired of the whole matter, and without specific comment, have given camphor a final grade of safe and effective in concentrations of 0.1 to 3 percent for use up to 6 times daily. For more on camphor, *see* pp. 124-129, and *see* CAMPHOR: SPECIAL NOTE.

- **JUNIPER TAR, 1 TO 5 PERCENT (EXTERNAL USE ONLY):** This is a dark red oil with a tar-like odor and a bitter taste; it also is called *oil of cade*. Juniper tar is a natural substance that has been used for thousands of years to relieve skin discomfort. There are no specific reports in the FDA record on its specific value for treating anorectal disorders. Nevertheless, based on long use, FDA rates it safe and effective for application up to 6 times daily. For more on juniper tar, *see* p. 562.

- **MENTHOL, 0.1 TO 1 PERCENT (EXTERNAL USE ONLY):** It is hard to believe that as little as one part per thousand of this minty alcohol will make much difference, but the FDA has approved it nonetheless as safe and effective. It has a long-established cooling effect, which may distract one from other unpleasant anal sensations. The FDA's approval appears to be based on menthol's general record of safety and effectiveness when used on other parts of the body. (*See* p. 562.)

CONDITIONALLY APPROVED ITCH-PAIN RELIEVING ACTIVE INGREDIENTS

None.

DISAPPROVED ITCH-PAIN RELIEVING ACTIVE INGREDIENTS

None.

Skin-Peeling Agents (Keratolytics)

A drug that loosens and removes the outer, horny, keratin-containing layer of skin cells is called a *keratolytic*, or skin-peeling, agent. Several types of chemicals have this ability. They are for the most part used on warts and corns and for other conditions where an overgrowth of dry, keratin-rich outer skin cells exist. These drugs reduce itching and may also expose deeper skin layers to medication.

Their value in treating perianal skin disorders—where the skin is usually moist, not dry—is less clear. The consumer should note that the FDA's approval applies only to *external* application of these drugs to the perianal area, not to intrarectal use, since there are no keratin-containing cells in the rectal mucosa.

 ## Claims for Skin Peelers

Accurate
• "For the temporary relief of the discomfort associated with hemorrhoids and other anorectal disorders"
• "Helps relieve anorectal itching"
  • "Gives temporary relief of itching of piles (hemorrhoids)"

APPROVED SKIN-PEELING ACTIVE INGREDIENTS

• *ALCLOXA (EXTERNAL USE ONLY):* This aluminum compound, which also is called *aluminum chlorhydroxy allantoinate,* is a form of *allantoin,* a safe and effective compound that is widely used to soothe irritated skin. A traditional skin remedy, *comfrey root,* which contains a natural chemical predecessor of allantoin, has been known for several centuries to soften and protect skin.

   Like other forms of allantoin, alcloxa has never been shown to harm the skin. Furthermore, it does relieve itching, although how this happens remains unclear. Its skin-peeling capacity appears to be based on its ability to break the chemical bonds that hold together the skin's outer layer. Despite a lack of clarity about how it acts, and a paucity of studies on its activity in the anorectal area, evaluators say alcloxa is safe and effective for adults in concentrations of 0.2 to 2 percent when used up to 6 times in 24 hours.

• *RESORCINOL (EXTERNAL USE ONLY):* Despite some doubts, this phenol-like alcohol was judged by the majority of Panel members to be safe for use as an anorectal skin-peeling and skin-softening agent. The FDA agreed. A number of studies indicate that resorcinol is effective in softening and removing the scales of psoriasis and other conditions in which the perianal skin has become thickened. The drug is safe and effective in concentrations of 1 to 3 percent. Apply up to 6 times daily.

CONDITIONALLY APPROVED SKIN-PEELING ACTIVE INGREDIENTS

None.

DISAPPROVED SKIN-PEELING ACTIVE INGREDIENTS

None.

Corticosteroids

These drugs deserve a special mention because they are very effective in relieving itching and irritation and have been approved for "anal itching" by the FDA under its rule-making for external analgesics. They also are approved, *for prescription use*, to relieve inflammation and swelling. (*See* Hydrocortisone in ITCH AND PAIN RELIEVERS APPLIED TO THE SKIN.)

    The FDA nevertheless seems to have some lingering doubts about over-the-counter marketing of hydrocortisone for hemorrhoidal symptoms. The agency is still mulling over its final word on hydrocortisone and hydrocortisone acetate's place in hemorrhoidal products. However, with the reservation that they are for external use only, the FDA has approved hydrocortisone and hydrocortisone acetate for the relief of anal itching in concentrations of up to 1 percent, for adults and children over 2 years of age, up to 4 times daily. For younger children, consult a physician.

OTHER INGREDIENT

The FDA still has not decided about one remaining ingredient. It is only conditionally approved:

- LIVE YEAST-CELL DERIVATIVE (EXTERNAL AND INTRARECTAL USES): It is claimed by a manufacturer, and some researchers, that the live yeast cells, when applied to a sore or injured area, stimulate oxygen uptake, which in turn speeds healing. Some studies suggest, too, that this ingredient promotes healing by helping to build new connective tissue in wounds that have been contaminated with bacteria.

Products containing live yeast-cell derivative have been widely and successfully marketed for decades. Nevertheless, the FDA is not convinced of either these products' safety or their effectiveness. The agency has told the manufacturer of two of these products that it "has evaluated...studies...for anorectal use [of this substance] and finds that they are unacceptable to demonstrate the effectiveness of live yeast-cell derivative for relief of hemorrhoidal symptoms of pain, itching, burning or irritation." The FDA went on to say that the studies "do not contain data to support the claim" that this substance causes "shrinking [of the] swelling of hemorrhoidal tissue caused by inflammation."

So the current (1992) evaluation is: not proved safe or effective.

Safety and Effectiveness: Active Ingredients in Over-the-Counter Products for the Treatment of Hemorrhoids and Other Anorectal Conditions

Active Ingredient	Assessment: Safe and Effective When Applied Externally to Perianal Area	Assessment: Safe and Effective When Applied Intrarectally
Local Anesthetics		
benzocaine	yes	no
benzyl alcohol	yes	no
dibucaine	yes	no
dibucaine hydrochloride	yes	no
dyclonine hydrochloride	yes	no
lidocaine	yes	no
pramoxine hydrochloride	yes	no
tetracaine	yes	no
tetracaine hydrochloride	yes	no
Vasoconstrictors		
ephedrine sulfate	yes	yes
epinephrine	yes	no
epinephrine hydrochloride	yes	no

phenylephrine hydrochloride	yes	yes
Protectants		
aluminum hydroxide gel	yes	yes
calamine	yes	yes
cocoa butter	yes	yes
cod-liver oil	yes	yes
glycerin	no	yes
hard fat	yes	yes
kaolin	yes	yes
lanolin	yes	yes
mineral oil	yes	yes
petrolatum, white petrolatum	yes	yes
shark-liver oil	yes	yes
topical starch	yes	yes
zinc oxide	yes	yes
Itch-Pain Relievers		
camphor	no	yes
juniper tar	no	yes

Safety and Effectiveness: Active Ingredients in Over-the-Counter Products for the Treatment of Hemorrhoids and Other Anorectal Conditions (contd)

Active Ingredient	Assessment: Safe and Effective When Applied Externally to Perianal Area	Assessment: Safe and Effective When Applied Intrarectally
menthol	yes	no
Astringents		
calamine	yes	no
hamamelis water (witch hazel)	yes	no
zinc oxide	yes	no
Skin Peelers		
alcloxa	yes	no
resorcinol	yes	no
Other Ingredients		
hydrocortisone*	yes	no
hydrocortisone acetate*	yes	no
live yeast-cell derivative	not proved safe or effective	not proved safe or effective

*As evaluated by the OTC Panel on Topical Analgesics.

Safety and Effectiveness: Combination Products Sold Over-the-Counter to Treat Hemorrhoids and Other Anorectal Conditions

---

Safe and Effective

2, 3, or 4 approved protectants, constituting, in all, at least 50% of the product (aluminum hydroxide gel and kaolin may be combined only with topical starch, calamine and/or zinc oxide)

1 to 4 protectants as above + 1 local anesthetic

1 to 4 protectants as above + 1 vasoconstrictor

1 to 4 protectants as above + 1 itch-pain reliever

1 to 4 protectants as above + 1 astringent

1 to 4 protectants as above + 1 skin peeler

1 local anesthetic + 1 vasoconstrictor

1 local anesthetic + 1 astringent

1 local anesthetic + 1 skin peeler

1 vasoconstrictor + 1 astringent

1 itch-pain reliever + 1 astringent

1 itch-pain reliever + 1 skin peeler

1 astringent + 1 skin peeler

1 local anesthetic + 1 vasoconstrictor + 1 astringent

1 local anesthetic + 1 astringent + 1 skin peeler

1 vasoconstrictor + 1 itch-pain reliever + 1 astringent

1 itch-pain reliever + 1 astringent + 1 skin peeler

any of the previous 11 combinations + 1 to 4 protectants (except that aluminum hydroxide gel and kaolin can be combined only with topical starch, calamine and/or zinc oxide)

Conditionally Safe and Effective

None

Unsafe or Ineffective

contains hydrocortisone or hydrocortisone acetate, when used internally

Hemorrhoid Medication and Other Anorectal Applications: Product Ratings

Product and Distributor	Dosage of Active Ingredients	ANESTHETIC PRODUCTS Rating for External Use in Perianal Area*	Rating for Use Intrarectally*	Comment
benzocaine in polyethylene				
Americaine First Aid (Fisons)	ointment: 20%	A	C	no pain receptors in rectum so pain reliever ineffective
dibucaine				
Dibucaine hydrochloride (generic)	ointment: 1%	A	C	no pain receptors in rectum so pain reliever ineffective
Nupercainal (Ciba)		A	C	
Nupercainal (Ciba)	cream: 0.5%	A	C	
lidocaine				
Xyclocaine (Astra)	ointment: 2.5%	A	C	no pain receptors in rectum so pain reliever ineffective
pramoxine hydrochloride				

Fleet Relief Anesthetic Hemorrhoidal (Fleet)	ointment: 1%	A	C	no pain receptors in rectum so pain reliever ineffective
Itch-X (Ascher & Co.)	gel: 1%	A	C	
ProctoFoam (Reed & Carnrick)	aerosol foam: 1%	A	C	
Tronolane (Ross)	cream: 1%	A	C	
Tronothane (Abbott)	cream: 1%	A	C	
tetracaine				
Pontocaine (Sanofi Winthrop)	ointment: 0.5% tetracaine	A	C	no pain receptors in rectum so pain reliever ineffective
	cream: 1% as hydrochloride	A	C	

Hemorrhoid Medication and Other Anorectal Applications: Product Ratings (contd)

STEROID PRODUCTS FOR ITCH, INFLAMMATION, AND SWELLING

Product and Distributor	Dosage of Active Ingredients	Rating for External Use in Perianal Area*	Rating for Use Intrarectally*	Comment
hydrocortisone				
Anusol-HC (Parke-Davis)	ointment: 1%	A	C	℞ to OTC switch; safety for internal use undetermined
Cortizone-5 (Thompson)	ointment: 0.5%	A	C	
Cortizone-10 (Thompson)	ointment: 1%	A	C	
Cortril (Pfizer)	ointment: 1%	A	C	
Dermolate Anti-Itch (Schering-Plough)	cream: 0.5%	A	C	
Maximum Strength Cortaid (Upjohn)	ointment, cream: 1%	A	C	

Product and Distributor	Dosage of Active Ingredients	Rating for External Use in Perianal Area*	Rating for Use Intrarectally*	Comment
Tegrin-HC (Block)	ointment: 1%	A	C	
hydrocortisone acetate				
CaldeCort (Fisons)	cream: 0.5% hydrocortisone equivalent	A	C	Rx to OTC switch; safety for internal use undetermined
Cortaid (Upjohn)	ointment and cream: 0.5% hydrocortisone equivalent	A	C	
Lanacort-5 (Combe)	ointment, cream: 0.5%	A	C	
Lanacort-10 (Combe)	ointment, cream: 1% hydrocortisone equivalent	A	C	

PROTECTANT PRODUCTS

Product and Distributor	Dosage of Active Ingredients	Rating for External Use in Perianal Area*	Rating for Use Intrarectally*	Comment
cocoa butter				
cocoa butter (generic)	cream	A	A	

Hemorrhoid Medication and Other Anorectal Applications: Product Ratings (contd)

Product and Distributor	Dosage of Active Ingredients	Rating for External Use in Perianal Area*	Rating for Use Intrarectally*	Comment
mineral oil				
Mineral oil (generic)	liquid	A	A	
petrolatum, white				
Vaseline Pure Petroleum Jelly (Chesebrough-Ponds)	ointment: 100%	A	A	

ASTRINGENTS

Product and Distributor	Dosage of Active Ingredients	Rating for External Use in Perianal Area*	Rating for Use Intrarectally*	Comment
Hamamelis water (witch hazel)				
Witch hazel (generic)	solution	A	C	

see also: Perianal Hygeine Products, further on

COMBINATION PRODUCTS

Product and Distributor	Dosage of Active Ingredients	Rating for External Use in Perianal Area*	Rating for Use Intrarectally*	Comment

Product	Ingredients			Comments
A-Caine Rectal (A.V.P.)	**ointment:** 0.25% diperodon hydrochloride + 0.1% pyrilamine maleate + 0.25% phenylephrine hydrochloride + 0.2% bismuth subcarbonate + 5% zinc oxide + cod-liver oil + petrolatum	C	C	diperodon not approved; pyrilamine maleate not submitted to or assessed as anorectal; phenylephrine is an Rx to OTC switch
Anuprep Hemorrhoidal (Great Southern)	**suppositories:** 2.25% bismuth subgallate + 1.75% bismuth resorcin compound + 1.2% benzyl benzoate + 1.8% peruvian balsam + 11% zinc oxide	—	C	bismuth disapproved
Anusol (Parke-Davis)	**suppositories:** 0.25% phenylephrine hydrochloride + 88.7% hard fat	—	A	Rx to OTC switch (phenylephrine)
Gentz (Philips Roxane)	**wipes:** 1% pramoxine hydrochloride + 0.2% alcloxa + 50% Hamamelis water	A	A	—

Hemorrhoid Medication and Other Anorectal Applications: Product Ratings (contd)

Product and Distributor	Dosage of Active Ingredients	Rating for External Use in Perianal Area*	Rating for Use Intrarectally*	Comment
Hemocaine (Mallard)	**ointment:** 0.25% diperodon hydrochloride + 0.1% pyrilamine maleate + 0.25% phenylephrine hydrochloride + 0.2% bismuth subcarbonate + 5% zinc oxide + cod-liver oil + petrolatum	C	C	diperodon not approved; pyrilamine maleate not submitted to or assessed as anorectal; phenylephrine is an Rx to OTC switch
Pazo Hemorrhoid (Bristol-Myers Squibb)	**suppositories:** 15.4 mg benzocaine + 3.8 mg ephedrine sulfate + 42 mg camphor + 77 mg zinc oxide	—	C	benzocaine disapproved for internal use; Rx to OTC switch (ephedrine)
Preparation H (Whitehall)	**ointment:** live yeast-cell derivative supplying 2000 units skin respiratory factor per ounce + 3% shark-liver oil	B		live yeast-cell derivative not proved safe or effective

Product	Ingredients			Comments
	suppositories: live yeast-cell derivative supplying 2000 units skin respiratory factor per ounce + 3% shark-liver oil	—	B	live yeast-cell derivative not proved safe or effective
Rectagene II (Pfeiffer)	**suppositories:** 2.25% bismuth subgallate + 1.75% bismuth resorcin compound + 1.2% benzyl benzoate + 1.8% peruvian balsam + 11% zinc oxide	—	C	bismuth disapproved
Tronolane (Ross)	**suppositories:** 5% zinc oxide + 95% hard fat	—	A	

PERIANAL HYGIENE PRODUCTS

Product	Ingredients		
Tucks (Parke-Davis)	**pads:** 50% Hamamelis water + 10% glycerin	A	—
	cream: 50% Hamamelis water	A	—

*Author's interpretation of FDA criteria. Based on contents, not claims.

Hormone Skin Creams and Oils

Vanity of vanities; all is vanity.

-Ecclesiastes I:2

It is the female hormone *estrogen*, and to a lesser extent *progesterone*, that transforms a girl into a woman at puberty. Later, as she grows older, her skin begins to lose its smooth, pliable, youthful feeling and appearance. A woman then may be tempted by seductive advertisements to try to rejuvenate her skin by treating it with supplements of these hormones in skin creams, oils, lotions, and other cosmetically appealing preparations.

These products, which contain only low doses of hormones, have been judged safe. But they do not produce visible changes in the skin; they are not effective.

HORMONE SKIN CREAMS AND OILS is based on the report "Topically Applied Hormone-Containing Drug Products for OTC Human Use" by the FDA's Advisory Review Panel on OTC Miscellaneous External Drug Products and the agency's Tentative Final Rule on these products.

Claims

All claims are disapproved.

Hormone Preparations

The Panel's assessment of these preparations is summarized in the Safety and Effectiveness table that concludes this Unit. All are disapproved, primarily on grounds that they are ineffective.

The FDA thus is likely, sooner or later, to ban the sales of hormone-containing creams as drugs.

Will this have much influence on the marketing of these anti-wrinkle and anti-aging skin creams, a business that has been estimated to be worth several hundred million dollars a year in the U.S.? Not likely. The reason is that many of these products also are sold as *cosmetics*, not drugs, and the rules governing cosmetic products are much looser than those for drugs. Manufacturers still will be able to include the hormones, although they may not be able to label them as such, since as the FDA says, the word "hormone" implies a medicinal claim.

The agency may be able to limit, somewhat, the promotional statements for these products, since it interprets claims like "prevent, postpone and minimize the effect of the aging process," and "recreate the structure of a young skin," that have been used for them as drug claims: *Any* claim that a product changes the function or structure of skin or any other body organ or tissue is a drug claim, according to the FDA—and federal law.

Manufacturers thus will have to stop calling these hormones "hormones." (But even under the cosmetics regulations they must list the specific names of the hormones on the label, which is likely to make this labeling more confusing, rather than less. Manufacturers could still say "contains natural estrogen and progesterone.")

It should be added that these products are not absolutely safe. In an article on estrogens in cosmetics, published after the Panel's report, the *Medical Letter on Drugs and Therapeutics* (vol. 27, pp. 54-55, 1985) described side effects of these products. In several cases, boys and men experienced breast enlargement and darkening of the nipples, penis, and surrounding skin after using hair lotions or creams containing estrogens. Breast growth and related hormonal changes also have been reported in girls as young as 10 months of age who were exposed to these products. Older, post-menopausal women have begun bleeding again following use of hair products containing high concentrations of estrogen. In short, while the FDA accepted the Panel's findings—and manufacturers' claims—that these products are safe, they can on occasion cause embarrassing, even frightening, body changes.

APPROVED ACTIVE INGREDIENTS IN HORMONE PREPARATIONS

None.

CONDITIONALLY APPROVED ACTIVE INGREDIENTS IN HORMONE PREPARATIONS

None.

DISAPPROVED ACTIVE INGREDIENTS IN HORMONE PREPARATIONS

• ESTROGENS: ESTRADIOL, ESTROGEN, ESTROGENIC HORMONES, NATURAL ESTROGENIC HORMONES, NATURAL ESTROGENS, AND ESTRONE: These hormones are produced naturally by a woman's ovaries and, during pregnancy, by the placenta. They ready her body for conception and are necessary to sustain pregnancy. Natural and synthetic estrogens are widely used medicinally, principally in oral contraceptives. Estrogens also are formulated into skin creams meant to soften and rejuvenate the skin.

The outer layer of the skin (epidermis) becomes thinner with advancing age. In one study, the use of an estrogen preparation resulted in a doubling of epidermal thickness. However, this increase in number and size of skin cells could be detected only by microscope. Furthermore, other studies have failed to confirm these changes. Some reduction in wrinkling has also been reported from the use of estrogen skin products. But evaluators say wrinkling results from degeneration of the inner skin layer (dermis) and not from the drying out and thinning of the epidermis. So the reviewers strongly doubt that these reports are valid.

It is the Panel's judgment that estrogen in concentrations of up to 10,000 international units (IU) per ounce is safe. Higher concentrations are not. But there is no scientifically acceptable evidence that a product containing up to 10,000 IU of estrogen per ounce of cream is any more effective than the same product without it.

In sum: Although safe in low doses, estrogen preparations for the skin are not effective. At higher doses, they are unsafe because, once absorbed through the skin, they may upset the body's natural hormonal balance. The Panel recommends that these products be banned from the over-the-counter drug market. The FDA plans to do so.

• *PROGESTERONES: PREGNENOLONE ACETATE AND PROGESTERONE:* Progesterones are put into skin products because they are thought to stimulate the sebaceous glands to produce more sebum—a natural skin lubricant—and thus soften the skin. In the concentration in which these hormones are marketed (5 mg of progesterone per ounce of cream or oil), the Panel says they seem to be free of side effects.

Progesterone has been shown to increase sebum secretions in female and castrated male rats, but not in women. In one study, progesterone-treated sides of women's faces were compared with the opposite, untreated sides. Skin samples taken failed to show even microscopic differences. (The male hormone *testosterone* may stimulate sebum production, but the female hormone progesterone will not, the Panel says.)

Evaluators conclude that 5 mg of progesterone per ounce of cream, oil, or lotion is safe but not effective—and they recommend that such products be barred over-the-counter. The FDA plans to do so.

Note: Some progesterone products have been claimed to stimulate breast development. Young women who fear they are underendowed may be tempted to try these preparations. The Panel said, in a rough draft report, that progesterone creams are *not effective* as breast developers.

Let the Buyer Beware!

"Most cosmetics contain ingredients that are promoted with exaggerated claims of beauty or long-lasting effects to create an image .... Image is what the cosmetics industry sells through its products, and it's up to the consumer to believe it or not!"

—John E. Bailey, Ph.D.
Director, FDA division of color and cosmetics

Safety and Effectiveness: Active Ingredients in
Over-the-Counter Hormone Skin Treatments*

Active Ingredient	Assessment
estradiol	not effective
estrogen	not effective
estrogenic hormones	not effective
estrone	not effective
natural estrogenic hormones	not effective
natural estrogens	not effective
pregnenolone acetate	not effective
progesterone	not effective

*Aside from being ineffective, estrogens

Hormone Skin Creams and Oils: Product Ratings

The FDA's judgment is that no hormonal ingredient in a skin cream or oil has discernible benefit to the skin. So all products containing the relatively low concentrations of these hormones that are sold over-the-counter must be rated "C."

Ingrown-Toenail Relievers

An ingrown toenail is like a train that has jumped its track. The nail, which protects the tip of the toe from injury, normally grows slowly outward along track-like grooves at the edge of the nail bed. But if the nail gets dislocated a bit—if it "jumps the track"—it digs into the nail bed and groove. This causes pain, inflammation, and swelling. Infections, blood poisoning, and other serious damage may follow.

The Panel that assessed drugs to relieve this condition said that the term *ingrown toenail* is a misnomer. The nail does not actually grow into the flesh but rather becomes embedded in it.

 ### Claims

Accurate if one or more ingredient is shown to be safe and effective—which none as yet has been
- "For the temporary relief of discomfort from ingrown toenails"

INGROWN-TOENAIL RELIEVERS is based on the report "Ingrown Toenail Relief Drug Products for OTC Human Use" by the FDA's Advisory Review Panel on OTC Miscellaneous External Drug Products and the FDA's Tentative Final Monograph on these products.

False or Misleading
• "Fast pain relief" (treatment may require several days)

WARNING:

 Do not use for more than 7 days unless directed by a doctor. Consult a doctor if no improvement is seen after 7 days. If you have diabetes or poor circulation, see a doctor for treatment of an ingrown toenail. Do not apply this drug to open sores. If redness and swelling of a toe increases, or if a discharge is present around a nail, stop treatment and see your doctor.

Pedicure for Prevention

Toe-pinching shoes, tight hosiery, and too-tight bed clothing all can force the side edge of the nail into the softer toe tissue. Even walking may cause poorly pedicured nails to become enclosed in this way.

Careful and correct nail-cutting will forestall ingrown toenails. The *incorrect* way to cut is to create a crescent-like curve, as one does with fingernails. This creates tapered corners below the end of the nail groove. These corners may then get pushed up against the groove and embedded in it.

The *correct* method to prevent this condition is to cut the toenails straight across. The corners will then be square and they will also be out beyond the ends of the nail grooves. That way there is no chance that a sharp or ragged edge can cut into a groove, nail bed, or other soft tissue. Using this pedicure method should prevent most ingrown toenails, according to the Panel.

Drugs to Treat Ingrown Toenails

If caught early enough, there may be merit in self-treatment with a non-prescription drug that can harden the nail groove so it will resist further injury or will shrink the soft tissue to provide more space for the nail to resume its normal position—to get back on track. If self-treatment with drugs does not free the nail, or if the area becomes sore, swollen, or painful, then medical help should definitely be sought.

Evaluators assessed the ingredients of two products sold to treat ingrown toenails and reviewed several other ingredients that have been used for this purpose in the past. It classified two ingredients—isopropyl alcohol and trolamine—as inactive. Three others were considered pain killers and referred to another Panel, which judged the ingredients as follows:

benzocaine	safe and effective
chlorobutanol	not proved effective
dibucaine	safe and effective

The Panel appeared to sanction combinations that contain pain-relieving drugs along with ingredients that relieve ingrown toenails. But the FDA thus far has shown no enthusiasm for such products.

APPROVED ACTIVE INGREDIENTS

None.

CONDITIONALLY APPROVED ACTIVE INGREDIENTS

• *SODIUM SULFIDE:* The rationale for using this drug is that it softens the keratin (horny material) in the nail and adjacent callused skin. This allegedly relieves the pressure and pain caused by contact between embedded nail and skin.

Tests in rats show that you would have to drink a large amount of a sodium-sulfide ingrown-toenail remedy to poison yourself. Other tests, in rabbits, show that it is only slightly irritating to the skin. The Panel judges sodium sulfide to be safe.

The results of a study done with 100 ingrown-toenail patients seem to show that the sodium sulfide produced relief in most subjects within 3 to 7 days, whereas a dummy drug given to some of the patients did not. But in analyzing these findings, the Panel concluded that the test had been conducted in a sloppy manner and stipulated that either this study must be redone or another one designed and carried out if the manufacturer hopes to show that sodium sulfide really works as an ingredient that provides relief from an ingrown toenail. In short, effectiveness remains to be proved.

• *TANNIC ACID:* This compound is believed to harden the skin surrounding the nail and shrink the adjacent soft tissue, making room for the nail to resume its normal position. Another Panel that evaluated tannic acid for treating burns and other skin injuries found that it has little effect— good or bad—on intact skin. This led the present Panel to conclude that it is safe enough for consumers to use, a few drops at a time, to treat sore toes but also led it to doubt the compound's effectiveness.

The one published study that the present evaluators reviewed indicates that tannic acid along with a pain reliever and alcohol proved to be "an excellent aid in helping restore the nail to its proper relationship to the soft tissue of the toe." But it is not clear whether it was the alcohol (which would counteract infection) or the tannic acid that was mainly responsible for these good results.

More recent studies in mice, whose skins were treated with tannic acid and then punctured with needles, support the notion that this substance turns live skin more leathery. But the Panel said a scientifically sound study must be conducted on humans with sore toes from ingrown nails before the substance can be considered effective for relieving this condition.

DISAPPROVED ACTIVE INGREDIENTS
None.

Safety and Effectiveness: Active Ingredients in Over-the-Counter Ingrown Toenail Relievers

Active Ingredient	Assessment
sodium sulfide	safe, but not proved effective
tannic acid	safe, but not proved effective

Ingrown-Toenail Relievers: Product Ratings

Product and Distributor	Dosage of Active Ingredients	Rating*	Comment
Dr. Scholl's Ingrown Toenail Reliever (Schering-Plough)	liquid: 5% tannic acid + 5% chorbutanol	B	neither ingredient proved effective
Outgro (Whitehall)	liquid: 25% tannic acid + 5% chlorobutanol	B	neither ingredient proved effective

*Author's interpretation of FDA criteria. Based on contents, not claims.

Insect Repellents and Bite and Sting Treatments

For a few individuals who are highly allergic to insects' venom, stings by bees, wasps, or hornets can be life-threatening emergencies. For most other persons, such stings and bites are simply a pain in the neck—or wherever else they are struck.

People who are highly sensitive to insect venom may already know their vulnerability. They should be under the care of an allergist, who may be administering desensitizing shots. These highly susceptible individuals may also have been advised to purchase and carry pen-like hypodermic needles that are pre-loaded with *epinephrine*. This substance counteracts *anaphylactic shock*, a condition that may cause death when highly allergic persons are restung by insects to which they are especially sensitive.

Three approaches have been available for combating insects.

INSECT REPELLENTS AND BITE AND STING TREATMENTS is based on the report "OTC Insect Bite Neutralizer Drug Products" by the FDA's Advisory Review Panel on OTC Miscellaneous External Drug Products, the FDA's Tentative Final Monograph on External Analgesic Drug Products for OTC Human Use, the report "Insect Repellent Drug Products for OTC Oral Human Use" by the Advisory Review Panel on OTC Miscellaneous Internal Drug Products, and the FDA's Tentative Final and Final Rules on these products.

The first is to prevent bites and stings by wearing insect helmets, netting, or other such devices, or by using insect repellents. Most repellents marketed for direct application to the skin are not classified as drugs; one of them, oil of citronella, was judged by the Panel (in a preliminary assessment) to be ineffective. Vitamin B$_1$, also known as *thiamin hydrochloride*, has been marketed as an *internal* insect repellent—a repellent to be taken orally. The Panel that reviewed this ingredient assessed it as being ineffective for this purpose. The FDA agreed and banned it. Other, nondrug approaches must be sought for *prevention*. One is described in the section When Further Relief Is Needed at the end of this Unit.

The second approach to insect stings and bites is to treat them after they occur, with the aim of reducing the swelling and pain and relieving the itching and other discomfort. The idea is to use substances that specifically neutralize the venom. However, the ingredients that manufacturers say have this effect are currently listed as "not proved effective" by the FDA.

Therefore, a more fruitful path to relief may be to use the drugs that act in general and non-specific ways to relieve itching and pain of the skin. Many of these ingredients are formulated into products that are safe and effective for treating insect bites. They are listed here. Readers who want more information about them should turn to the Unit ITCH AND PAIN REMEDIES APPLIED TO THE SKIN (pp. 557-565).

- *BENZOCAINE*
- *BENZYL ALCOHOL*
- *BUTAMBEN PICRATE*
- *CAMPHOR*
- *CAMPHORATED METACRESOL*
- *DIBUCAINE*
- *DIBUCAINE HYDROCHLORIDE*
- *DIMETHISOQUIN HYDROCHLORIDE*
- *DIPHENHYDRAMINE HYDROCHLORIDE*
- *DYCLONINE HYDROCHLORIDE*
- *HYDROCORTISONE*
- *HYDROCORTISONE ACETATE*
- *JUNIPER TAR*
- *LIDOCAINE*
- *LIDOCAINE HYDROCHLORIDE*
- *MENTHOL*
- *PHENOL (0.5 TO 1.5 PERCENT)*
- *PHENOLATE SODIUM (0.5 TO 1.5 PERCENT PHENOL)*
- *PRAMOXINE HYDROCHLORIDE*
- *RESORCINOL*
- *TETRACAINE*

- *TETRACAINE HYDROCHLORIDE*
- *TRIPELENNAMINE HYDROCHLORIDE*

Drugs to Neutralize Insect Venom

Since the reviewers do not believe that any of these ingredients is a safe and effective neutralizer, they were not able to grant full approval to any claim that such products will actually neutralize insect venom.

 Claims

Approved
None.

Unproved
- "For the temporary relief of stings caused by wasps, hornets, bees, mosquitoes, spiders, fleas, chiggers, ticks, and ants"

APPROVED INSECT VENOM-NEUTRALIZING ACTIVE INGREDIENTS
None.

CONDITIONALLY APPROVED INSECT VENOM-NEUTRALIZING ACTIVE INGREDIENTS

- **AMMONIUM HYDROXIDE:** This ingredient neutralizes acids very effectively. (*See* ANTACIDS.) But insect toxins are chemically complex, and they are not all acids. So the Panel had reservations about the effectiveness of this substance. The FDA agrees: It says that while ammonium hydroxide is safe, the data submitted by manufacturers to show that it neutralizes insect venom is inadequate. For now, ammonium hydroxide is safe but not proved effective for this purpose.
- **TROLAMINE (TRIETHANOLAMINE):** This chemical penetrates the skin to reach poisons deposited there by insect stings or bites. The amount absorbed into the body from this self-treatment is too small to be dan-

gerous, the Panel says, so it concludes that trolamine is safe.

The drug is highly alkaline (pH 10 to 11), which may be why manufacturers formulate it into neutralizing preparations for treating insect stings and bites. The Panel notes that *some* venoms contain acids, but they also contain other, nonacidic irritants. So trolamine's effectiveness cannot come solely from its alkalizing capability.

In the one double-blind study submitted for review, trolamine was compared with a dummy preparation of salt water. Bee stings were simulated by injecting tiny amounts of bee venom under participants' skin. When the subjects began to feel pain, they were given swabs containing either trolamine or the salt water. A full 40 percent of the subjects (13 out of 26) felt relief or elimination of pain within 2 minutes when they used trolamine, but only 23 percent (6 of 26) reported comparable relief when they applied the salt-water swabs. Neither the active drug nor the salt water reduced the redness and swelling.

The Panel thought these findings were interesting but not persuasive. It granted conditional approval, pending further testing, and the FDA agreed. Trolamine is judged safe but not proved effective as an insect sting and bite neutralizer.

DISAPPROVED INSECT VENOM-NEUTRALIZING ACTIVE INGREDIENTS

The Panel, the FDA, or both disapproved of 19 compounds because they could find little or no data on them; *see* the Safety and Effectiveness table, further on in this unit.

When Further Relief Is Needed

Since neither the specific preventive drugs nor the one repellent designed to be taken internally (thiamin hydrochloride) show much promise, other means must be sought. With regard to prevention, the gold standard for insect repellents is called *deet*. Deet is the chemical nickname for N,N-diethyl-m-toluamide, which is what, more often than not, shows up on the product label. *Consumer Reports* (July 1987) says deet "is generally regarded as the most effective repellent compound you can buy"—a judgment that has not been seriously challenged since that report. The product rating magazine says specifically that deet is more effective than *Rutgers 6-12* and other currently marketed repellent ingredients. Other, less-effective compounds include citronella and a cosmetic bath oil (*Skin-So-Soft*, Avon), which experts say is richer in users' endorsements than it is in supportive scientific data.

Deet does not kill insects. It appears to jam their sensory receptors so they cannot home in on the skin they need to bite: Their signals become crossed. Deet is effective against mosquitoes, chiggers, biting flies including black flies, fleas, and ticks, including *Ixodes dammini*, which transmit Lyme disease, or Lyme arthritis as it also is called. But deet is *not* effective against wasps, bees, hornets, or ants.

Deet is an extremely potent chemical. It is absorbed through the skin. Products come in a wide range of strengths. Side effects, including allergic and toxic responses have been reported, and brain damage (toxic encephalopathy) has been reported several times in the medical literature when high concentrations of deet were used in young children or when the repellent was used for a prolonged period of time. Authorities at the *Medical Letter on Drugs and Therapeutics* (May 19, 1989) and elsewhere caution that low concentrations of this compound, in the range of 10 to 15 percent, should suffice for most uses, particularly on children indoors. On the other hand, a man or woman who hopes to concentrate on trout fishing rather than black-fly swatting in the North Woods in June may be well advised to use the deepest "deep woods" deet preparations, which contain up to 100 percent deet.

As a second line of defense in heavy mosquito, tick, and fly territory, sprays containing deet or, alternatively, 0.5 percent permetherin are sold for spraying one's clothing. In one test, summarized in the *Medical Letter*, a one-minute spray treatment of clothing provided 100 percent protection against *I. dammini*, compared with 86 to 92 percent protection with one-minute applications of 20 percent and 30 percent deet.

WARNING:

 After being bitten or stung, if you suddenly feel faint, sweaty, nauseous, or otherwise ill, or if, later, the available over-the-counter itch-pain remedies do not provide adequate relief, go to the nearest hospital emergency room.

Insect venom is not to be trifled with, particularly if you are particularly sensitive to it. Emergency room teams have a number of methods to relieve itching and pain and safeguard your health against insect toxins.

Safety and Effectiveness: Active Ingredients in Over-the-Counter Products for the Prevention and the Specific Relief of Insect Bites and Stings

Active Ingredient	Assessment
alcohol	not safe and effective
ammonium hydroxide	safe, but not proved effective
ammonia solution, strong	not safe and effective
benzalkonium chloride	not safe and effective
calamine*	
camphor	not safe and effective
colloidal oatmeal*	
ergot fluid extract	not safe and effective
ethoxylated alkyl alcohol	not safe and effective
ferric chloride	not safe and effective
menthol*	
obtundia surgical dressing	not safe and effective
peppermint oil	not safe and effective
polyvinylpyrrolidone-vinylacetate copolymers	not safe and effective
pyrilamine maleate	not safe and effective

For many safe and effective ingredients and products that will relieve the itching and pain of insect bites and stings, see ITCH AND PAIN REMEDIES APPLIED TO THE SKIN. For many safe and effective ingredients and products that will cover, protect and help dry out welts and rashes from insect bites and stings, See UNGUENTS AND POWDERS TO PROTECT THE SKIN.

Safety and Effectiveness: Active Ingredients in Over-the-Counter Products for the Prevention and the Specific Relief of Insect Bites and Stings (contd)

Active Ingredient	Assessment
sodium bicarbonate*	
sodium borate	not safe and effective
thiamin hydrochloride (vitamin B_1), taken orally	not safe and effective
trolamine	safe, but not proved effective
turpentine oil	not safe and effective
zinc oxide*	
zirconium oxide	not safe and effective

*Safe and effective as a nonspecific itch and pain reliever or skin protectant.

Insect Bite and Sting Treatments: Product Ratings*

NEUTRALIZERS FOR USE ON SKIN

Product and Distributor	Dosage of Active Ingredients	Rating†	Comment
Aspercreme Cream (Thompson)	cream: trolamine 10%	B	not proved effective
Skeeter Stik (Triton)	liquid: 4% lidocaine + 2% phenol	B	a bit too much phenol; probably o.k. in small amounts
Sting-Kill (Kiwi)	swabs: 18.9% benzocaine + 0.9% menthol	C	no data to show that menthol is safe and effective for neutralizing insect venom, but menthol, and menthol in combination with benzocaine, well may provide non-specific relief for itch and pain

*For safe and effective itch and pain relievers see Itch and Pain Remedies Applied to the Skin: Product Ratings, on pp. 571-575.
†Author's interpretation of FDA criteria. Based on contents, not claims.

Insulin for Diabetics

By Thomas G. Watkins

Insulin is among the most powerful drugs you can buy in the United States without a prescription. In many other countries it is available by prescription only.

In nondiabetics, insulin is released from cells in the pancreas called beta cells. They are clustered together in what are called the islets of Langerhans. Under the microscope, these clusters look like islands. The word insulin is derived from the Latin, *insula*, for "island." Its physiological and medical function is to help sugar get into the body's cells to be burned as energy. The condition for which supplements are needed is the disease *diabetes*.

About 14 million Americans have diabetes, according to the American Diabetes Association. Fewer than 10 percent of them require insulin therapy. The majority are treated with dietary restriction, exercise, and with prescription drugs that lower blood sugar levels.

INSULIN FOR DIABETICS is based on standard medical and pharmacological sources, including interviews with manufacturers' professional representatives.

Ready access to insulin can be crucial: Deprived of it, 20 million people in the world would die, many within a few days. *No one else should buy or use insulin.*

Too much insulin can be as dangerous as too little. As the prosecution pointed out in its unsuccessful case against Claus Von Bulow, for allegedly trying to murder his wife, Sonny, the drug can also bring about intentional death. (The movie based on the case is *Reversal of Fortune*.) Insulin helps sugar pass from the blood into the cells. Too little sugar in the blood leaves the brain without fuel, which can, in rare cases, cause convulsions and death.

In nondiabetics, insulin is released by the pancreas, a large gland near the stomach, in response to a rise in glucose in the blood. (Starchy foods turn into this simple sugar as they are digested.) Insulin stimulates the formation and movement of glucose transporters to the cell membrane, and activates them to move glucose molecules out of the bloodstream and into the cell where they are burned as energy or converted to fat. In non-diabetics, this process keeps blood sugar levels within a narrow range. In diabetics, however, the pancreas cannot secrete enough insulin and, as a result, cannot get sugar into the cells. Instead, diabetics burn their fat reserves, leaving in the blood a residue of organic compounds called ketoacids. High blood sugar, dehydration, and ketoacids can induce coma and death.

This was the usual course of events for insulin-requiring diabetics until 1922, when the lifesaving hormone was discovered. Injected frequently, insulin stimulates glucose metabolism and restricts the wasting of fat reserves and muscle tissue.

But insulin is no cure: A shot or two a day can keep diabetics out of coma. Yet this still leaves many of them susceptible to complications associated with poor blood sugar control. Years of too much sugar in the blood are blamed for the higher risk of heart attacks, atherosclerosis, kidney failure, nerve damage, and blindness that face diabetics. Thus, many doctors recommend several shots a day, in an attempt to keep blood sugars within normal limits round-the-clock.

 Claims

Accurate
- "For the treatment of insulin-requiring diabetes"

WARNING:

 Insulin reaction (too little sugar in the blood, also called *hypoglycemia)* can be brought about by

1. Taking too much insulin

2. Missing or delaying meals

3. Exercising or working hard without compensating by reducing insulin or eating first.

4. A change in the body's need for insulin

The first symptoms of insulin reaction may come on suddenly. They may include hunger, fatigue, nervousness or shakiness, headache, rapid heartbeat, blurred vision, and a cold sweat.

Eating sugar or a sugar-sweetened product will correct the condition and prevent more serious symptoms.

Makers

Two companies make all the insulin sold in the United States: the Bagsvaert, Denmark manufacturer Novo-Nordisk, and Indianapolis-based Eli Lilly. (Lilly has most of the U.S. market; Novo-Nordisk has most of the world market.) There appears to be little reason to choose one product over the other. Both companies' prices are about the same in the United States, and neither maker is willing to say its product is better than the other's. Thus, their advertising tends to be pretty tame; the competitors sometimes even collaborate at diabetes meetings, cohosting parties for physicians and research scientists.

Lilly and Novo-Nordisk both promote a combination medium-acting insulin called NPH (Neutral Protamine Hagedorn) as a "human insulin." Though the insulin itself is indeed structurally equivalent to human insulin, protamine is added to slow its absorption. Protamine is extracted from salmon sperm. In rare cases, it can cause severe allergic reactions. The combination was discovered by researcher H.C. Hagedorn to prolong the period of action of insulin. John A. Galloway, M.D., a Lilly clinical research fellow, acknowledged that "it does occasionally cause antibodies [to form]," but added that the protamine used today is so pure that such occurrences are "exceedingly rare." (Lente insulin, which has similar action, contains zinc instead of protamine.

Lente is the French word for "slow.")

Route of Administration

Commercially available insulins must be injected. If ingested, stomach acids destroy the insulin protein before it can make its way to the bloodstream. However, researchers now are working on insulins to be taken in pill form, that would be protected from gastric acids. Insulins that could be given in eye drops or nasal sprays also are in the works.

Storage and Handling

Care must be taken to ensure that insulins that are safe and effective at the factory remain that way until they are used. According to representatives from Lilly and Novo-Nordisk, bottles stored in the refrigerator at between 36° and 46° will last 18 months to two years.

A user's current vial can be kept at room temperature for up to a month. Afterward, it can lose potency.

What is room temperature? Though the package insert cites 86°, Lilly's Dr. Galloway considers anything above 80° too high. "Anything over ought to be refrigerated most of the time." Novo-Nordisk recommends an upper limit of 77°. At higher temperatures, insulin may aggregate. On rare occasions, allergic reactions may result. Lente insulin is less stable than other insulins, according to Dr. Galloway, and should be refrigerated "when possible."

Freezing causes long-acting (cloudy) insulins to resuspend unevenly after thawing, making it difficult to withdraw accurate doses. Vibration and exposure to bright light can also diminish insulin's potency.

Precautions

All insulins are subject to *flocculation*, or frosting on the vial, which indicates a loss of insulin potency. Check vials for changes in the appearance of the contents. Discard or consult your doctor about any that appear different.

Dr. Richard K. Bernstein, author of *Diabetes Type II* (Prentice Hall, 1990) recommends that long-acting insulins be used only down to the bottom of the label, in order to guard against the chance that, if the contents are not well mixed, the concentration of zinc or protamine will change, upsetting the insulin's control of blood sugar. Lilly's Dr. Galloway calls such precautions unnecessary. "[The concentration] won't change if the patient carefully follows the instructions," he says.

Lilly's instructions say that long-acting insulin vials should be rolled between the palms to mix them. Lilly cautions against shaking the vial: Air might mix with the insulin, resulting in an inaccurate dose being drawn into the syringe. Dr. Bernstein disagrees, saying that foam floats above the syringe, and that shaking is the best way to ensure the insulin is well mixed. Novo-Nordisk says it does not have a position. A spokesperson said, "It [shaking] probably doesn't do anything at all."

All insulins bear a warning that patients should consult their physicians before changing brands or types. Changes may result in a change of dosage required.

In a small place, such as tubing or the cannula of a syringe, insulin molecules tend to combine with other insulin molecules. A little bit of this polymerized insulin can act as a nidus for further polymerization. Thus, if polymerized insulin is repeatedly re-injected into a vial (as may occur when a syringe is reused a few hours later), the contents can eventually become useless. Lilly's Dr. Galloway said, however, that polymerization should not be a concern: "It's theoretically possible, but [it's] never presented to me as an issue."

Exposure to carbon dioxide can cause insulin to precipitate out of solution. This can be a problem when insulin is shipped with vaccines, which typically are packed in dry ice.

Treatment Considerations

Insulins differ in four respects:
* **PURITY:** Are there any contaminants that may affect the user?
* **CONCENTRATION:** How much is needed to lower blood sugar a given amount?
* **SOURCE:** Is it made from cow pancreases, pig pancreases, or by genetic engineering?
* **TYPE:** When does it start lowering blood glucose, when does it peak, and when does it stop?

Purity

Impurities in insulin can cause immunological reactions and can cause the fat under the injection site to waste away, leaving an indentation. But the purity of insulins has improved in recent years, and such cases are rare. Swelling at the site of injection has also been blamed on impurities, even among people using human insulin. This, too, is rare.

Proinsulin, a biological precursor of insulin, is the marker for insulin impurity. Early insulins contained up to 30,000 parts per million (ppm) of this impurity. By the early 1970s, advances in manufacturing dropped the level of this impurity to 10 ppm for standard insulins. Insulins labeled "purified" contain less than 3 ppm of proinsulin.

According to Novo-Nordisk, their human insulins contain less than 1 ppm of impurities; Lilly says the proinsulin levels in its human insulins are "unmeasurable."

Concentration

All insulins sold for injection in the United States and Canada are in concentrations of U-100, or 100 units per ml. (A unit is one-third the amount of insulin required to lower the blood sugar of a rabbit starved for 24 hours to 45 mg/dl, the point at which convulsions occur, within 5 hours.) Beware, though. Other countries still sell insulin in U-40 and U-80 concentrations.

They should be used only with U-40 or U-80 syringes.

Some pediatricians prefer U-40 for children who only require small amounts of insulin. They say it is easier to measure fractions of units using the less-concentrated insulin. But, according to Lilly's Dr. Galloway, "it's just a matter of time before [U-40] disappears."

Self-Treatment Problems

Insulin is available without a prescription in the United States and Canada. But this is not always the case in other countries. Diabetic travelers abroad are advised to carry along a back-up supply and a prescription. Although U.S. lawmakers agree that insulin is of such importance that no diabetic should be denied access to the drug simply because he or she lacks a prescription, this thinking does not extend to needles: A prescription for needles and syringes is required in 39 of the 50 states.

A U-500 insulin is made for use in implantable pumps. It packs the same blood sugar lowering punch as U-100, in one-fifth the space.

Source

All insulins once were made from animals: primarily pig and cow pancreases obtained from slaughterhouses. There is nothing special about pigs or cows; they just happened to be the most plentiful sources. In Japanese-occupied Shanghai, when the pharmacies were shut during World War II, a diabetic woman and her husband processed water buffalo pancreases in a crude lab to keep her and hundreds of other diabetics alive for years. Sheep, fish, and whale insulin have also been used.

Insulin from pigs and cows was the standard from 1922 until 1983, when human insulin was first sold. Porcine insulin differs from human insulin by just one amino acid; bovine insulin differs by three. As a result, beef insulin is slightly more *antigenic* (antibody-stimulating) than porcine.

Unlike insulins made from animal pancreases, human insulins rarely cause immunological reactions. In 1983, Novo and Nordisk introduced a human insulin that was called "semi-synthetic" because it was made by altering the one amino acid in porcine insulin that distinguishes it from human insulin.

A few months later, Lilly brought out its version of human insulin, made through recombinant DNA technology: The insulin gene is inserted into the bacterium *E. coli*, which then acts as a tiny factory, churning out exact copies of human insulin.

Recently, Novo-Nordisk (the product of the 1990 merger of two firms that each made insulin since the 1920s) started making its human insulin by inserting the genes that produce it into baker's yeast. Novo-Nordisk says that baker's yeast is "milder," but a company representative would not say if that confers any clinical advantage.

The recombinant DNA insulins are about 30 percent cheaper than porcine insulin. But for most diabetics, the clinical value of human insulin seems to be minimal in terms of efficacy. "Compared to the discovery of insulin, it's a relatively small advance," says Dr. John K. Davidson, author of *Clinical Diabetes Mellitus—A Problem-Oriented Approach* (Thieme, 1991).

In many people, antibodies form and latch onto animal insulins, and then release them at unpredictable times. This makes blood sugar control somewhat erratic when these animal insulins are used. Some individuals have an increased number of low blood sugar episodes when they switch from animal insulin to human insulin. Possibly, with fewer antibodies to lock up the insulin molecules, less insulin is needed. Thus, diabetics who switch from animal insulin to human insulin should beware: They may need less insulin.

Type

Because Regular insulin (fast-acting) peaks within 2 to 4 hours, several injections daily were needed in the first years of insulin therapy, when this was the only kind of insulin available. In 1936, the addition of zinc and protamine to Regular insulin was found to delay its action.

Today, there are three types of insulin:

1. Fast-acting (clear), or Regular.
2. Intermediate-acting (cloudy), such as NPH (which contains protamine) and Lente (which contains zinc).
3. Prolonged-acting (cloudy), or Ultralente, which also contains zinc.

BR is Regular insulin that has been buffered. It is intended for use in insulin pumps. Lilly says it is less likely to polymerize in the tubing, clogging the device, than are other insulins.

How long an injection will continue to lower blood sugar depends on

1. Injection site: One study found absorption was 39 percent faster when injected into the abdomen than when injected into the arm.
2. Blood sugar at the time of injection: High blood sugar can slow insulin's action.
3. Depth of injection: Insulin injected into the muscle gets into the blood more quickly than insulin injected into fat just beneath the skin.
4. Exercise of the muscle under the injection site: This can speed insulin absorption.
5. Temperature at the injection site: Blood circulation—and insulin absorption—increase with temperature.

Mixing Insulins

Regular and Lente insulin should not be mixed in the same syringe: Excess zinc quickly converts regular into long-acting insulin, according to Dr. Bernstein.

The conversion does not occur so fast when Regular is mixed with NPH. But if these two insulins are allowed to remain in a syringe for more than a few minutes, protamine from the NPH can mix with the Regular, turning some of the Regular into long-acting insulin.

Studies that showed doctors and nurses often made mistakes when mixing Regular with NPH led insulin-makers to come out with premixed versions that are 70 percent NPH and 30 percent Regular (*Humulin 70/30* and *Mixtard 70/30*). In 1992, Lilly introduced *Humulin 50/50* to the U.S. market. Other percentages already are available abroad.

NOTE: The fast-acting component of a premixed insulin may take longer to kick in than the usual wait with a shot of Regular, experts acknowledge.

Specialized Means of Delivery

Novo-Nordisk has been selling devices called *Novopens*. This is an insulin-containing cartridge that is inserted into a pen-like barrel, to which disposable needles can be attached. The pens are intended to make it more convenient and easy for diabetics to mimic the body's release of insulin by injecting Regular insulin just before each meal. The advantage is that patients need not carry a fat bottle of insulin and several syringes.

Needle-less injectors also can be a problem: They may shorten insulin's activity and increase its apparent potency. So patients who opt to try these devices should stay in touch with their doctor during the transition.

Insulins Available Without Prescription in the United States

Duration/Source	Product	Manufacturer	Peak Activity (hr)	Strength
Short-Acting				
human	Humulin R	Lilly	2-4	U-100
	Humulin BR	Lilly	2-4	U-100
	Novolin R	Novo-Nordisk	2.5-5	U-100
	Velosulin Human R	Novo-Nordisk	1-3	U-100
pork	Iletin II Regular	Lilly	2-4	U-100, U-500
	Regular	Novo-Nordisk	2.5-5	U-100
	Purified Pork Regular	Novo-Nordisk	2.5-5	U-100
	Velosulin	Novo-Nordisk	1-3	U-100
beef	Iletin II Regular	Lilly	2-4	U-100
	Semilente	Novo-Nordisk	5-10	U-100
beef/pork	Iletin I Regular	Lilly	2-4	U-100
	Iletin I Semilente	Lilly	3-8	U-100
Intermediate-Acting				
human	Humulin L	Lilly	6-12	U-100

Insulins Available Without Prescription in the United States (contd)

Duration/Source	Product	Manufacturer	Peak Activity (hr)	Strength
	Humulin N (NPH)	Lilly	6-12	U-100
	Novolin L (Lente)	Novo-Nordisk	7-15	U-100
	Novolin N (NPH)	Novo-Nordisk	4-12	U-100
	Insulatard NPH Human	Novo-Nordisk	4-12	U-100
pork	Iletin II Lente	Lilly	6-12	U-100
	Iletin II NPH	Lilly	6-12	U-100
	Purified Pork Lente	Novo-Nordisk	7-15	U-100
	Purified Pork NPH	Novo-Nordisk	4-12	U-100
	Insulatard NPH	Novo-Nordisk	4-12	U-100
beef	Iletin II Lente	Lilly	6-12	U-100
	Iletin II NPH	Lilly	6-12	U-100
	Lente	Novo-Nordisk	7-15	U-100
	NPH	Novo-Nordisk	4-12	U-100
beef/pork	Iletin I NPH	Lilly	6-12	U-100
	Iletin I Lente	Lilly	6-12	U-100

Long-Acting

human	Humulin U (Ultralente)	Lilly	8-20	U-100
beef	Ultralente	Novo-Nordisk	6-30	U-100
beef/pork	Iletin I Ultralente	Lilly	14-24	U-100

Fixed Combinations (all are U-100, NPH/Regular insulins)

human	Humulin 70/30	Lilly	2-12	70/30
	Novolin 70/30	Novo-Nordisk	2-12	70/30
	Mixtard Human 70/30	Novo Nordisk	4-8	70/30
pork	Mixtard	Novo Nordisk	4-8	70/30
human	Humulin 50/50	Lilly	2-6	50/50

Itch and Pain Remedies
Applied to the Skin

Some skin irritations are caused by external factors; others are symptoms of diseases originating within the skin itself or deeper in the body. Many remedies have been developed for these complaints, and Panel reviewers found a wide selection of safe and effective active ingredients that will temporarily relieve pain and itching of the skin. Many of these drugs have been sold in over-the-counter preparations for decades. They generally act by directly or indirectly blocking or reducing the activity of sensory nerve receptors in the skin.

On the Panel's recommendation, the FDA has allowed preparations of two potent drugs from the class called *corticosteroids* to be sold without prescription for the first time. They are *hydrocortisone* and *hydrocortisone acetate*. Previously all corticosteroids were available only by prescription. But the evaluators judged these preparations safe and effective for self-treatment of minor skin irritations as well as

ITCH AND PAIN REMEDIES APPLIED TO THE SKIN is based on the report on External Analgesic Drug Products, prepared by the FDA's Advisory Review Panel on OTC Topical Analgesic, Antirheumatic, Otic, Burn and Sunburn Prevention and Treatment Drug Products and on the FDA's Tentative Final Monograph on these products. It also is based on documents in the rulemaking for OTC hydrocortisone products.

for treating the itching and rashes—but *not* the pain—caused by eczema, dermatitis, insect bites, poison ivy-oak-sumac, soaps, detergents, cosmetics, and jewelry, and for itchy genital and anal areas.

The antihistamine that once was most commonly formulated into over-the-counter itch remedies is methapyrilene. When it was removed from the market as a possible cancer-causing agent, manufacturers substituted other antihistamines, including phenyltoloxamine dihydrogen citrate and pyrilamine maleate. The FDA has not yet stated its position on their safety or effectiveness as over-the-counter drugs.

Hydrocortisones and antihistamines may help *cure* a rash or other skin irritation. But most of the other drugs described here provide only the relief of symptoms. If the condition does not improve or vanish in a week, show it to a doctor.

 Claims

Accurate for all products and ingredients except hydrocortisone and hydrocortisone acetate
- "For the temporary relief of pain and itching associated with minor burns, sunburn, minor cuts, scrapes, insect bites or minor skin irritations"

Accurate for hydrocortisone preparations
- "For the temporary relief of itching associated with minor skin irritations, and rashes due to eczema, seborrheic dermatitis, insect bites, poison ivy-oak-sumac, soaps, detergents, cosmetics and jewelry, and for itchy genital and anal areas, and for other uses only under the advice and supervision of a doctor"

WARNING:

 If the condition worsens, or if symptoms persist for more than 7 days, or clear up and occur again within a few days, discontinue use, and do not begin use of any other hydrocortisone product unless you have consulted a doctor. Do not use for the treatment of diaper rash.

Why We Itch

Feelings of itchiness are close to feelings of pain, the Panel said. Both are produced by the same sensory nerve endings in the skin. Weak stimulation of these nerve fibers causes itching; strong stimulation causes pain. The response, however, is different: We withdraw from a painful stimulus but we attend to an itch by scratching it. Recent research suggests, however, that some skin receptors may be specific for itching.

An itch can be produced directly, by an irritative chemical or other foreign substance, or it may result indirectly, from the body's defensive reaction against a certain substance. The latter response is an allergic reaction. The redness and swelling is caused by the release into the skin of *histamine,* an irritating chemical that is made by the body.

An itch sometimes can be relieved by gently touching the skin with a clean pin, about an inch away from a source of discomfort such as a mosquito bite; scratching gently at this distance also may help. But scratching *on* the bite—or on poison ivy or other rashes—may release more of the irritative substances into the skin, intensifying the itch and even transforming it into out-and-out pain.

The technical name for an itch is *pruritus,* so a drug that relieves itch is an *anti-pruritic.* Small itchy areas can be self-treated. Large areas, including generalized itching all over the body, require medical care.

Superficial Pain

Pain originating in the skin and tissue layers immediately beneath it differs little from other pain — with the important exception that skin discomfort appears not to be relieved by aspirin or chemically related salicylates. Because of this, there is no merit to product-label claims that aspirin or other salicylates in drugs applied to the skin will relieve the pain of sunburn or shallow cuts and scrapes.

Types of Medications

All over-the-counter topical drugs used to relieve itching and pain are characterized by the Panel—somewhat confusingly—as "external analgesics," meaning pain relievers that act on body surfaces.

A drug that acts specifically to block the nerve receptors for pain in the skin is a *topical analgesic.* But since pain and itch travel the same nerve routes, these preparations may also relieve itching. A drug that acts more generally to block all sensation in the skin, causing numbness, is called a *topical anesthetic*. It may block pain and itch sensations as well as feelings of hot, cold, or external pressure.

The medications assessed in the accompanying table may act as analgesics by relieving pain, as anesthetics by causing numbness or as anti-pruritics by relieving the itch. They may provide two or all three of these benefits. Some act only on damaged skin, where they have easy access to the nerve endings. Others penetrate unbroken skin as well.

Pharmacological Class

The Panel attempted to categorize the two dozen active ingredients in external analgesics by pharmacological class.

- *Group 1* includes *anesthetics* whose names end in the suffix - *caine* or are -*amine compounds* that resemble them in chemical structure. The -*caines* tend to be stronger and provide faster relief than the -*amines*, but they also are more toxic.

- *Group 2* includes *alcohols* and *ketones* (compounds chemically related to alcohols). They act like the amines, but their therapeutic routes and toxic properties are different.

- *Group 3* are *antihistamines*. They work principally against itching but are also mildly anesthetic.

- *Group 4* are *salicylates*—aspirin-type compounds.

- *Group 5* consists of the *corticosteroids*. They are treated separately because they act against itching but not pain.

General Properties

Taken as a class, the external analgesics tend to be safe as well as effective. Reviewers rejected only one ingredient, chloral hydrate, as unsafe. However, these judgments are less well grounded in scientific data than those of some of the other Panels—largely because the self-limiting nature of these skin problems makes it almost impossible for investigators to conduct meaningful experiments. Thus the evaluators relied to a large extent on less-definitive kinds of reports, and on manufacturers' data showing that products made with these ingredients have been popular with consumers (effective) and have elicited few complaints of adverse reactions (safe).

Benefits of Approved Itch- and Pain-Relieving Active Ingredients*

Active Ingredient	Induces Numbness	Stops Pain	Stops Itching	Effective on Damaged Skin	Effective on Intact Skin
benzocaine	yes	yes	yes	yes	yes
benzyl alcohol	yes	yes	yes	yes	yes
butamben picrate	yes	yes	yes	yes	no
camphor	yes	yes	yes	yes	yes
dibucaine	yes	yes	yes	yes	yes
dibucaine hydrochloride	yes	yes	yes	yes	no
dimethisoquin hydrochloride	maybe	yes	yes	yes	maybe
diphenhydramine hydrochloride	feebly	no	yes	yes	no
dyclonine hydrochloride	yes	yes	yes	yes	no
hydrocortisone	no	no	yes	yes	yes
hydrocortisone acetate	no	no	yes	yes	yes

juniper tar	no	unclear	yes	apparently	apparently
lidocaine	yes	yes	yes	yes	yes
lidocaine hydrochloride	yes	yes	yes	yes	no
menthol	no	yes	yes	yes	yes
phenol	yes	yes	yes	yes	yes
phenolate sodium	yes	yes	yes	yes	yes
pramoxine hydrochloride†	yes	yes	yes	yes	no
resorcinol	no	no	yes	yes	yes
tetracaine	yes	yes	yes	yes	yes
tetracaine hydrochloride	yes	yes	yes	yes	no
tripelennamine hydrochloride	yes	no	yes	yes	unclear

* Author's interpretations, based on Panel's report.

† Pramoxine hydrochloride may relieve pain in unbroken skin, but it does not produce numbness and may not relieve itching unless the deeper layers of skin are exposed.

Side Effects

The most severe risk posed by external analgesics is also fortunately a rare one: when large amounts of some of the *-caine* preparations are applied to wide areas of bruised or otherwise damaged skin, much of the drug will be absorbed into the body. In some cases reported in the medical literature this has caused life-threatening (and even lethal) toxic reactions. Convulsions and paralysis of the nervous system can occur. The heart may slow down or even stop beating. Reviewers stressed, however, that these complications do not occur when moderate amounts of these drugs are used. It is worth noting, too, that these effects apparently cannot occur with one of the principal *-caine* drugs, benzocaine, because it is insoluble in body fluids. This explains why benzocaine is so widely used and accepted. The more common and less severe side effects of external analgesics are rashes, hives, and other skin eruptions—the very symptoms these products are intended to relieve! The reactions usually abate when use of the drug is discontinued.

The skin is a sensitive organ. So adverse reactions may occur more frequently when analgesic medications are applied to it than they do when the same drugs are taken internally. Persons allergic to a large number of foods and other substances should be especially careful in using these drugs.

The location of a rash or other lesion—as well as the skin's condition—can influence a drug's action. Some drugs are more readily absorbed through thin than through thick skin. Most are better absorbed, and so are more effective, on mucous membranes like the lips, nostrils, and anus than they are on ordinary skin, but they also may be more toxic when applied to these delicate and absorbent surfaces.

External analgesics have varying degrees of solubility in water and body fluids. A compound that is insoluble in water may be relatively worthless when placed on unbroken skin, yet may be quite effective when used on cut or broken skin since it then can reach underlying nerve endings. Many external analgesics are soluble in fats and so can reach underlying layers through fatty parts of the skin barrier.

Consumers should keep in mind that newborn babies' skin absorbs drugs very readily. A stable, "adult" absorbency level is reached by about 6 months of age, but to provide an added margin of safety, experts recommend that external analgesics *not* be used on children under 2 years of age except on the advice of a physician.

These drugs all can be used 3 or 4 times daily, or oftener if recommended by a doctor.

Finally, the assessment of the safety and effectiveness of external analgesics is complicated by the formulation of most—as creams, sprays, or lotions—with inactive ingredients that influence the active drug's ability to reach and remain in contact with the skin. The concentration of the active ingredient also varies from product to product. Consumers may need some trial and error to find the preparations that best meet their own and their families' needs.

Combination Products

Many external analgesic products include two or more active ingredients. The Panel took an equivocal stand on combination products: They maintained that single active ingredients are preferable, but they also said they are "strongly convinced that there is a need for combination products."

A dissenting minority of two members of the Panel addressed itself to this contradiction and claimed (1) that approval of combination products as safe and effective is spurious and unscientific, and (2) that consumers should use external analgesics containing a single active ingredient wherever and whenever possible.

The FDA took the majority's side—and approved several combination of active ingredients. The rules for combining pain and itch relievers are summarized in the Safety and Effectiveness: Combination Products to Relieve Itch and Pain table at the end of this Unit.

Topical Itch and Pain-Relieving Medications

Reviewers evaluated many active ingredients that are applied to the skin to relieve pain and itch. The majority were found to be safe and effective. (*See* the Safety and Effectiveness: Active Ingredients table at the end of this Unit, which also lists approved concentrations and dosage information.)

APPROVED ACTIVE INGREDIENTS

• *BENZOCAINE:* When properly formulated (preferably in propylene glycol), and in adequate concentration (at least 5 percent), this anesthetic is an effective and very safe remedy for pain and itch on the skin. It has been used successfully by tens of millions of people since the turn of the century; over 1.5 million pounds of it are sold in the United States each year.

Benzocaine is relatively insoluble in water; thus very little penetrates the skin to enter the bloodstream. So the serious side effects in the body reported occasionally for other *-caine* drugs do not occur. For the same reason, benzocaine's beneficial activity occurs almost wholly within the skin and mucous membranes, where it blocks the pain-conducting nerve endings. The drug also provides long-acting relief; a single application may quell pain and itching for 4 to 6 hours.

However, a small percentage of users experience some irritation or sensitivity reactions from benzocaine. While serious side effects have been reported in the medical literature, reviewers believe they are far rarer—and the drug far safer—than sometimes has been suggested. Verdict: safe and effective.

• BENZYL ALCOHOL: This substance, which is found naturally in oil of jasmine, is usually synthesized for commercial sale. It has a faint aromatic odor and a sharp, burning taste. It relieves itching, burning, and irritation due to cuts, abrasions, and insect bites, but it is not as effective as benzocaine, and its therapeutic action is briefer. When applied to a cut on the lip or other mucous membrane, for example, benzyl alcohol provides relief within 2 minutes—but this effect lasts less than a half-hour.

While benzyl alcohol will kill some bacteria, it is not reliable for this purpose. But it is a very safe drug. For example, the convulsions and heart problems that have been reported with some *-caine* anesthetics do not occur. Even mild skin sensitization is rare. Conclusion: safe and effective.

• BUTAMBEN PICRATE: This compound, insoluble in water, does not readily penetrate the skin's outer layer. So while it relieves pain and itching where the skin has been cut or bruised, it is not very effective on undamaged skin. It works less well than benzocaine (*see* previously) and has the added disadvantage of forming a yellow stain on the skin, on bandages, and on clothing.

Available data indicate that butamben picrate is nontoxic and quite safe to use, although skin sensitization and other allergic responses have been reported. The compound is made in part of picric acid, which has been used as a burn dressing. But because picric acid is no longer considered a wise choice for burn therapy, butamben picrate has no special value for treating burns, although it appears to be safe and effective for pain and itch. Conclusion: safe and effective.

- *CAMPHOR:* This natural extract of the East Asian camphor tree, an evergreen, also is now made synthetically for drug products. In low concentrations, of 0.1 to 2.5 percent, it has a mild warming, numbing effect on the skin. This action relieves itching and burning feelings due to sunburn, insect bites, allergic reactions, and other problems. Camphor's characteristic pine-like aroma is also often associated with healing, which may contribute to its therapeutic value.

  Camphor's ability to relieve itch has been widely reported in the medical literature but has not been confirmed by controlled tests. Its long history of successful use confirms its effectiveness and safety when applied to the skin in the approved low doses. Higher doses can be harmful, and when taken orally, camphor can be a deadly poison. Nonetheless, in the recommended dosages, camphor is considered safe and effective for topical use.

- *CAMPHORATED METACRESOL:* This ingredient is a combination of camphor and metacresol, which is a form of *phenol*, or *carbolic acid*. Therefore, its pluses and minuses are very much like those of these other two ingredients. Although it has been marketed for half a century, evaluators could find little data on its safety or its effectiveness in relieving pain and itching. But based on its long record of use, and similarity to camphor and phenol, the FDA has rated it safe and effective.

- *DIBUCAINE:* Made synthetically, dibucaine is an extremely potent and long-acting topical anesthetic. It was first introduced a half-century ago. When applied to the skin, dibucaine begins to relieve pain and itch within 15 minutes. If it is formulated in an effective base that keeps it moist and in touch with the skin surface, dibucaine may continue to provide relief for up to 4 hours. When the drug is removed, the noxious sensations return within 15 minutes.

  Dibucaine is 15 times stronger than procaine, the reference drug of the *-caine* group; it is a half-dozen times stronger than cocaine. With this degree of potency, very small amounts of dibucaine are required. It should not be used over large areas of the body or applied to badly bruised or cut skin because it is readily absorbed. This could slow the heartbeat and cause convulsions or even death. The drug may also be fatal if swallowed—particularly by children— and it should not be applied in large quantities, especially on raw or blistered surfaces. Nonetheless, this Panel ranked this drug safe and effective.

- **DIBUCAINE HYDROCHLORIDE:** As one might assume, this drug is similar to dibucaine, just described. But it penetrates into skin so slowly that it is not effective unless the skin is cut or damaged. On the other hand, once through the skin, it is more soluble in water than dibucaine; thus it may pose an even greater hazard of generalized poisoning if too much is used. Used judiciously on small areas of unbroken skin, it is safe and effective in approved concentrations and dosages.

- **DIMETHISOQUIN HYDROCHLORIDE:** Long use indicates that this substance is a very safe -*caine* topical anesthetic. No serious nerve or heart complications have been reported; it rarely causes skin reactions; and there are few reports of systemic side effects after accidental ingestion. But while studies have demonstrated dimethisoquin hydrochloride's effectiveness in relieving pain and itching on the skin (850 of 1000 patients obtained relief in one study), it appears to do so less reliably than some other drugs of its class. Investigators are still not clear, for example, if dimethisoquin hydrochloride will penetrate intact skin; it is known to reach and quiet painful nerve endings when the skin is bruised or cut. The Panel's conclusion: safe and effective.

- **DIPHENHYDRAMINE HYDROCHLORIDE:** Diphenhydramine hydrochloride is an antihistamine whose role as an over-the-counter oral drug has been controversial, in part because it makes some users sleepy. The evaluators found that drowsiness and other side effects are rare or nonexistent when diphenhydramine hydrochloride is applied directly to the skin, where it acts protectively by blocking the sites at which the irritating body substance *histamine* binds to cells in the skin, inducing itching. However, it does not penetrate unbroken skin and so cannot relieve itching in such a case. (An oral dose—*prescribed by a doctor*—may be helpful under these circumstances.) Also, because diphenhydramine hydrochloride can lose its effectiveness after it has been used for several days, and may eventually cause a skin reaction, the experts reiterate that it be used no longer than a week, except under a doctor's supervision. Evaluation: safe and effective.

- **DYCLONINE HYDROCHLORIDE:** This anesthetic is chemically different from the -*caine* drugs with which it is grouped, so it does not produce the convulsions and severe cardiovascular symptoms for which many of these -*caine* drugs are noted. Thus, like benzocaine, it is a very safe drug in its class. Even mild side effects are rare: In one set of trials of 5656 patients, only 2 developed skin sensitivity to this drug.

Dyclonine hydrochloride is particularly effective in relieving pain and itching on mucous membrane and bruised and damaged skin. (It will not pass through undamaged skin.) About one-half to two-thirds of patients with severe pain and itching find it helpful. It is fast-acting (within 2 or 3 minutes) but affords relief only for about half an hour. Conclusion: safe and effective.

• *HYDROCORTISONE AND HYDROCORTISONE ACETATE:* These anti-itch drugs are natural extracts of the cortex of the adrenal glands, and also made synthetically. They are extremely potent, relieving itching and inflammation—but not pain—owing to a variety of causes. Their mode of action is not fully understood.

Hydrocortisone, which is also called *cortisol,* was introduced as a prescription drug more than 30 years ago. Efforts have been repeated since then to have it approved for nonprescription use, culminating in the present Panel's recommendation that it be sold over-the-counter. The FDA did not object—though it still might do so—and over-the-counter marketing of hydrocortisone preparations began in 1980. A year later, the FDA said it had not seen any problems as a result of this change.

Despite its great potency—which is one reason for the FDA's reluctance to permit it to be marketed without prescription—hydrocortisone has been shown to be an extremely safe drug in many scientifically controlled animal and human studies. In fact, aside from aspirin, it may be the best-studied external analgesic ingredient. Hydrocortisone is particularly safe in the relatively weak concentrations for which over-the-counter sale now is authorized. One report reviewed 90 different clinical trials on 12,000 human subjects, among whom only 222 adverse reactions were cited. All were mild and, for the most part, were caused by the base in which the drug was formulated or were due to some contaminant. No case of skin irritation or sensitivity was found.

The hydrocortisone preparations are very effective. The Panel says unequivocally: "Hydrocortisone and hydrocortisone acetate are two of the most potent and effective agents for the treatment of many common skin diseases." In a wide variety of studies on the treatment of contact dermatitis, itchiness of the vulva and anus, eczema, and other skin conditions, the majority of patients experience improvement or total relief of symptoms.

In the low concentrations approved for over-the-counter use, hydrocortisone and hydrocortisone acetate can be used for the temporary relief of minor skin irritations, itching, and rashes due to eczema, dermatitis, insect bites, poison ivy-oak-sumac, detergents, cosmetics, and jewelry and for itchy genital and anal areas. They are safe and effective.

- **JUNIPER TAR:** A pungent, oil extract from the wood of the juniper tree, this is a traditional "folk" remedy that has a number of exotic names, including *oil of cade*, *Haarlem oil*, *bili-drops*, *Holland balsam*, and *silver balsam*. It is dark brown in color, with a smoky aroma and an acrid, slightly aromatic bitter taste.

    Although juniper tar can be harmful if accidentally swallowed, localized application is of value in relieving minor skin irritation and itching. Despite scanty scientific data, long use persuaded the Panel to judge the ingredient safe and effective for topical use.

- **LIDOCAINE:** A topical anesthetic of the *-caine* type, lidocaine has been widely used by doctors and first-aiders. It is very safe when applied to small areas of wounded or itchy skin, and irritation and sensitization of the skin are rare. The ingredient is especially effective in treating itchiness, irritation, and pain of the mucous membranes. However, *large* amounts applied to wide areas of bruised or broken skin can cause severe—even fatal—damage to the heart and arteries and the nervous system. Label warnings should caution consumers not to use lidocaine in large quantities, especially over raw or blistered surfaces. Consumers should heed these warnings.

    Lidocaine is effective as a topical anesthetic if judiciously used, and, in a suitable base (vehicle), it will penetrate both broken and unbroken skin. It may start to act within minutes, and its benefit can continue for several hours if the base keeps the active ingredient in touch with the skin. Verdict: safe and effective.

- **LIDOCAINE HYDROCHLORIDE:** This compound is very similar to lidocaine (just described) except that it cannot penetrate unbroken skin. So its use is not recommended when the skin remains intact. Neither should it be used in large quantities over raw or blistered skin. However, when used in the recommended manner, the ingredient is judged safe and effective.

- **MENTHOL:** A minty-smelling alcohol, menthol is extracted from natural peppermint or manufactured synthetically. At relatively high concentrations of 1.25 to 16 percent it is stimulating and mildly irritating to the skin and is used as an ingredient in liniments and rubs. When used in low concentrations of 0.1 up to 1 percent, menthol—which is usually combined with camphor or other external analgesic ingredients—is a safe and effective means of relieving itching and pain. Menthol will penetrate unbroken as well as injured skin to reach sensory nerve endings.

- **PHENOL:** A coal-tar derivative, phenol is sometimes called *carbolic acid.* It is the source of what many people have come to think of as *the* "medicinal smell." Phenol easily penetrates the outer layers of the skin and acts somewhat as the *-caine* drugs do, relieving pain and deadening feeling. It also makes itching subside.

     The problem with phenol is that a relatively weak concentration—say 5 percent—can cause serious skin burns and even internal injury if it is absorbed. Mixed with water, even a 2 percent solution is too irritating to be applied to the skin. However, somewhat stronger concentrations are judged to be safe if the substance is dissolved in glycerin, or in mineral oil, along with camphor.

     Despite questions about phenol's capacity to irritate skin and some National Cancer Institute studies that conceivably might lead the FDA to ban the substance as a nonprescription ingredient, the Panel says phenol is safe and effective when used as directed and in the proper concentrations. (*See* the Safety and Effectiveness of Active Ingredients table at the end of this Unit.) The FDA concurs at this time. Experts warn that phenol should be applied only to the smallest possible areas of skin and should *never* be covered with a compress or bandage; covering the phenol may cause it to burn the skin. *This substance thus should never be used to treat diaper rash in babies.* It also is dangerous if swallowed and must be kept away from children. Conclusion: safe and effective when used as directed.

- **PHENOLATE SODIUM:** As the name suggests, phenol is the active part of this compound, which may also be called *sodium phenoxide, sodium phenate, sodium carbolate,* or *phenol sodium.* It has much the same ability to relieve pain and itching as phenol (*see* the preceding entry) but also shares that substance's risks. In fact, it may be even more risky, because the sodium hydroxide in phenolate sodium is caustic.

     Despite these problems, this compound is rated safe on the basis of its wide and apparently safe use. On similar grounds, it is also judged effective in relieving pain and itching. Phenolate sodium rarely is sold as the sole active ingredient in over-the-counter products; it is usually combined with other active ingredients.

- **PRAMOXINE HYDROCHLORIDE:** Also called *pramocaine* and *proxazocain*, this topical anesthetic nevertheless is chemically different from the *-caine*-type of drug, and it appears to be essentially free of their systemic side effects. It irritates some mucous membranes and produces a burning sensation in the eyes, but it does not irritate the skin.

Evaluators say there are studies documenting the effectiveness of pramoxine hydrochloride as a nonprescription analgesic for injured skin but not unbroken skin. Their assessment: safe and effective.

• *RESORCINOL:* This compound, also known as *resorcin*, is a phenol-like alcohol that has the advantage of being less toxic than phenol. In the concentrations that are safe and effective for nonprescription use, it relieves itching but not pain. Resorcinol is readily absorbed through the skin. This enhances its medicinal value but it also means that—to avoid internal poisoning—it must be used only on small areas of skin.

The drug's safety record is difficult to interpret. On one hand, toxic reactions (even death) have been reported when resorcinol has been swallowed or, has even been applied to the skin of young babies. On the other hand, the Panel reviewed one product that has been marketed for 78 years without any report of substantial toxicity. So approval was granted.

WARNING:

 Do not apply resorcinol to large areas of the body.

• *TETRACAINE:* A potent *-caine*-type of anesthetic, tetracaine relieves itching and pain on both damaged and undamaged skin. It is a half-century-old drug, which is also called *amethocaine*, *pantocaine*, *decicaine*, *certacaine*, and *anethicaine*. The Panel bases its approval of tetracaine on a few scientific studies and on this ingredient's wide use and clinical acceptance.

Like other *-caine* drugs, tetracaine could interfere with brain and heart function if large amounts were applied to wide areas of injured skin and were absorbed. But this risk is remote if the drug is applied to the relatively small skin areas that a first-aider would treat without a doctor's help. Adverse skin reactions are rare.

Water-based (aqueous) tetracaine solutions lose their potency within months. So products should be replaced if they have been stored for long in the medicine chest.

Tetracaine penetrates both intact and injured skin, relieving itching and pain. When the skin is damaged, it induces numbness, too. The drug provides relatively long-lasting relief.

WARNING:

 Do not use in large quantities, particularly on raw surfaces or blistered areas.

• *TETRACAINE HYDROCHLORIDE:* This compound has pharmaceutical properties very similar to tetracaine (as described in the preceding paragraphs). The shelf life is known to be less than one year, so products that have been stored in the medicine cabinet may no longer be effective.

When applied to the mucous membrane, tetracaine hydrochloride is converted to tetracaine and rapidly absorbed. However, this conversion does not occur on unbroken skin, which tetracaine hydrochloride penetrates too slowly to be of medicinal value. It is effective only when the skin is scraped or otherwise broken.

Tetracaine hydrochloride is capable of causing convulsions and slowed heart rate if large amounts are absorbed. Therefore it never should be used over wide areas of damaged skin. However, standard first-aid use of this ingredient has not led to toxicity reports in the medical literature, even though less serious, allergic reactions have been documented. Verdict: safe and effective.

• *TRIPELENNAMINE HYDROCHLORIDE:* This substance is an antihistamine that will cause numbness, thus relieving itching in the skin due to allergic and irritative eruptions of poison ivy, bee sting, and similar causes that may be the result of histamine's release in the body.

When taken orally, tripelennamine hydrochloride can cause drowsiness. But too little of the drug is absorbed through the skin from topical ointments and creams to cause this problem. Users eventually may, however, become sensitive to this medication, for which reason it should not be applied longer than a week except under medical supervision. Conclusion: safe and effective.

CONDITIONALLY APPROVED ACTIVE INGREDIENTS

Evaluators assessed several other anti-itch, anti-pain agents and could find no solid evidence that they actually work.

• *GLYCOL SALICYLATE:* This ingredient is related chemically to aspirin. A label reader may find it variously listed as *glycol monosalicylate, monoglycol salicylate, ethylene glycol monosalicylate,* or *2-hydrox-*

yethyl salicylate. Long use, together with a paucity of reports on adverse effects, indicates that the ingredient is safe. But on the matter of relieving superficial pain or itching when applied to the skin, the Panel noted that no significant topical pain-relieving or numbing activity can be demonstrated. Conclusion: not proved effective.

• TROLAMINE SALICYLATE (TRIETHANOLAMINE SALICYLATE): A salicylate, like aspirin, this compound has been used in topical preparations for years. It appears to be harmless. But there is not enough evidence to show that it works when applied to the skin. Conclusion: not proved effective.

DISAPPROVED ACTIVE INGREDIENTS
None.

UNCATEGORIZED ACTIVE INGREDIENTS

• PHENYLTOLOXAMINE DIHYDROGEN CITRATE: The FDA authorized manufacturers to use this antihistamine in topical preparations in place of methapyrilene, which was withdrawn from the market because it may cause cancer. No assessment of the safety and effectiveness of phenyltoloxamine dihydrogen citrate has as yet been published within the context of the OTC Drug Review.

• PYRILAMINE MALEATE: The FDA authorized manufacturers to formulate this antihistamine into external analgesic products after methapyrilene was removed from the market because of its cancer-causing risk. The agency has not yet published an assessment of pyrilamine maleate's effectiveness for over-the-counter topical use within the context of the OTC Drug Review.

When Greater Relief Is Needed

For the relief of itching, hydrocortisone and hydrocortisone acetate are listed by drug evaluators (AMA *Drug Evaluations Annual*, 1991, p. 1027) as only *mildly potent.* Prescription corticosteroids range upward in strength to *super potent*, which is to say that they are much, much stronger. So, much greater relief is available from a doctor. Similarly, for pain, far stronger topical anesthetics are available on prescription (℞).

Safety and Effectiveness: Active Ingredients in Over-the-Counter Itch and Pain Relievers

Active Ingredient*	Pharmacological Group	Approved Concentration (%)	Assessment†
benzocaine	1	5-20	safe and effective
benzyl alcohol	2	10-33	safe and effective
butamben picrate	1	1	safe and effective
camphor	2	0.1-3	safe and effective
camphorated metacresol	2	camphor 3-10.8%, metacresol 1-3.6%	safe and effective
dibucaine	1	0.25-1	safe and effective
dibucaine hydrochloride	1	0.25-1	safe and effective
dimethisoquin hydrochloride	1	0.3-0.5	safe and effective
diphenhydramine hydrochloride	3	1-2	safe and effective
dyclonine hydrochloride	1	0.5-1	safe and effective
glycol salicylate	4		safe but not proved effective
hydrocortisone	5	0.25-1	safe and effective
hydrocortisone acetate	5	0.25-1	safe and effective

Safety and Effectiveness: Active Ingredients in Over-the-Counter Itch and Pain Relievers (contd)

Active Ingredient*	Pharmacological Group	Approved Concentration (%)	Assessment†
juniper tar	2	1-5	safe and effective
lidocaine	1	0.5-4	safe and effective
lidocaine hydrochloride	1	0.5-4	safe and effective
menthol	2	0.1-1	safe and effective
phenol	2	0.5-1.5	safe and effective
phenol + camphor in light mineral oil	2	phenol 4.7 + camphor 10.8	safe and effective
phenolate sodium	2	0.5-1.5	safe and effective
phenyltoloxamine dihydrogen citrate	3		not assessed
pramoxine hydrochloride	1	0.5-1	safe and effective
pyrilamine maleate	3		not assessed
resorcinol	2	0.5-3	safe and effective
tetracaine	1	1-2	safe and effective
tetracaine hydrochloride	1	1-2	safe and effective

(trolamine salicylate) triethanolamine salicylate	4		safe but not proved effective
tripelennamine hydrochloride	3	0.5-2	safe and effective

* Group 1, amines and chemically related -caine drugs; group 2, alcohols and ketones; group 3, antihistamines; group 4, salicylates; group 5, hydrocortisone preparations.

† For persons over the age of 2 years; use on younger children should be supervised by a physician.

Safety and Effectiveness: Combination Products Sold Over-the-Counter to Relieve Itching and Pain

Safe and Effective Combinations

may include a safe and effective combination of these safe and effective ingredients

    1 -caine drug or amine + 1 alcohol

    1 alcohol or ketone + 1 antihistamine

    camphor + menthol

    camphor + menthol + any one other alcohol or ketone

    camphor 10.8% + phenol 4.1% in light mineral oil

    any approved single ingredient or combination + any approved single protectant or combination of protectants (*See* pp. 568-575).

    any approved single ingredient or combination + any approved single first-aid antiseptic or approved combination of first-aid antiseptics

Conditionally Safe or Conditionally Effective Combinations

a combination is only conditionally approved if it

    contains any conditionally approved active ingredient

    contains any approved ingredient at less than an effective concentration

Unsafe or Ineffective Combinations

a combination is considered unsafe or ineffective if it

    contains any unsafe or ineffective ingredient

    contains hydrocortisone + any other itch-pain relieving active ingredient

    contains any ingredient that has not been evaluated by a panel or the FDA, or has been found unsafe, ineffective, or irrational by another panel

    contains a salicylate + a sunscreen active ingredient (the pain reliever may mask the symptoms of oncoming sunburn)

    contains any active ingredient for relieving itch and pain + any counterirritant active ingredient, since the former depresses and the latter stimulates nerve endings in the skin, the combination is irrational.

By checking this Unit's Safety and Effectiveness table, label readers can determine the pharmacological group to which any single compound belongs. For example, dimethisoquin hydrochloride is a -caine drug and diphenhydramine hydrochloride is an antihistamine. In most cases, the pharmacological group is fairly obvious from the compound's name. For example, benzyl alcohol is an alcohol; tetracaine is a -caine drug; triethanolamine salicylate is a salicylate.

Itch and Pain Remedies Applied to the Skin: Product Ratings

SINGLE-INGREDIENT PRODUCTS*

Product and Distributor	Dosage of Active Ingredients	Rating†	Comment
benzocaine			
Americaine Topical Anesthetic (Fisons)	spray, ointment: 20%	A	
butamben picrate			
Butesin Picrate (Abbott)	ointment: 1%	A	
dibucaine			
Dibucaine Hydrochloride (generic)	ointment: 1%	A	
Nupercainal (Ciba)	ointment: 1%	A	
Nupercainal (Ciba)	cream: 0.5%	A	
diphenhydramine hydrochloride			
Benadryl (Parke-Davis)	cream, spray: 1%	A	
Maximum strength Benadryl (Parke-Davis)	cream, spray: 2%	A	

Itch and Pain Remedies Applied to the Skin: Product Ratings (contd)

Product and Distributor	Dosage of Active Ingredients	Rating†	Comment
hydrocortisone			
Bactine Hydrocortisone (Miles)	**cream:** 0.5%	A	℞ to OTC switch
Cortizone-5 (Thompson)		A	
Dermolate Anti-Itch (Schering)		A	
Cortizone-5 (Thompson)	**ointment:** 0.5%	A	℞ to OTC switch
CaldeCort Anti-Itch (Fisons)	**spray:** 0.5%	A	℞ to OTC switch
Cortizone-10 (Thompson)	**cream:** 1%	A	℞ to OTC switch
Maximum Strength Cortaid (Upjohn)	**cream, ointment, spray:** 1%	A	℞ to OTC switch
Anusol-HC (Parke-Davis)	**ointment:** 1%	A	℞ to OTC switch
Cortizone-10 (Thompson)		A	
Tegrin-HC (Block)		A	
hydrocortisone acetate			
CaldeCort (Fisons)	**cream:** 0.5% hydrocortisone equivalent	A	℞ to OTC switch

Lanacort 5 (Combe)	cream: 0.5%	A	℞ to OTC switch
Extra Strength Gynecort 10 (Combe)	cream: 1%	A	℞ to OTC switch
Lanacort 10 (Combe)	ointment, cream: 1%	A	℞ to OTC switch
lidocaine			
Solarcaine (Schering-Plough)	cream: 0.5%	A	
Xylocaine (Astra)	ointment: 2.5%	A	
pramoxine hydrochloride			
Prax (Ferndale)	cream: 1%	A	
Tronothane (Abbott)		A	
tetracaine			
Pontocaine (Winthrop)	cream: 1% as hydrochloride	A	
	ointment: 0.5%	C	too weak
trolamine salicylate (triethanolamine salicylate)			
Mobisyl Creme (Ascher)	cream: 10%	B	not proved effective
Myoflex Creme (Fisons)		B	not proved effective

*Products are arranged by dosage form and strength of active ingredients.
†Author's interpretation of FDA criteria. Based on contents, not claims.

Itch and Pain Remedies Applied to the Skin: Product Ratings (contd)

ANESTHETIC-BASED COMBINATION PRODUCTS—PRINCIPALLY FOR PAIN

Product and Distributor	Dosage of Active Ingredients	Rating*	Comment
Bicozene (Sandoz)	cream: 6% benzocaine + 1.67% resorcinol	A	
Campho-Phenique (Sterling Health)	liquid: 4.7% phenol + 10.8% camphor in light mineral oil	A	
Dermoplast (Whitehall)	lotion: 8% benzocaine + 0.5% menthol	A	
	spray: 20% benzocaine + 0.5% menthol	A	
Feminine Gold (Au Pharmaceuticals)	lotion: 3% menthol + 2.5% camphor	C	too much menthol
Foille Plus (Blistex)	spray: 5% benzocaine + 0.6% chloroxylenol + 57% alcohol	B	chloroxylenol not proved safe or effective
Itch-X (Ascher)	gel: 1% pramoxine hydrochloride + 10% benzyl alcohol	A	
Lanacane (Combe)	spray: 20% benzocaine + 0.1% benthzethonium chloride	A	

Product and Distributor	Dosage of Active Ingredients	Rating	Comment
Lanacane (Combe)	**spray:** 20% benzocaine + 0.1% benthzethonium chloride	A	—
Solarcaine (Schering-Plough)	**spray:** 20% benzocaine + 0.13% triclosan	B	triclosan not proved safe or effective as antimicrobial
Unguentine Plus (Mentholatum)	**cream:** 2% lidocaine + 2% chloroxylenol + 0.5% phenol	B	chloroxylenol not proved safe or effective as antimicrobial

ANTIHISTAMINE-BASED COMBINATION PRODUCTS—PRINCIPALLY FOR ITCHINESS

Product and Distributor	Dosage of Active Ingredients	Rating*	Comment
Caladryl Cream (Parke-Davis)	**cream:** 1% diphenhydramine hydrochloride + 8% calamine	A	
Caladryl Lotion (Parke-Davis)	**lotion:** 1% diphenhydramine hydrochloride + 8% calamine	A	

*Author's interpretation of FDA criteria. Based on contents, not claims.

Jock Itch, Athlete's Foot, and Ringworm Cures

Several of the most modern and effective nonprescription drugs introduced in recent decades are topical antifungal agents used to treat jock itch, athlete's foot, and some forms of ringworm. The Panel described these drugs' effectiveness enthusiastically and succinctly when it said that "unlike other OTC products, [they] treat disease rather than symptoms." That is to say, they are *curative* drugs.

 Claims

Accurate
- "For the treatment of athlete's foot (*tinea pedis*)"
- "Cures jock itch (*tinea cruris*)"
- "Clears up athlete's foot, jock itch, and ringworm"

JOCK ITCH, ATHLETE'S FOOT, AND RINGWORM CURES is based on the report "Topical Anti-fungal Drug Products for OTC Human Use" by the FDA's Advisory Review Panel on OTC Antimicrobial Drug Products (Antimicrobial II Panel) and the FDA's Tentative Final Monograph on these products.

- "Proven clinically effective in the treatment of ringworm (*tinea corporis*)"
- "Treats athlete's foot, jock itch, and ringworm"
- "Proven to kill dermatophytic fungi and yeast" (causes of athlete's foot)
- "Prevents," or "helps prevent athlete's foot with daily use," or "guards against athlete's foot with daily use" is accurate *only* for the drug tolnaftate, when used against athlete's foot, *not* against jock itch or ringworm.

WARNING:

 These drugs should not be used on children under 2 years of age except under the advice and supervision of a doctor. They should be used by children under 12 years old only under parental supervision.

What is Fungus?

The funguses (or *fungi*) that cause human skin diseases are microorganisms that belong to a primitive group of plant-like organisms that lack the green pigment chlorophyll. For this reason they must derive their life energy from other living things, rather than from the rays of the sun. The fungal molds that cause jock itch and athlete's foot obtain their vital energy by breaking down *keratin,* the horny substance that provides strength and structure to hair, nails, and skin. Molds and yeasts are both funguses, and so, of course, are mushrooms. Most of the funguses that cause jock itch, athlete's foot, and ringworm on the body are molds.

The common skin-disease funguses that afflict people normally grow in the soil. But they can also thrive on human bodies, especially in warm, moist areas like the crotch, toe webs, and underarms and in protected and concealed places in the hair or under the nails. They may also cause infection in normal, dry skin.

Fungal Infections

Fungal infections are typically itchy and red. They may become quite painful, particularly if the skin cracks so that bacteria can enter and start secondary infections. The tissue may look and smell decayed or rotten. In some fungal attacks there is a secondary eruption elsewhere on the body, called a *dermatophytid reaction*. It may consist of hard pimples that tend to arise around hair follicles, bruise-like lesions, hives, or ring-shaped red rashes. The cause of these eruptions—which may be accompanied by fever, malaise, and loss of appetite—is unclear. They are not secondary fungal infestations but rather appear to be defensive over-reactions, in which the white blood cells attack noninfected skin in much the same way that they attack the moldy skin at the infection site.

More than 200,000 funguses have been discovered and described in the scientific literature. Only very few, fortunately, cause human diseases, albeit some of these diseases are grotesquely disfiguring, incurable, and eventually lethal. The funguses that cause jock itch and athlete's foot are much less worrisome and now can be treated much more successfully than in the past. Yet anyone who has suffered from these disorders knows they can be tenaciously annoying and frustratingly difficult to cure.

Jock itch and athlete's foot tend to be caused by the same funguses, particularly *Trichophyton rubrum*, *T. mentagrophytes*, and *Epidermophyton floccosum*. The first is more commonly found on the feet, the last, more commonly in the groin. Ringworm of the body is commonly caused by *Microsporum canis*, which, as its name implies, is transmitted by dogs (but also by cats).

A number of different diseases may create itchy, unpleasant-appearing lesions that look a lot like jock itch or athlete's foot. Bacterial infections can cause itchy scaling and redness between the toes. Psoriasis, a scaly disease of unknown cause, creates itchy patches in the toe webs and groin that look very much like fungus. *See* PSORIASIS LOTIONS. Allergic responses to shoe material, sock dyes, or other footwear components sometimes are mistaken for athlete's foot.

If you are in doubt, or if self-treatment with a nonprescription drug does not quickly relieve the itching and pain and begin to clear up the skin, then seek a dermatologist's help. Simple tests are available to pinpoint the cause of distressing skin complaints in the groin or on the feet.

Athlete's Foot

This skin disease is technically called *tinea pedis*, which means foot fungus. Soldiers who suffer severe cases of it in the tropics call it "jungle rot."

The characteristic "cheesy" smell, however, is not caused by the fungi themselves, but rather by tag-along bacteria called *Brevibacterium.* They break the amino acid *methionine* in the skin down to the metabolite methanethiol, which is the gas that gives cheddar cheese its characteristic odor.

Athlete's foot usually originates in the toe webs, the areas between the toes. The rash is itchy, red, and scaling; the toe webs may appear white and soggy. The white scale is particularly common between the fourth and fifth toes. Cracks commonly appear. Blisters and pimples may erupt on the soles of the feet, so that walking becomes painfully difficult at best. These disabling symptoms often occur because the original fungal infection has opened the skin up to bacteria. Sometimes the infectious molds invade and destroy the toenails.

Athlete's foot is more common in men than in women, and it occurs most frequently in men between the ages of 15 and 40 years. It may be picked up at summer camps or resorts, military bases or prisons, or other places where there are many bare or dirty feet. The offending funguses are everywhere, however, so the question of why some people get athlete's foot and others do not has not been satisfactorily answered. The Panel noted that many people who are plagued by recurrent fungal skin diseases also suffer from asthma, hay fever, or atopic eczema—conditions in which the body's protective immune mechanism appears to be somewhat defective.

The standard recommendations for preventing athlete's foot or limiting its spread once it has occurred are to wash the feet once or twice daily with soap and water, keep them dry, and, if possible, cool. Each foot has 125,000 sweat glands that produce moisture, especially when the feet are hot. For this reason, you also should select absorbent cotton socks and light, ventilated shoes that "breathe" rather than boots or other thick, heavy shoes.

"Curing" athlete's foot, insofar as that means clearing up all symptoms, may not end the problem. Some dermatologists believe the fungi can never be wholly eliminated, and that some fungal spores or cells will always remain hidden in skin cracks and nail beds. Then when conditions are again right for them, they regrow—even many summers later.

Since the body *can* build up a protective immunity against these funguses, the question is often asked: Why do these conditions recur?

The answer may be that the blood-borne antibodies that could destroy the funguses are unable to reach the outermost layers of the skin in which athlete's foot occurs.

Because of the risk of recurrences, reviewers see some value in using antifungal medication on a *preventive* basis once the original infection has been cleared up. However, only one nonprescription drug, tolnaftate, is approved as safe and effective for preventing athlete's foot.

Jock itch

This persistent and recurring fungal infection of the upper, inner thighs and groin is most common in men between the ages of 18 and 40 years. It is rare in children and uncommon in women. The technical name is *tinea cruris*, but it more likely to be recognized by the slangier names "crotch rot" and "dhobie itch." There does not seem to be a generally recognized name for these infections when they occur in women; the Panel suggests that the term *intertrigo,* which has the more general meaning of an inflammation or an eruption in a skinfold area, might serve.

Jock itch usually originates in the crease between the inner thigh and the scrotum. It may spread around the groin, down the thigh, and across the scrotum and penis. The rash is red, scaly, and quite itchy, and often has a ring-like curved margin along the thigh and the scrotum. This expanding margin may be raised and flaky while the center of the rash, having begun to heal, is stained a light brown color by blood and other breakdown products of inflammation.

No certain way is known to prevent jock itch. But cleanliness and the avoidance of tight, air-tight, or chafing underwear and outerwear undoubtedly help, since fungal infections usually start in warm, moist, damaged skin.

Body Ringworm

Itchy ring-shaped eruptions on children's bodies are very likely to be body ringworm, or *tinea corporis*. They commonly are caused by the fungus *M. canis*, carried by pets. The "rings" may be red, scaly, and quite itchy, while the areas inside the rings heal rather quickly. Despite the name *ringworm*, this disorder is a fungus infection. *Ringworm is not caused by or associated with worms of any kind.*

Scalp Ringworm and Nail Ringworm

The technical names for scalp ringworm and nail ringworm are *tinea capitis* and *tinea unguium*: fungal infection of the head and of the "claws" (nails), respectively. The ring shape of the lesion is a strong indication that it is caused by a fungus: No worm of any kind is involved.

These fungal infections may be hard to self-diagnose and they are certainly very hard to self-treat, since antifungal powders, sprays, and liquids penetrate only poorly to the hair roots and nail beds where the funguses have set up housekeeping. Systemically applied medication prescribed by a doctor will probably be needed.

Evaluators warn that the topical drugs described in this Unit are not effective for treating ringworm of the scalp and the nails. Persons who think they are suffering such an infection should see their doctor for diagnosis and treatment.

Candidiasis

Not all crotch and toe fungal diseases are caused by molds. Certain yeasts, which are also funguses, can cause horrific itching and other symptoms that may be indistinguishable from those caused by the aforementioned molds.

The best-known—and very likely the least loved—of these yeasts is a species called *Candida albicans*. The disease it causes is called *candidiasis*, or *monilia*, or *moniliasis*, or simply "yeast."

Like the molds, *C. albicans* thrives in warm, moist body areas like the toe webs and groin. On the feet, it causes redness, toe rot, and cracking between the toes. In the groin it produces bright, red, weepy rashes with many pimple-like bumps along their outer edge. These eruptions are extremely itchy. In men, they often spread to the scrotum and the outside of the rectum. In women the pattern may be similar, but the disorder is usually associated with what experts call *extreme* itching of the vulva, as well as with a characteristic white, unpleasant-smelling vaginal discharge. (Women who suspect that they have candidiasis should consult the Unit 'YEAST' KILLERS FOR FEMININE ITCHING.)

These eruptions may also occur on other parts of the body. The yeast appears to be everywhere in the human environment, yet most people resist it most of the time. Risk factors include diabetes, pregnancy, obesity, profuse sweating, and the use of certain drugs, particularly birth-control pills, oral corticosteroid drugs, and broad-spectrum antibiotics.

Rapid tests, which can be conducted in a dermatologist's or a gynecologist's office, will differentiate yeast infections from the molds that more often are the cause of jock itch, athlete's foot, and ringworm. This diagnostic step is important because most drugs used against molds are not comparably effective against yeast. A few special antifungals, however, will kill both molds and yeast.

Given that the victim of these infections may not be able to tell which organism is causing his or her grief, the Panel felt that there is a therapeutic advantage can be gained by using either a broad-spectrum antifungal or a drug that acts against *both* molds and yeast.

The FDA takes a more cautious view of self-treatment of candidal infections. It insists that candidiasis must be diagnosed originally by a doctor, and preferably treated under his or her supervision at first. Later, when a person has become aware of the symptoms, and the drugs that will relieve the condition, self-diagnosis and self-treatment with over-the-counter drugs is appropriate, the agency says.

Treatment

Though it may seem surprising, since they occur at very different parts of the anatomy, jock itch, athlete's foot, and ringworm of the body respond to the same drugs. This is because most cases are caused by very similar species of molds or yeasts.

Many people routinely self-treat jock itch and athlete's foot with medicated powders and sprays. However, as several available drugs will limit fungal growth but will not kill all residual fungus cells, the conditions constantly recur. Sufferers become accustomed to them and come to regard them as an unavoidable annoyance rather than as diseases that can be treated aggressively and very possibly cured.

Fatalistic acceptance of fungal afflictions can have two dangerous consequences. At a moment when the body defenses for some reason are suddenly weakened, a minor fungal condition can explode into a serious—even life-threatening—illness. Moreover, continuous use of antifungal drugs, particularly on injured or broken-down skin, can lead to the body's absorbing dangerous amounts of these compounds.

The Panel believed that stand-offs between fungus and hosts are dangerous and should not be allowed to continue. The Panel recommended that sufferers of these conditions use only those drugs that have the potential for *eradicating* the fungus rather than for just holding it in abeyance. The antifungal agents listed as approved have this capacity, although none has been shown to cure every case for which it is used. For this reason, if the condition has not been cleared up after a reasonable period of time—two weeks for jock itch and feminine itching; a month for athlete's foot and ringworm of the body—it may be wise to switch to a product that contains a different active ingredient, or better yet, visit a doctor.

Infected areas always should be washed with soap and water and dried thoroughly before the medicine is applied. Two applications daily, morning and night, should suffice, unless more frequent treatment is recommended by a doctor.

Dosage Forms

Antifungal active ingredients are formulated in a variety of bases that includes ointments, creams, powders, liquids, and aerosol sprays. The Panel believed that a soluble form is the most effective; these preparations include rapidly evaporating liquids (like alcohol-acetone solutions) and aerosol sprays. They dry quickly and leave the antifungal agent in close contact with the skin. It may be much more difficult for the active drug to reach the skin and fungus cells when it is formulated in an ointment, cream, or powder.

Drying Agents

Many antifungal preparations are formulated in a starch, alcohol, or other substance that dries the skin. Drying is useful, but the Panel considered drying agents to be inactive ingredients.

Combination Products

In order for a combination of two or three antifungals to be approved as safe and effective, each active ingredient must be safe and effective and must be present in the approved dosage. Each must contribute to the product by broadening the range of funguses against which the drug is effective. The FDA says no such combination is currently marketed over-the-counter.

Comparison of Safe and Effective Anti-Fungal Active Ingredients

Ingredient	Can Cure Jock Itch, Athlete's Foot, Ringworm of Body	Can Cure Yeast Infections (C. albicans)	Proved Safe and Effective for Preventing Athlete's Foot
clioquinol (3%)	yes	no	no
clotrimazole (1%)	yes	yes	no
miconazole nitrate (2%)	yes	yes	no
povidone-iodine (10%)	yes	yes	no
tolnaftate (1%)	yes	no	yes
undecylenates (10-25%) undecylenic acid, calcium undecylenate, copper undecylenate, and zinc undecylenate	yes	no	no

Evaluators also recommended the approval of several combinations of an antifungal agent with approved active ingredients of other classes. They appear particularly to approve combinations of 0.5 percent hydrocortisone or hydrocortisone acetate with one of the recently developed antifungals. Hydrocortisone acts quickly to relieve inflammation and to reduce itching, burning, and pain. Meanwhile, the antifungal attacks and kills the fungus—which takes a longer time.

Hydrocortisone and the new antifungals seem to act in a complementary fashion. The Panel reported that double-blind clinical studies demonstrate that hydrocortisone with miconazole or with clioquinol produces a significantly higher rate of cures than either hydrocortisone or one of the antifungals used alone. In one study done in South America with soldiers who had jock itch or athlete's foot, a combination of miconazole (2 percent) and hydrocortisone (1 percent) cured 97 percent of the men in 14 days. This result compared with a cure rate of 82 percent for miconazole alone and 6 percent for the hydrocortisone alone. According to the investigator who conducted the tests, these results were particularly impressive, because the subjects lived under the "worst conditions of heat, humidity, and poor hygiene."

However, the FDA has safety concerns about the combination of hydrocortisone and an antifungal in an over-the-counter product. None is approved as safe and effective.

The Panel also recommended approval of combinations of antifungal agents with one other active ingredient that has been approved as safe and effective as an antiperspirant or as a skin-peeling agent. However, the FDA is less enthusiastic about these combinations, which it says are not proved effective. It will not permit them to be sold over-the-counter. The combinations are listed in the Safety and Effectiveness: Combination Products table at the end of this Unit. Conditional approval was granted to a traditional antifungal preparation called Whitfield's ointment. This ointment is a combination of benzoic and salicylic acids in polyethylene glycol; its effectiveness has never been convincingly demonstrated.

Another widely used combination, called *carbol-fuchsin* solution (sometimes known as *Castellani's paint* or *Magenta paint BPC*), appears to be effective against several types of fungal disease. But most studies concerned with proving the merit of this mix used methods the Panel questioned. Worse, carbol-fuchsin contains carbolic acid (phenol) at dangerously high concentrations (4.5 percent), while the fuchsin, a red dye, is suspected to cause cancer. Given these risks, the evaluators assessed carbol-fuchsin as unsafe for over-the-counter sales and self-treatment, although it may be appropriate for use when supervised by a doctor.

Antifungal Drugs

APPROVED ANTIFUNGAL ACTIVE INGREDIENTS

The Panel identified six individual ingredients and one group of ingredients that it believed are safe and effective for self-treatment of jock itch, athlete's foot, and ringworm of the body. Clioquinol, clotrimazole, miconazole nitrate, povidone-iodine, tolnaftate, and the undecylenates (undecylenic acid and calcium, copper, or zinc undecylenate)—are already available over-the-counter. Haloprogin is a prescription drug that the evaluators recommended switching to nonprescription status. All of them have the virtue of being effective against yeasts, including *C. albicans*.

• CLIOQUINOL: This active ingredient effectively combats the molds that cause jock itch, athlete's foot, and ringworm of the body as well as some bacteria that may be responsible for secondary infections in persons suffering these itchy conditions. This drug was developed in the 1960s and has been carefully tested in animals and people, under stringent drug-approval standards. In the small amounts used on the skin clioquinol appears to be safe, although very large doses taken internally have been identified as the cause of a severe neurological disorder called *subacute myelooptic neuropathy*. The Public Citizen Health Research group petitioned the FDA, requesting that clioquinol be banned. The agency decided that the group's evidence showing that the drug could be absorbed through the skin in dangerous amounts was unreliable. Used as directed, the FDA said, clioquinol is safe.

Clioquinol cures between one-half and two-thirds of fungal infections, the evaluators reported. It seems from the Panel's comments that it is less effective than some of the other nonprescription antifungals. It is not useful against *C. albicans* yeast infections.

The safe and effective dose of clioquinol is a 3 percent concentration in a cream or other base applied twice daily to the toe webs, groin, or other body sites of adults and children over 2 years of age. Children under 12 years should have parental supervision when using the drug.

WARNING:

 Do not use on children under 2 years of age. Do not use for diaper rash.

• **CLOTRIMAZOLE:** This is an effective antifungal agent, which long was available only by prescription (℞). The FDA switched it to nonprescription status in 1989 on the manufacturer's petition, outside of the OTC Drug Review. It is effective against *C. albicans* "yeast" infections as well as the funguses that cause athlete's foot, jock itch, and ringworm. Chemically, clotrimazole is closely related to miconazole. (*See* further on.)

The *AMA Drug Evaluations Annual* 1991 calls clotrimazole a "useful" drug. Two to four weeks of treatment may be needed to cure a fungal infection with it, the AMA says. It adds: Side effects may include redness, stinging, blistering, and itching.

If athlete's foot is not cleared up within 4 weeks, or jock itch within 2 weeks, seek a doctor's help.

The approved dosage is 1 percent clotrimazole in a lotion or cream twice daily for adults and children over 2 years old. For younger children, ask the pediatrician. Children under 12 years old should be supervised in this use of clotrimazole products.

• **MICONAZOLE NITRATE:** This broad-spectrum antifungal works effectively against the yeast *C. albicans* as well as against the molds that cause jock itch, athlete's foot, and body ringworm.

Miconazole was approved by the FDA in the 1970s under the tight requirements in force at that time for all new drugs. It is one of a very few over-the-counter drugs about which an expert body like the present Panel can say: "Adequate, well-controlled animal and human toxicity studies were conducted." It is, in short, safe at manufacturers' recommended dosages.

Careful and well-controlled double-blind clinical tests (in which neither the investigator nor the patient knew who was receiving the active medication and who a dummy drug), have shown that miconazole is highly effective—even under difficult conditions. Among patients at an Air Force hospital in Mississippi, for example, 93 percent of the men who received the active drug were cleared of all signs and symptoms of their fungal disease. This compares very favorably with just 19 percent whose conditions cleared up on the dummy medication. No effort was made to induce these servicemen to bathe more often, dress differently, or change their habits in any other way. The miconazole also provided *fast* relief: Itching and burning had subsided in three-quarters of the men by the end of the third day.

In another test, in a crowded Florida prison, three-quarters of the inmates treated with the active drug experienced relief of itching within a week, compared with only one-tenth of those who applied the dummy medications to their toe webs, groins, or bodies. There was only one recurrence of fungal infection in the prisoners successfully treated with miconazole nitrate. These results indicate that in most such cases the drug successfully eliminates the causative organisms. Miconazole also is effective against the yeast infection *C. albicans* as well as against several bacterial infections that mimic jock itch and athlete's foot.

The safe and effective dosage is 2 percent miconazole nitrate in cream or another base, applied twice daily, for adults and children over 2 years old. For younger children, consult a physician. Youngsters under 12 years of age should be overseen by adults when they use this medication.

• POVIDONE-IODINE: The povidone in this complex binds iodine and then releases it onto the skin. When an iodine molecule is absorbed from the povidone onto the skin, or into a fungus, a fresh iodine molecule replaces it at the interface with the skin in a tiny fraction of a second. Animal and human studies persuaded the Panel and the FDA that povidone-iodine is safe.

Clinical studies have established its effectiveness. In one double-blind study (meaning that neither the users nor their doctors knew whether the user was applying 10 percent povidone-iodine or a dummy medication), two-thirds of athlete's foot sufferers were cured after a month of treatment. Less than half as many who used the dummy preparations were cured.

The FDA's decision, then, is that 10 percent povidone-iodine is safe and effective for athlete's foot, jock itch, and ringworm. Apply twice daily for children over age 2 years and adults. For younger children, consult a doctor. Children under 12 years old should be supervised by an adult. Jock itch should clear up within 2 weeks, athlete's foot, within a month. If not, show the condition to a doctor. Povidone-iodine is effective against yeast infections.

• TOLNAFTATE: An antifungal introduced in the 1960s, tolnaftate was shown to be both safe and effective in many studies conducted under the very demanding guidelines then required by the FDA and comparable agencies. In the Panel's view, these studies demonstrated that tolnaftate is safe and effective for treating jock itch, athlete's foot, and ringworm of the body. (Tolnaftate is not effective against bacteria or against *Candida albicans* and other yeasts.)

Tolnaftate is the only nonprescription drug that has been proved safe and effective for *preventing* athlete's foot. But, because the groin is a much more sensitive area than the feet, reviewers do not approve the ongoing use of the drug to prevent jock itch.

In recent years, tolnaftate has become the standard drug against which other topical antifungals are compared. It has a 90 percent cure rate in patients with athlete's foot.

The safe and effective dose for the treatment of jock itch, athlete's foot, and ringworm of the body is 1 percent tolnaftate twice daily in adults and children over 2 years of age; for younger children, consult a physician. Children under 12 years old should be supervised in their use of this drug. One or two applications daily are recommended when tolnaftate is used preventively against athlete's foot.

• UNDECYLENIC ACID AND ITS SALTS: CALCIUM UNDECYLENATE, COPPER UNDECYLENATE, AND ZINC UNDECYLENATE: Although they are only 40 years old, these are granddaddies among the approved antifungal agents. They are less potent than the new agents discussed above, and the cure rates, which in most studies run around 50 percent, also are lower.

The Panel described a fair number of animal and human tests that indicate that undecylenic acid and its compounds cause little irritation or other toxicity, so safety is not in question. The various undecylenates appear roughly comparable with each other in effectiveness, and they are often combined in products used to treat jock itch, athlete's foot, and ringworm of the body. These compounds do not work against yeast infections caused by *C. albicans*; neither will they cure bacterial infections.

A concentration of from 10 to 25 percent of one or more undecylenates is safe and effective for adults and children over 2 years old; for children under 2 years, consult a doctor. Children up to 12 years of age should be supervised when they use this medication.

CONDITIONALLY APPROVED ANTIFUNGAL ACTIVE INGREDIENTS

A wide range of standard over-the-counter drugs—many of them used for a variety of other purposes—are claimed to be beneficial in treating jock itch, athlete's foot, and ringworm of the body. Many are safe in the recommended dosages, according to the Panel. But for most of them, the evidence that allegedly proves that they work is weak or deficient in some way. Since there are several quite effective antifungal drugs that will cure a fair proportion of these infections, the less convincing medications will be described only cursorily.

- **ALUMINUM PREPARATIONS: ALCLOXA, ALUMINUM SULFATE, AND POTASSIUM ALUM:** These drugs are widely used as astringents and antiperspirants, and are generally regarded as safe. Low doses kill funguses in lab dishes, but higher doses are required to kill them between a person's toes. Tests conducted in an effort to prove effectiveness were questioned on grounds of poor methodology. In short, these aluminum preparations are safe but not proved effective.

- **BASIC FUCHSIN:** This red dye is suspected of causing cancer, so the Panel questioned its safety. It *does* kill bacteria and has been used for years to combat both bacteria and funguses. But there are no studies demonstrating its value against the specific funguses that are known to cause jock itch, athlete's foot, and ringworm of the body. So the Panel said basic fuchsin's safety and effectiveness remain to be proved. The FDA agreed.

- **BENZETHONIUM CHLORIDE:** This Panel, along with several others, found that this ingredient, a quaternary ammonium compound, is of doubtful safety, except when used for very brief periods. Furthermore, no data are available showing that it is effective when used alone against fungal infections. Conclusion: Both the safety and effectiveness of benzethonium chloride as an antifungal remain to be proved.

- **BENZOIC ACID:** A widely used over-the-counter medicine that is applied to the skin, benzoic acid is accepted as safe. In one study it was found to be almost as effective as undecylenic acid in treating jock itch and related fungal disorders. But reviewers say this study was flawed, and they want to see a first-rate clinical test done to determine how well benzoic acid actually works. The Panel's assessment of benzoic acid is: safe but not proved effective.

- **BORON COMPOUNDS: BORIC ACID AND SODIUM BORATE (BORAX):** These are common components of athlete's-foot powders. While borates have been used medicinally for over a thousand years, serious doubts have recently been raised about both their safety and effectiveness.

    In concentrations of under 5 percent, the Panel believed borates are safe, because only very small amounts are absorbed into the bloodstream. However, their effectiveness remains much in doubt: Only one test has been conducted to assess boric acid as an active ingredient against athlete's foot. The results were not convincing to the evaluators. Wanting better evidence, the Panel said that up to 5 percent boric acid or sodium borate is safe but not proved effective. Concentrations over 5 percent are not safe. The FDA concurred.

- CAPRYLATES: SODIUM CAPRYLATE AND ZINC CAPRYLATE: These compounds are derived from caprylic acid. This fatty acid occurs naturally in human sweat and has been found to inhibit fungal growth. The caprylates may cause some irritation, but clinical studies and long marketing experience—during which few adverse effects have been reported— persuaded the Panel that they are safe.

   Some old but rather well-conducted studies strongly indicate that these compounds are effective against jock itch, athlete's foot, and ringworm of the body. The Panel believed these compounds can be proved to be effective if rigorous scientific methods are used. Until this is done, however, it assessed them as safe but not proved effective.

   The caprylates have also been used experimentally and clinically against yeast infections caused by *C. albicans*. The results seem promising, but pending a double-blind controlled study in which caprylates are compared with a dummy medication, the Panel granted them only conditional approval for use against yeast infections.

- CHLOROTHYMOL: Although chlorothymol is a phenol-like drug, it is less toxic dose for dose than phenol. (*See* Phenolates: Phenol and Phenolate Sodium, further on in this section.) However, it is strongly irritating to the skin and mucous membranes, and so the Panel said chlorothymol's safety has yet to be established. As to effectiveness, the substance is strongly active against bacteria and has been shown to possess powerful antifungal properties in lab dishes. But it has not been established clinically whether chlorothymol relieves jock itch, athlete's foot, or ringworm of the body. In short: Chlorothymol has not been proved safe or effective.

- CHLOROXYLENOL: This Panel concluded that in the low doses (under 3 percent) used in a topical antifungal drug, chloroxylenol is safe. However, while chloroxylenol appears to kill funguses, well-devised double-blind studies that might confirm this supposition are yet to be done. Until they are, the Panel assessed the drug as safe but not proved effective.

   A study subsequently submitted to the FDA by a manufacturer was found to be methodologically faulty, so efficacy remains to be proved.

- CRESOLS: CAMPHORATED METACRESOL, M-CRESOL AND SECONDARY AMYLTRICRESOLS: These coal-tar derivatives are structurally related to phenol and share its toxic properties. Many cases of cresol toxicity have occurred, and chronic poisoning can result from application of cresols to the skin. Cresols effectively kill bacteria, and some studies show them to have antifungal properties as well. But only two studies—both uncontrolled—have been conducted on cresols' effectiveness against athlete's foot. One was done at an army base; the other, in a prison. Neither satisfactorily proved cresols effective. So the Panel decided that cresols are not proved safe or effective against the funguses that cause athlete's foot and related disorders.

- *DICHLOROPHEN:* This substance, commonly called *G-4*, is a phenol-like drug that has been used for flea powders, worm medicines, and other treatments for pets and farm animals. It is not marketed for oral human use in the United States but it is in Britain, where it is used against tapeworm. Dichlorophen is chemically related to the antiseptic hexachlorophene, which has been banned for nonprescription use because it is a nerve poison that has killed babies. The Panel was concerned about the risk of its use and wants its safety carefully studied.

  Dichlorophen is a fairly effective anti-bacterial. It appears to be less effective against funguses, and most studies to prove its effectiveness are poorly documented. Verdict: not proved safe or effective.

- *OXYQUINOLINES: BENZOXIQUINE, OXYQUINOLINE, AND OXYQUINOLINE SULFATE:* There is some evidence that these compounds may cause cancer, which worried the Panel. Studies that purport to show that the drugs are effective against fungal diseases were criticized for poor and unscientific design. Wanting better evidence on both counts—that is, safety and effectiveness—the Panel assessed the oxyquinolines as only conditionally approved as antifungal agents.

- *PARABENS: METHYLPARABEN AND PROPYLPARABEN:* These substances are widely used as drug preservatives at concentrations of 0.4 percent or lower. This is considered too low a level to cure jock itch or athlete's foot. Yet at therapeutic concentrations of 0.5 to 5 percent, the safety of the parabens has not been well established. Neither has their effectiveness been assessed in a systematic and scientific way, although one promising report was published back in 1944 on 5 percent methylparaben as an athlete's-foot medication. Lacking definitive evidence, evaluators concluded: not proved safe or effective.

- *PHENOLATES: PHENOL AND PHENOLATE SODIUM:* These coal-tar and benzene derivatives are among the drugs with a characteristically medicinal smell; they have been widely used as antiseptics and disinfectants for over a century. The Antimicrobial I Panel decided that at concentrations under 1.5 percent phenol may be safe. The FDA remains undecided, based on the evidentiary record. Mild to severe signs of body-system poisoning have been reported following applications of higher, 2 or 3 percent aqueous solutions of phenol to open wounds. Evidence for the phenolates' effectiveness as antifungals for treating athlete's foot, jock itch, and ringworm also is wanting. The FDA's tentative verdict: not proved safe or effective. Also, concentrations of *under* 1.5 percent are likely to be ineffective.

- **PHENYL SALICYLATE:** Also known as *salol*, this substance has been around for a century. Despite this long history of medicinal use, manufacturers failed to present the Panel with evidence to prove the substance's safety or effectiveness in treating jock itch or athlete's foot. So, until acceptable data are available, phenyl salicylate is listed as not proved safe or effective.

- **PROPIONIC ACID AND ITS SALTS: SODIUM PROPIONATE AND ZINC PROPIONATE:** Many studies have demonstrated that these compounds are essentially non-toxic. Also, a number of studies demonstrate the ability of the propionates to quell or prevent athlete's-foot infections. But a carefully controlled, double-blind study on a meaningfully large group of patients has yet to be done. Until it is, the Panel's verdict—and FDA's—is: safe but not proved effective.

- **SALICYLIC ACID:** In concentrations of 3 percent or less, salicylic acid applied to the skin is safe. Higher concentrations may be risky, the Panel said. Test data to show that salicylic acid effectively combats athlete's foot and similar fungal infections are inadequate. So pending more definitive results, the judgment is that salicylic acid is safe at concentrations up to 3 percent but not effective against fungal disorders.

- **SULFUR:** Hippocrates, the Father of Medicine, kept sulfur in his doctor's bag. This elemental substance has been used for a variety of illnesses since then. Sulfur can irritate the skin, and its safety when applied to the skin has virtually never been studied! Yet, the Panel hesitantly accepts sulfur as safe because of the drug's almost universal acceptance by dermatologists.

  There are no controlled studies demonstrating that sulfur effectively works against fungal diseases in humans. So the Panel had little choice but to mark it as safe but of unproved effectiveness.

- **TRIACETIN:** This compound releases glycerin and acetic acid when it is exposed to enzymes produced by some athlete's-foot funguses. Both breakdown products are non-injurious to the skin; accordingly, the Panel judged that triacetin, too, is non-injurious. The drug appears to be effective against the funguses *T. mentagrophytes* and *E. floccosum*, which produce a soggy-toe web form of athlete's foot, but supporting studies are still needed. Triacetin does not seem to be effective against *T. rubrum*, a fungus that produces a drier form of toe web trouble. Also, its value against jock itch and ringworm of the body remain to be determined. Pending new evidence to show that triacetin works, the drug is judged safe but not proved effective. The Panel noted that the drug should be used only against athlete's foot of the soggy, wet form.

DISAPPROVED ANTIFUNGAL ACTIVE INGREDIENTS

A number of compounds that have been labeled for use against fungal infections of the skin are dismissed by the Panel as unsafe or ineffective.

• *CAMPHOR:* Although considerable concern exists about camphor's safety, the low dosages used in treating athlete's foot are not likely to be hazardous. A mixture of camphor and phenol was used for years in the treatment of athlete's foot. Although it seems to have been relatively effective, careful and controlled scientific studies were never done. No evidence of effectiveness was or is available on the antifungal properties of camphor as a single active ingredient. The Panel classified it as not effective.

• *COAL TAR:* This is a blackish-brown distillation product from soft coal. The Panel was worried because coal contains chemicals that may cause cancer, and it also is a skin irritant. Furthermore, no adequate studies have shown that the substance is effective against funguses. The Panel judged coal tar as not safe for treating jock itch or athlete's foot.

• *MENTHOL:* Can this minty alcohol relieve athlete's foot or other fungal infections? There is no evidence that it can.

• *RESORCINOL:* A phenol-like compound, resorcinol appears to be more toxic even than phenol (*See* Phenolates, previously discussed.) The one marketed product containing resorcinol that was submitted contained 10 percent of the drug: The Panel considered this level in excess of what might be needed to achieve antifungal treatment goals. Worse, the evaluators could find no well-conducted clinical studies demonstrating that the drug really works against athlete's foot, jock itch, ringworm of the body, or any other superficial fungus—whether at low dose or high. So the Panel said that resorcinol's effectiveness has not been proved and that lack of safety is a matter of record. Conclusion: not safe.

- *TANNIC ACID:* Although this substance has been shown to be a potent liver poison, it reacts quickly with surface protein when applied to the skin: Little if any is likely to be absorbed unchanged into the body. The Panel, therefore, regarded it as safe. But because the Panel knew of no studies demonstrating that tannic acid has an antifungal property, it said: not effective.
- *THYMOL:* Thymol is irritating to the skin, so the Panel was not convinced of its safety. Does it work? The one controlled study done indicated that thymol is not effective against athlete's foot.

Safety and Effectiveness: Active Ingredients in Over-the-Counter Medications for Treating Jock-Itch, Athlete's Foot, and Ringworm

Active Ingredient	Assessment
alcloxa (*see* aluminum preparations)	
aluminum preparations: alcloxa, aluminum sulfate, potassium alum	safe but not proved effective
aluminum sulfate (*see* aluminum preparations)	
basic fuchsin	not proved safe or effective
benzethonium chloride	not proved safe or effective
benzoic acid	safe but not proved effective
benzoxiquine (*see* oxyquinolines)	
boron compounds: boric acid and sodium borate (borax) 　under 5%	safe but not proved effective
over 5%	not safe
boric acid (*see* boron compounds)	
calcium undecylenate (*see* undecylenic acid and its salts)	
camphor	not effective
camphorated metacresol (*see* cresols)	
caprylates: sodium caprylate and zinc caprylate	safe but not proved effective

Safety and Effectiveness: Active Ingredients in Over-the-Counter Medications for Treating Jock-Itch, Athlete's Foot, and Ringworm (contd)

Active Ingredient	Assessment
chlorothymol	not proved safe or effective
chloroxylenol	safe but not proved effective
clioquinol	safe and effective
clotrimazole	safe and effective
coal tar	not safe
copper undecylenate (*see* undecylenic acid and its salts)	
cresols: camphorated metacresol, *m*-cresol and secondary amyltricresols	not proved safe or effective
dichlorophen	not proved safe or effective
m-cresol (*see* cresols)	
menthol	safe but not proved effective
methylparaben (*see* parabens)	
miconazole nitrate	safe and effective
oxyquinolines: benzoxiquine, oxyquinoline, and oxyquinolinesulfate	not proved safe or effective
oxyquinoline sulfate (*see* oxyquinolines)	
parabens: methylparaben and propylparaben	not proved safe or effective
phenol (*see* phenolates)	
phenolates: phenol and sodium phenolate under 1.5%	safe but not proved effective
over 1.5%	not safe
phenyl salicylate	not proved safe or effective
potassium alum (*see* aluminum preparations)	

Safety and Effectiveness: Active Ingredients in Over-the-Counter Medications for Treating Jock-Itch, Athlete's Foot, and Ringworm (contd)

Active Ingredient	Assessment
povidone-iodine	safe and effective
propionic acid and its salts: sodium propionate and zinc propionate	safe but not proved effective
propylparaben (*see* parabens)	
resorcinol	not safe
salicylic acid (up to 3%)	safe but not proved effective
secondary amyltricresols (*see* cresols)	
sodium borate (*see* boron compounds)	
sodium caprylate (*see* caprylates)	
sodium phenolate (*see* phenolates)	
sodium propionate (*see* propionic acid and its salts)	
sulfur	safe but not proved effective
tannic acid	safe but not effective
thymol	not proved safe and not effective
tolnaftate	safe and effective
triacetin	safe but not proved effective
undecylenic acid and its salts: calcium undecylenate, copper undecylenate, and zinc undecylenate	safe and effective
zinc caprylate (*see* caprylates)	
zinc propionate (*see* propionic acid and its salts)	
zinc undecylenate (*see* undecylenic acid and its salts)	

Safety and Effectiveness: Combination Products Sold Over-the-Counter to Treat Funguses

---

Safe and Effective

None

Conditionally Safe and Effective

includes any conditionally approved ingredient contains an approved active ingredient at less than the minimal effective dose

1 anti-fungal + 1 antiperspirant

2 or 3 approved anti-fungals

1 or more anti-fungals + 1 skin-peeling agent

includes an antibacterial agent

Whitefield's ointment (benzoic acid 6 percent + salicylic acid 3 percent in polyethylene glycol)

Unsafe or Ineffective

contains any active ingredient disapproved by the FDA

contains 4 or more anti-fungal active ingredients

contains any local anesthetic, such as benzocaine

carbol-fuchsin

Jock Itch, Athlete's Foot, and Ringworm Cures: Product Ratings

SINGLE-INGREDIENT PRODUCTS

Product and Distributor	Dosage of Active Ingredients	Rating *	Comment
clioquinol			
Vioform (Ciba)	cream, ointment: 3%	A	
clotrimazole			
Lotrimin AF (Schering-Plough)	cream, solution, lotion: 1%	A	Rx to OTC switch
Mycelex (Miles)		A	Rx to OTC switch
miconazole nitrate			
Micatin (Ortho Pharm.)	cream, spray, powder: 2%	A	Rx to OTC switch
povidone-iodine			
Betadine (Purdue-Frederick)	spray and ointment: liberates about 10% iodine on skin	A	
tannic acid			
Zilactin Medicated (Zila)	gel: 7%	B	not proved effective
tolnaftate			
Aftate (Schering-Plough)	gel, powder, spray: 1%	A	

Jock Itch, Athlete's Foot, and Ringworm Cures: Product Ratings (contd)

Product and Distributor	Dosage of Active Ingredients	Rating *	Comment
Aftate for Jock Itch (Schering-Plough)	gel, powder: 1%	A	
Tinactin (Schering-Plough)	cream, powder, solution: 1%	A	
Tolnaftate (generic)	cream, powder, solution, spray: 1%	A	
undecylenic acid and its salts			
Cruex (Fisons)	powder: 10% calcium undecylenate, powder; aerosol: as undecylenic acid + zinc; cream: 20%	A	
Desenex (Fisons)	ointment: 22% as undecylenic acid + zinc undecylenate	A	
Desenex (Fisons)	powder: 19% as undecylenic acid + zinc undecylenate	A	

COMBINATION PRODUCTS

Product and Distributor	Dosage of Active Ingredients	Rating *	Comment
Blis-To-Sol (Chattem)	liquid: undecylenic acid + salicylic acid	B	conditionally approved combination; salicylic acid not proved effective

| Whitfield's (generic) | ointment: 6% benzoic acid + 3% salicylic acid | B | not proved safe |

*Author's interpretation of FDA criteria. Based on contents, not claims.

Kidney and Bladder Drugs: Preliminary Report

Several nonprescription preparations are marketed for the purpose of relieving kidney or bladder irritation and pain, and also for easing the flow of urine. One drug is also marketed for the treatment of benign prostatic hypertrophy (a nonmalignant enlargement of the prostate gland). However, it is unwise to attempt self-treatment of kidney, bladder, or prostate conditions without asking a doctor for his or her advice.

The over-the-counter drugs sold for the relief of urinary-tract problems were to have been evaluated by the FDA's Advisory Review Panel on Miscellaneous Internal Drug Products. The Panel was terminated before this task was started. At some point, the FDA or a new Panel may undertake the review. The FDA and its over-the-counter drug reviewers take a generally dim view of self-diagnosis of self-treatment of problems in major internal organs. It is surprising, therefore, that these products continue to be listed in drug compendia and are

KIDNEY AND BLADDER DRUGS: PRELIMINARY REPORT is based on FDA status reports on the OTC Drug Review.

readily available on druggists' shelves. Yet they are seemingly unregulated and ignored by the agency, which even has deleted these uses of these ingredients from its current status report on OTC drug ingredients.

The active ingredients in some of these nonprescription drugs intended for relief of kidney and bladder irritation are:

- *BENZOIC ACID*
- *METHENAMINE*
- *PHENAZOPYRIDINE HYDROCHLORIDE*
- *SALICYLAMIDE*
- *SODIUM SALICYLATE*

Laxatives

Constipation is defined by the standard *Dorland's Medical Dictionary* simply as "infrequent or difficult evacuation of the feces." Laxatives are drugs used to relieve this condition. These definitions are endorsed by the Panel—which comments that constipation is far less common and needs far less treatment than is often believed: "Preoccupation with the bowel seems to be the concern of a significant proportion of our population, judging from the inordinately large number of laxative agents available, and by the significant expenditure for over-the-counter laxatives."

An industry publication has reported that Americans spend more than $700 million yearly for laxatives and other elimination aids. Panel members believed that there is widespread overuse of laxatives and said that the pharmaceutical industry has contributed to the false impression that serious and health-endangering consequences will occur if the bowel is not evacuated daily.

LAXATIVES is based on the report of the FDA's Advisory Review Panel on OTC Laxative, Antidiarrheal, Emetic, and Antiemetic Drug Products and the FDA's two Tentative Final Monographs on these products.

Normal Bowel Function

Many people believe there is a need for one bowel movement a day. This is a myth.

What *is* normal bowel function? Reviewers found several recent studies that shed light on this question. In one study it was shown that, on the average, test subjects passed stools each 27 hours and 36 minutes, with a range of 9 hours to 57 hours. In another study, researchers found that 99 percent of adults fall within a range from three bowel movements per day down to three bowel movements per week. The Panel believes this is the normal range. So unless one is having fewer than three bowel movements weekly—or more than three each day—experts see no need for medications that either increase or decrease their number.

Constipation

Most often, constipation is caused by poor diet, particularly inadequate intake of dietary fiber or too little water and other fluids. Lack of exercise can also slow the bowels. Traveling, which imposes the need to use unfamiliar toilets, inhibits some people from defecating, and constipation may result.

The cures in these instances are fairly obvious: more roughage in the diet; intake of more water and other beverages; exercise; and a prompt response to the urge to defecate when it first is felt.

The use of laxatives should be, at most, a temporary measure. They should not be used on a regular basis, nor should they be used for any extended period of time. Experts say there are few reasons to take laxatives for more than a week, unless you are directed to do so by a physician.

Prolonged use of laxatives can seriously impair normal bowel function: People become dependent on laxatives. Serious consequences also may follow if laxatives are used when you have a stomachache, nausea and vomiting, or gastrointestinal symptoms related to conditions other than simple constipation. Any sudden change in bowel habits that persist for 2 weeks should prompt you to consult a doctor—*not* to reach for a laxative. The cause could be the onset of a serious disease.

Types of Laxatives

Several words are used to describe drugs that evacuate the bowels. *Cathartics* and *purgatives* are strong; they act rapidly to soften the stool or evacuate the bowel and should be used only under a doctor's supervision. *Laxatives* are supposed to be milder and act less precipitously, though a large dose may have a cathartic effect.

There are several different kinds of laxatives, and in this unit they are grouped according to these drug actions:

- **BULK-FORMING LAXATIVES:** Promote evacuation by increasing the stools' bulk volume and water content.
- **STIMULANT LAXATIVES:** Act directly on the intestinal wall to promote *peristalsis* (waves of muscular contraction that result in defecation).
- **SALINE LAXATIVES:** Draw water into the bowel, promoting movement.
- **HYPEROSMOTIC LAXATIVES:** Increase the water content of the stool.
- **STOOL SOFTENERS:** Penetrate and soften the stool.
- **LUBRICANT LAXATIVES:** These make the intestinal tract and fecal matter more slippery.
- **CARBON DIOXIDE-RELEASING LAXATIVES:** Suppositories that contain ingredients that release carbon dioxide in the rectum, creating gentle pressure that promotes bowel movement.

The Safety and Effectiveness table at the end of this Unit indicates which of these categories each laxative active ingredient belongs in, and records the FDA's present assessment of each ingredient's safety and effectiveness.

Before choosing a laxative, it would be well for the person who believes he is constipated to ask himself if he is trying to achieve an unnecessary regularity in bowel movements. He then should ask himself *what* the problem is—for example, too few bowel movements over a week's time, or alternatively, difficulty in passing a well-formed stool. Then he—or she—can select a product that contains an active ingredient that can relieve the specific complaint. The reviewers add one more guideline:

"The smallest dose of a laxative that is effective is the optimal dose to use."

The Panel found no evidence that any particular type of laxative is particularly advantageous for any set group of people (for example, older persons, younger ones, men, women), with one exception: Persons whose diets are low in fiber content may benefit from using bulk-forming laxatives.

Claims

Accurate
- "For the relief of occasional constipation (irregularity)"

The label should also state the product's mode of action. A bulk-forming laxative, for example, should say that it promotes the evacuation of the bowel by increasing bulk volume and water content of the stools.

WARNINGS:

 Do not use laxative products when abdominal pain, nausea, or vomiting are present unless directed by a doctor.

If you have noticed a sudden change in bowel habits that persist over a period of two weeks, consult a doctor before using a laxative.

Laxative products should not be used for a period longer than one week unless directed by a doctor.

Rectal bleeding or failure to have a bowel movement after using a laxative may indicate a serious condition. Discontinue use and consult your doctor.

Combination Products

The fewer active ingredients there are in any over-the-counter medicine, the better. For laxatives, which can waste body fluids and salt and cause cramping and loss of normal bowel function, the least-is-best rule is particularly appropriate.

Reviewers were stymied by a lack of data on the minimal effective doses for most laxative ingredients. In formulating its policy for combination products, the Panel therefore stipulated that each active ingredient be present in an amount *no lower* than the minimal approved dose when the ingredient is used alone. By the same token, there should be *no more* of each ingredient than the maximal approved dose when it is used alone. But these standards would still allow a consumer to take a combined dose that had almost twice the maximal laxative effect of either of 2 ingredients used by itself. To prevent this, the evaluators proposed a formula ensuring that no combination delivers more than 100 percent of a maximal effective dose. This formula is on p. 627, in footnote of table.

Bulk-Forming Laxatives

Bulk-forming laxatives increase the bulk volume and the water content of stools, which softens them, and makes them easier to evacuate. Some of the ingredients in this class are available as a dietary substance, *bran*, as well as in medicinal form. Experts view bulk-forming laxatives as one of the safest types of laxative.

Bulk-forming laxatives generally provide bowel movement in 12 to 72 hours.

Note: Users should always drink an 8-ounce glass of water when taking a bulk-forming laxative. This provides the liquid that the active ingredient needs to soften and expand the stools. The water also guards against the rare possibility that the laxative might become impacted in the digestive tract.

APPROVED BULK-FORMING LAXATIVE ACTIVE INGREDIENTS

• *BRAN:* Whole-wheat bread, which contains 1 to 2 grams of bran per slice, and bran-rich breakfast cereals, which contain from 2.7 to 6.5 grams per 100 grams of bran flakes, are convenient sources of dietary crude fiber, the beneficial component of bran. This bran is usually obtained from the milling of wheat, though it may come from other grains and plant foods. As an alternative, or supplement to dietary bran, which is classified as *food*, bran is available in *medicinal form* as, for example, bran tablets.

Bran acts by attracting water into the stool. It also acts—through mechanisms that remain unclear—directly on the large intestine to prompt it to void its contents.

Reviewers say that up to 14 grams (half an ounce) of bran—half an ounce—each day is safe and effective for laxation for adults and children over 12 years of age. The daily dose for children 6 to 12 years old is 7 grams; for children 2 to 6 years, 3.5 grams. The daily dose should be divided into two doses taken at different times of the day.

- **CELLULOSE DERIVATIVES: METHYLCELLULOSE AND SODIUM CARBOXYMETHYLCELLULOSE:** These substances are safe and effective in the amounts usually ingested: 4 to 6 grams daily for adults and children over 12 years old; or 1 to 1.5 grams daily for children over 6 years old. You must drink water when taking these laxatives. The daily dose should be divided into two separate doses taken at different times in the day.

   The water is absorbed by the cellulose to form a syrupy liquid. When it reaches the colon, some of the fluid is lost, which causes the remaining cellulose and water to form a gel that increases the bulk of the stool and promotes its evacuation.

- **KARAYA (STERCULIA GUM):** A vegetable gum, karaya gum is indigestible, but it does absorb water. It has little effect on the body as a whole, but some people may be allergic to the gum.

   The safe and effective dose is up to 14 grams daily for adults and children over 12 years old. For younger children, consult a doctor. The daily dose should be divided into two separate doses taken at

Laxatives' Speed Is Gauged

Different types of laxatives have significantly different response times. The FDA offers these estimates of what can be generally expected:

Bulk laxatives	12 to 72 hours
Hyperosmotic laxatives	15 minutes to 1 hour
Lubricant laxatives	
By mouth	6 to 8 hours
Rectal dosages	2 to 15 minutes
Saline laxatives	
By mouth	30 minutes to 6 hours
Rectal dosages	2 to 15 minutes
Stimulant laxatives	
By mouth	6 to 12 hours
Rectal dosages	15 minutes to 1 hour
Stool-softener laxatives	
By mouth	12 to 72 hours
Rectal dosages	2 to 15 minutes
Carbon dioxide-releasing suppositories	5 to 30 minutes

different times in the day. Water must be drunk *immediately* after taking karaya in order to avoid the risk of bowel obstruction.

• MALT SOUP EXTRACT: Malt soup extract is a powder prepared from partially germinated barley grains. It contains 73 percent maltose, 7 percent protein, and 1.5 percent potassium, plus lesser amounts of calcium and other minerals. The Panel classifies malt soup as a bulk-forming laxative but says that it seems to have other laxative actions as well—a matter that merits further study. Malt soup makes the gut acidic, but it is not clear how this might promote evacuation. There is no proof that malt soup extract relieves anal itching, as has been claimed.

The safe and effective dosage for adults and children over 12 years old is up to 64 grams daily with water; for children 6 to 12 years old it is up to 32 grams daily with water; for children aged 2 to 6 years it is up to 16 grams daily with water; for children under 2 years of age, consult a doctor. The daily dose should be divided into two separate doses taken at different times in the day.

• POLYCARBOPHIL: Of all the bulk-forming ingredients, polycarbophil absorbs the most liquid: It can bind and absorb 60 times its weight in water. It holds water and other fluids in the stool and in the hollow inside of the colon. In tests, polycarbophil held 120 cubic centimeters of digestive juices per gram of polycarbophil, compared with 36 for methylcellulose, 30 for psyllium preparations, and 14 for agar. Tests in animals indicate that polycarbophil is nontoxic and that it has no undue effects on nutritional status, digestive enzymes, or digestion itself. Tests in humans confirm the safety and effectiveness of the substances.

The dose for adults and children over 12 years of age is up to 4 grams per day; for children 6 to 12 years old, it is 2 grams per day; for children 2 through 6 years, it is 1 gram per day; and for children under age 2, a physician should be consulted. The daily dosage should be divided into 4 individual doses taken at different times during the day. You should drink a full glass of water with each dose.

• PSYLLIUM PREPARATIONS: PLANTAGO OVATA HUSKS, PLANTAGO SEED, PSYLLIUM (HEMICELLULOSE), PSYLLIUM HYDROPHILIC MUCILLOID (PSYLLIUM HYDROCOLLOID), PSYLLIUM SEED, PSYLLIUM SEED (BLOND), AND PSYLLIUM SEED HUSKS: These substances are widely used derivatives of the seeds and husks of plants from the plantain family. An indigestible hemicellulose in these seeds and husks binds and holds water. Some psyllium preparations may cause color changes in the kidney tubules. Other—apparently harmless—biological changes also have been discovered in humans and in animals dosed with these medications. But evaluators concluded that these side effects are minor and that more serious ones—like obstruction of the esophagus or the intestines—are too rare to preclude approval.

So psyllium preparations are judged to be both safe and effective in the amounts usually taken orally, with water. Dosages are up to 30 grams per day for adults and children over 12 years old; for children 6 to 12 years old, it is up to 15 grams per day; for children under age 6, consult a doctor. The daily dosages should be divided into 4 individual doses to be taken at different times in the day.

CONDITIONALLY APPROVED BULK-FORMING LAXATIVE ACTIVE INGREDIENT

• **ALPHA-CELLULOSE:** This is a semi-synthetic cellulose very similar to methylcellulose, which is safe and effective. But the studies to demonstrate the safety and effectiveness of alpha-*cellulose* simply have not been done, the FDA says.

DISAPPROVED BULK-FORMING LAXATIVE ACTIVE INGREDIENTS

None.

Stimulant Laxatives

Here the Panel's principal message is: *caution.* These laxatives act directly on the walls of the large intestine, small intestine, or both. They stimulate the slow, wavelike intestinal contractions (peristalsis) that move fecal matter along toward excretion. Some stimulant laxatives may act by irritating the intestinal wall. Others may act by stimulating the nerves that start peristalsis. These pathways of action are as yet not clearly established.

What *is* clear is that stimulant laxatives can be hard on the user. As the *Handbook of Nonprescription Drugs* (9th ed.) 1990, a guidebook for pharmacists, warns: "All stimulant laxatives produce griping [severe spasmodic bowel pain], increased mucus secretion, and, in some people, excessive evacuation of fluid."

Reviewers warn that stimulant laxatives should not be used daily for more than a week (except on the advice of a physician), and that overdosage or persistent use can produce serious side effects. These include a dependence on the laxative that inhibits or blocks a person's ability to move his or her bowels without use of the drug. Body fluids and essential body salts (electrolytes) may be depleted.

The Panel assessed a number of stimulant laxatives and found many of them safe and effective as long as the consumer keeps in mind the specific limitations cited. The FDA largely concurs with the Panel's judgment but tends to be a little less concerned about the risks of these ingredients.

Oral doses of stimulant laxatives generally produce bowel movement within 6 to 12 hours. Rectal dosing works faster—within 15 minutes to an hour.

APPROVED STIMULANT LAXATIVE ACTIVE INGREDIENTS

• ANTHRAQUINONES: ALOE, CASCARA SAGRADA PREPARATIONS, AND SENNA PREPARATIONS: These safe and effective substances all are plant derivatives. The anthraquinones act mainly in the large intestine, but the precise mechanism through which they stimulate bowel movements are not known. They all may discolor the urine, turning acid urine yellowish-brown and alkaline urine reddish-violet; these effects that are considered harmless. The senna products are more potent than cascara, according to the authorities, and they may cause greater abdominal discomfort. At least one senna laxative is available as a suppository.

• BISACODYL: This substance, which can be taken orally or inserted in a suppository, produces brief but very strong evacuatory movements in the large intestine. When the drug is applied intrarectally, this action occurs within 15 minutes to an hour. Bisacodyl appears to act on the mucous membranes or underlying nerves, but it may also cause water to be secreted into the bowel or to be held there.

Although bisacodyl is a very effective laxative, it may be risky to use: Excessive use or overdosage can lead to severe diarrhea and the loss of vital body fluids and body salts. Muscle weakness and tremor may result. It can cause abdominal discomfort, faintness, rectal burning, and mild cramps. When given orally, bisacodyl must be swallowed, not chewed, and people who cannot swallow the tablet whole should not take the drug in its oral form. However, the drug

Approved Daily Dosage of Laxatives Containing Anthraquinones

Anthraquinone Ingredient	USUAL ORAL DOSES	
	Adults	Children
aloe	120-250 mg	under 6 years: consult a doctor ages 6-8 years: 40 to 80 mg ages 8-15 years: 80 to 120 mg
cascara sagrada preparations aromatic cascara fluid extract	2-6 ml	under age 2 years: consult a doctor ages 2-12 years: 1 to 3 ml
casanthranol	30-90 mg	under age 2 years: consult a doctor ages 2-12 years: 15 to 45 mg
cascara sagrada bark	300 mg-1 gram	under age 2 years: consult a doctor ages 2-12: 150 to 500 mg
cascara sagrada extract	200-400 mg	under age 2 years: consult a doctor ages 2-12 years: 100 to 200 mg
cascara sagrada fluid extract	0.5-1.5 ml	under age 2 years: consult a doctor ages 2-12 years: 0.25 to 0.75 ml
sennosides A and B preparations:	12-50 mg sennosides A and B once or twice daily	under age 2: consult a doctor ages 2-6: 3 to 12.5 mg sennosides A and B, once or twice daily ages 6-12: 6 to 25 mg sennosides A and B, once or twice daily

Approved Daily Dosage of Laxatives Containing Anthraquinones (contd)

Anthraquinone Ingredient	Adults	Children
senna fluid extract	see previous comment	see previous comment
senna fruit extract		
senna leaf powder		
senna pod concentrate		
senna syrup		
sennosides A and B crystalline		

was assessed as safe when taken in oral doses of 5 to 15 mg daily for adults and children older than 12 years of age, or 5 mg for children aged 6 to 12 years. For younger children, consult a physician. Suppository dosage is generally 10 mg for adult use and 5 mg for children 6 to 12 years old. When used judiciously, bisacodyl can be safe as well as effective.

• *CASTOR OIL:* A traditional plant remedy, castor oil more than meets modern standards: One dose of 15 to 60 mg will completely clear out the lower bowel. This is the approved dose for adults and children over 12 years. The dose for children aged 2 to 12 years is 5 to 15 ml, which is 1 to 3 teaspoonfuls of the unpleasant-tasting oil. For children under 2 years old, consult a doctor.

The laxative effect of castor oil comes from ricinoleic acid, a substance that is not produced until the oil reaches the small intestine. There the castor oil is broken down by a pancreatic enzyme called *lipase*. Exactly how the acid product acts to evacuate the bowel remains unclear; what is known is that the colon secretes both water and electrolytes in response to its presence.

While safe and effective in appropriate doses, continued use of castor oil can result in excessive—and dangerous—loss of water and essential body salts. So evaluators warn against overuse.

• *DEHYDROCHOLIC ACID:* This substance is derived from cholic acid, a natural bile acid. Its presence significantly increases the water content of bile, which is a mixture of digestive juices. How this helps evacuate the stool is not known for sure; the dehydrocholic acid may stimulate the secretion of sodium bicarbonate and water from the colon or inhibit their absorption by it. Dehydrocholic acid does not relieve "indigestion," "excessive belching," or the "sensation of abdominal fullness," as has been claimed. But tests in animals, as well as in humans, show that it is quite nontoxic. It was judged safe and effective at doses of 250 to 500 mg, 3 times daily. But it should not be used by children under 12 years of age without a doctor's recommendation.

• *PHENOLPHTHALEIN, WHITE OR YELLOW:* These compounds act in the colon and possibly in the small intestine. They apparently prevent water and salt from being reabsorbed from the gut into the body. Yellow phenolphthalein is claimed to be more potent than white. The substances may temporarily turn the urine pink. More seriously, they can lead to excessive laxation and a loss of body salts. They should be used only occasionally and should not be given to children under 2 years old, except as recommended by a doctor.

Nevertheless, phenolphthalein compounds were judged safe and effective when used infrequently by adults and older children and in the correct amounts. Dosages are 30 to 270 mg per day for adults and children over 12 years old in one or two doses; 30 to 60 mg for children 6 to 12 years old in one or two doses daily; and 15 to 30 mg for children 2 through 6 years of age, in one or two doses daily. For younger children, consult a doctor.

CONDITIONALLY APPROVED STIMULANT LAXATIVE ACTIVE INGREDIENTS

None.

DISAPPROVED STIMULANT LAXATIVE ACTIVE INGREDIENTS

None.

Saline Laxatives

Saline refers to salt. Saline laxatives—magnesium, phosphate, and tartar salts—were long believed to pull water into the gut by the membrane-penetrating process of osmosis. They may indeed work this way, but investigators believe other, as yet not understood, mechanisms may also be involved. Saline laxatives generally produce bowel movement within 2 to 6 hours when taken by mouth. Rectal enemas act much more quickly, within 2 to 15 minutes. Since serious loss of normal body salts can result from use of saline laxatives, these substances should be used only occasionally.

APPROVED SALINE LAXATIVE ACTIVE INGREDIENTS

• MAGNESIUM SALTS: MAGNESIUM CITRATE ORAL SOLUTION USP, MAGNESIUM HYDROXIDE (MILK OF MAGNESIA), AND MAGNESIUM SULFATE: These magnesium salts draw water into the gut by osmosis, just as salt water will draw plain water through a semi-permeable membrane. But they also appear to act through at least one other route as well: They stimulate the release of a hormone called CCK-PZ into the gut. This action stimulates motor and secretory activity that may help move stubborn stools along.

(Magnesium hydroxide acts as an antacid. (*See* ANTACIDS.) But its ability to neutralize acid in no way contributes to its value as a laxative; acid secretion and constipation are not related.)

The Panel cites no instances of untoward effects in users of these laxatives when taken as recommended and says they are safe and effective. But it indicates that persons with kidney disease should check label warnings, as should persons who need to limit their intake of salt.

Approved Daily Dosage of Laxatives Containing Magnesium

	DAILY DOSAGE*		
Age	Magnesium Citrate	Magnesium Hydroxide	Magnesium Sulfate
adults	11-25 gm	2.4-4.8 gm	10-30 gm
children 6-12 years	5.5-12.5 gm	1.2-2.4 gm	5-10 gm
children 2-5 years	2.7-6.25 gm	0.4-1.2 gm	2.5-5 gm
children under 2 years		consult a physician	

* Daily dosages given can be divided into 2 or 3 individual doses to be taken at different times during the day.

•PHOSPHATE SALTS: SODIUM PHOSPHATE, SODIUM BIPHOSPHATE, SODIUM PHOSPHATE/SODIUM BIPHOSPHATE SOLUTION: As with the compounds just described, these substances draw water into the gut. They tend to be fast-acting.

Persons with kidney disease should avoid these laxatives, except when approved by a doctor. Also, products that contain phosphate salts should not be given orally to children under 5, years of age, or in enemas or other rectal doses to children under 2 years of age, except on a doctor's orders. Used with these precautions in mind, and taken as recommended, the phosphate-salt laxative ingredients are judged to be safe and effective.

The daily dosages, which should be taken as a single dose, are as follows:

- Sodium phosphate taken by mouth: adults and children over 12 years old, 3.42 to 7.56 grams; children 10 to 12 years old, 1.71 to 3.78 grams; and children 5 to 9 years old, 0.86 to 1.89 grams; for children under 5 years of age, only as recommended by a doctor.

- Sodium biphosphate taken by mouth: adults and children over 12 yaers old, 4.5 to 20.2 grams; children 10 to 12 years old, 2.25 to 10.1 grams; children 5 to 9 years old, 1.12 to 5.05 grams; children under 5 years of age, only as directed by a doctor.

- Sodium phosphate/sodium biphosphate taken by mouth: adults and children over 12 years old, 3.42 to 7.56 grams sodium phosphate and 9.1 to 20.2 grams sodium biphosphate; children 10 to 12 years old, 1.71 to 3.78 grams sodium phosphate and 4.5 to 10.1 grams sodium biphosphate; and children 5 to 9 yaers old, 0.86 to 1.89 grams sodium phosphate and 2.2 to 5.05 grams sodium biphosphate; for children under 5 years of age, as directed by a doctor.

Sodium phosphate/sodium biphosphate taken rectally in an enema: adults and children over 12 years old, 6.84 to 7.56 grams sodium phosphate and 18.24 to 20.16 grams sodium biphosphate; and children 2 to 12 years old, 3.42 to 3.78 grams sodium phosphate and 9.12 to 10.08 grams sodium biphosphate; for children under 2 years old, consult a doctor.

CONDITIONALLY APPROVED SALINE LAXATIVE ACTIVE INGREDIENTS

None.

DISAPPROVED SALINE LAXATIVE ACTIVE INGREDIENTS

None.

Hyperosmotic Laxatives

A hyperosmotic laxative attracts water into the stool. It thus acts in much the same way as the saline laxatives, with the clear difference that it is less likely to cause serious imbalances in body salts and so is likely to be safer. These laxatives are approved for *intrarectal* administration only. They generally yield results in between 15 and 60 minutes.

APPROVED HYPEROSMOTIC LAXATIVE ACTIVE INGREDIENTS

- **GLYCERIN:** This clear, syrupy substance will attract and hold large amounts of water. It may act by bringing water into the large intestine where it can soften hardened fecal matter. Glycerin also may irritate the rectal mucosa, promoting defecation. A third laxative action may also occur: Glycerin's water-absorbing activity may dry the rectal mucosa, which in turn stimulates defecation by a reflex action. For whichever of these reasons, a glycerin rectal suppository usually promotes defecation within half an hour in adults and in children. The side effects tend to be minimal but may include rectal discomfort, burning, and spasmodic bowel pain or stomach cramps. Some rectal bleeding or discharge also may occur.

  Glycerin has been administered orally to promote defecation. Evaluators say that the amounts needed to produce this effect could be toxic, so oral usage is disapproved.

  When administered intrarectally, however, glycerin is safe and effective for adults and children over 6 years old, in dosages of 2 to 3 grams per suppository or 5 to 15 milliliters in an enema. For children under 6 years old, the dosage is 1 to 1.7 grams in suppository form or 2 to 5 ml in an enema. For children under 2 years of age, consult a doctor.

- **SORBITOL:** An alcohol derived from sugar, sorbitol is effective as a laxative when given either orally or intrarectally. But the Panel says the effective oral dose is too large to be considered a safe medication without prescription, so only rectal use is approved. Administered this way, sorbitol appears to produce similar, but less troublesome, side effects than glycerin. Sorbitol should be used only occasionally. The safe and effective dose for adults is 120 ml as a 25 to 30 percent solution; for children 2 years of age and over, it is 30 to 60 ml in the same percent solution.

CONDITIONALLY APPROVED HYPEROSMOTIC LAXATIVE ACTIVE INGREDIENTS

None.

DISAPPROVED HYPEROSMOTIC LAXATIVE ACTIVE INGREDIENTS

None.

Stool Softeners

The active ingredients characterized by the Panel as stool softeners may be particularly helpful when the stools are hard and dry or when hemorrhoids or other anorectal disorders make it difficult to pass a solid stool. Stool softeners should be used only occasionally and not for longer than a week on a daily basis. This precaution must be observed because these substances can interfere with the absorption of vitamins and other nutrients into the body. If relief is not obtained within a week, experts say, you should consult a physician. Stool softeners taken by mouth usually yield bowel movements within 12 to 72 hours. Rectal dosages act more quickly—usually within an hour.

The Panel approved 3 stool softeners. However, unlike the other laxatives described in this Unit, the FDA has not completed or announced its preliminary assessment of stool softeners. The hold-up is data, from animals, suggesting that compounds used in stool softeners might cause birth defects. As of this writing, this has *not* been confirmed.

APPROVED STOOL-SOFTENING ACTIVE INGREDIENTS

All 3 safe and effective stool-softening agents belong to a single group of drugs, the *sulfosuccinates*, which were assessed together.

• SULFOSUCCINATE PREPARATIONS: DOCUSATE CALCIUM (DIOCTYL CALCIUM SULFOSUCCINATE), DOCUSATE POTASSIUM (DIOCTYL POTASSIUM SULFOSUCCINATE), DOCUSATE SODIUM (DIOCTYL SODIUM SULFOSUCCINATE, DSS): It is not clear how these compounds soften the stool. They may have a detergent action, according to reviewers. In other words, sulfosuccinate preparations may lower surface tension at interfaces between oil and water. As the result, more oil and more water may be absorbed from the gut into the fecal matter, which softens it. One or more of these substances also may stimulate the secretion of water and body salts into the colon. This would also soften the stool. By whichever means they work, these substances are effective, as has been demonstrated by published scientific reports.

Few side effects have been attributed to sulfosuccinate preparations. They appear to be partially absorbed from the gut into the body, with unknown consequences. This action could enhance the absorption of mineral oil, a common lubricant laxative. Since mineral oil may be quite toxic if it escapes the gut, evaluators warn that it should *never* be used at the same time you are taking a sulfosuccinate. The Panel urges that these ingredients be used only in the smallest possible amounts and their use limited to brief periods.

Approved Daily Dosage of Laxatives Containing Sulfosuccinates

Age	Docusate Calcium (Dioctyl Calcium Sulfo-succinate) Oral use only	Docusate Potasium (Dioctyl Potassium Sulfo-succinate) Rectal use only	Docusate Sodium (Dioctyl Sodium Sulfo-succinate, DSS) Oral use only
adults	50-360 mg	50-250 mg	50-360 mg
children 2-11 years	50-150 mg	100 mg	50 mg
children under 2 years	25 mg	not approved	20 mg

CONDITIONALLY APPROVED STOOL-SOFTENING ACTIVE INGREDIENTS

None.

DISAPPROVED STOOL-SOFTENING ACTIVE INGREDIENTS

None.

Lubricant Laxatives

The time-honored intestinal lubricant is mineral oil, which may be taken orally or inserted into the rectum. It tends to produce bowel movement within 6 to 8 hours when taken by mouth. Inserted rectally, bowel movement may occur within 2 to 15 minutes.

- MINERAL OIL: This compound is widely used to facilitate bowel evacuation and is safe and effective if properly used. Mineral oil is a clear, tasteless, petroleum by-product that smooths the intestinal tract and softens and lubricates fecal material. It is not irritating, is not absorbed from the gut, and is not broken down by gastrointestinal enzymes. So it is quite safe, although it may impair absorption of vitamins and other necessary nutrients. Consequently, mineral oil should be taken orally only at bedtime. It should not be used daily for more than a week and should never be used if you are taking a sulfosuccinate (*see* Stool Softeners, p. 620.)

    Persistent use of mineral oil can lead to leakage of fecal material between bowel movements and to skin reactions. Except under medical supervision, it should not be taken orally by children under 6 years of age, or by pregnant women, or by persons who have difficulty swallowing. These restrictions do not apply to intrarectal use of mineral oil, which is safer in the sense that when taken this way it cannot affect digestion or nutrient uptake. Neither can it get into the lungs and cause trouble as it might when swallowed.

Safe and Effective Daily Dosages of Mineral Oil

Age	Administered Orally	Administered Intrarectally
adults	15-45 ml	120 ml
children over 6 years	5-15 ml	60 ml
children 2 to 6 years	consult a doctor	60 ml
children under 2 years	consult a doctor	consult a doctor

Carbon Dioxide-Releasing Laxatives

The Panel assessed one laxative that works by releasing carbon dioxide gas into the rectum, thereby increasing pressure inside the rectum and gently forcing out its contents. The FDA assessed a second such product. Both are judged to be safe and effective. They produce bowel movement in 5 to 30 minutes. The two products are

- COMBINATION OF SODIUM BIPHOSPHATE ANHYDROUS + SODIUM ACID PYROPHOSPHATE + SODIUM BICARBONATE: This preparation is formulated as a rectal suppository. When wetted, then inserted into the rectum, the solid ingredients react with the water; this gives off about 230 ml of carbon dioxide gas. The expanding gas gently increases pressure inside the rectum and the enhanced sense of fullness in turn promotes a bowel movement.

    These suppositories are safe and effective when used once daily. They should not be used in children under 12 years of age, except as directed by a doctor. The approved preparations contain 1.2 to 1.5 grams sodium biphosphate anhydrous, 0.04 to 0.05 gram sodium acid pyrophosphate, and 1 to 1.5 grams sodium bicarbonate. The suppositories should not be lubricated with mineral oil or petrolatum before insertion, as these greasy substances may retard the release of gas.

- COMBINATION OF SODIUM BICARBONATE + SODIUM BITARTRATE: This carbon dioxide-releasing suppository formulation contains 0.6 gram sodium bicarbonate and 0.9 gram potassium tartrate. It releases only 90 ml of carbon dioxide, considerably less than the aforementioned combination. Hence, two insertions a day may be needed. FDA rules this combination safe and effective for adults and children over 12 years of age. For younger children, ask a doctor.

When Greater Relief Is Needed

See a *proctologist*—a specialist in diseases of the anorectal organs—if your intestines become so impacted that you cannot move your bowels. Straining to defecate is dangerous. It is safer and less painful to seek professional help.

Safety and Effectiveness: Active Ingredients in Over-the-Counter Laxatives

Active Ingredient	Type of Laxative	Panel's Assessment
aloe	stimulant	safe and effective

Safety and Effectiveness: Active Ingredients in Over-the-Counter Laxatives (contd)

Active Ingredient	Type of Laxative	Panel's Assessment
alpha-cellulose	bulk-forming	safe, but not proved effective
bisacodyl	stimulant	safe and effective
bran	bulk-forming	safe and effective
carboxymethylcellulose sodium	bulk-forming	safe and effective
cascara sagrada preparations:		
aromatic cascara fluid extract	stimulant	safe and effective
casanthranol	stimulant	safe and effective
cascara sagrada bark	stimulant	safe and effective
cascara sagrada extract	stimulant	safe and effective
cascara sagrada fluid extract	stimulant	safe and effective
castor oil	stimulant	safe and effective
dehydrocholic acid	stimulant	safe and effective
docusate calcium (dioctyl calcium sulfosuccinate)	stool softener	safe and effective
docusate potassium (dioctyl potassium sulfosuccinate)	stool softener	safe and effective
docusate sodium (dioctyl sodium sulfosuccinate)	stool softener	safe and effective
DSS (See docusate sodium, immediately above)		
glycerin	hyperosmotic	safe and effective
karaya (sterculia gum)	bulk-forming	safe and effective
magnesium citrate	saline	safe and effective

Safety and Effectiveness: Active Ingredients in
Over-the-Counter Laxatives (contd)

Active Ingredient	Type of Laxative	Panel's Assessment
magnesium hydroxide	saline	safe and effective
magnesium sulfate	saline	safe and effective
malt soup extract	bulk-forming	safe and effective
methylcellulose	bulk-forming	safe and effective
mineral oil	lubricant	safe and effective
phenolphthalein, white	stimulant	safe and effective
phenolphthalein, yellow	stimulant	safe and effective
phosphate preparations:		
sodium biphosphate	saline	safe and effective
sodium phosphate	saline	safe and effective
plantago ovata husks	bulk-forming	safe and effective
plantago seed	bulk-forming	safe and effective
polycarbophil	bulk-forming	safe and effective
psyllium, hemicellulose	bulk-forming	safe and effective
psyllium, hydrophilic mucilloid (psyllium hydrocolloid)	bulk-forming	safe and effective
carbon dioxide	carbon dioxide-releasing	safe and effective
psyllium seed	bulk-forming	safe and effective
psyllium seed, blond	bulk-forming	safe and effective
psyllium seed husks	bulk-forming	safe and effective
sennosides A and B:		
senna fluid extract	stimulant	safe and effective
senna fruit extract	stimulant	safe and effective
senna leaf powder	stimulant	safe and effective

Safety and Effectiveness: Active Ingredients in Over-the-Counter Laxatives (contd)

Active Ingredient	Type of Laxative	Panel's Assessment
senna pod concentrate	stimulant	safe and effective
senna syrup	stimulant	safe and effective
sennosides A and B, crystalline	stimulant	safe and effective
sorbitol	hyperosmotic	safe and effective
sulfosuccinate preparations dioctyl calcium sulfosuccinate (*See* docusate calcium)		
dioctyl sodium sulfosuccinate (DSS) (*See* docusate potassium)		
dioctyl sodium sulfosuccinate (DSS) (*See* docusate sodium)		
DSS (*See* docusate sodium)		

Safety and Effectiveness: Combination Products Sold Over-the-Counter as Laxatives

Safe and Effective Combinations

An approved amount of any of the following 2 ingredients formulated in such a way that the combined effective dosage range does not exceed 100%.*

Oral Dosage Forms

docusate sodium + casanthranol
docusate sodium + phenolphthalein
casanthranol + aloe
cascara sagrada + magnesium hydroxide
cascara sagrada extract + phenolphthalein
malt soup extract + psyllium seed, blond
   malt soup extract + psyllium seed husks
mineral oil + casanthranol
mineral oil + cascara sagrada extract

Safety and Effectiveness: Combination Products Sold Over-the-Counter as Laxatives (contd)

mineral oil + cascara sagrada fluid extract
mineral oil + magnesium hydroxide
mineral oil + phenolphthalein
mineral oil + psyllium seed
plantago ovata husks + methylcellulose
psyllium (hemicellulose) + crystalline sennosides
psyllium seed (blond) + casanthranol
senna concentrate + docusate sodium
carboxymethycellulose sodium + docusate sodium

Rectal Dosage Forms

glycerin + docusate potassium
sorbitol + docusate potassium

Conditionally Safe and Effective Combinations

one or both ingredients are present in less than the minimum approved dosage
one or both ingredients are conditionally approved by the Panel as single
    active laxative ingredients
karaya gum + cascara sagrada

Unsafe or Ineffective Combinations

psyllium + bran
contains 3 or more active laxative ingredients
docusate sodium + mineral oil, plain (the former may enhance the latter's
    absorption into the body)
contains any disapproved active ingredient
contains the maximum dosage set by the panel for 1 ingredient + more than the
    minimum dosage for the second ingredient
the sum of the percentage amounts of each ingredient exceeds 100%*
the combination contains any laxative active ingredient not reviewed by the
    Panel or the FDA
magnesium hydroxide + simethicone
the combination contains any non-laxative active ingredient for which a
    treatment claim is made

---

* To encourage the use of ingredients in amounts at the minimum end of the dosage range (rather than at the maximum end of the range), the Panel devised a formula to express the sum of the percentage amounts of the effective dosage range (EDR) of each ingredient. The EDR of the 2 ingredients must not exceed 100. In this formula L max d is the labeled maximum daily dosage listed in the labeling information for the product, EDR (min) is the minimum effective dosage range set by the Panel, and EDR (max) is the maximum effective dosage range set by the Panel.

$$\frac{L \max d - EDR (min)}{EDR (max) - EDR (min)} \times 100 = \% \ EDR \ of \ each \ ingredient$$

Laxatives: Product Ratings

SINGLE-INGREDIENT PRODUCTS: BULK-FORMING LAXATIVES

Product and Distributor	Dosage of Active Ingredients	Rating *	Comment
cellulose derivatives, semisynthetic			
Citrucel (Marion Merrell Dow)	**powder:** 2 grams methylcellulose per rounded tablespoonful	A	
Unifiber (Dow B. Hickam)	**powder:** 3 grams methylcellulose per tablespoonful	A	
malt soup extract			
Maltsupex (Wallace)	**tablets:** 750 mg nondiastatic barley malt extract; also in powder and liquid	A	
polycarbophil			
FiberCon (Lederle)	**tablets:** 500 mg (as calcium polycarbophil)	A	
Mitrolan (A. H. Robins)	**chewable tablets:** 500 mg (as calcium polycarbophil)	A	
psyllium preparations			
Hydrocil, Instant (Reid-Rowell)	**powder:** 3.5 grams psyllium hydrophilic mucilloid per dose	A	

Product and Distributor	Dosage of Active Ingredients	Rating*	Comment

Konsyl-D (Lafayette) — **powder:** 3.4 grams psyllium hydrophilic mucilloid per rounded teaspoonful — A

Metamucil (Procter & Gamble) — **powder:** 3.4 grams psyllium hydrophilic mucilloid per rounded teaspoonful — A

Metamucil Wafers (Procter & Gamble) — **wafers:** 1.7 grams psyllium hydrophilic mucilloid per wafer — A

Reguloid (Rugby) — **powder:** 3.4 grams psyllium mucilloid per rounded tablespoonful — A

Siblin (Warner-Lambert) — **granules:** 2.5 grams blond psyllium seed coatings per rounded teaspoonful — A

SINGLE-INGREDIENT PRODUCTS: STIMULANT LAXATIVES

ANTHRAQUINONES

Product and Distributor	Dosage of Active Ingredients	Rating*	Comment
cascara sagrada			
Cascara sagrada (generic)	**tablets:** 325 mg	A	
Cascara sagrada aromatic fluid extract (generic)	**liquid**	A	

Laxatives: Product Ratings (contd)

Product and Distributor	Dosage of Active Ingredients	Rating *	Comment
senna			
Senna Black-Draught (Chattem)	tablets: 600 mg senna equivalent	A	
Senexon (Rugby)	tablets: 187 mg senna concentrate	A	
Senokot (Purdue Frederick)	tablets: 187 mg standardized senna concentrate	A	
	granules: 326 mg standardized senna concentrate per teaspoonful	A	
Senolax (Schein)	tablets: 187 mg senna concentrate	A	
sennosides A and B, calcium salts of			
Ex-Lax Gentle Nature (Sandoz)	tablets: 20 mg	A	

OTHER STIMULANT LAXATIVES

Product and Distributor	Dosage of Active Ingredients	Rating *	Comment
bisacodyl			
Bisacodyl (generic)	tablets: enteric coated: 5 mg	A	
	suppositories: 10 mg	A	
Bisco-Lax (Raway)	suppositories: 10 mg	A	

Ducolax (Boehringer Ingelheim)	**tablets:** enteric coated: 5 mg	A
	suppositories: 10 mg	A
Fleet Laxative (Fleet)	**suppositories:** 10 mg	A
castor oil		
Castor oil (generic)	**liquid**	A
Emulsoil (Paddock)	**emulsion:** 95% + emulsifying agents	A
Neoloid (Lederle)	**emulsion:** 36.4% + emulsifying agents	A
Purge (Fleming)	**liquid:** 95%	A
dehydrocholic acid		
Cholan-HMB (Pennwalt)	**tablets:** 250 mg	A
Decholin (Miles)	**tablets:** 250 mg	A
phenolphthalein, yellow and white		
Evac-U-Gen (Walker)	**chewable tablets:** 97.2 mg yellow phenolphthalein	A
Ex-Lax (Sandoz)	**chewable tablets:** 90 mg yellow phenolphthalein	A
	pills: 90 mg yellow phenolphthalein	A

Laxatives: Product Ratings (contd)

Product and Distributor	Dosage of Active Ingredients	Rating*	Comment
Feen-a-Mint (Schering-Plough)	**tablets:** 97.2 mg yellow phe-nolphthalein	A	
Phenolax (Upjohn)	**wafers:** 64.8 mg phenolphthalein	A	
Prulet Liquitab (Mission)	**tablets:** 60 mg white phenolph-thalein	A	

SINGLE-INGREDIENT PRODUCTS: SALINE LAXATIVES

Product and Distributor	Dosage of Active Ingredients	Rating*	Comment
magnesium salts			
Citrate of magnesia (generic)	**liquid:** magnesium citrate	A	
Citro-Nesia (Century)	**liquid:** magnesium citrate	A	
Epsom salt (generic)	**powder:** magnesium sulfate	A	
Milk of magnesia (generic)	**liquid:** magnesium hydroxide	A	
Milk of magnesia – Concentrated (generic)	**liquid:** magnesium hydroxide	A	
Phillips' Milk of Magnesia (Glenbrook)	**liquid:** magnesium hydroxide	A	

SINGLE-INGREDIENT PRODUCTS: HYPEROSMOTIC LAXATIVES

Product and Distributor	Dosage of Active Ingredients	Rating*	Comment
glycerin			
Fleet Babylax (Fleet)	liquid: 4 ml per applicator	A	
Glycerin, USP (generic)	suppositories	A	

SINGLE-INGREDIENT PRODUCTS: STOOL-SOFTENERS

Product and Distributor	Dosage of Active Ingredients	Rating*	Comment
docusate calcium			
Docusate calcium (generic)	capsules: 240 mg	A	
Sulfax Calcium (Major)	capsules: 240 mg	A	
Surfak (Hoechst-Roussel)	capsules: 50 mg, 240 mg	A	
docusate potassium			
Dialose (J&J-Merck)	capsules: 100 mg	C	not approved by Panel or FDA for oral use
Kasof (J&J-Merck)	capsules: 240 mg	C	not approved by Panel or FDA for oral use
docusate sodium, or DSS			

Laxatives: Product Ratings (contd)

Product and Distributor	Dosage of Active Ingredients	Rating*	Comment
Colace (Mead Johnson)	**liquid:** 20 mg per teaspoonful	A	
	syrup: 20 mg per tablespoonful	A	
	capsules: 100 mg	A	
Docusate Sodium (Roxane)	**capsules:** 50 mg	A	
	syrup: 50 mg per teaspoonful	A	
Docusate sodium (generic)	**capsules:** 100 mg	A	
	capsules: 250 mg	A	
Dok (Major)	**capsules:** 250 mg	A	
D-S-S (Warner Chilcott)	**capsules:** 100 mg	A	
Modane (Adria)	**capsules:** 100 mg	A	
Regutol (Schering-Plough)	**tablets:** 100 mg	A	

SINGLE-INGREDIENT PRODUCTS: LUBRICANT LAXATIVES

Product and Distributor	Dosage of Active Ingredients	Rating*	Comment
mineral oil			
Mineral oil (generic)	**liquid:** liquid petrolatum	A	
mineral oil, emulsified			

Kondremul Plain (Fisons)	emulsion: mineral oil	A	

COMBINATION PRODUCTS: CARBON-DIOXIDE RELEASING PRODUCTS

Product and Distributor	Dosage of Active Ingredients	Rating*	Comment
Ceo-Two (Beutlich)	suppositories: sodium bicarbonate + potassium bitartrate	A	

COMBINATION PRODUCTS: TABLETS AND CAPSULES

Product and Distributor	Dosage of Active Ingredients	Rating*	Comment
Correctol (Schering-Plough)	tablets: 100 mg docusate sodium + 65 mg phenolphthalein	A	
Disolan Forte (Lannett)	capsules: 100 mg docusate sodium + 30 mg casanthranol + 400 mg sodium carboxymethyl-cellulose	A	
D-S-S plus (Warner-Chilcott)	capsules: 100 mg docusate sodium + 30 mg casanthranol	A	
Nature's Remedy (SmithKline Beecham)	tablets: 150 mg cascara sagrada + 100 mg aloe	A	
Peri-Colace (Mead Johnson)	capsules: 100 mg docusate sodium + 30 mg casanthranol	A	

Laxatives: Product Ratings (contd)

Product and Distributor	Dosage of Active Ingredients	Rating*	Comment
Senokot S (Purdue-Frederick)	**tablets:** 50 mg docusate sodium + 187 mg senna concentrate	A	

COMBINATION PRODUCTS: LIQUIDS

Product and Distributor	Dosage of Active Ingredients	Rating*	Comment
Docusate sodium with casanthranol (generic)	**syrup:** 20 mg docusate sodium + 10 mg casanthranol per teaspoonful	A	
Haley's M-O (Glenbrook)	**liquid:** 900 mg magnesium hydroxide + 1.25 ml mineral oil per teaspoonful	A	
Kondremul with Phenolphthalein (Fisons)	**emulsion:** 55% mineral oil + 50 mg phenolphthalein per teaspoonfulful	A	
Peri-Colace (Mead Johnson)	**syrup:** 20 mg docusate sodium + 10 mg casanthranol per teaspoonful	A	

COMBINATION PRODUCTS: POWDERS AND GRANULES

Product and Distributor	Dosage of Active Ingredients	Rating *	Comment
Perdiem (Rhone-Poulenc Rorer)	**granules:** 3.25 grams psyllium + 740 mg senna per rounded teaspoonful	A	
Syllamalt (Wallace)	**powder:** 4 grams malt soup extract + 3 grams psyllium seed husks per rounded teaspoonful	A	

*Author's interpretation of FDA criteria. Based on contents, not claims.

Liniments and Poultices for Aches and Pains

When a dentist starts to drill a tooth, many people dig their fingernails into the palms of their hands. The self-inflicted pain, which they control, blocks the drilling pain—which they do not control. Liniments and comparable preparations that are applied to the skin work in roughly the same way; they produce counterirritation, distracting you from more deep-seated pain. These countervailing feelings may be warm—or cool—and so also may soothe the soreness.

 Claims

Accurate
- "For the temporary relief of minor aches and pains of muscles and joints, which may be associated with simple backache, arthritis, strains, bruises, and sprains"

LINIMENTS AND POULTICES FOR ACHES AND PAINS is based on the report "External Analgesic Drug Products for OTC Human Use" by the Advisory Review Panel on OTC Topical Analgesic, Antirheumatic, Otic, Burn, and Sunburn Prevention and Treatment Drug Products and the FDA's Tentative Final Monograph on these products.

- "Provides penetrating pain relief"
- "Provides warming pain relief"
- "Provides cooling pain relief"

What They Are and How They Work

Counterirritating substances are formulated in different ways:

- A *liniment* is a liquid that is rubbed gently onto the skin.

- A *rub* may require more vigorous massage.

- A *poultice* is a damp, doughy, or porridge-like mixture that may be spread on a cloth laid over a sore spot.

- A *plaster* is a thicker, self-sticking mixture.

- *Balms* describe those applications concocted of aromatic plant resins and juices so that they smell sweet.

These preparations mildly stimulate nerve endings in the skin that respond to warmth, coolness, or pain. This drug action blocks or distracts you from a more bothersome pain that is deep-seated in muscles, bones, and even viscera (internal organs). To reach the nerve endings, the irritating ingredients in liniments must be absorbed through the protective upper skin layers (the epidermis). Most of this absorption occurs directly through the epidermis—some via hair follicles, which explains why it occurs most readily in hairy areas. Although absorption happens more rapidly if the protective outer layers of skin have been broken or scraped, these preparations should *not* be used in such an instance for fear of damaging underlying tissues.

Oils, water, and other substances are actively absorbed by the skin, which is why counterirritant active ingredients are dissolved in them. Wetting the skin can further enhance absorption, as can heat. Covering the skin with a tight dressing will also significantly increase absorption, but this can increase the risk of damaging the skin after you have applied irritating substances.

Doctors today rarely prescribe or propose these remedies. Liniments nevertheless have been a part of traditional medical practice and folk healing for thousands of years.

Relatively few scientific studies have been conducted to demonstrate that these substances are really effective. So the Panel decided to judge them by less rigorous standards than have been applied to many other classes of drugs in the OTC Drug Review. It took into account popular appeal, as expressed in sales, as one criterion of effectiveness, and also noted that complaints about these products have been rare and the problems mild.

WARNINGS:

 Do not apply to wounds or damaged skin. Do not apply over large areas of the body.

All liniments and poultices are for external use only and should be kept out of children's reach, since they may be quite poisonous if swallowed. Because these substances are irritating, they should be kept away from the eyes. Liniments and poultices can be used for self-treatment for adults and children over the age of 2 years, but should be used for younger children only if recommended by a doctor. Do not use more often than 3 or 4 times daily.

Pain and Counterirritation

The deep-lying pains that can be successfully treated with counterirritants tend to be *dull* rather than sharp in feeling. They may originate at the place where they are felt, or they may be *referred* pains, which means that a hurt felt in one place may emanate from damaged tissue that is some distance away.

A recent theory may help explain how a poultice applied to the skin can relieve a charley horse deep in the muscle. This *gate theory* was developed to explain how acupuncture—the traditional Chinese therapy in which thin needles are stuck into the body—can relieve pain at other body sites. The theory says that stimulating nerve pathways in one place can cause other pathways to close, like a gate. This prevents other, more painful impulses from entering these pathways en route to the brain.

The nervous system thus can be thought of as a railroad, with trunk lines leading to the brain. When irritating—but tolerable—impulses generated by a liniment flow onto the trunk line from a branch line to the skin, the system closes switches (or "gates") that lead on from other branch lines to the muscles and bones. Pain impulses from these areas then cannot enter the trunk and so are not received or registered by the brain for as long as the counterirritating impulses continue.

Liniments and rubs are not the only topical remedies for deep-seated pain. Ice packs, heat lamps, hot water bags, and warm or hot baths also act as counterirritants. Heat acts directly to relax painfully tense muscles. The warmth of a hot tub does not directly penetrate more than a fraction of an inch beneath the skin surface. But it warms and relaxes blood vessels in the skin, which enhances blood flow through them to deeper tissues. This warming action may also help carry off plasma and other irritating substances that have accumulated in muscle tissues.

Liniments are designed to be rubbed onto the skin. This massage provides part (some experts say *most*) of the benefit of the treatment. Massaging the skin stimulates blood flow; dexterous fingertips can loosen tight muscles. Massage also is a pleasant-feeling counterirritation—and feeling good, even for a few moments, may break the vicious cycle of pain, tension, and more pain. In the same way, the comforting warmth and agreeably sweet and pungent odors of liniments and balms may contribute to the relief that they bring.

"There is no doubt," the Panel said, "that the action of counterirritants has a psychic component as well as a drug-induced therapeutic component."

Over-the-counter oral drugs that relieve pain and inflammation also may be helpful. (*See* PAIN, FEVER, AND ANTI-INFLAMMATORY DRUGS TAKEN INTERNALLY.)

When counterirritants fail to bring relief within a week, a doctor should be consulted. Doctors can provide a variety of more potent prescription medications that may effectively relieve arthritic pain and other nagging, deep-seated discomfort. They also have treatment devices, including diathermy and ultrasound machines, that can beam warming impulses into sore spots in the body.

Types of Counterirritants

Reddeners

As their name implies, these substances redden the skin and also warm it. They tend to be strong counterirritants. This group includes *allyl isothiocyanate* preparations (in plain language, *mustard plasters*) and methyl salicylate, turpentine oil, and stronger ammonia water.

Nonreddeners

These are red-pepper preparations that irritate the skin but do not cause it to redden. They are roughly as potent as reddeners.

Coolants

These agents produce a cooling sensation and yet may stimulate warming and tingling sensations in the skin as well. Counterirritants in this class are camphor and menthol, both of which stimulate the sense of taste and smell, which also may enhance feelings of well-being.

Blood-vessel expanders

These agents—technically called *vasodilators*—widen the capillaries in the skin, which increase blood flow through them. The two vasodilators used in over-the-counter counterirritants are *histamine dihydrochloride* and *methyl nicotinate*.

Combination Products

Many counterirritant products are combinations of several active ingredients. Since the Panel interpreted the FDA's Drug Regulations on combinations in a liberal way, many liniments can continue to be marketed without proof that each of the several ingredients they contain provides a well-defined therapeutic benefit.

A safe and effective amount of an approved counterirritant from one of the four aforementioned groups may be combined with a comparably safe and effective amount of an approved ingredient from one, two, or three other groups. The coolants camphor and menthol can be combined, and *both* can be used, with one ingredient in each of the three other groups, so that approved products may have as many as five active ingredients. But: No ingredient is allowable if it diminishes the effectiveness or the safety of any other.

A combination that contains less than an effective concentration of any other ingredient, rates only conditional approval. A combination containing an active ingredient that had not been assessed by one of the review Panels would be disapproved.

Two Panel members raised strenuous objections to the majority's proposals. They objected to the combining of two or more counterirritants, because the potential hazards of blending them have not been carefully studied. The only justification for such a combination, these experts said, would be if it provided some well-defined therapeutic advantage that was not present when one ingredient was used alone. They added: "The minority of the Panel is not impressed by the statements appearing in manufacturers' submissions, such as 'marketing experience has been favorable,' or 'no complaints have been reported.'"

Counterirritant Ingredients

As noted earlier, standards for the approval of these products were less rigorous scientifically than those used by some other review Panels. In particular, they are less exacting than the standards used by reviewers who evaluated aspirin and other drugs taken internally to relieve aches and pains similar to those for which liniments and poultices are applied externally. (*See* PAIN, FEVER, AND ANTI-INFLAMMATORY DRUGS TAKEN INTERNALLY.)

APPROVED ACTIVE INGREDIENTS

• ALLYL ISOTHICOCYANATE (MUSTARD OIL): This volatile oil is a powerful irritant. It stimulates nerve endings in the skin. It is the active ingredient in mustard plasters (considered to be *poultices*), which consist of powdered mustard seed and flour fixed to a cloth or paper backing that can be dampened and pressed to the skin. Body heat releases the allyl isothiocyanate from the powdered mustard. It produces a decided warmth and reddening of the skin within 5 minutes.

In one test of 9 reddening counterirritants, allyl isothicocyanate was one of the few that both reddened *and* warmed the skin.

Blistering of the skin may occur in some instances. But manufacturers' data show that in a recent 11-year period, during which 15 million package units were sold, only 43 complaints, all minor, were received. This translates into a ratio of one complaint per 350,000 packages. On the basis of these data, the Panel and the FDA say that allyl isothicocyanate—in 0.5 to 5 percent concentrations and applied no more often than 4 times daily—is a safe and effective counterirritant ingredient for the self-treatment of aches and pains in adults and children over 2 years old.

• *AMMONIA, STRONG SOLUTION:* This peculiarly named colorless solution is, in fact, stronger than ordinary household ammonia. But it is diluted for use in liniments and is safe when formulated in 1 to 2.5 percent concentrations.

Ammonia irritates the skin because it is strongly corrosive. But stronger ammonia solution liniments, which are formulated as soaps by combining them with oleic acid and sesame oil, have caused few adverse reactions, according to marketing data. Without citing any scientific study on their effectiveness, the Panel concluded (and the FDA agreed) that stronger ammonia solution is effective as well as safe for use on adults and children over 2 years of age, as long as it is not applied more than 4 times daily.

• *CAMPHOR:* At low dosage, camphor has a cooling, numbing effect on skin receptors and is used to relieve pain and itching. But, paradoxically, in somewhat higher concentrations it produces a warming sensation that helps to block and relieve aches and pains. Camphor's persistent, pungent odor may well contribute to the sense of relief people experience.

Taken orally, camphor can be a deadly poison. It is absorbed through both intact and injured skin, and the Panel on Miscellaneous External Drugs has declared it unsafe in concentrations over 2.5 percent. This Panel disagrees, saying it is unaware of any poisonings attributable to applying camphor to the skin and believes such application is safe.

Camphor usually is mixed with other irritating substances in liniments and related products. Although the report cites no published scientific data, camphor—in concentrations of 3 to 10.8 percent plus 1 to 3.6 percent metacresol, in a 3 to 1 ratio, used no more than 4 times a day by adults and children over 2 years of age—was judged by this Panel to be safe and effective for use as a counterirritant.

• *CAPSICUM PREPARATIONS: CAPSAICIN, CAPSICUM, AND CAPSICUM OLEORESIN:* These counterirritant ingredients are derived from a variety of red peppers. Paradoxically, while they create a warm, even burning, feeling on the skin, they do *not* redden it. They do not raise skin temperature or dilate superficial blood vessels to enhance blood flow. Neither do they cause blistering, although they may feel intolerably hot.

How these capsicum preparations do work and their therapeutic effectiveness have not been adequately studied. Yet the sense of warmth they produce is gratefully accepted by users. These preparation do not appear dangerous. Two companies that were selling more than 4 million product units annually in the early 1970s reported only 16 customer complaints, all of them minor, in one of those years.

In most of these products, red-pepper extract is mixed with other counterirritant ingredients. Insofar as the pepper is concerned, the safe and effective concentration is 0.025 to 0.25 percent capsaicin. Also approved is its equivalent in less refined form, such as capsicum, which is the whole ground dried red pepper, or capsicum oleoresin, which is obtained by percolating the whole pepper in volatile solvents. These preparations are approved as safe and effective for use up to 4 times daily on adults and children over 2 years old.

Cautionary note: Liniments are intended mostly to relieve transitory aches and pains. One capsaicin product is intended as a counterirritant to more severe pains of arthritis, and the nerve pains of diabetic neuropathy and *herpes zoster* (as the product's name—*Zostrix GenDerm*—indicates). It has previously been available as a single-ingredient 0.025 percent cream. The maker now markets a three-times stronger (0.075 percent concentration), as *Zostrix-HP*. These drugs may be effective against significant pain, but analysts for the *Medical Letter on Drugs and Therapeutics* (June 26, 1992) are skeptical. They point out, too, that burning and redness—as side effects—might continue for weeks after use. The *Zostrix-HP* formulation is far above the limit stipulated by the FDA in the OTC Drug Review. These preparations appear not to be designed for weekend warriors' aches and pains.

• HISTAMINE DIHYDROCHLORIDE: Histamine is naturally present, in a bound and inactive form, in most body cells. When released, it stimulates smooth muscle; increases the heart rate, blood flow, and metabolic rate; and causes a generalized flushing and feeling of warmth around the head and neck. In the same way, when histamine is vigorously massaged into intact skin or simply *applied* to broken skin, it penetrates to the underlying layers. There it dilates small blood vessels and increases the blood flow through them. A warming effect results. At the low doses in which histamine dihydrochloride is used in nonprescription medications there have been few (and only minor) side effects reported. The Panel cited no published studies to show that histamine is therapeutically effective at these low levels. Yet it says it is effective, as well as safe, at concentrations of 0.025 to 0.10 percent when applied no more often than 3 to 4 times daily to the skin of adults and children over 2 years of age.

• MENTHOL: This aromatic substance is sometimes called *peppermint camphor*. When rubbed vigorously onto the skin, relatively high concentrations of menthol produce an intense feeling of coolness, even though the skin temperature in the treated area is likely to be warmer than the surrounding skin. The chemical seems to stimulate the nerves for cold perception. This cool feeling often is followed by a sense of warmth. Menthol also depresses the activity of nerve receptors for pain, so it can be effectively used in low doses to treat pain and itching. (*See* Menthol, pp. 673-674.)

Menthol penetrates both unbroken and broken skin. But there are few reports of toxicity when it is rubbed onto the skin. Neither do the sharply aromatic menthol vapors appear to harm the lungs. Some 32 million dosage units of mentholated counterirritant products are sold each year, and manufacturers report no more than one to three complaints per million dosage units—none of them serious.

The Panel concluded that menthol is safe and effective as a counterirritant alone or in combination products at concentrations of 1.25 to 16 percent, if the preparation is applied no more than 3 or 4 times daily and its use is confined to adults and to children over 2 years old. The FDA agrees.

• *METHYL NICOTINATE:* Judging by the Panel's assessment, this derivative of the vitamin niacin is both widely used and poorly studied as a reddening counterirritant. Approval was based on a handful of scientific studies and on marketing reports that show, for example, that in one recent year three companies that sold 2.7 million product units received only 16 customer complaints, all about minor problems.

Methyl nicotinate rapidly penetrates the skin's protective barrier and stimulates underlying sense receptors. These receptors, in turn, trigger return impulses from the brain that expand small blood vessels in the skin, increasing blood flow. This warms and reddens the skin. In doses of 0.25 to 1 percent, applied no more than 4 times daily, methyl nicotinate was evaluated as a safe and effective counterirritant for self-treatment by adults and children over 2 years of age.

• *METHYL SALICYLATE:* This sweet- and pungent-smelling chemical, a member of the aspirin family, is one of the most widely used counterirritant active ingredients; it is also one of the better studied. It is sometimes called *wintergreen oil.*

If eaten, methyl salicylate is quite poisonous, and it now must be sold in childproof containers. Even so, products that contain it should be kept out of reach of children.

Despite methyl salicylate's toxic risk, however, a three-year search of records of the National Clearinghouse for Poison Control

Centers in Bethesda, Maryland, revealed no fatal cases and only a few serious ones resulting from accidental ingestion of methyl salicylate in the forms used as counterirritants for aches, pains, and bruises. Ten manufacturers who sold 35 million packages of these products in one recent year also reported no serious customer complaints and only about one minor complaint for each half-million packages sold.

Methyl salicylate's effectiveness has been tested in controlled scientific studies. They show subjectively experienced pain relief and objectively measured reduction in muscle tension after treatment with lotions that contained the active ingredient.

When applied to the skin of adults and children over 2 years of age, no more than 4 times daily, methyl salicylate is safe and effective in concentrations of 10 to 60 percent.

• TURPENTINE OIL: Medicinal-grade turpentine oil, the Panel says, is of better quality than hardware-store turpentine sold as paint thinner, but it still shares its pungent odor and irritant properties. The use of turpentine for aches and pains has become a part of American folklore. It appears to be safe as well as effective. One company that sold 40 million bottles of a turpentine-oil liniment annually for 80 years claimed it had received no reports of customer problems; another manufacturer, who sold 9 million ounces of it in 1972, reported only two minor problems.

Turpentine is a potent skin irritant. It also causes allergic reactions in 5 to 10 percent of its users.

Although no scientifically controlled studies have been conducted, wide acceptance by consumers and doctors led the Panel and FDA evaluators to declare turpentine oil safe and effective when applied up to 4 times a day on adults and children over 2 years of age and in concentrations of 6 to 50 percent.

CONDITIONALLY APPROVED ACTIVE INGREDIENTS
None.

DISAPPROVED ACTIVE INGREDIENTS
None.

Safety and Effectiveness: Active Ingredients in
Over-the-Counter Liniments and Poultices

Active Ingredient	Mode of Action	Assessment
allyl isothiocyanate (mustard oil)	reddener	safe and effective
ammonia solution, strong	reddener	safe and effective
camphor	coolant	safe and effective
capsicum preparations (capsaicin, capsicum, capsicum oleoresin)	non-reddener	safe and effective
histamine dihydrochloride	blood-vessel expander	safe and effective
menthol	coolant	safe and effective
methyl nicotinate	blood-vessel expander	safe and effective
methyl salicylate	reddener	safe and effective
turpentine oil	reddener	safe and effective

Liniments and Poultices for Aches and Pains: Product Rating

SINGLE-INGREDIENT PRODUCTS

Product and Distributor	Dosage of Active Ingredients	Rating*	Comment
menthol			
Ben-Gay Warming Ice (Pfizer)	gel: 2.5%	A	
Eucalyptamint (Ciba)	ointment: 15%	A	
Extra Strength Absorbine Jr. Liquid (W.F. Young)	liquid: 4%	A	
Flex-all 454 (Chattem)	gel: 7%	A	
Therapeutic Mineral Ice (Bristol-Myers)	gel: 2%	A	
Therapeutic Mineral Ice Exercise Formula (Bristol-Myers)	gel: 4%	A	
methyl salicylate			
Exocaine Medicated Rub (Commerce)	ointment: 25%	A	
Exocaine Plus Rub (Commerce)	ointment: 30%	A	

Liniments and Poultices for Aches and Pains: Product Rating (contd)

COMBINATION PRODUCTS: GELS, CREAMS, AND OINTMENTS

Product and Distributor	Dosage of Active Ingredients	Rating*	Comment
Ben Gay Original Ointment (Pfizer)	**ointment:** 18.3% methyl salicylate + 16% menthol	A	
Ben Gay Ultra Strength Cream (Pfizer)	**cream:** 30% methyl salicylate + 10% menthol + 4% camphor	B	too much camphor
Extra Strength Icy Hot (Richardson-Vicks)	**stick:** 30% methyl salicylate + 10% menthol	A	
Icy Hot Cream (Chattem)	**cream:** 30% methyl salicylate + 10% menthol	A	
Musterole Deep-Strength Rub (Schering-Plough)	30% methyl salicylate + 0.5% methyl nicotinate + 3% menthol	A	
Musterole Extra Strength Ointment (Schering-Plough)	**ointment:** 5% camphor + 3% menthol	B	too much camphor
Odor Free ArthriCare Rub (Commerce)	1.25% menthol + 0.25% methyl nicotinate + 0.025% capsaicin	A	
Tiger Balm (Drug Houses of Australia)	**ointment:** camphor + menthol	B	dosages not listed

COMBINATION PRODUCTS: LOTIONS, LINIMENTS, AND SPRAYS

Product and Distributor	Dosage of Active Ingredients	Rating*	Comment
Banalg Hospital Strength Lotion (Forest)	lotion: 14% methyl salicylate + 3% menthol	A	
Banalg Lotion (Forest)	lotion: 4.9% methyl salicylate + 2% camphor + 1% menthol	B	too little menthol
Ben Gay Lotion (Pfizer)	lotion: 15% methyl salicylate + 7% menthol	A	
Heet Liniment (Whitehall)	liniment: 15% methyl salicylate + 3.6% camphor + 0.025 capsaicin as capsicum oleoresin	B	too much camphor
Heet Spray (Whitehall)	spray: 25% methyl salicylate + 3% camphor + 1% methyl nicotinate + 3% menthol	A	
Panalgesic Liniment (E.C. Robins/Poythress)	liniment: 55% methyl salicylate + 3.1% camphor + 1.25% menthol	B	too much camphor (Panel's upper limit was 3%, FDA's is 2.5%)

*Author's interpretation of FDA criteria. Based on contents, not claims.

Louse Poisons

In recent decades, lice that suck human blood have been on the rise in the United States and perhaps elsewhere as well. Officials at the federal Centers for Disease Control (CDC), in Atlanta, confirm sharp increases of *pediculosis* (louse infestations) in all socioeconomic classes. The reasons for this upsurge of lice are not clearly known. The increase of *pubic lice*—or *crabs*, as they often are called—has been attributed to less-restrained sexual activity. The trend toward transient group living arrangements may favor *body lice*, which thrive where large groups of people live in close quarters. These changes cannot, however, account for the epidemic rise in *head lice*, which particularly afflict school children; children live now much as they did a few decades ago when lice were only rare classroom visitors. After reviewing the available nonprescription pediculicides (louse killers), the Panel decided that one combination of two ingredients—a poison + a booster, or an adjuvant—will effectively control these insects. Subsequently, the FDA switched a potent prescription head louse-killer to nonprescription sta-

LOUSE POISONS is based on report "Pediculicide Drug Products for OTC Human Use" by the FDA's Advisory Review Panel on OTC Miscellaneous External Drug Products, the FDA's Tentative Final Monograph on these products, and the monograph on permethrin in Drug Facts and Comparisons, 1992.

tus, based on a manufacturer's New Drug Application (NDA).

 Claims

Accurate

- "For the treatment of head, pubic (crab), and body lice" (pyrethrins + piperonyl butoxide)
- "For the treatment of head lice" (permethrin)

WARNING:

 Use with caution on persons allergic to ragweed. For external use only. Do not use near eyes or permit contact with mucous membranes. If the product gets into the eyes, immediately flush with water. Consult a doctor if eyebrows or eyelashes are infested with lice.

Types of Infestation

Three kinds of lice attack humans. All create the same symptom: itchiness. These louse species have different life styles, which must be taken into account in de-lousing efforts. All, however, are vulnerable to the same insect poisons.

Head Lice

Technically called *Pediculus humanus capitis*, head lice are 1 to 2 mm long. They rarely are seen because they fade quickly into thick areas of hair, where they escape searching eyes and fingers. What is more likely to be spotted—during what school nurses call *lice inspection*—are the shiny, whitish or silvery egg cases, called *nits*. Female lice attach their nits to a hair shaft, within a quarter-inch of the scalp. Using a strong light, a magnifying glass, and a fine-toothed comb, you can look for them on the short hairs behind the ears or on the nape of the neck. Nits may also be found near the base of the combed-out hairs.

The clue to lice is always the itching. Any time a school child suddenly starts scratching his or her head, lice are suspect. (Boils and other crusty or bloody scalp sores also may occur as the result of infections caused by the scratching.) Lice feed on human blood. The itching is provoked by their saliva, which they leave in the skin while eating. The bitten area reddens and wells up like a tiny mosquito bite.

Head lice are as common in short hair as in long, so giving children short haircuts will not prevent these lice from occurring. According to recent government data, boys appear less vulnerable than girls, and blacks have a relative immunity to head lice.

School authorities should be informed of head-lice cases, since the insects are often transmitted by scarves, hats, coats, and other garments hung together in school cloakrooms. Lice also move from person to person by hiding out in bedding, clothing, or towels.

All suspect clothing and bedding should be disinfected by machine washing in hot water and drying on the dryer's hot cycle for at least 20 minutes. Alternatively, clothing and personal items can be disinfected by dry cleaning or by sealing them in a plastic bag for at least two weeks, until the last louse and last egg die. As a third alternative, spray products now are available that will kill lice and nits concealed on and in personal objects. Brushes and combs and other grooming items should be soaked in hot water (above 130°F) for 5 to 10 minutes. Bedrooms and also all the common rooms of a dwelling should be thoroughly vacuumed.

Pubic Lice

Commonly called *crabs*, the technical name for pubic lice is *Phthirius pubis*. This louse has two pairs of greatly enlarged claw-like legs; it looks like a crab when inspected with a magnifying glass or microscope. Pubic lice are spread mainly by sexual contact, but they may be picked up from bedding, toilet seats, or shared towels. Crab lice favor the pubic and anal-area hairs, although they sometimes are found elsewhere on the body (especially in eyelashes and eyebrows). Their bites raise pale, bluish-gray blotches on the skin, which may be mildly or intolerably itchy. Pubic lice are easier to get rid of than head lice, since they survive only a day when not on a human body. Elaborate disinfecting procedures are not needed.

Body Lice

This louse, technically called *Pediculus humanus corporis*, is generally found where many people live together under crowded conditions. It lives in and lays its eggs in clothing seams and bites skin areas where clothing rubs along the body (for example, at the waistline and in the armpits). The bites cause itching, reddish blotches, and hive-like eruptions as well as raised red bumps like mosquito bites.

Body lice can survive hungry in clothing for up to 10 days, and their eggs remain viable for a month. The disinfectant steps described above for head lice must be followed rigorously. In addition, heat sterilization or insecticides rather than storage in plastic should be used on clothing and other personal belongings. Body lice can carry typhus and other illnesses; anyone who has these lice should probably visit a doctor, particularly if they were picked up in a tropical or semi-tropical area outside the United States.

Louse Killers (Pediculicides)

Insecticides that kill lice are called *pediculicides*. The Panel assessed a dozen insecticides, but approved only one over-the-counter regimen, pyrethrins + piperonyl butoxide. A more effective insecticide, gamma benzene hexachloride (also called *Lindane*) is available by prescription (℞). Because it can be a systemic poison, it must be used very carefully and only once or twice, as directed by a doctor.

In 1990, the FDA approved a 1 percent cream rinse of permethrin as safe and effective for treating head lice but not pubic lice or body lice.

APPROVED ACTIVE INGREDIENTS

• PERMETHRIN (1 PERCENT): This drug is a synthetic form of the insect-killing natural plant poison *pyrethrin*, which tropical chrysanthemum flowers produce to protect themselves from being eaten by bugs. It is a potent nerve poison that paralyzes lice, mites, and other insects, and thus quickly kills them.

Permethrin has an advantage over other nonprescription louse killing drugs in that it kills both living insects *and* their eggs (nits).

The result is that only a single application is necessary rather than two applications, as is the case with the other approved nonprescription treatment, pyrethrins + piperonyl butoxide. (*See* further on.) The conservative *Medical Letter on Drugs and Therapeutics* (March 6, 1992) lists permethrin as the treatment of choice for all three types of louse infestation, although the FDA's approval is specifically limited to head lice and does not include pubic lice or body lice.

The safety of permethrin has been carefully considered by FDA. Based on manufacturers' information, the agency believes that only a very tiny amount will be absorbed through the human skin during the recommended 10-minute application of the drug. Mild and passing itching, stinging, tingling, numbness, and other discomfort may occur.

A single application of permethrin clears up 97 to 99 percent of hair-louse infestations, according to researchers' reports. On this basis, FDA approved 1 percent permethrin, in a liquid cream-rinse formulation, as safe and effective for adults and children over 2. One application should suffice.

• **PYRETHRINS + PIPERONYL BUTOXIDE (LIQUID):** This is a combination of the insecticide pyrethrins with a booster called *piperonyl butoxide*. Piperonyl butoxide enhances pyrethrins' effectiveness because it inhibits the natural detoxification system lice have to combat these poisons. Pyrethrins are natural substances derived from chrysanthemum flowers: They protect the plants from insects. Pyrethrins ruin the insects' nervous systems. They are fast-acting, often killing within minutes.

Both the insecticide and the adjuvant are poorly absorbed through intact human skin, so they pose little risk of systemic toxicity. However, both are slightly irritating, and persons allergic to ragweed may also be allergic to pyrethrins, and so should not use them. Generally speaking, however, the reviewers found that this combination is safe for the self-treatment of lice.

A number of studies have demonstrated this preparation's effectiveness against lice. Two or three applications of pyrethrins with piperonyl butoxide will kill all the lice on most individuals. Itching usually stops after the initial treatment. While the clinical trials of pyrethrins did not meet the Panel's preferred standards, the panelists were impressed enough by the available data to declare pyrethrins with piperonyl butoxide effective as well as safe. However, this mixture does not kill nits, so it must be used a second time—7 to 10 days after the first application—to kill newly hatched lice. The approved dosages are 0.17 to 0.33 percent pyrethrins with 2 to 4 percent piperonyl butoxide.

CONDITIONALLY APPROVED ACTIVE INGREDIENTS

* PYRETHRINS + PIPERONYL BUTOXIDE (AEROSOL): The spray form of this treatment was not submitted to the Panel. The FDA later assessed manufacturers' studies and concluded that while the aerosol is safe, the evidence as yet is insufficient to say that it is effective.

DISAPPROVED ACTIVE INGREDIENTS

As shown in the Safety and Effectiveness table that concludes this Unit, one ingredient (isobornyl thiocyanoacetate) was rejected as unsafe and ineffective. Eleven ingredients were summarily disapproved for want of any data about effectiveness or safety.

* ISOBORNYL THIOCYANOACETATE: This chemical has been used in a nonprescription preparation to kill crab, head, and body lice. But virtually no toxicity data were reported to the Panel. In laboratory tests, isobornyl thiocyanoacetate was not quite so effective as pyrethrins + piperonyl butoxide. Furthermore, it appears that no clinical tests were available to the Panel for its assessment. So isobornyl thiocyanoacetate is judged not safe or effective.

What To Do about Mites

Intense itching of the skin may result from mites rather than lice. The most common culprit is the bite of *Sarcoptes scabiei*, also known as *scabies*. This mite burrows under the top layer of skin, causing intense itching and inflammation. Favored spots are the fingerwebs, wrists, penis, buttock, and underarms; unlike the situation with lice, the head and neck are rarely attacked.

Some experts claim cleanliness keeps mites away. Once mites are present, the Panel said in a rough-draft report, they can be controlled with the use of topical sulfur ointments and lotions containing 5 to 10 percent sulfur. The far better choice would be to visit a doctor, and ask for a prescription drug that will kill scabies. The *Medical Letter* lists 5 percent permethrin as the drug of choice.

Safety and Effectiveness: Active Ingredients in
Over-the-Counter Louse Killers

Active Ingredient	Assessment
aqueous coconut-oil soap	summarily disapproved
benzocaine	summarily disapproved
benzyl alcohol	summarily disapproved
benzyl benzoate	summarily disapproved
dichlorodiphenyl trichlormethane (DDT)	summarily disapproved
dioctyl sodium sulfosuccinate	summarily disapproved
isobornyl thiocyanoacetate	not safe or effective
permethrin 1%	safe and effective
propylene glycol	summarily disapproved
picrotoxin	summarily disapproved
pyrethrins + piperonyl butoxide (liquid)	safe and effective
pyrethrins + piperonyl butoxide (aerosol)	safe, but not proved effective
sabadilla alkaloids	summarily disapproved
sublimed sulfur	summarily disapproved
thiocyanoacetate	summarily disapproved

Louse Poisons: Product Ratings

Product and Distributor	Dosage of Active Ingredients	Rating*	Comment
A-200 (SmithKline Beecham Consumer)	**shampoo and gel:** 0.33% pyrethins + 4% piperonyl butoxide	A	
Barc (Commerce Drug)	**liquid:** 0.18% pyrethrins + 2.2% piperonyl butoxide		
Blue (generic)	**gel:** 0.3% pyrethrins + 3% piperonyl butoxide	A	
Nix (Burroughs Wellcome)	**liquid:** 1% permethrin	A	℞ to OTC switch
Pyrinyl (generic)	**liquid:** 0.2% pyrethrins + 2% piperonyl butoxide	A	
RID Shampoo (Pfizer)	**liquid:** 0.3% pyrethrins + 3% piperonyl butoxide	A	
Pronto (Del)	**shampoo:** 0.33% pyrethrins + 4% piperonyl butoxide	A	
R + C (Reed & Carnrick)	**shampoo:** 0.3% pyrethrins + 3% piperonyl butoxide	A	

*Author's interpetation of FDA criteria. Based on contents, not claims.

Medicaments for Sore Gums, Mouths, and Throats

The *oral cavity*—the subject of this Unit—means, more simply, the mucous membrane surfaces of the gums, mouth, and throat. These internal surface areas, called the *oral mucosa*, start with the lips and move inward and downward to just past the Adam's apple. (Drug products specifically for the teeth and for bad breath are treated elsewhere, in the units MOUTHWASH FOR ORAL HYGIENE; TEETHING EASERS; TOOTHACHE RELIEVERS; FLUORIDE TOOTHPASTES AND RINSES FOR CAVITY PREVENTION; and TEETH: ANTI-PLAQUE PRODUCTS.)

The mucous membranes that line the mouth and throat, unlike the skin that covers most of the rest of our bodies, must be bathed constantly by saliva and other fluids in order to remain healthy. The mucous membranes differ from ordinary skin in another important respect: They readily absorb drugs and other chemicals to which they are exposed. These substances are picked up and carried throughout

MEDICAMENTS FOR SORE GUMS, MOUTHS AND THROATS is based on the reports of the FDA's Advisory Review Panel on OTC Oral Cavity Drug Products and the Advisory Review Panel on OTC Dentifrice and Dental Products. Later sources are the FDA's several Tentative Final Monographs on these products.

the body in the lymph and in the blood.

This capacity for absorption means that some drugs, like the pain-reliever *dibucaine*, that are safe for use on the skin cannot be used safely inside the mouth. However, this absorption through the mucous membranes is not a consistent or reliable method for medicating the body internally. The FDA has decided—tentatively—that aspirin in chewing-gum form probably does not act directly on sore mucous membranes of the throat, as has been suggested by a manufacturer of such products. Rather, the agency says, insofar as these preparations work, they do so by reaching the brain after absorption through the oral mucosa. But the effectiveness of this drug-taking route has yet to be proved, the FDA has ruled.

The different parts of the oral mucosa and the health problems that occur in them—some self-diagnosable and self-treatable, some not—are considered briefly in the following sections. Then the types of drugs that are available over-the-counter to medicate the self-treatable conditions are categorized, described, and evaluated.

The Gums

Few body tissues weather as much stress and strain as the gums, or *gingiva*. Over-laying our jawbones and ensheathing our teeth, the gums are scalded and chilled by food and drink, assaulted by hard and sharp food substances and other objects that are stuck into the mouth, and subjected to extreme pressure when we chew. Moreover, infections can arise from the bacteria that thrive on food that becomes lodged between gums and teeth and then decays. Gingival infections may also be caused by bacteria, viruses, and other microorganisms deposited in the gums by infections elsewhere in the body, or transported to the nose and mouth in the air we breathe.

Gum problems often are closely related to the teeth. Teething is the first cause of sore gums for most babies. In childhood tooth-straightening braces can be irritating and painful. Later in life, the buildup of bacteria-laden dental plaque is a principal cause of the persistent gum soreness called *gingivitis*. False teeth (dentures) often cause gum pain. So, too, do tooth extractions and other dental procedures.

Minor gum sores and irritations soon heal. This natural healing perhaps can be assisted—and the soreness certainly can be relieved—by a variety of drugs that can be applied to the gums. Reviewers caution, however, that many dental products sold for gum care contain ingredients that are useless or even harmful. Some claims made for them are extravagant. Also, seriously and persistently painful gums should not be self-treated, says the Dental Panel. A dentist should be consulted.

Gingivitis

The Dental Panel makes a critical distinction between minor gum disorders and gingivitis. The former refers to inflammation, irritation, and injuries caused principally by "mechanical" forces, such as newly erupting teeth and poorly fitting dentures, and might also include overzealous tooth-picking, burns from hot food or utensils, and other types of injury (trauma). These are conditions that can be successfully self-treated with over-the-counter dental-care products.

The second type of gum inflammation, gingivitis, often is a more serious condition. But it is less amenable to self-treatment with nonprescription drugs, or, for that matter, with available prescription drugs. *Gingivitis* is defined as inflammation in the contact areas where gums and teeth meet. It is caused by bacterial plaque, the sticky, gel-like mass of food particles, tissue secretions, and bacteria and their breakdown products that build up on the teeth. Plaque is the principal cause of dental cavities. *See* TEETH: ANTI-PLAQUE PRODUCTS.

The bacteria in plaque secrete acids and other substances that cause chronic redness, swelling, and soreness of the gum. Besides being extremely irritating, plaque may cause the gums to recede from the teeth, which then become loose in their sockets. They eventually may fall out or require extraction. For these reasons, the Dental Panel says: "Dental plaque and gingivitis represent two of the leading dental-health problems in the country today." Some bacterial plaque can be removed by tooth-brushing. But even very diligent brushing can leave behind significant plaque deposits because tooth alignment and related factors block the bristles' action.

The Dental Panel believes that none of the currently marketed preparations promoted for use against plaque have been demonstrated to be safe and effective. Such drugs may include cetylpyridinium chloride and domiphen bromide, which have been reported to yield a 30 to 40 percent reduction in plaque when used regularly, as well as more traditional antimicrobial agents like thymol and eucalyptol.

The Dental Panel, like the Panel on Oral Cavity Drug Products, is particularly worried about antimicrobials in mouthwashes that are recommended for daily use. This routine use may be hazardous. Therefore, these reviewers have rejected as unproved, untrue, or misbranding all claims that antiseptic mouthwashes and gum-care drugs will reduce or prevent plaque or gingivitis. However, they strongly endorse self-treatment with fluoride toothpastes, rinses, and gels for preventing tooth decay. (*See* FLUORIDE TOOTHPASTES AND RINSES FOR CAVITY PREVENTION). The regular use of dental floss to remove food particles between the teeth may help, too. But the most effective method for removing plaque and preventing gingivitis is periodic cleaning and polishing of the teeth by a dentist or an oral hygienist, and, when necessary, curettage (scraping under the gum line).

Sore Throat

Most sore throats are a symptom of some underlying infection or other illness. They are particularly common in sufferers of colds and other upper-respiratory infections that produce thick secretions that adhere to and irritate the throat's mucous membranes. The streptococcal bacteria that cause scarlet fever and rheumatic fever (most often in children) may first make themselves felt as a sore and reddened "strep throat." Other serious illnesses—such as Vincent's disease (an ulcerating infection that kills gum tissue), oral gonorrhea, measles, and some cancers—also produce sore-throat symptoms. Fish bones, glass, or other sharp objects ingested with food can injure the throat so that pain and infection may follow.

The discomfort of mild sore throat can be successfully treated with over-the-counter drugs. Reviewers warn, however, that these drugs provide only *temporary* relief of symptoms. They do not correct the underlying conditions.

Sore Mouth

Unlike sore throat, few sore-mouth problems lend themselves either to self-diagnosis or self-treatment. Yet labels on many nonprescription oral health-care products make treatment claims that the Oral Cavity Panel would ban. Immediately following are descriptions of several common mouth infections and other conditions and information about whether the Panel and the FDA think they can be self-diagnosed and treated with nonprescription preparations.

Mouth Infections

Candidiasis

This is a common fungal infection of the mouth. It is characterized by white bumps and reddish, inflamed patches on the mucous membrane. This infection can only be diagnosed by a physician or a dentist through laboratory tests.

Canker Sores (aphthous stomatitis, Behçet's syndrome)

These sores, or *ulcers*, appear suddenly in the movable, soft tissues of the mouth. There may be one, two or more, or one or more groups of them. They tend to recur, and often are quite painful.

Most canker sores are a quarter inch across or smaller, and most heal by themselves, within two weeks, without residual scarring. Larger such sores take longer to heal, and may leave scars behind.

The cause of canker sores is unclear. They may be due to an immunological defect, or vitamin or iron deficiency. Stress and minor injury also may be a factor. Canker sores are commoner in women than in men.

The Dental Panel did not think canker sores can be reliably self-diagnosed or self-treated, and instead wanted sufferers of this condition to seek medical help. The FDA disagrees. The agency has ruled that "canker sores can be recognized by the consumer, and the pain associated with canker sores is amenable to self-treatment with OTC pain-relieving active ingredients." However, canker sores, or *any* other sores or bumps in the mouth that do not disappear within a week or two should be shown promptly to a dentist or doctor.

Gonococcal Sores of the Mouth

A diagnosis of venereal disease can be made only by a doctor, and only a doctor can provide appropriate treatment.

Herpangina

A common disease in young children, herpangina is especially prevalent in late summer. Tiny ulcers appear at the back of the mouth and in the throat. They soon rupture, causing a burning sensation or pain. The pain can be excruciating. Herpangina must be treated by a dentist or a doctor.

Primary Herpetic Stomatitis

This is a viral illness that causes extremely painful blisters on the cheek, tongue, palate, and floor of the mouth. The gums may be swollen, bright red, and may bleed easily. A dentist or a doctor must diagnose and treat this ailment.

Secondary Herpetic Infections

These recurrent herpes attacks are caused by the same virus as primary herpetic stomatitis (*see* immediately preceding). The sores usually erupt on the roof of the mouth or on the lips, where they cause a burning sensation or pain. The Oral Cavity Panel failed to say whether it believed consumers can self-diagnose and self-treat this condition.

Syphilis

Sore mouth and throat can occur in the early, delayed, or late stages of this venereal disease. If the infection results from oral sex, the primary ulcer (chancre) may appear in the mouth. Wherever the disease starts, the second stage—beginning about 6 weeks after onset—is often characterized by sore throat, possibly by sore mouth, and by grayish mucous patches. This disease cannot be self-diagnosed or self-treated with over-the-counter products.

Tuberculosis Lesions

A chronic ulcer or sore on the tongue or inside the cheek may be caused by this serious lung disorder, or a form of it that originates within the mouth. Self-diagnosis and treatment are simply not possible. Medical supervision is the answer.

Vincent's Disease (acute necrotizing ulcerative gingivitis)

This infection produces sores between teeth that secrete a grayish, pus-like substance. The gums bleed easily. A doctor's or a dentist's diagnosis and antibiotic therapy are usually needed to relieve the symptoms and to clear up the infection.

Cough

Some lozenges and other over-the-counter products used to treat sore throat and sore mouth contain drugs intended to loosen thick mucus and relieve throat irritation and coughing. Most coughs can be more effectively treated with cough suppressors, decongestants, or expectorants that are taken internally. (See Cough Suppressors and Expectorants in COLD AND COUGH MEDICINES). But there may also be some value in treating the throat directly with topical drugs.

Effective Ways to Use Oral Cavity Medication

Over-the-counter drugs that are applied directly to the mucous membranes for relief of sore gums, sore mouth, sore throat and coughs are classified as *oral health-care products*. They are intended for brief use, over a few days, to relieve specific symptoms of injury or disease. The FDA has reserved the alternative phrase *oral hygiene products* to describe mouthwashes, rinses and sprays that are recommended for routine daily use. (See MOUTHWASH FOR ORAL HYGIENE).

Oral health-care products are made in a variety of ways for application inside the mouth. Some are formulated to be swished around the mouth, and then spat out. Others are applied from spray bottles, which is a particularly effective way to get medication to the back of the mouth and the throat.

A gargling solution—or, simply, a *gargle*—is used to rinse or bathe the upper part of the throat. The best way to gargle is to take some of the fluid into the mouth, tilt the head back, and then force air from the lungs up through the liquid to splash it around before spitting it out. A useful trick is to try "singing" through the rinse.

The Oral Cavity Panel, however, does not think gargling is an effective way of medicating the throat. Tests with dyes and X-rays show that gargled liquids often do not reach the back of the throat where the soreness is likely to occur, and the liquids may bathe even the front of the throat only briefly. The evaluators said sprays are more effective.

The trouble with mouthwashes, rinses, and sprays is that saliva quickly washes them away. For treating small, discrete areas in the mouth, it may be more effective to swab the medication onto the sore spot with a clean cotton applicator. For wider soreness, the most effective method may be to use candy-like lozenges (troches), which dissolve slowly and bathe the irritated areas with the medicine for 5 or 10 minutes or more. The Panel added, however, that it had not seen well-controlled studies that really prove the advantage of this method.

The Dental Panel pointed out that some pain-relief products are sold in *poultices*, small porous sacks that hold drugs that have been formulated in a slow-release base. Poultices can be a very effective method for self-medicating the inside of the mouth, the Panel said, adding this word of caution:

WARNING:

 Be sure to take the poultice out before going to sleep, lest you inadvertently swallow it and choke.

Some products are formulated to adhere to the mucosa. Pain relievers, for example, are mixed with a denture adhesive and so may keep the medication effectively in touch with the sore area for longer than mouth rinses or lozenges are able to.

Types of Active Ingredients

Several different kinds of drugs are formulated into products meant to be swished around, sprayed on, or dissolved inside the mouth:

• *ANESTHETICS/ANALGESICS:* Temporarily relieve pain or discomfort.

• *ANTIMICROBIALS:* Kill or inhibit infectious microorganisms.

• *ASTRINGENTS:* Bind and remove irritating protein-type substances.

• *DEBRIS REMOVER/WOUND CLEANSERS:* Loosen and remove mucus and debris and cleanse the sore, irritated or injured area.

• *DEMULCENTS—OR "SOOTHERS":* Coat and protect sore spots.

• *MUCOSAL PROTECTANTS:* Form a temporary protective coating over sore and irritated areas.

Saliva Substitutes for Dry Mouth

A dry mouth—caused by inadequate salivation—is a fairly common problem: The older you get, the more likely you are to suffer from it. The technical name for dry mouth is *xerostomia*.

Besides being unpleasant, inadequate salivation increases the frequency of tooth decay (since saliva contains substances that kill tooth-destroying bacteria and the saliva itself also washes the bacteria away). It also produces distressing swelling inside the mouth, inflammation, pain and persistent sores. Food tastes different, and oral functions—such as talking, chewing, and swallowing—may be affected.

Xerostomia is caused by a variety of illnesses, one of which is Sjögren's syndrome. X-rays and drugs, including antihistamines and anticholinergics, also can dry out the mouth. Persons who feel that their mouths are drier than normal should see a doctor, who can determine if there is a problem and offer medical or other remedies.

Doctors tell dry-mouth patients to drink water frequently or suck on pieces of ice. For some sufferers, chewing stimulates salivary flow. They also are encouraged to nibble on carrots, celery, and other chewy foods or to chew sugarless gum (which will not cause dental cavities).

For many sufferers of this complaint, saliva substitutes may be the only recourse other than frequently sipping water. Several drug preparations are available without prescription to provide this transient relief. Some are water-based or glycerin-based fluids or sprays. Others contain polymers such as sodium carboxymethylcellulose or hydroxymethylcellulose that bind and hold moisture. These saliva substitutes also may contain other ingredients, including vital mineral salts (electrolytes).

Saliva substitutes are not part of the FDA's Over-the-Counter Drug Review. Carboxymethylcellulose sodium, which is the common ingredient in several of them, is described on p. 390.

The individual drugs for sore gums, mouth, and throat are described here under these general headings, and the two Panels' findings, as amended by the FDA, are summarized in the Safety and Effectiveness table at the end of this Unit. Any active ingredient that has not been specifically judged by a panel or the FDA is automatically listed as disapproved when used to relieve sore-throat and sore-mouth symptoms.

Combination Products

Reviewers expressed caution about combination products, even though they are extremely popular with over-the-counter oral-health-care product makers—and apparently with consumers, too. Most of the currently approved combination products contain one safe and effective anesthetic/analgesic + one safe and effective ingredient from a second class of ingredients, such as a demulcent, an astringent, a mucosal protectant, or a denture adhesive. The Panels' and the FDA's specific decisions are summarized in the Safety and Effectiveness: Combination Products table at the end of this Unit.

Anesthetics/Analgesics

Pain relief is the most clear-cut benefit that can be obtained from over-the-counter oral health-care products. Many commonly used ingredients are safe and effective for this purpose. Some are powerful enough to inhibit all sensory impulses from the mucous membranes, including not only pain but also feelings of coldness, warmth, touch, and pressure. Less potent ingredients relieve or dampen pain but spare the other senses. The former effect is technically called *anesthesia* (numbness); the latter, *analgesia* (pain relief).

The anesthetics/analgesics fall into three pharmacological groups:

• NITROGENOUS ANESTHETICS: Most of these drugs are recognizable because their names end in the suffix -*caine*, as in lidocaine, or in -*ine*. They are the most potent but also potentially the most dangerous pain relievers formulated into nonprescription oral health-care products. They act by temporarily short-circuiting sensory nerve receptors in the mucosa so that "pain messages" cannot be transmitted toward the brain.

When absorbed into the system, stronger nitrogenous anesthetics affect the central nervous system. They can cause convulsions, coma, and death. They slow the heartbeat and may cause it to stop altogether. These serious side effects, fortunately, have been extremely rare.

• *ALCOHOL-TYPE ANESTHETICS:* These are older drugs, such as menthol, some of which have been used over the ages in folk medicine. They tend to be less potent than the nitrogenous anesthetics. But they are also safer, because they do not carry the risk of central nervous system side effects.

• *SALICYLATES:* This group includes aspirin and related drugs. Salicylates do not block nerve impulses as the nitrogenous and alcoholic anesthetics do. They act on pain centers in the brain, the FDA says, but do not act directly to relieve inflammation and pain when applied to mucosal tissue in the throat and mouth.

 ## Claims for Anesthetics/Analgesics

Accurate

• "For the temporary relief of occasional minor irritation, pain, sore mouth and sore throat or injury of soft tissue of the mouth"

• "...temporary relief of pain due to minor dental procedures"

• "...temporary relief of pain due to minor irritation of the mouth and gums caused by dentures [false teeth] or orthodontic appliances [braces]"

• "...temporary relief of pain associated with canker sores"

WARNING:

 When used for sore gums or mouth:

If symptoms do not improve in 7 days, see your dentist or doctor promptly.

When used for sore throat:

If sore throat is severe, persists for more than 2 days, or is accompanied or followed by fever, headache, rash, nausea, or vomiting, consult a doctor promptly.

APPROVED ANESTHETIC/ANALGESIC ACTIVE INGREDIENTS

Several ingredients are approved as safe and effective for relieving discomfort and pain due to sore gums, mouth, or throat. They are

- BENZOCAINE: A widely used -*caine* type of anesthetic, benzocaine is extremely safe because—unlike others in its class—it is quite insoluble in water. This means that when it is applied to the skin or mucous membranes of the mouth or throat, very little of the drug is absorbed into the body. So there is almost no risk of injury to the nervous system, heart, or other vital organs.

  Wide and varied studies as well as case reports attest to benzocaine's safety and effectiveness. When it is applied to the mucous membranes of the mouth and throat in a lozenge or a spray, it produces pain relief in 30 to 60 seconds. Given the normal dilution and washout by saliva, each application should block pain for 5 to 10 minutes; continuous application in lozenges will produce continuing relief.

  Benzocaine acts only on the sensory receptors of the mucous membranes. It does not penetrate into these membranes, and so will not relieve deep-seated inflammatory pain or dental pain originating deep in the teeth or gums.

  The approved dosage for adults and children over age 2 years is 5 to 20 percent benzocaine in a gel or spray for use not more than 4 times daily, or in lozenges taken not oftener than every 2 hours for up to 2 days for sore throat or 7 days for sore gums or mouth. Each lozenge should contain 2 to 15 mg benzocaine. Children under 12 years old should be supervised by an adult when using this drug. It should not be used in children under 2 years of age except as recommended by a doctor. *But*: Parents of new babies should note that benzocaine is one of the two drugs that is safe enough, in small amounts, to be used to relieve teething pain. *See* TEETHING EASERS.

- BENZYL ALCOHOL: This alcoholic anesthetic does not carry the risk of central nervous system and cardiac complications that are a problem with some nitrogenous anesthetics. Evaluators judged it safe largely on the basis of long use and the rarity of reported side effects.

  While benzyl alcohol is less potent than benzocaine, it is nevertheless effective in relieving irritation and soreness in the mouth and throat. It takes 2 minutes to produce pain relief that may then last for 5 to 10 minutes. In pure form, benzyl alcohol is irritating to the mucous membranes and so must be diluted.

For adults and children over age 2 years, the safe and effective dose is 0.05 to 10 percent benzyl alcohol as a rinse, a mouthwash, drops, or sprays, used no more than 4 times daily for up to 2 days for sore throat or 7 days for sore gums or mouth. Lozenges may be taken up to once every 2 hours. Each lozenge should contain 100 to 500 mg of benzyl alcohol. For children under 2 years of age, consult a dentist or a doctor.

• *BUTACAINE SULFATE:* This effective analgesic has been used by dentists for a long time and is intended for use on the gums and mouth, not for sore throat. The Dental Panel recommended that it be made available without prescription. Several researchers who have studied butacaine sulfate concur that it is very effective in relieving pain after dental work and also in reducing the soreness and discomfort caused by braces and dentures. The only approved dose is 30 mg.

The trouble with butacaine, as with similar nitrogen-based pain relievers, is that it can be highly toxic. It can cause convulsions, coma, slowed heartbeat, heart failure, and death *if* large enough quantities are absorbed through the lining of the mouth and reach the central nervous system or heart. To forestall this hazard, the FDA requires manufacturers to clearly indicate how consumers can be sure they are getting only the appropriate 30-mg dose.

Butacaine should *not* be used for teething in infants, or for any other reason in children under age 12, except under a dentist's or a doctor's supervision.

The safe and effective dose is 30 mg (0.75 gram of a 3 percent ointment) to be used at no less than 3-hour intervals, up to 3 times daily. Persons allergic to procaine or other *-caine* analgesics should not use this drug.

• *DYCLONINE HYDROCHLORIDE:* Of the several nitrogenous anesthetics, this is the most effective drug that can be safely used in the mouth and throat. It has been modified chemically from a *-caine* to an *-ine* compound—a step that eliminates the risk of convulsions and other central nervous system side effects that are present with many of the *-caine* drugs (although not benzocaine) when they are absorbed through the mucous membranes into the body.

A variety of animal and human tests indicate that dyclonine hydrochloride is safe for use in the mouth, reviewers say. Studies are available that show, too, that it is quite an effective anesthetic when used on mucosal surfaces. According to one investigator, 2 to 3 minutes after application a 1 percent concentration of this drug produces numbness that lasts almost half an hour. Used as a rinse or gargle, it may provide an hour's relief. When it is sucked from a lozenge, relief may last longer.

The FDA says the safe and effective dosage for adults and children over age 2 years is a 0.05 to 0.1 percent solution of dyclonine hydrochloride in a rinse, a mouthwash, a gargle or a spray, used not more than 4 times daily. The approved dosage for lozenges is one lozenge every 2 hours for up to 2 days. Each lozenge should contain 1 to 3 mg dyclonine hydrochloride. For children under 2 years of age, consult a dentist or doctor.

• *HEXYLRESORCINOL:* This is a sharp-tasting, aromatic alcohol that has been used as an anesthetic (as well as for other medicinal purposes) for more than 40 years. It is chemically related to phenol but is less irritating to skin and mucous membranes than phenol. Animal tests and long marketing experience, with few reports of allergic reactions or other complications, led evaluators to rank hexylresorcinol as safe.

The data on hexylresorcinol's effectiveness is less impressive. It appears to be less potent than benzocaine and shorter-acting than dyclonine hydrochloride (*see* previously). Nevertheless, the Oral Cavity Panel found that hexylresorcinol is effective as well as safe for adults and for children over age 3 years, when used every 4 hours for up to 2 days for sore throat or 7 days for sore gums or mouth. Dosages should be 0.05 to 0.1 percent in rinses, gargles, sprays, and mouthwashes and 2 to 4 mg per lozenge. Lozenges containing 2 to 4 mg of hexylresorcinol may be taken as often as once every 2 hours. For children under 2 years of age, use only as directed by a dentist or a doctor.

• *MENTHOL:* A pepperminty alcohol, menthol is now more likely to be manufactured synthetically than extracted from mint plants. Its wide use in candies and other foods, as well as in medicines, persuades evaluators that menthol is safe. The Panel warns, however, that menthol products should not be given to children under 2 years of age because they have been known to choke some infants and toddlers.

No well-controlled studies are available to document menthol's effectiveness in quelling irritation and soreness in the throat and mouth. But reviewers believed its wide use, its acceptance by doctors and consumers, and the paucity of reports on adverse effect permit its classification as a safe and effective ingredient. In liquid preparations, relief usually lasts no longer than 5 to 10 minutes; lozenges may extend this time.

The safe and effective dosage of menthol for adults and children over 2 years of age is 0.04 to 2 percent concentrations of menthol in rinses, mouthwash, gargles or sprays to be used not more than 3 or 4 times daily for up to 2 days for sore throat or 7 days for sore gums or mouth. For lozenges, the dosage is one lozenge with 2 to 20 mg menthol, taken up to once every 2 hours if necessary. For children under 2 years old, consult a dentist or doctor.

- *PHENOL PREPARATIONS (PHENOL AND PHENOLATE SODIUM):* An alcohol, this coal-tar derivative has been used in medicine for more than a century, and its safety has been carefully studied. Although the drug can be quite toxic in higher doses, evaluators regard it as safe in the low doses approved for use inside the mouth.

  Phenol penetrates the sensory nerve endings in the mucosal surfaces of the mouth and throat, temporarily blocking transmission of impulses for pain and other sensations. This blockage begins in 1 to 2 minutes and may go on for 5 to 10 minutes—or longer if the phenol is being continuously released from a lozenge. As the drug is washed away by saliva, the numbness recedes and the pain may return.

  The FDA approves as safe and effective for persons over age 6 years water-based (aqueous) solutions of from 0.5 to 1.5 percent phenol or its phenolate sodium equivalent, not oftener than every 2 hours, for no longer than 2 days for sore throat or 7 days for sore gums or mouth. Children 6 to 12 years old need adult supervision. Rinses (mouthwashes) should not be used by children under age 6 unless recommended by a doctor or dentist. The Oral Cavity Panel warned that aqueous solutions of phenol stronger than 2 percent can be dangerously irritating to the mucous membranes. (Stronger mixtures of phenol in glycerin are claimed to be safe because the glycerin releases phenol only slowly.)

  The safe and effective dose of phenol in lozenges is 10 to 50 mg per lozenge, to be taken as often as once every 2 hours if necessary. For children under 12 years of age, adult supervision is required; for children under 6 years old, use only as directed by a dentist or a doctor.

- *PHENOLATE SODIUM (SODIUM PHENOLATE):* The active material in this ingredient is phenol discussed in the preceding paragraphs. Its safety and effectiveness are comparable.

- *SALICYL ALCOHOL:* Except for over-the-counter preparations, this pain-damping alcohol is no longer widely used, and there are few scientific studies that indicate it is safe and effective. Going by what is known, however, the Oral Cavity Panel said that the drug "appears" to have no adverse effects on the mucous membranes in concentrations under

6 percent, and the FDA has concurred with this judgment. The Panel assessed salicyl alcohol as an effective—albeit short-acting—anesthetic. Relief comes within 2 to 3 minutes and lasts 5 to 10 minutes when liquid dosage forms are used; lozenges may afford longer relief.

The safe and effective dosage of salicyl alcohol is 1 to 6 percent concentrations in aqueous solutions in the form of mouth rinses, mouthwash, gargles, or sprays, to be used up to 2 days for sore throat or 7 days for sore mouth. It is safe and effective self-medication for adults and for children over 2 years old to use a lozenge containing 50 to 100 mg of salicyl alcohol every 2 hours for 2 days for sore throat, or for up to 7 days for sore mouth.

CONDITIONALLY APPROVED ANESTHETIC/ANALGESIC ACTIVE INGREDIENTS

Only a conditional approval has been granted to several of the pain-relieving drugs that are applied topically to sore throats and mouths. Most are safe. The unanswered question usually is: Are they effective?

• *ASPIRIN IN CHEWING GUM:* Aspirin, which belongs to the class of drugs called *salicylates*, is the most widely used medicinal ingredient. A mountain of data indicates that it is safe and effective when swallowed in a tablet. In the doses in which aspirin is usually formulated into chewing-gum products, it is also safe, unless the inside of the mouth or throat is highly inflamed, cut, or torn. In that case, aspirin may induce bleeding. The Oral Cavity Panel also warned that persons with underlying bleeding problems should not use topical aspirin products.

However, there is no convincing scientific evidence shows that aspirin is at all effective when applied directly to mouth-throat mucosal surfaces. It does not block nerve transmission of pain, as nitrogenous anesthetics do. Whatever pain-relieving benefit the drug may offer when used locally is said to result from its absorption through the mucosal lining of the gastrointestinal tract and into the bloodstream, from whence it is carried to the brain.

• *CHLOROPHYLLINS, WATER-SOLUBLE:* These preparations are derivatives of chlorophyll, the plant material that is responsible for photosynthesis (the process that uses sunlight to convert basic materials into the carbohydrates that support most life on earth). On a label, the drug may be called *potassium-sodium-copper chlorophyllin*. Chlorophyllins appear not to belong to any of the groups of pain-relieving drugs described above. But chlorophyllins have been used medicinally—both as topical and as systemic drugs—for a variety of medical problems, and they have not been reported to have caused toxicity (poisoning). Animal studies also suggest these substances are safe—a judgment in which the Oral Cavity Panel concurs.

Chlorophyllins have been used to control odor and bacteria, and to speed healing of wounds and ulcerated sores. (*See* DEODORANTS FOR INCONTINENCE AND OSTOMIES.) But the evidence that they relieve pain is scant. The FDA says that more definitive, well-controlled scientific work remains to be done.

• *CRESOL:* This is a phenol-like compound that can be highly irritating to skin and mucous membranes. Dilute solutions are used therapeutically, but the Dental Panel could find no evidence to show that they are safe.

Although studies in humans and animals indicate that cresol does have some local analgesic activity, these reviewers found no adequately controlled scientific studies to demonstrate cresol's effectiveness as a pain reliever for the gums. In sum, cresol has not been proved safe or effective.

• *THYMOL PREPARATIONS: THYMOL AND THYMOL IODIDE:* These substances are toxic in large doses, but apparently are safe in the tiny doses for which they may be used to treat sore gums. They are used by dentists to relieve gingival pain, but scant scientific documentation demonstrates their effectiveness for this purpose. So the thymols are, for now, judged safe but not proved effective.

DISAPPROVED ANESTHETIC/ANALGESIC ACTIVE INGREDIENTS

On the basis of the available evidence, the Panels have recommended that the following active ingredients that have been formulated into oral health-care products be banned.

• *CAMPHOR:* Despite its long use, concern persists about this substance's toxicity. Lacking data showing that camphor is effective on the mucous membranes of the throat and mouth, evaluators judged it both unsafe and ineffective.

• *METHYL SALICYLATE:* The pleasant wintergreen aroma and taste of this aspirin-like drug tend to conceal that it is highly toxic. It is also extremely irritating to the gums. The Dental Panel says it is both unsafe and ineffective.

Antimicrobials

An antimicrobial kills or inhibits the growth and spread of bacteria and other microorganisms. These drugs are also known as *antiseptics* or *germ killers*. Antimicrobials are present in many oral-health-care products sold to relieve sore throat and mouth. Evaluators say, however, that there is little evidence that they really work, and they may interfere with the healing of both clean and infected wounds.

Each of the antimicrobial agents available in over-the-counter products is effective against only a relatively few disease-producing organisms. Most are wholly ineffective against viruses, which are a principal cause of sore throat associated with colds. Health-care consumers have no way to decide which organisms are causing their complaint—since medical tests are required for this purpose—and so they cannot make an informed choice about which antimicrobial to use. This means that self-treating sore throat or mouth conditions with antimicrobials is likely to be ineffective, according to the experts.

Swishing an antimicrobial around in your mouth—even if it happens to be one that acts against the offending "germ"—is likely to be fruitless for some other reasons, too. The drug probably cannot penetrate into the deeper layers of the mucous membranes where holed-up microorganisms are causing inflammation and pain. In addition, no sooner is the antimicrobial gone from the mouth than the microorganisms reproduce their numbers anew.

Most antimicrobials, what is worse, kill *useful* microorganisms as well as harmful ones. Repeated self-dosing thus may encourage the growth of resistant breeds that may be more difficult to control—and so more dangerous—than the ones that originally were there. Antimicrobial drugs may also counteract the action of the body's natural protective mechanisms.

For these reasons, antimicrobials should never be used for preventive purposes, particularly not on a routine, daily basis as some manufacturers advise. (*See* MOUTHWASH FOR ORAL HYGIENE.) Since none of the antimicrobial active ingredients in these products have been demonstrated to be safe and effective for relieving sore throat or sore mouth, the Oral Cavity Panel suggests that they not be used for that purpose. Instead of antimicrobials, evaluators suggest that small wounds or sores in the mouth or sore throats be treated by gently swishing clean, cool water over the inflamed area, and then spitting out the water. (A cotton swab can be used to remove foreign matter from a wound.) Or you might use a gentle water spray.

 Claims for Antimicrobials

Accurate

• "For the temporary relief of minor sore mouth and sore throat by decreasing the germs in the mouth" (*if* any were safe and effective, which none is)

APPROVED ANTIMICROBIAL ACTIVE INGREDIENTS

None.

CONDITIONALLY APPROVED ANTIMICROBIAL ACTIVE INGREDIENTS

• *BENZALKONIUM CHLORIDE:* This chemical is a quaternary ammonium compound (quat). It is a white to yellowish powder or gel, that is soluble in both water and alcohol. It has been shown to be safe in a variety of studies, although few of these investigations involved use on mucous membranes of the throat and mouth. No acceptable evidence is available concerning the safety of long-term, day-to-day use. Nor is it known if the chemical may cause cancer, birth defects, or genetic damage when used in this way. The Oral Cavity Panel nevertheless rates benzalkonium safe when used—very briefly—in an attempt to kill organisms that can cause sore throat and sore mouth.

However, benzalkonium chloride controls only a limited range of these microorganisms. It is of dubious value when applied to the surface of an infected area. So, while this agent is designated safe, reviewers say its effectiveness in relieving sore throat and sore mouth remains to be proved.

• *BENZETHONIUM CHLORIDE:* This compound is similar to benzalkonium chloride (*see* immediately preceding). It is absorbed into the bloodstream when it is applied to the mucous membranes of the mouth and throat. Since the results, if any, of this absorption remain to be determined, evaluators ranked this agent's safety as unproved, although, generally speaking, benzethonium chloride is not highly toxic.

The drug has been shown to be highly effective against bacteria and other microorganisms in many infectious settings. But its value in killing microorganisms when applied directly to the mouth or throat has yet to be proved. What is worse, it may increase rather than decrease inflammation. In sum: both the safety and effectiveness of benzethonium chloride are yet to be proved.

• **BENZOIC ACID:** This ingredient is widely used in medicines, and as a food preservative. A number of studies have shown that benzoic acid is relatively nontoxic to humans, and the Oral Cavity Panel said it is safe. These experts note, however, that it may be mildly irritating to the mucous membranes of the throat and mouth.

Benzoic acid kills microorganisms under many laboratory and real-life conditions. But by and large it does not work against the organisms that are responsible for sore throat and sore mouth. Results cited by manufacturers in support of the ingredient were found to be both outdated and unconvincing. So the Panel's verdict is that benzoic acid is safe, but its effectiveness needs to be shown.

• **CARBAMIDE PEROXIDE IN ANHYDROUS GLYCERIN (UREA PEROXIDE):** Anhydrous (water-free) glycerin is a vehicle that keeps the carbamide peroxide dry. When the carbamide peroxide is exposed to saliva and enzymes in the mouth, it breaks down to hydrogen peroxide. This, in turn, breaks down into bubbling, foaming oxygen and water. The oxygen released in this way is alleged to kill bacteria.

Reviewers noted, however, that most organisms are relatively resistant to the action of peroxides, and they doubted that the bacteria and viruses that cause sore throats and sore mouths are much affected by these preparations. But since the breakdown products—urea, oxygen, and water—all occur naturally in the body, the Oral Cavity Panel accepts carbamide peroxide as safe. Conclusion: safe but not proved effective.

• **CETALKONIUM CHLORIDE:** This is another quaternary ammonium compound that disrupts the cell surfaces of many bacteria and funguses. So it is employed to control both kinds of microorganisms. In the dilute form in which this compound is used in mouthwashes and other oral health-care products, it is odorless and practically tasteless. It may be mildly irritating, the Oral Cavity Panel says, but not to a harmful degree. However, cetalkonium chloride's effectiveness against the microorganisms that cause sore throat and sore mouth is questionable. Because their tests were poorly constructed, results submitted by manufacturers who hoped to show that the substance rapidly kills bacteria in human saliva were rejected by the Panel. So while cetalkonium chloride is safe, it remains to be shown that it is effective.

• *CETYLPYRIDINIUM CHLORIDE:* Yet another quaternary ammonium compound, this drug was introduced into clinical use in 1942. Since that time, it has been shown to kill or inhibit some species of bacteria and fungus and some other microorganisms as well. However, many important questions have never been resolved: long-term and cumulative effects, metabolism, and information on excretion. Furthermore, the compound works against only a limited number of bacteria, and its lethal effect on these organisms can be blocked by natural or introduced chemicals present in the mouth. Finally, even if the drug does reduce bacterial counts, it remains doubtful whether curative effects are achieved. The Oral Cavity Panel ruled that both the safety and the effectiveness of cetylpyridinium chloride for mouth-throat use must be proved.

• *CHLOROPHYLL:* Since chlorophyll is a major part of food, experts ruled it reasonable to assume that the substance is safe in the amounts present in oral health-care products. Some forms of chlorophyll marginally inhibit bacterial growth, but no evidence shows that this is really useful. (Chlorophyll has been shown to relieve bad breath in dogs—but not in people.) Verdict: safe but not proved effective in combating the bacteria and viruses that cause sore throat and mouth.

• *DEQUALINIUM CHLORIDE:* This quaternary ammonium compound is believed to be relatively nontoxic. However, few toxicologic test results were submitted, so the reviewers could not certify that its use in oral health-care products is safe. Dequalinium chloride kills both bacteria and funguses, but it is not effective against very many species of bacteria. Even the limited activity that it does have may be easily compromised, since the drug is neutralized by natural body secretions, debris in the mouth, and other materials that may be introduced into the mouth by the preparation itself. Both the safety and the effectiveness of dequalinium chloride remain to be proved.

• *DOMIPHEN BROMIDE:* A compound that has been widely tested in animals and in humans, domiphen bromide appears to cause few if any toxic reactions in the dosages recommended for mouth and throat products.

But studies that might rule out the risk that it can cause cancer, birth defects, or genetic damages appear not to have been done. Evaluators therefore regard its safety as unproved.

According to manufacturers' data, this chemical will kill the bacteria present in dental plaque. But the reviewers say this does not establish its ability to kill bacteria that are on or embedded in nearby mucous membranes. Like other quaternary ammonium compounds, domiphen bromide is inactivated by tissue debris and body fluids. To really work, it may require far longer exposure to infected surfaces than is realistically possible, given that saliva rapidly dilutes drugs applied to the mouth. Also, currently marketed mouthwashes contain 1:20,000 dilutions of domiphen bromide, which may be too weak to kill significant numbers of bacteria under any circumstances. For these reasons, the Oral Cavity Panel says the safety and effectiveness of domiphen bromide have yet to be demonstrated.

• ETHYL ALCOHOL: Although use of this alcohol is safe in the concentrations—up to 35 percent—that are used in over-the-counter oral health products, these relatively low concentrations have not been shown to be effective against bacteria. Higher concentrations, which *are* effective, cause burning and intense discomfort, making them too irritating to be used to treat sores and inflammation in the mouth or throat. The Oral Cavity Panel concludes: Ethyl alcohol is safe but of unproved effectiveness in relieving sore throat and mouth.

• EUCALYPTOL: An oil obtained by boiling fresh eucalyptus leaves, eucalyptol has a pungent smell and a spicy, cooling taste. It is widely used in folk and nonprescription medicines, and long marketing experience indicates that small amounts of it probably are not harmful. The reviewers could find little information about which bacteria eucalyptol may kill or how, or how rapidly it might do so. One manufacturer submitted data showing that a mixture of eucalyptol and several other agents will kill more microbes than will the same mixture without the eucalyptol. The reviewers say this does not prove that eucalyptol is an effective antimicrobial agent when used by itself. Verdict: Eucalyptol is safe but its effectiveness as an antimicrobial agent must be demonstrated.

• GENTIAN VIOLET: This greenish-purple dye will kill some bacteria, funguses, and other microorganisms. Currently, it is less widely used than it once was because more effective drugs have been developed and because doubts have been raised about its safety. Gentian violet has the added disadvantage that it stains false teeth and other dental appliances as well as mucous membranes. The Panel decided that 1 percent gentian violet is safe. But there is little or no evidence from controlled scientific studies to show that it acts effectively as an antimicrobial, compared with other agents that are available, or that it really relieves sore throat and mouth. So the Oral Cavity Panel rated gentian violet safe but of still-unproved effectiveness.

• *HYDROGEN PEROXIDE:* Basing their decision on another panel's analysis, the Oral Cavity Panel accepts this bitter-tasting substance as being safe for brief, occasional use in the mouth at concentrations up to 3 percent (*see* Hydrogen Peroxide, p. 692). It warns, however, that continuing use of hydrogen peroxide can damage the calcium in teeth.

High concentrations of hydrogen peroxide will kill bacteria. But these concentrations may also be dangerous, and evaluators say it is difficult to imagine the circumstances under which the compound will kill bacteria without injuring mucous membranes of the throat and mouth. Lower concentrations have been shown to be bactericidal, too, but only if they remain in contact with the microorganisms for relatively long periods—say, for an hour. Because of natural salivary dilution, it seems unlikely that a safe dose of the drug will remain in the mouth in effective amounts for this length of time. The Oral Cavity Panel accepts hydrogen peroxide as safe but is skeptical about its antimicrobial effect in treating sore throat and mouth.

• *IODINE:* This element has been used medicinally since 1819, and it is an extremely potent antimicrobial agent that works against bacteria, viruses, and funguses. The major difficulty with iodine is its toxicity. It is deadly if swallowed in large amounts. Even lesser amounts, if used repeatedly, can lead to a chronic poisoning called *iodism*. (The principal symptom is pain or a sense of heaviness in the sinuses around the nose.) Iodine also stings, irritates, and inflames the skin, and its effects on mucous membranes in the mouth and throat are even more severe.

Despite iodine's potent germicidal effect, the Panel says studies have yet to be done to obtain proof that it works effectively as an oral-cavity drug to relieve sore throat and mouth. Thus iodine is "on probation" both in terms of safety and effectiveness.

• *MENTHOL:* A fragrant alcohol obtained from oil of peppermint and other mint oils, menthol is a common ingredient in candy and other foods as well as medicines. Few serious adverse effects have been reported, so the Panel assessed it as safe.

Menthol is germicidal, but little or no data are available on *which* germs it kills or how rapidly it kills them. One manufacturer submitted test results that showed that a mix of aromatic substances— including thymol, menthol, camphor, and methyl salicylate—had more antimicrobial power than the same mixture without the menthol. The Oral Cavity Panel dismisses this finding, saying the test does not establish the antimicrobial value of menthol used as a single ingredient. At this time, therefore, menthol is categorized as safe but in need of proof about effectiveness.

• METHYL SALICYLATE: This aspirin-like compound has the fragrance and taste of wintergreen and teaberry. Its taste appeal has been a problem: A number of accidental poisonings have occurred because children ate methyl salicylate products. Newer safety packaging requirements have greatly reduced this risk, so the Panel calls it safe. But no controlled scientific study demonstrates that methyl salicylate has useful antimicrobial action when used in over-the-counter drugs applied to the mucous membranes of the throat and mouth. The Panel's verdict: The effectiveness of this pleasant-smelling compound still needs to be established.

• OXYQUINOLINE SULFATE (8-HYDROXYQUINOLINE): Also known as *oxine, quinphenol-8-hydroxyquinoline*, and *bioquin*, this drug is widely used in industry because of its ability to bind to metals. Medicinally, its action is believed to involve picking up and binding copper from body tissues. The copper bound to the oxyquinoline sulfate in this way readily enters bacterial cells. Once inside these cells, the copper is released and it kills the bacteria.

Oxyquinoline and related compounds have seen wide use as antimicrobials. But they pose two problems: First, they are toxic, although oxyquinoline sulfate may be less poisonous than some others. Second, scientific data that clearly establish the effectiveness of the chemicals is lacking. The Oral Cavity Panel says it received no results from well-controlled scientific studies to show oxyquinoline sulfate's value as a broad spectrum antimicrobial agent. Its value in relieving sore throat and mouth is similarly unclear. The judgment: Both the safety and the effectiveness of this compound remain to be demonstrated.

• PHENOL: This compound has been widely used in over-the-counter medications to relieve pain and control microorganisms. The Oral Cavity Panel finds phenol in very low concentrations safe. But its effectiveness as an antimicrobial *is* in question. While this drug, which also is known as *carbolic acid*, is the antiseptic that was used over a century ago to prove that antiseptic practices reduce post-operative infections, phenol has by and large been replaced in this use by more effective antiseptics. As for its efficacy against the microorganisms that cause sore throat or mouth, phenol's supporters provided no specific evidence to the Panel. So the verdict is: safe (in very low concentrations) but not proved effective.

• PHENOLATE SODIUM: Similar to phenol (*see* immediately preceding), this compound has comparable actions. Approved as a pain reliever, phenolate sodium also possesses "germ-killing" properties. But reviewers said they received insufficient evidence to show that the chemical effectively kills the specific microorganisms responsible for sore throat and sore mouth. In sum: safe but not proved effective for over-the-counter oral-health-care products.

• POVIDONE-IODINE: Because iodine is extremely irritating to the skin and mucous membranes, manufacturers have combined it with other substances, like povidone, in order to reduce the amount of free iodine that reaches the body surface at any one time. The povidone is practically nontoxic, the Oral Cavity Panel said, and experimental and marketing data indicate that 1 or 2 applications of povidone-iodine to the throat or mouth are also safe. But the compound's safety on a regular-use, long-term basis has not been established. Also, the rate at which povidone-iodine is absorbed into the bloodstream from the mouth and throat is not known.

The compound's efficacy remains in question, even though a number of studies on its use on the skin and in the mouth have been published. In particular, it is not clear how much of the iodine's germicidal effect is lost when its activity is inhibited by the presence of povidone. It is not clear, either, whether povidone-iodine slows or actually enhances wound healing. Conclusion: Neither the safety nor the effectiveness of povidone-iodine has been confirmed.

• SECONDARY AMYLTRICRESOLS: Secondary amyltricresols are phenol-like compounds that are a hundred or more times more potent than phenol itself against some bacteria. They have been used in medicine for half a century.

Animal studies show that secondary amyltricresols are slightly irritating to mucous membranes. Evaluators were given only one study concerning the use of these substances for human mouth wounds. No clear signs of toxicity were noted, but the report contained no information about rate of absorption from the mucous membranes, mucosal irritation, or the breakdown and excretion of the drug from the body. The Oral Cavity Panel says it knows too little to declare secondary amyltricresols safe for use in the mouth and throat. Further, no data were submitted demonstrating that secondary amyltricresols are effective in combating bacteria responsible for mouth or throat soreness. Conclusion: Both safety and effectiveness must be shown.

- *Sodium caprylate:* Sodium caprylate is a fatty acid that has been demonstrated to work against fungal infections of the mouth and of the skin (including athlete's foot and jock itch). Although there is little scientific evidence that it is safe when used as an oral drug, the Oral Cavity Panel notes that fatty acids are major components of many of our foods, and they appear to cause no harm. The Panel assumes the substance is safe.

    Effectiveness is another matter. While the dental literature contains several reports of dramatic cures of thrush—a disease that raises painful white bumps in the mucous membranes of the throat and mouth—there are no properly conducted studies to show that sodium caprylate kills the microorganism responsible for sore throats and mouths. The judgment: safe but not proved effective.

- *Thymol:* Standard toxicology tests and long use indicate that serious side effects are very rare when thymol, a pleasant-smelling alcohol, is taken in the doses commonly available in over-the-counter preparations. The Oral Cavity Panel puts it into the "safe" category, noting, however, that thymol can irritate mucous membranes. Thymol has been shown to kill both bacteria and funguses, but its potency is reduced when it interacts with the natural organic material that is always present in the mouth and throat. Little contemporary data is available to demonstrate thymol's effectiveness in relieving sore throat and mouth. The Panel rejected one study that seemed to demonstrate greater antimicrobial potency of a thymol-containing mixture compared with the same mixture minus the thymol. In short: Thymol is safe, but effectiveness needs to be shown.

- *Thymol iodide:* A combination of thymol and iodine—also known as *dithymol diiodide*—thymol iodide is a red-yellow or red-brown powder. It is often dissolved in peanut oil for application inside the mouth. The Panel expressed doubts about the safety of thymol iodide when the substance is applied topically in the mouth. They also said they received no reliable test results demonstrating that thymol iodide effectively limits or destroys the microorganisms responsible for sore throat and mouth. Conclusion: Both safety and effectiveness remain unproved.

• *TOLU BALSAM:* This sap extract has a pleasant, vanilla-like aroma and has been used medicinally for many years. But its therapeutic properties have rarely been assessed according to acceptable scientific standards. Although it is not considered to be dangerous, it also is not thought to be very effective in killing or inhibiting the growth of microorganisms that cause sore throat and sore mouth. Verdict: safe but not proved effective.

DISAPPROVED ANTIMICROBIAL ACTIVE INGREDIENTS

• *BORIC ACID:* This drug is derived from the non-metallic element *boron*—a potent nerve poison. Skin can block boric acid's absorption but mucous membrane cannot. The early signs of boron or boric-acid poisoning are nausea, vomiting, diarrhea, and stomach pain.

      Boric acid is only weakly effective, at best, in killing microorganisms in the mouth and throat. The Oral Cavity Panel therefore classifies boric acid—and the related compounds sodium borate and borax—as both unsafe and ineffective.

• *BOROGYLCERIN GLYCERITE:* As its name suggests, this is a compound of boric acid and glycerin. No convincing scientific evidence is available on its worth in the case of sore throat and sore mouth, and it also shares the toxic risk of boric acid (*see* immediately preceding). The Panel's verdict: not safe and effective.

• *CAMPHOR:* Serious safety questions have been raised about this aromatic substance. Since it is easily absorbed through the mucous membranes of the mouth and throat, the Oral Cavity Panel rates it unsafe. Neither was any valid scientific study submitted to demonstrate that camphor works as an antimicrobial when used in the mouth and throat. Thus it is judged to be both unsafe and ineffective.

• *CRESOL:* This is a phenol derivative that may be more irritating to body surfaces than phenol itself is. Cresol is readily and rapidly absorbed into the body through mucous membranes and produces local damage to tissues even in dilute solutions. For these reasons, it was declared unsafe. It is more active against some bacteria than is phenol, but the Panel did not rule on cresol's effectiveness. It disapproved of cresol wholly on grounds of safety.

• *FERRIC CHLORIDE:* An iron salt that is reddish or brownish in color, ferric chloride is irritating to the mucosal lining of the gastrointestinal tract. It is fairly toxic, and large doses, accidentally swallowed, could cause death. Therefore, the Panel ruled it unsafe. Also, since they were provided no data indicating that ferric chloride effectively combats the microorganisms that cause sore throat and mouth, the Oral Cavity Panel declared ferric chloride ineffective as well as unsafe.

• **MERALEIN SODIUM:** This substance, commonly called *merodicein*, is a mercury derivative that may vary in color from green to dark red. It can poison the kidneys, and one expert cited by the Oral Cavity Panel rates it as being highly toxic. Meralein sodium slows bacterial growth and reproduction. But it requires many hours to kill the bacteria, which means that swabbing it once onto sore spots in the mouth and throat is not likely to be of much therapeutic value; the saliva quickly dilutes and washes away drugs applied in this way. Verdict: unsafe and not effective.

• **NITROMERSOL:** Although like meralein sodium (*see* previous paragraph), this drug is derived from mercury, its different chemical nature makes it more active against bacteria and less irritating and less toxic. This difference does not, however, persuade the Oral Cavity Panel that nitromersol is safe for self-use in nonprescription oral health-care products. On the contrary, the reviewers categorized it as unsafe because of the damage that even small amounts of mercury can do to the fine, inner structures of the kidney after it has been absorbed through the mucous membranes. Besides these risks, there was no evidence to convince the Panel that nitromersol effectively kills or inhibits the microorganisms specifically responsible for sore throat and mouth. Verdict: unsafe and ineffective.

• **POTASSIUM CHLORATE:** According to the experts, chlorate poisoning was common when this drug enjoyed widespread medicinal use after its introduction as a seemingly innocuous substance. Potassium chlorate specifically damages the gastrointestinal tract, kidneys, and red blood cells. Furthermore, chlorates show no germ-killing activity when studied in the test tube, and the reviewers were puzzled as to how such drugs ever came to be used as antimicrobials. The Oral Cavity Panel judges potassium chlorate as both unsafe and ineffective.

• **SODIUM BICHROMATE AND SODIUM DICHROMATE:** Both sodium bichromate and sodium dichromate are derivatives of the element chromium. As ingredients, both are exceedingly dangerous because they are corrosive to skin and to mucous membranes. They can cause violent stomach pain, circulatory collapse, dizziness, headaches, muscle cramps, coma, and even death. The Oral Cavity Panel's verdict is that chromium derivatives should have *no* use as therapeutic agents because of this tremendous danger of toxic reactions. In short: unsafe.

- *TINCTURE OF MYRRH:* The ancients used this gum resin as a medicine and as a component of embalming mixtures. Myrrh is irritating to the skin and to mucous membranes. In recent years it has been dropped from major drug reference books, and the Oral Cavity Panel could find no sound scientific data to show that the substance kills the microorganisms that cause sore throat and sore mouth. The Panel disapproved myrrh on counts of safety and effectiveness.

Astringents

An *astringent* is a chemical that will bind to or hold proteins that are present in saliva and other body fluids and then pull them out of these solutions. When swished around the mouth, astringent preparations briefly form a thin layer on mucosal cell surfaces. They draw together proteins on these cells' surfaces (causing a puckery sensation) that briefly protects the tissue from painful and irritating substances.

Used in recommended doses, an astringent acts only on the surface of the outer layer of these mucosal cells. It does not penetrate into the cells' interiors or into deeper layers of tissues, so it carries little or no risk of systemic poisoning. (More highly concentrated astringent solutions—which are *not* recommended for use without prescription—may, however, reach and damage cell interiors and internal organs.)

 Claims for Astringents

Accurate
- "For temporary relief of occasional minor irritation, pain, sore mouth, and sore throat"

APPROVED ASTRINGENT ACTIVE INGREDIENTS

Two astringents are rated safe and effective by the FDA:

- *ALUM:* As its name implies, alum is a preparation of the metallic element *aluminum*. Three different aluminum compounds are sold as alum. The most common is *potassium aluminum sulfate*. Other forms include *sodium aluminum sulfate* and *ammonium aluminum sulfate*. These three preparations have essentially the same therapeutic properties.

Alum is widely used in foods; for example, it is a part of baking powder. Extremely large doses may irritate the stomach lining or produce diarrhea, but side effects are rare or nonexistent when recommended dose levels are maintained. So the Oral Cavity Panel and the FDA say alum is safe.

Although the Oral Cavity Panel cited no specific studies that demonstrate alum's effectiveness as an oral astringent, it called dilute solutions workable aids in relieving sore throat or mouth because the drug provides a protective layer over irritated areas. The evaluators said that these drugs do not cure: They provide relief only.

The safe and effective dosage for adults and for children over 2 years of age is 0.2 to 0.5 percent alum in water-based rinses, gargles, sprays, or swabs, applied to the affected site up to 4 times daily; for children under 2 years old, consult a doctor or a dentist. Children under 12 should be supervised by an adult. The excess drug should be spit out, and such preparations should not be used longer than 7 days.

• ZINC CHLORIDE: This water-soluble zinc compound is sometimes called *butter of zinc*. Like other forms of zinc, it is quite harmless when swallowed; zinc is an essential nutritional ingredient and is present in many foods. For these reasons, evaluators judged zinc chloride safe—in the recommended medicinal dosages—for use to relieve sore throat and mouth. As is the case with alum (*see* the preceding discussion), no scientific studies are cited, but the substance is said to effectively relieve— not cure—mouth and throat soreness.

The approved astringent dosage of zinc chloride for adults and for children over age 12 years is a 0.1 to 0.25 percent concentration applied up to 4 times daily in rinses, in mouthwashes, or on cotton swabs. Children under 12 years of age need adult supervision in using this drug; for children under 2 years old, use only when and if directed by a doctor.

CONDITIONALLY APPROVED ASTRINGENT ACTIVE INGREDIENTS

None.

DISAPPROVED ASTRINGENT ACTIVE INGREDIENT

• *TINCTURE OF MYRRH:* This aromatic, bitter-tasting plant product can be highly irritating, and there is no evidence to support its use as an astringent. The Panel's verdict: unsafe and ineffective.

Debris Removers/Wound Cleansers

Colds and other conditions that cause sore throat or irritation and soreness in the mouth may produce an accumulation of mucus, phlegm, and other secretions that stick to and build up on the mucous membranes. These secretions can be irritating and are apt to cause coughing. They may also cause pain.

Effective drugs are available to remove these unpleasant exudates: Technically they are called *debriding agents.* They act in several ways. Some release tiny bubbles of oxygen that lift the offending matter off the tissue surface. Other mineral-containing compounds may act mechanically to wash the gunk away. Gargling with sodium bicarbonate—ordinary baking soda—seems to help in this way. Sodium bicarbonate also increases the alkalinity of mucus and appears to soften and loosen it so that it is easier to swallow, cough up, or blow out through the nose. Salt water also is widely used as a debris remover. The salt draws water out of the mucous membranes, which dilutes mucus and acts to cleanse the membrane surfaces. The Oral Cavity Panel stresses, however, that debriding agents work only briefly; they do not cure the underlying condition.

The same ingredients can be helpful in removing foreign matter, including food and dirt, from small wounds in the mouth and gums.

Many dentists recommend these drugs to their patients for relieving gum and mucosal injuries and for cleansing the mouth. The Dental Panel says that the "wound-cleansing action appears to be a result of this foaming activity, which physically removes debris from the wound." And it adds that evidence for these products' effectiveness comes mostly from clinical impressions rather than from scientific study.

 ## Claims for Debris Removers/Wound Cleansers

Accurate

• "Aids in the removal of phlegm, mucus or other secretions

associated with occasional sore mouth"

- "For temporary use in cleansing minor wounds or minor gum inflammation resulting from minor dental procedures, dentures, orthodontic appliances, accidental injury, or other irritations of the mouth and gums"
- "For temporary use to cleanse canker sores"
- "Assists in the removal of foreign material from minor wounds"
- "Physically removes debris from oral wounds"

WARNING:

 These preparations should not be used for more than a week at a time without a dentist's or a physician's supervision. See your dentist or doctor promptly if irritation, pain, or redness persists or worsens, or if swelling, rash, or fever develops.

APPROVED DEBRIS-REMOVER/WOUND-CLEANSER ACTIVE INGREDIENTS

- **CARBAMIDE PEROXIDE IN ANHYDROUS GLYCERIN:** When put in the mouth, where it is wet, carbamide peroxide quickly breaks down to about 70 percent urea and 30 percent hydrogen peroxide. The hydrogen peroxide further separates into water and oxygen. The effervescent action of the oxygen bubbles released by the hydrogen peroxide provides the cleansing action—and does so effectively. The glycerin acts as a stabilizing agent.

  Currently marketed products contain 10 to 15 percent carbamide peroxide and yield about 3 percent hydrogen peroxide, which the FDA says is safe. The glycerin and urea by-products are also generally considered to be safe. The approved dose is several drops of the preparation applied directly to the affected areas of the mouth.

  The medication should remain in place at least one minute, then be spat out. It can be used 4 times daily—after meals and before bedtime or as directed by a dentist or physician. Children under 12 years of age should be supervised by their parents in the use of this preparation, and it should not be used on babies under age 2 years, even if they are teething, except with the advice and supervision of a dentist or a pediatrician.

Alternatively, the product can be used as a mouthwash: Place 10 to 20 drops on the tongue, mix with saliva, and swish around in the mouth over the sore or irritated area for a minute or longer. Then spit the medication out. Use up to 4 times daily, or use more often if advised to by a dentist or a physician. Children under 12 years of age require supervision. Do not use for children under 2 years old without medical advice.

• *HYDROGEN PEROXIDE 3 PERCENT, IN AN AQUEOUS SOLUTION:* The Panel's decision that this preparation is safe and effective for temporary use is supported by studies in animals and by considerable medical and dental experience with human patients. Salivary enzymes in the mouth release oxygen bubbles that provide the cleansing action. The assessment "safe and effective" also is upheld by manufacturers' marketing data, which show that many, many bottles of this preparation are sold but few complaints are received.

The approved concentration is 3 percent hydrogen peroxide. Higher levels, particularly if used over a long period of time, can injure the gums and cause a condition that researchers graphically describe as "black hairy tongue." Even at the approved dosages, repeated use may irritate the gums, so hydrogen peroxide should not be used routinely.

The safe and effective dosage for adults and for children over age 2 years is several drops of 3 percent hydrogen peroxide, when it is formulated as drops to put onto the affected area of the mouth, or somewhat more of the liquid when it is to be used as an oral rinse that is diluted by half and swished around the teeth and mouth. In either case, the drug should be applied for at least 1 minute, then spat out. Children under 12 years of age should be supervised in their use of this preparation, and it should not be used on babies under age 2 years, even if they are teething, except with the advice and supervision of a dentist or a pediatrician.

• *SODIUM BICARBONATE:* This debris remover and wound cleanser is old-fashioned baking soda—found in most kitchens. Since it is widely used as food, the Oral Cavity Panel had little trouble deciding that it is safe. This Panel also declared that sodium bicarbonate is safe for removing debris from the mouth and for cleansing small wounds when the powder is diluted to a 10 to 15 percent concentration in water, even though they cited no specific studies to support this judgment.

Sodium bicarbonate is highly alkaline (for which reason many people use it as an antacid. (*See* ANTACIDS.) The theory is that this alkalinity softens the gums and oral mucosa so that mucus deposits and other sticky debris can be dislodged by rinsing or gargling.

For adults and for children over 2 years of age, prepare a solution of one teaspoon sodium bicarbonate in a half glass (4 ounces) of water. Swish around in the mouth over affected areas for at least a minute, then spit the medication out. Repeat up to 4 times daily. Children under 12 years old should be supervised, and children under 2 years old should not be treated with sodium bicarbonate unless it is recommended by a doctor or dentist.

• *SODIUM PERBORATE MONOHYDRATE:* This preparation releases a small amount of hydrogen peroxide into the mouth. It also contains the mineral boron, which is toxic. Reviewers worried that if a 1.2-gram package of sodium perborate monohydrate were used 4 times daily, as the manufacturer suggests, and if the material were swallowed instead of being spat out, as the manufacturer also advises, this usage would deliver several times the amount of boron that can safely be ingested in a day.

Judging by the preparation's taste when swallowed, this observer believes that users would not go on swallowing sodium perborate monohydrate for very long! The FDA, similarly, decided that the reviewers' fears were excessive, based on an examination of published safety studies. The agency calls sodium perborate monohydrate safe, and also rules that it is effective. The approved dose is one 1.2-gram package, dissolved in one ounce of water, swished around in the mouth over the affected area for one minute, and then spit out. This oral cleanser can be used up to 4 times daily by adults and children over 6. Children 6 to 12 years of age need adult supervision. Use only as directed by a doctor for children under 6 years old.

CONDITIONALLY APPROVED DEBRIS-REMOVER/ WOUND-CLEANSER ACTIVE INGREDIENTS

None.

DISAPPROVED DEBRIS REMOVER/WOUND-CLEANSER ACTIVE INGREDIENTS

None.

Demulcents (Soothers)

Thick, syrupy, soothing substances are formulated into oral health-care products such as lozenges, mouth rinses, and gargling solutions to cover and protect sore tissues in the throat and mouth. They also offer protection from chemicals, fluids, air, and other irritants. Some of these soothers, which are technically called *demulcents*, will bind and hold irritating substances, thereby neutralizing them.

Demulcents are largely or wholly inert (chemically inactive); their major benefit rests in their soothing physical properties. They are not absorbed through the mucous membranes, or, if absorbed, are excreted unchanged. No breakdown products are produced that might prove toxic to internal organs. As a result these drugs cause few, if any, adverse reactions.

 Claims for Demulcents

Accurate
• "For temporary relief of minor discomfort and protection of irritated areas in sore mouth and sore throat"

APPROVED DEMULCENT ACTIVE INGREDIENTS

• *ELM BARK:* This traditional remedy, obtained from the dried inner bark of the slippery-elm tree, is harvested in spring. When boiled, it produces a gluey substance with a curry-like aroma. Not much information is available on its safety. But since the bark breaks down into a variety of harmless sugars and since, too, there have been no reports of adverse effects from using it, the Oral Cavity Panel has judged the substance safe. When sucked from troches and lozenges, the elm-bark mucilage appears to cover and protect inflamed and irritated mucous membranes in the throat and mouth. This may temporarily help relieve sore throat or sore mouth. Elm bark has no curative or pain-killing properties.

The safe and effective dosage consists of lozenges or troches that contain 10 to 15 percent elm bark in agar or another water-soluble gum base. Adults and children over 2 years old can suck 1 or 2 of these lozenges every 2 hours as needed. For children under age 2 years, consult a physician.

• *GELATIN:* Because the substance is widely used in foods as a jelling agent, the FDA judges it to be safe for occasional medicinal use.

Gelatin will provide a protective coating over irritated or ulcerated areas in the mouth and throat. It also will inhibit the ability to feel cold, warmth, pressure, or pain, although it has no curative or wound-healing powers. A special dosage form called an *absorbable gelatin sponge* may be used to medicate the upper throat and insides of the cheeks.

The safe and effective dosage for adults and children over age 2 years is 5 to 10 percent gelatin in aqueous (water) solutions. It can be used as a rinse, a gargle, or a spray or with a swab as often as needed. On a specific sore area, the gelatin may be applied with the tip of the finger; use enough to form a solid or semi-solid layer over the affected tissue.

• *GLYCERIN:* This is a clear, colorless, syrupy liquid used to protect the skin as well as the mucous membranes. A century of medicinal use with no reported adverse effects persuades the Oral Cavity Panel that glycerin is safe as a topical drug. When applied to the mouth in a rinse, a wash, or a spray or on a swab, it forms a thin protective layer that adheres to the mucous membranes. It insulates sensory nerve endings from hurtful stimuli, but it does not promote healing or "cure" the wound.

Glycerin should be diluted with 2 or 3 parts of water before use. It can be applied freely, as often as necessary.

• *PECTIN:* The fruit extract that makes fruit jellies jell, pectin has a long record of use in foods and medicines, and no record of known adverse effects. This convinces the FDA that pectin is safe. Forming a protective covering over raw or ulcerated areas in the mouth and throat, it protects the sensory receptors from further stimulation and the tissue from further irritation. Pectin does not, however, enhance healing or actually cure the soreness in the tissue it is covering. The substance is safe and effective, used as often as necessary, in rinse, gargle, spray, lozenge, or gel form. A thick enough preparation should be used to form a solid or semi-solid coating over the irritated tissue. Use as needed. For children under 2 years old, ask a doctor.

CONDITIONALLY APPROVED DEMULCENT ACTIVE INGREDIENTS

In general, most lozenges are made mostly of sugar. In some tests, plain lozenges without *any* other medicinal ingredient have been shown to be as effective as look-alike *medicated* lozenges in briefly relieving sore throat.

This discovery has prompted one or two manufacturers to propose that the various sugars be approved by the FDA as safe and effective demulcents. The agency's answer, in essence, is that it would consider the request, but that it believed it unnecessary, since the label on a package of lozenges made up mostly of sugar—as an *inactive* ingredient—could claim to contain "a drug product formulated in a soothing sugar (or sorbitol) base."

Nevertheless, the FDA agreed to classify the following sugars as conditionally safe and effective, pending manufacturers' production of scientifically sound clinical tests demonstrating their soothing capabilities—in which case they will become approved medicinal active ingredients. These are the sugars that are now conditionally approved in this way:

• **SORBITOL:** This is a sugar derived from alcohol. It is widely used in food processing and in making drugs. It is obviously safe. What manufacturers must now do is to prove that it is medicinally active and effective in soothing sore throats.

• **SUGARS (SUCROSE, DEXTROSE, FRUCTOSE, DEXTRINS):** These are widely known and widely used food sugars. Most people know that sucking a hard candy will sooth a sore throat and may relieve coughing as well. These are demulcent effects. Whether scientific proof can be obtained to show that these sugars are medicinally effective remains to be seen. Sugars will certainly go on providing soothing relief, whether they are labelled as *candy* or as *nonprescription drugs*.

DISAPPROVED DEMULCENT ACTIVE INGREDIENTS

None.

Mucosal Protectants

A *protectant* is a pharmacologically *inert* substance; that is, it is chemically inactive. Protectants help by adhering to the gums and other mucosal surfaces to provide a protective-coating that insulates a sore area against further irritation. Some protectants form fairly rigid covering layers; others are flexible.

 ### Claims for Mucosal Protectants

Accurate

- "Forms a coating over a wound"
- "Protects against further irritation"
- "For temporary use to protect wounds caused by minor irritations or injury"
- "For protecting recurring canker sores"

APPROVED MUCOSAL-PROTECTANT ACTIVE INGREDIENTS

- **BENZOIN PREPARATIONS: BENZOIN TINCTURE AND COMPOUND BENZOIN TINCTURE:** These are preparations that dentists have used for years to cover and protect small wounds in the gums, lips, and other soft tissues in the mouth. Benzoin is a pine-tree resin with a vanilla-like aroma and slightly acrid taste. Benzoin tincture contains 20 percent benzoin in alcohol. Compound benzoin tincture contains 10 percent benzoin, 2 percent aloe, 8 percent storax, 4 percent tolu balsam, and 74 to 80 percent alcohol.

  These preparations are relatively toxic, largely because of their high alcohol content. But in the tiny amounts that are required to treat small sores in the mouth, the Dental Panel says they are safe.

  No really thorough studies have been conducted to confirm that benzoin preparations are effective when used on the oral mucosa. But a host of clinical reports, plus the long history of benzoin's use by dentists convinced reviewers that these compounds are effective for covering and thus easing the pain of chemical or thermal burns, minor injuries, and irritations. They also are sometimes applied to canker sores. The Panel believed they should be used for this purpose only under a doctor's supervision.

Experts urge that these preparations always be used at full strength—*not* diluted—in order to preserve their protectant effectiveness. Before application, dry the affected tissue. Then put a few drops of the medicine on with a cotton swab.

For adults and for children over 6 months of age, the safe and effective dosage is a few drops, used no more often than once every 2 hours. For infants, use only as recommended by a doctor or a dentist.

CONDITIONALLY APPROVED MUCOSAL-PROTECTANT ACTIVE INGREDIENT

• MYRRH FLUID EXTRACT: This dressing is obtained from a tree resin that the ancient Egyptians used to embalm the dead. The Dental Panel could find no reports of toxicity following the use of small amounts of myrrh on the gums. Neither, however, could it find much data to establish the extract's safety when it is used in this way.

As to effectiveness, these evaluators could not find any studies in humans to demonstrate that this preparation is of value as a protectant to injured gums. Both the safety and the effectiveness of this resin remain to be proved.

DISAPPROVED MUCOSAL-PROTECTANT ACTIVE INGREDIENTS

None.

Safety and Effectiveness: Active Ingredients in Over-the-Counter Medicaments for Sore Gums, Mouths, and Throats

ANESTHETICS/ANALGESICS

Active Ingredient	Assessment
aspirin (in chewing gum)	safe, but not proved effective
benzocaine	safe and effective
benzyl alcohol	safe and effective
butacaine sulfate	safe and effective
camphor	not safe or effective
chlorophyllins	safe, but not proved effective
cresol	not proved safe or effective
dyclonine hydrochloride	safe and effective
hexylresorcinol	safe and effective
menthol	safe and effective
methyl salicylate	not safe or effective
phenol	safe and effective
phenolate sodium (sodium phenolate)	safe and effective
salicyl alcohol	safe and effective
thymol preparations	safe, but not proved effective

ANTIMICROBIALS

benzalkonium chloride	safe, but not proved effective
benzethonium chloride	not proved safe or effective
benzoic acid	safe, but not proved effective
boric acid	not safe or effective
boroglycerin glycerite	not safe or effective
camphor	not safe or effective
carbamide peroxide in anhydrous glycerin (urea peroxide)	safe, but not proved effective

Safety and Effectiveness: Active Ingredients in Over-the-Counter Medicaments for Sore Gums, Mouths, and Throats (contd)

Active Ingredient	Assessment
cetalkonium chloride	safe, but not proved effective
cetylpyridinium chloride	not proved safe or effective
chlorophyll	safe, but not proved effective
cresol	not safe
dequalinium chloride	not proved safe or effective
domiphen bromide	not proved safe or effective
ethyl alcohol	safe, but not proved effective
eucalyptol	safe, but not proved effective
ferric chloride	not safe or effective
gentian violet	safe, but not proved effective
hydrogen peroxide	safe, but not proved effective
iodine	not proved safe or effective
menthol	safe, but not proved effective
meralein sodium (merodicein)	not safe or effective
methyl salicylate	safe, but not proved effective
nitromersol	not safe or effective
oxyquinoline sulfate (8-hydroxy-quinolone)	not proved safe or effective
phenol	safe, but not proved effective
phenolate sodium	safe, but not proved effective
potassium chlorate	not safe or effective
povidone-iodine	not proved safe or effective
secondary amyltricresols	not proved safe or effective
sodium bichromate	not safe
sodium caprylate	safe, but not proved effective

Safety and Effectiveness: Active Ingredients in Over-the-Counter Medicaments for Sore Gums, Mouths, and Throats (contd)

Active Ingredient	*Assessment*
sodium dichromate	not safe
thymol	safe, but not proved effective
thymol iodide	not proved safe or effective
tincture of myrrh	not safe or effective
tolu balsam	safe, but not proved effective
ASTRINGENTS	
alum	safe and effective
tincture of myrrh	not safe or effective
zinc chloride (butter of zinc)	safe and effective
DEBRIS REMOVERS (DEBRIDING AGENTS, WOUND CLEANSERS)	
carbamide peroxide	safe and effective
hydrogen peroxide	safe and effective
sodium bicarbonate (baking soda)	safe and effective
sodium perborate monohydrate	safe and effective
DEMULCENTS (SOOTHERS)	
elm bark	safe and effective
gelatin	safe and effective
glycerin	safe and effective
pectin	safe and effective
sorbitol	safe, but not proved effective
sugars (sucrose, dextrose, fructose)	safe, but not proved effective
MUCOSAL PROTECTANTS	
benzoin tincture	safe and effective
compound benzoin tincture	safe and effective

Safety and Effectiveness: Combination Products Sold Over-the-Counter for Sore Gums, Mouths, and Throats

Safe and Effective

(Each active ingredient must be present within the dosage range approved by a panel and/or the FDA)

1 approved anesthetic/analgesic + 1 approved demulcent

1 approved anesthetic/analgesic + 1 approved decongestant (*see* COLD AND COUGH MEDICINES)

1 approved anesthetic/analgesic + 1 approved mucosal protectant

1 approved anesthetic/analgesic + 1 approved debris remover/wound cleanser

1 approved anesthetic/analgesic + 1 safe and effective denture adhesive

1 approved anesthetic/analgesic + 1 approved astringent

benzocaine + menthol in approved amounts

benzocaine + phenol in approved amounts

Conditionally Safe and Effective

any approved ingredient is present in less than the approved dose

1 or more of the approved ingredients is only conditionally approved

2 or more approved ingredients are included from the same drug class, but the combination has not been proved to have a therapeutic advantage (e.g., to be safer, more effective, better-accepted by consumers, or to have some other clear advantage over each of the active ingredients, individually, at full therapeutic doses)

1 anesthetic/analgesic + 1 mucosal protectant

1 anesthetic/analgesic + 1 antimicrobial

1 debris remover/wound cleanser + 1 antimicrobial

any 2 approved or conditionally approved ingredients from the same pharmacological group, acting by different mechanisms, provided both are present within the effective dosage range. (Does not apply to anesthetic/analgesics.)

1 anesthetic/analgesic + 1 counterirritant

1 mucosal protectant + 1 anesthetic/analgesic claimed to have a prolonged action (the protectant may hold the anesthetic/analgesic in contact with the affected area for an extended period of time)

1 mucosal protectant + 1 antimicrobial

Unsafe or Ineffective

contains any disapproved ingredient

contains any ingredient at more than the maximum allowed dose

contains any active ingredient that has not been reviewed by an OTC advisory panel or the FDA

contains active ingredients from 2 pharmacological groups but a significant population requiring the concurrent therapy does not exist is "irrational"*

contains drugs that are dangerous or neutralize each other when combined contains 1 mucosal protectant + 1 toothache relief agent ("irrational" and dangerous)

contains 1 mucosal protectant + 1 counterirritant ("irrationally counterproductive")

contains 1 mucosal protectant + 1 tooth desensitizer ("irrational")

contains 1 toothache relief agent + 1 counterirritant ("irrational")

contains 1 toothache relief agent + 1 tooth desensitizer ("irrational")

contains 2 chemically similar anesthetic/analgesics

contains 1 anesthetic/analgesic + 1 tooth desensitizer ("irrational")

contains 2 counterirritants

contains 1 counterirritant + 1 tooth desensitizer

contains 2 tooth desensitizers

contains 1 mucosal protectant + 1 debris remover/wound cleanser ("irrational")

contains 1 toothache relief agent + 1 debris remover/wound cleanser ("irrational")

contains 1 anesthetic/analgesic + 1 debris remover/wound cleanser ("irrational")

contains 1 counterirritant + 1 debris remover/wound cleanser ("irrational")

contains 1 tooth desensitizer + 1 debris remover/wound cleanser ("irrational")

contains 1 toothache relief agent + 1 antimicrobial ("irrational")

contains 1 counterirritant + 1 antimicrobial ("irrational")

contains 1 tooth desensitizer + 1 antimicrobial ("irrational")

contains 1 debris remover/wound cleanser + 1 tooth desensitizer ("irrational")

contains a debris remover/wound cleanser formulated as a dentifrice (brushing can aggravate a wound)

1 or more approved antimicrobials + expectorant (since the expectorant will dilute or diminish the contact time of the antimicrobial) (*See* COLD AND COUGH MEDICINES.)

1 or more antimicrobials + 1 debris remover/wound cleanser (since the debris remover/wound cleanser will dilute or wash the antimicrobial from the diseased surface)

1 or more approved antimicrobials + 1 approved expectorant + 1 approved debris/wound cleanser (since the combination drug will tend to be washed away from the mucous-membrane surface)

1 approved anesthetic/analgesic + 1 approved debris remover/wound cleanser (since the anesthetic/analgesic will be washed away, diluted, or mixed with the debris raised by the debris remover and will be inactivated)

1 or more approved anesthetics/analgesic + 1 approved expectorant (since the drug will be diluted and removed from the site of action)

1 or more approved anesthetic/analgesics ingredients + 1 approved expectorant + 1 or more debris removers/wound cleansers (since the anesthetic/analgesic will be diluted or removed from the intended site) (*See* COLD AND COUGH MEDICINES.)

Safety and Effectiveness: Combination Products Sold Over-the-Counter for Sore Gums, Mouths, and Throats (contd)

1 or more approved astringents + 1 or more approved debris removers/wound cleansers (since the latter will prevent the former from exerting its effect on protein matter)

1 or more approved astringents + 1 expectorant (since the expectorant will dilute and wash away the astringent) (*see* COLD AND COUGH MEDICINES)

1 or more approved decongestants + 1 approved expectorant + 1 or more approved debris remover/wound cleansers (since these drugs will nullify and wash each other away) (*see* COLD AND COUGH MEDICINES)

1 or more decongestants + 1 expectorant (because the expectorant would dilute or nullify the decongestant) (*see* COLD AND COUGH MEDICINES)

----

* By "irrational" the evaluators mean a combination that makes no sense because the effects counteract one another, may interfere with specific treatment, or could mask a condition so that it becomes worse or otherwise prove unworkable.

Sore Throat and Mouth Medicines: Product Ratings

MEDICATED GUM

Product and Distributor	Dosage of Active Ingredients	Rating*	Comment
aspirin			
Aspergum (Schering-Plough)	chewable gum tablets: 227.5 mg	B	not proved effective

MOUTHWASH, SPRAYS, AND GARGLES

See pp. 752, 753, Product Ratings in MOUTHWASH FOR ORAL HYGIENE

MEDICATED GELS, PASTES & OTHER APPLICATIONS—MOSTLY FOR PAIN RELIEF

Product and Distributor	Dosage of Active Ingredients	Rating*	Comment
benzocaine			
Orabase-O (Colgate-Hoyt)	gel: 20%	A	
Orajel (Commerce)	gel: 10%	A	
Maximum Strength Anbesol (Whitehall)	gel, liquid: 20%	A	
Maximum Strength Orajel (Commerce)	gel: 20%	A	
Rid-A-Pain (Pfeiffer)	gel: 10%	A	

Sore Throat and Mouth Medicines: Product Ratings (contd)

COMBINATION PRODUCTS

Product and Distributor	Dosage of Active Ingredients	Rating*	Comment
Anbesol (Whitehall)	**gel, liquid:** 6.3% benzocaine + 0.5% phenol	A	
Benzodent (Vick's)	**ointment:** 20% benzocaine + 0.1% oxyquinoline sulfate + 0.4% eugenol	B	second and third ingredients not proved safe and effective
Orabase with Benzocaine (Colgate/Hoyt)	**paste:** 20% benzocaine + gelatin + pectin	B	too many demulcents—but both are harmless
Orajel Mouth Aid (Commerce)	**gel:** 20% benzocaine + 0.12% benzalkonium chloride + 0.1% zinc chloride	B	benzalkonium chloride not proved effective
S.T. 37 (Menley & James)	**liquid:** 0.1% hexylresorcinol + 28.2% glycerin	A	

LOZENGES AND TROCHES

Product and Distributor	Dosage of Active Ingredients	Rating*	Comment
Cepacol Troches (Marion Merrell Dow)	**lozenges:** 0.3% benzyl alcohol + 0.07% cetylpyridinium chloride	B	latter ingredient not proved safe or effective

Product and Distributor	Dosage of Active Ingredients	Rating*	Comment
Cepastat (Marion Merrell Dow)	lozenges: 1.45% phenol + 0.12% menthol	A	
Children's Chloraseptic (Richardson-Vicks)	lozenges: 5 mg benzocaine	A	
Chloraseptic (Richardson-Vicks)	lozenges: 6 mg benzocaine + 10 mg menthol	A	
Conex (Forest)	lozenges: 5 mg benzocaine + 0.5 mg cetylpyridinium chloride	B	latter ingredient not proved effective
Listerine Antiseptic (Warner-Lambert)	lozenges: 2.4 mg hexylresorcinol	A	
Sucrets Maximum Strength (SmithKline Beecham)	lozenges: 3 mg dyclonine hydrochloride	A	
Sucrets Regular Strength (Smithkline Beecham)	lozenges: 2.4 mg hexylresorcinol	A	
T-Caine (Schein)	lozenges: 5 mg benzocaine	A	℞ to OTC switch

GINGIVAL PROTECTANTS

benzoin preparations

Benzoin (generic)	tincture: 20%	A	

Sore Throat and Mouth Medicines: Product Ratings (contd)

Product and Distributor	Dosage of Active Ingredients	Rating*	Comment
Benzoin Compound (generic)	tincture: 10% benzoin + 2% aloe + 8% storax + 4% tolu balsam + 75-83% alcohol	A	

DEBRIS REMOVERS (DEBRIDING AGENTS)

Product and Distributor	Dosage of Active Ingredients	Rating*	Comment
carbamide peroxide in anhydrous glycerin			
Gly-Oxide (Marion Merrell Dow)	drops: 10%	A	
Proxigel (Reed & Carnrick)	gel: 11%	A	
hydrogen peroxide			
Hydrogen Peroxide 3% (generic)	solution: 3%	A	
Perimed (Olin)	rinse: 1.5% hydrogen peroxide + 5% povidone-iodine	B	conditionally approved combination
PerOxyl Mouth Rinse (Colgate-Hoyt)	solution: 1.5%	A	
sodium bicarbonate			
Arm & Hammer Baking Soda (Church & Dwight)	powder	A	grocery store item

Sodium Bicarbonate (generic)	**powder**	A
sodium perborate		
Amosan (Oral-B)	**powder:** 1.7 g per packet	A

SALIVA SUBSTITUTES

Product and Distributor	Dosage of Active Ingredients	Rating*	Comment

Note: The FDA has not yet assessed these products in the OTC Drug Review. Most if not all are based on carboxymethylcellulose sodium. This active ingredient has been proved to be safe and effective in the eye, which is more sensitive than the mouth, and has also been approved as a bulk laxative. In saliva substitutes, carboxymethylcellulose sodium is an inert substance. One product listed in the 1992 *PDR for Nonprescription Drugs* is *Salivart Saliva Substitute* (Gebauer).

---

*Author's interpretation of FDA criteria. Based on contents, not claims.

Menstrual Distress Preparations

Many women experience bloating and other unpleasant physical and emotional changes in the week before their menstrual periods. Many, too, experience cramping and other discomfort once they start to bleed. No single cause has been identified for either of these situations. But fortunately, a few nonprescription and prescription drugs have been developed that will effectively relieve them.

Reviewers say that the nonprescription drugs should be used only for the *mildest* symptoms of premenstrual distress or painful menstruation (technically called *dysmenorrhea*). Severely disturbing or disabling pain and other serious symptoms should prompt a woman to visit her gynecologist or family physician. Recent discoveries have opened new ways for successfully treating menstrual distress with prescription drugs.

MENSTRUAL DISTRESS PREPARATIONS is based on the report "OTC Orally Administered Menstrual Drug Products" by the FDA's Advisory Review Panel on OTC Miscellaneous Internal Drug Products and on the FDA's Tentative Final Monographs on these products and on internal analgesic and antirheumatic products.

Why Some Women Suffer Monthly

The Panel tried to differentiate between two conditions: premenstrual syndrome (occurring in the week before menstruation) and dysmenorrhea (which occurs during menstruation). But their several symptoms—including weight gain, pain, and jangled nerves—may occur during one or both. So the evaluators found it difficult to draw sharp lines between these two conditions, and the FDA decided that, from the point of view of self-medication, they are indistinguishable from one another.

The principal symptoms of premenstrual syndrome, the Panel said, are water retention (edema), weight gain, abdominal bloating and pain, tender breasts, headache, fatigue, and feelings of depression, irritability, tension, and anxiety.

The symptoms of *dysmenorrhea* consist primarily of sharp, cramping pelvic pain, which may radiate to other parts of the body. Related symptoms include nausea, vomiting, diarrhea, headache, dizziness, and fatigue.

Many theories have been advanced to explain these conditions. Two facts stand out in the reviewers' report:

- The key premenstrual symptom for many women is water retention. Relieving this condition allows the pain, irritability, and other symptoms to subside. A woman may be able to do this without recourse to drugs simply by decreasing fluid load in the week before menstruation. Besides drinking less fluid, a woman can try to avoid salt- and sodium-rich foods like potato chips, pickles, sodas, and table salt on her three or four preperiod days, since salt and sodium hold water in the body tissues.

- Women who suffer premenstrual distress and painful periods tend to have high levels of body chemicals called *prostaglandins* when they menstruate. When these women are treated for a few days each month with nonprescription and prescription drugs called *prostaglandin inhibitors*, many experience remarkable symptomatic relief. Aspirin and related salicylates are prostaglandin inhibitors, as is the nonprescription non-steroidal anti-inflammatory drug ibuprofen. (*See* p. 779)

Drugs For Relief

Most nonprescription menstrual-relief products contain one or more of the following ingredients:

- **PAIN RELIEVERS:** These drugs, also called analgesics, act on the nervous system to block sensations of pain and discomfort.
- **ANTIHISTAMINES:** These drugs block the activity of irritating substances called *histamines*, which the body may produce in excess during menstruation. Antihistamines also have a mild pain-relieving effect, and they may counteract anxiety, tension, and irritability. But their exact contribution was not clearly spelled out by the Panel, which has doubts about the value of antihistamines for menstrual relief.
- **DIURETICS:** These drugs act on the kidney or on other organs to eliminate excess water that has accumulated in the body.
- **SMOOTH-MUSCLE RELAXANTS:** These drugs may relieve cramping by relaxing the muscles of the uterus, where the pain appears to originate. But their effectiveness has not been proved.
- **BOTANICAL OR VEGETABLE COMPOUNDS:** Extracts from plants have been formulated into menstrual drugs for at least a century, and possibly for thousands of years. But they appear to lack real medicinal value. (It may be the alcohol in which these ingredients are formulated that provides some symptomatic relief.)
- **VITAMINS:** The value of these nutritional ingredients in treating menstrual distress remains to be proved.

The Panel reviewed the active ingredients in menstrual products according to the categories described above; so this Unit is organized accordingly. Many other ingredients were not categorized or assessed, for want of any meaningful data; they are simply listed as "summarily disapproved" in the first of the two Safety and Effectiveness tables that conclude this Unit. In this welter of ingredients, only the following few compounds in products evaluated by the Panel, the FDA, or both are graded safe and effective:

- *Pain relievers:* acetaminophen, aspirin, carbaspirin calcium, choline salicylate, ibuprofen, magnesium salicylate, sodium salicylate
- *Diuretics:* ammonium chloride, caffeine, pamabrom.

Combination Products

Since premenstrual syndrome and dysmenorrhea cause a variety of symptoms, it made sense to the Panel (as it has to manufacturers and to women who use their products) that the symptoms be treated concurrently, with combination products. The Panel suggests that for premenstrual relief a woman should choose a diuretic, supplemented perhaps by an antihistamine, a pain reliever, or both. Once bleeding—and cramping—have started, a pain reliever is likely to be the best drug, supplemented perhaps by a smooth-muscle relaxant.

Naturally, the claims that can legitimately be made for menstrual relief products depend on their specific ingredients. For example, a claim for the relief of bloatedness or other signs of fluid retention can be made only if a diuretic is included. Pain-relief claims require that aspirin or another safe and effective pain reliever be present.

Pain Relievers

Drugs that relieve pain are principal ingredients in many combination products sold for the self-treatment of premenstrual and menstrual symptoms. Acetaminophen is the one that is most commonly used, according to the *Handbook of Nonprescription Drugs* (9th ed., 1990). It can, of course, be purchased as a single-entity drug far more cheaply than in combination products labeled for menstrual distress. An acetaminophen tablet or two and a cup of coffee provide essentially the same relief as the acetaminophen and caffeine in a tablet sold for menstrual pain (*See* STIMULANTS.)

 Claims for Pain Relievers

Accurate

- "For the temporary relief of minor aches and pains associated with the premenstrual and menstrual periods (dysmenorrhea)"
- "For the temporary relief of minor aches and pains associated with premenstrual and menstrual cramps"

APPROVED PAIN-RELIEVING ACTIVE INGREDIENTS

This Panel accepted the findings of the Advisory Review Panel on OTC Internal Analgesic and Antirheumatic Drug Products on the safety and effectiveness of over-the-counter pain relievers. Thus it approved the ingredients noted here. The FDA also has approved ibuprofen for menstrual relief. (These ingredients, as well as those conditionally approved or disapproved as pain relievers, are discussed more fully in the Unit PAIN, FEVER, AND ANTI-INFLAMMATORY DRUGS TAKEN INTERNALLY.)

- *ACETAMINOPHEN:* This ingredient is safe and effective in doses of 325 to 650 mg every 4 hours or 325 to 500 mg every 3 hours, or 650 to 1000 mg every 6 hours, up to 4000 mg in 24 hours.
- *ASPIRIN:* This ingredient is safe and effective in doses of 325 to 650 mg every 4 hours, or 325 to 500 mg every 3 hours, or 650 to 1000 mg every 6 hours, up to 4000 mg in 24 hours.
- *CARBASPIRIN CALCIUM:* This ingredient is safe and effective in doses of 414 to 828 mg every 4 hours, or 414 to 637 mg every 3 hours, or 828 to 1274 mg every 6 hours, up to 5096 mg in 24 hours.
- *CHOLINE SALICYLATE:* This ingredient is safe and effective in doses of 435 to 870 mg every 4 hours, or 435 to 669 mg every 3 hours, or 870 to 1338 mg every 6 hours, up to 6352 mg in 24 hours.
- *IBUPROFEN:* This ingredient is safe and effective for nonprescription use in doses of 200 to 400 mg every 4 to 6 hours, up to 1200 mg in 24 hours.
- *MAGNESIUM SALICYLATE:* This ingredient is safe and effective in doses of 377 to 754 mg every 4 hours, or 377 to 754 mg every 3 hours, or 754 to 1160 every 6 hours, up to 4640 mg in 24 hours.
- *SODIUM SALICYLATE:* This ingredient is safe and effective in doses of 325 to 650 mg every 4 hours, or 325 to 500 mg every 3 hours, or 650 to 1000 mg every 6 hours, up to 4000 mg in 24 hours.

CONDITIONALLY APPROVED PAIN-RELIEVING ACTIVE INGREDIENTS

One adjuvant, or helper drug, and two pain relievers are granted only tentative approval by the Panel.

- *CAFFEINE:* Manufacturers allege that caffeine relieves pain or enhances the effectiveness of pain relievers like aspirin. The Panel dismissed the notion that caffeine is itself a pain reliever but says it may enhance the effect of aspirin or acetaminophen. So the FDA grants caffeine conditional approval for this purpose; that is, the ingredient is safe but not proved effective. But, *See* p. 719.

- *POTASSIUM SALICYLATE:* This ingredient is similar, but not identical to aspirin and its approved salts, sodium salicylate, magnesium salicylate, and carbaspirin calcium. It may be the most widely used salicylate in menstrual relief products (*Handbook of Nonprescription Drugs*, 9th ed.) But no data was submitted to the FDA to support its use as a nonprescription pain reliever; the agency's provisional decision, therefore, is that it is not proved safe or effective.

- *SALICYLAMIDE:* This drug is promoted as a pain reliever, but neither its safety nor its effectiveness has been established. Therefore it merits only conditional approval.

DISAPPROVED PAIN-RELIEVING ACTIVE INGREDIENTS

None.

Antihistamines

Data are available on the two antihistamines that are used in menstrual remedies. Neither is rated as safe and effective. They are discussed here.

 ### Claims for Antihistamines

Accurate (if there were an approved antihistamine ingredient, but no antihistamine has been approved as safe and effective for menstrual relief as yet)

- "For the relief of emotional changes related to the premenstrual and menstrual periods"

- "For the relief of mood changes such as anxiety, nervous tension, and irritability related to the premenstrual and menstrual periods"

- "For the relief of water-retention symptoms related to the premenstrual and menstrual periods"

- "For the relief of temporary weight gain or swelling due to water retention during the premenstrual and menstrual periods"

• "For the relief of cramps and backache of the premenstrual and menstrual periods"

APPROVED ANTIHISTAMINIC ACTIVE INGREDIENTS

None.

CONDITIONALLY APPROVED ANTIHISTAMINIC ACTIVE INGREDIENTS

• PHENYLTOLOXAMINE CITRATE: This obscure antihistamine long has been used in a combination menstrual relief product. But it was overlooked in the early stages of the OTC Review, and the manufacturer failed to provide the FDA with data on its safety and efficacy. The agency thinks the long record of its use, without apparent problems, justifies the maker's claim that phenyltoloxamine is safe. But the agency wants to see data to prove that it is effective. Tentative verdict: safe but not proved effective. This drug only may be used in combination products when it is labeled for menstrual relief.

• PYRILAMINE MALEATE: Because of wide use over many years, this drug is judged safe, even though it may make the user drowsy. (*See* Pyrilamine maleate in ALLERGY DRUGS.)

The question of *how* pyrilamine maleate helps relieve premenstrual syndrome remains, in the Panel's word, "uncertain." A manufacturer claims that the initial discomfort is caused in part by the release of the body substance histamine, which is blocked by the drug—a theory that the Panel says is highly conjectural. Pyrilamine maleate, like other antihistamines, does have mild anesthetic (numbing) and analgesic (pain-killing) properties, and a sedative effect that may not be related to its effects on histamine.

In two recent controlled studies, pyrilamine maleate was shown to be significantly more effective than a dummy medication in relieving irritability, depression, and premenstrual tension. It also acted to reduce water retention. But the FDA found significant technical flaws in both studies and says pyrilamine maleate's effectiveness in relieving premenstrual and menstrual symptoms has yet to be proved.

None.

Diuretics

A *diuretic*—sometimes called a water pill—stimulates the kidneys or acts in other ways to remove excess water that has accumulated in body tissues. This fluid excess is called *edema;* why it occurs on premenstrual days is not known. Water is believed to be largely responsible for the bloated feeling that many women experience before their menstrual periods, and much of the other pain and discomfort that go with it. Removing water therefore relieves many of these symptoms.

Only very weak diuretics are formulated into over-the-counter preparations. But water pills alter key physiological functions that are intimately tied to water levels, which explains why almost all diuretics are prescription drugs, for use only under medical supervision.

Premenstrual syndrome is the *only* approved use for nonprescription diuretics. If you are using over-the-counter water pills for any other purpose, you should stop using them and see a doctor. Nonprescription diuretics are safe for treating premenstrual syndrome, the Panel says, "because [it] is self-diagnosable, limited in duration, occurs intermittently, disappears abruptly at the onset of the menstrual flow—and is not a sign of a potentially serious underlying disorder."

Damp Sheets

Dandelion is *not* approved as a safe and effective active diuretic ingredient for menstrual distress. But there *is* ample evidence, embedded in the French language, that it has this physiological effect: The current French root word for dandelion, *dent-de-lion*, or "lion's tooth," can be traced only to the eighteenth century according to one report (*New York Times*, Letters, May 16, 1992). But an earlier French name for dandelion, still found in the gastronomic literature, goes back much further: It is *pissenlit*. In French, *en lit* means "in bed."

Claims for Diuretics

Accurate
- "For the relief of temporary water-weight gain, bloating, swelling, and/or full feeling associated with the menstrual and premenstrual periods"

For caffeine only:
- "For the relief of fatigue associated with the premenstrual and menstrual periods"

APPROVED DIURETIC ACTIVE INGREDIENTS

- **AMMONIUM CHLORIDE:** This ingredient has seen many years of use for a variety of minor medical conditions. On that basis, the Panel accepts other reviewers' finding that the drug is safe in the low dosage that should be used for premenstrual relief. (In higher doses of 8 or more grams daily, ammonium chloride frequently causes nausea, vomiting, and stomachache.)

After the diuretic dose is swallowed and absorbed into the bloodstream, the ammonium and the chloride are separated from each other in the liver. The chloride combines with sodium—from sodium bicarbonate in the body—to form sodium chloride (salt). Loss of the sodium bicarbonate decreases the ability of the tissues to bind water, so both water and salt are free for elimination from the body. This reaction can be maintained by fresh doses of ammonium chloride for only a couple of days, after which the body blocks it, so there is no point in taking the drug for long periods of time.

Only one controlled study was available concerning ammonium chloride's use in the treatment of premenstrual edema. The drug was combined with caffeine, which also is a diuretic, so that the results were confounded. Nevertheless, on the basis of this study and wide clinical use, the Panel deemed ammonium chloride effective (as well as safe) in a dosage of 1 gram 3 times daily for up to 6 days for the relief of premenstrual syndrome. When a formal comment in the over-the-counter drug rule-making process challenged this decision, FDA trotted out several very old studies—one from 1925—to bolster the Panel's weakly supported decision in favor of ammonium chloride.

This brief is not the FDA's most convincing piece of reasoning.

WARNING:

 Do not use ammonium chloride if you have kidney or liver disease. This drug may cause nausea, vomiting and gastrointestinal distress.

- *CAFFEINE:* As the stimulant that is found in coffee, tea, chocolate, and many soft drinks, caffeine increases the rate at which the kidneys remove water from the blood and excrete it. The present reviewers accept the findings of another Panel that in customarily used doses the drug is safe. (*See* STIMULANTS.)

    Caffeine is a mild diuretic, the effectiveness of which is well established. The FDA found a study that indicates that caffeine equivalent to that in a cup of coffee increases urinary output by about one-third. The Panel and the FDA therefore approved it as effective for the relief of premenstrual and menstrual bloating at a dosage of 100 to 200 mg every 3 or 4 hours. The same effect can be obtained by drinking a cup of coffee every few hours. Caffeine has one benefit that other diuretics in OTC menstrual relief products lack: It is a mild stimulant, and so relieves the fatigue that may be associated with the menstrual period.

- *PAMABROM (2-AMINO-1-METHYL-PROPANOL-8-BROMOTHEOPHYLLINATE):* The safety of this compound by itself—and in combination with pyrilamine maleate, or pyrilamine maleate + pain relievers—was certified by the FDA back in the 1950s, when it licensed pamabrom as a new drug. Since then, no evidence of significant toxicity or adverse reactions has been reported, so the present Panel finds pamabrom safe.

    When given to healthy women when they are not accumulating fluid before menstruation, pamabrom doubles urinary output for at least one hour. When tested in the premenstrual week, however, the results are less persuasive. In one study of 194 subjects over several menstrual periods, the drug significantly lessened the women's pain, cramps, tension, irritability, and feelings of depression. But it did *not* significantly reduce the excess fluid. Despite these equivocal results, the Panel approved pamabrom as safe and effective. The FDA concurred. Dosage is set at 50 mg per dose 4 times a day, not to exceed 200 mg daily.

CONDITIONALLY APPROVED DIURETIC ACTIVE INGREDIENTS

- *THEOBROMINE SODIUM SALICYLATE:* This is a caffeine-like compound that simulates the kidneys to produce urine. Although it is safe, the drug is an especially weak diuretic and the Panel could find no evidence to show that it effectively relieves edema or other premenstrual symptoms. The FDA said: safe, but not proved effective.
- *THEOPHYLLINE:* While relatively potent as a diuretic, and in the same class as caffeine, theophylline also is occasionally toxic. So the Panel is not persuaded that the drug is safe. Reviewers decided at their very last meeting (which was also the last meeting of any Panel) that theophylline's safety and effectiveness for premenstrual syndrome remain to be established. The FDA agrees.

DISAPPROVED DIURETIC ACTIVE INGREDIENTS
None.

Smooth-Muscle Relaxants

The crampy pain of dysmenorrhea is attributed by many experts to spasmodic contractions of the smooth muscles that make up the wall of the uterus. So there may be merit in using a drug that will relax smooth muscle once bleeding has started, if not beforehand. Unfortunately, of the two smooth-muscle relaxants formulated into these products, the Panel could grant only a conditional approval to one product; it disapproved of the other.

 Claims for Smooth-Muscle Relaxants

No approved claims.

APPROVED SMOOTH-MUSCLE RELAXANT ACTIVE INGREDIENTS
None.

CONDITIONALLY APPROVED SMOOTH-MUSCLE
RELAXANT ACTIVE INGREDIENTS

• CINNAMEDRINE HYDROCHLORIDE: The safety of this compound as a single ingredient has not been studied. But in lab tests in mice, in which it was combined with other ingredients, it appeared to be relatively non-toxic. Moreover, in the first 35 years cinnamedrine was marketed in nonprescription menstrual products, only 23 instances of side effects were attributed to its use. This led the Panel to judge it safe.

But the evaluators could not find any clinical material that establishes the effectiveness of cinnamedrine hydrochloride—by itself—in treating cramps. One study shows that cinnamedrine combined with other ingredients works better than other combinations. This suggests some promising potential, but for the time being the Panel and the FDA assess cinnamedrine hydrochloride as safe but not proved effective.

DISAPPROVED SMOOTH-MUSCLE RELAXANT ACTIVE
INGREDIENTS

• HOMATROPINE METHYLBROMIDE: This is a belladonna derivative, sometimes used as a digestive aid. This Panel judged it safe for that purpose. Because even lower doses are used in menstrual products, the Panel judges the drug safe for such preparations. The problem is that these doses are probably too low to be effective. Worse, no evidence at all was available to demonstrate that homatropine methylbromide relieves menstrual cramps. In fact, one authority on this class of drugs states that the substance has very little effect on the uterus. So the verdict is: safe but not effective.

Botanical or Vegetable Compounds

Plant extracts, usually formulated in alcohol, were widely marketed in the last century for use when women were in what was then called "a delicate condition." Some of these products survive, if somewhat changed.

One preparation, sold both as an elixir and in tablet form, was submitted to the Panel. Reviewers judged that two of its ingredients—a bitter extract of the herb *Gentiana lutea* and licorice root *Glycyrrhiza glabra*—are simply flavoring, not active drugs. The Panel evaluated the five other plant substances in these products. Since it could not find any one of them that merited the "safe and effective" designation, it rejected as scientifically untenable or misleading all claims that these substances really combat the pain or distress of menstruation. A number of other botanical ingredients, for which no supportive data were submitted, also were disapproved.

 Claims for Plant Extracts

Approved
None.

False or Misleading
- "Relieve cramps and other distress of monthly periods"
- "Acts as a uterine sedative"

APPROVED PLANT-EXTRACT ACTIVE INGREDIENTS
None.

CONDITIONALLY APPROVED PLANT-EXTRACT ACTIVE INGREDIENTS
None.

DISAPPROVED PLANT-EXTRACT ACTIVE INGREDIENTS

- **ASCLEPIAS TUBEROSA (PLEURISY ROOT):** Drug reference books indicate that this compound has been used medicinally, for a variety of purposes, for almost a century. But records are nonexistent concerning its use for dysmenorrhea. No scientific studies of the safety of *Asclepias* for humans were submitted to the Panel, although women have taken the drug, apparently without hazard, for many decades. And no evidence indicates that this root extract effectively relieves cramps or other menstrual symptoms. The Panel judges *Asclepias* safe but ineffective.

- *CIMICIFUGA RACEMOSA (BLACK COHOSH):* This is a folk remedy that has been used for many purposes, one of which is *inducing* menstruation. The Panel is somewhat reassured about safety because of a 150-year history of the use of the drug. But it notes that *Cimicifuga* has been shown to be fairly toxic in animal tests, and its safety for human use has not been scientifically established. No studies have been done on its effectiveness in relieving menstrual discomfort. What is more, animal tests conducted a half-century ago indicate that the substance is therapeutically worthless. So evaluators conclude that *Cimicifuga* is neither safe nor effective.

- *PISCIDIA ERYTHRINA (JAMAICA DOGWOOD):* This tree is also called the *fish-poison tree*, because when its crushed bark, twigs, and leaves are dragged through water, fish become stupefied and float to the surface. Extracts of the bark have been promoted as a pain reliever for menstrual cramps. Although no safety studies have been conducted on humans, the Panel says that long use and studies on rats and mice indicate that *Piscidia* is safe. Some tests in animals show that the bark extract depresses uterine muscle tone; other tests do not. No studies have been done to specifically assess the effect of *P. erythrina* on menstrual cramps. Conclusion: safe but not effective.

- *SENECIO AUREUS (LIFE ROOT):* The manufacturer of the product that contains this material conceded back in 1975 that the drug's safety is questionable and said that the preparation would be reformulated. The Panel took the manufacturer at his word that *S. aureus* is unsafe. Furthermore, no data were submitted to show that the ingredient has medicinal value in treating menstrual distress. So the verdict is: not safe and not effective.

- *TARAXACUM OFFICINALE (DANDELION ROOT):* This bitter plant root has a lengthy history of medicinal use as a laxative. It also acts as a diuretic. (*See* box, p. 717.) Long use and a handful of animal tests persuaded the Panel that *T. officinale* is safe. But no scientific evidence was submitted that suggests a role for it in treating dysmenorrhea. The Panel concluded that the substance is safe but not effective. The FDA agrees.

The following ingredients were disapproved without comment as not safe and effective:

- *BUCHU EXTRACT*
- *CNICUS BENEDICTUS (BLESSED THISTLE)*
- *CORN SILK*
- *COUCH GRASS*
- *DOG GRASS EXTRACT*

- *HYDRASTIS CANADENSIS (GOLDENSEAL)*
- *JUNIPER OIL*
- *PIPSISSEWA*
- *TRITICUM*
- *UVA URSI EXTRACT*

Vitamins

A smattering of data is available to suggest that one vitamin might be of value in relieving premenstrual and menstrual distress. *How* it might do so remains wholly unclear.

APPROVED VITAMINS

None.

CONDITIONALLY APPROVED VITAMINS

- *PYRIDOXINE HYDROCHLORIDE (VITAMIN B6):* One of the B vitamins, this compound has been found to be safe and effective when given as a supplement to people who are deficient in it. One researcher has suggested that pyridoxine hydrochloride has an antispasmodic effect, which would relieve cramps. But the few studies cited to bolster this viewpoint cover only a few women and are not well enough constructed to be scientifically valid. One double-blind study failed to show that the B vitamin is any better at relieving menstrual symptoms than a dummy preparation. In view of all this, the Panel judged pyridoxine hydrochloride to be safe but not proved effective when used to relieve menstrual symptoms.

DISAPPROVED VITAMINS

None.

When Further Relief Is Needed

Gynecologists say that several nonsteroidal anti-inflammatory drugs that are available only by prescription are more effective than nonprescription products in relieving menstrual distress. Moreover, severe crampy pain during a woman's period may indicate that she is suffering from endometriosis or from some other condition for which medical care is required. It may be worthwhile to consult a gynecologist or an endocrinologist (hormone specialist) if you are suffering from menstrual distress.

Safety and Effectiveness: Combination Products Sold Over-the-Counter to Relieve Premenstrual and Menstrual Distress

---

Safe and Effective

    1 approved pain reliever or a combination of acetaminophen + another approved
       pain reliever + caffeine, or ammonium chloride, or pamabrom
    caffeine + ammonium chloride
    pamabrom + ammonium chloride

Conditionally safe and Effective

    aspirin + cinnamedrine hydrochloride + caffeine
    pyrilamine maleate + acetaminophen
    any other combination containing pyrilamine maleate
    phenyltoloxamine citrate + acetaminophen

Unsafe and/or Ineffective Combinations

    Piscidia erythrina + Asclepias tuberosa + Cimicifuga racemosa + Taraxacum
      officinale + Senecio aureus
    Cimicifuga racemosa + Senecio aureus + Taraxacum officinale + ferrous
      sulfate

Safety and Effectiveness:
Active Ingredients in Over-the-Counter Menstrual-Distress Preparations

Active Ingredient	Category	Assessment
acetaminophen	pain reliever	safe and effective
ammonium chloride	diuretic	safe and effective
Asclepias tuberosa (pleurisy root)	plant extract	safe, but not effective
aspirin	pain reliever	safe and effective
buchu extract	plant extract	not safe and effective
caffeine	as pain reliever	safe, but not proved effective
	as diuretic/stimulant	safe and effective
carbaspirin calcium	pain reliever	safe and effective
choline salicylate	pain reliever	safe and effective
Cimicifuga racemosa (black cohosh)	plant extract	not safe and effective
cinnamedrine hydrochloride	smooth-muscle relaxant	safe, but not proved effective
Cnicus benedictus (blessed thistle)	plant extract	not safe and effective
corn silk	plant extract	not safe and effective
couch grass	plant extract	not safe and effective

Substance	Type	Status
dog-grass extract	plant extract	not safe and effective
homatropine methylbromide	smooth-muscle relaxant	safe, but not effective
Hydrastis canadensis (goldenseal)	plant extract	not safe and effective
ibuprofen	pain reliever	safe and effective
juniper oil	plant extract	not safe and effective
magnesium salicylate	pain reliever	safe and effective
pamabrom (2-amino-1-methyl-1-propanol-8-bromotheophyllinate)	diuretic	safe and effective
phenyltoloxamine citrate	antihistamine	safe, not proved effective
pipsissewa	plant extract	not safe and effective
Piscidia erythrina (Jamaica dogwood)	plant extract	safe, but not effective
potassium salicylate	pain reliever	safe, not proved effective
pyridoxine hydrochloride (vitamin B6)	vitamin	safe, not proved effective
pyrilamine maleate	antihistamine	safe, not proved effective
salicylamide	pain reliever	not proved safe or effective
Senecio aureus (life root)	plant extract	not proved safe or effective
sodium salicylate	pain reliever	safe and effective
Taraxacum officinale (dandelion root)	plant extract/diuretic	safe, but not effective

Safety and Effectiveness:
Active Ingredients in Over-the-Counter Menstrual-Distress Preparations (contd)

Active Ingredient	Category	Assessment
theobromine sodium salicylate	diuretic	safe, but not proved effective
theophylline	diuretic	not proved safe or effective
triticum	plant extract	not safe and effective
uva ursi extract	plant extract	not safe and effective

Menstrual-Distress Preparations: Product Ratings

SINGLE-INGREDIENT PRODUCTS

Product and Distributor	Dosage of Active Ingredients	Rating*	Comment
ammonium chloride (diuretic)			
Ammonium chloride (generic)	tablets: 500 mg	A	approved for brief, monthly use only
	enteric coated tablets: 500 mg	A	approved for brief, monthly use only
Ammonium Chloride (Lilly)	enteric coated tablets: 500 mg	A	approved for brief, monthly use only
ibuprofen			
Midol IB (Sterling)	tablets: 200 mg	A	Rx to OTC switchonly
pamabrom			
Fluidex with Pamabrom (O'Connor)	capsules: 50 mg	A	approved for brief, monthly use only

COMBINATION PRODUCTS

Product and Distributor	Pain Reliever	Diuretic	Antihistamine	Other	Rating*	Comment
Aqua Ban Tablets (Thompson)		325 mg ammonium chloride		100 mg caffeine	A	

Menstrual-Distress Preparations: Product Ratings (contd)

Product and Distributor	Pain Reliever¹	Diuretic	Antihistamine	Other	Rating*	Comment
Maximum Strength Midol Multi-Symptom Menstrual Formula (Sterling)	500 mg acetaminophen		15 mg pyrilamine maleate	60 mg caffeine	B	pyrilamine maleate not proved effective
Midol Maximum Strength Premenstrual Syndrome Formula (Sterling)	500 mg acetaminophen	25 mg pamabrom	15 mg pyrilamine maleate		B	pyrilamine maleate not proved effective
Midol Regular Strength Multi-Symptom Formula (Sterling)	325 mg acetaminophen		12.5 mg pyrilamine maleate		B	pyrilamine maleate not proved effective
Pamprin Maximum Cramp Relief (Chattem)	500 mg acetaminophen	25 mg pamabrom	15 mg pyrilamine maleate		B	pyrilamine maleate not proved effective
PMS Tea (tea bags) (Traditional Medicines)		500 mg dandelion root		80 mg uva ursi leaf	C	not effective; may not be safe
Premenstrual Pain Formula (Sterling)	500 mg acetaminophen	25 mg pamabrom	15 mg pyrilamine maleate		B	pyrilamine maleate not proved effective

| Premsyn PMS (Chattem) | 500 mg acetaminophen | 25 mg pamabrom | 15 mg pyrilamine maleate | B | pyrilamine maleate not proved effective |

*Author's interpretation of FDA criteria. Based on contents, not claims.
†For ratings of other pain relievers, see pages 795-801; for ratings of caffeine products, see page 891.

Motion-Sickness Medicines

Severe nausea, and the realization that one is about to vomit, is one of the more dreadful conditions suffered by man!

— The Panel

Motion sickness occurs when our sense of what we are seeing with our eyes is out of sync with our sense of balance, which is maintained by sensitive organs of the inner ear. Trouble is particularly likely to arise as the head rotates and one becomes dizzy. Although some people may be less susceptible than others—astronauts, ice skaters, and ballet dancers are specially trained to overcome these effects—no one is wholly immune to this distress.

Fortunately, several nonprescription drugs are available that can be taken before departure, or during a trip, to quell the discomforting symptoms of airsickness, carsickness, seasickness, and other forms of motion sickness.

MOTION-SICKNESS MEDICINES is based on the report of the FDA's Advisory Review Panel on OTC Laxative, Antidiarrheal, Emetic, and Antiemetic Drug Products and on the FDA's Tentative Final and Final Monographs on Anti-emetic Drug Products for OTC Human Use.

Claims

Accurate

• "For the prevention and treatment of the nausea, vomiting or dizziness associated with motion sickness"

Products to Treat Motion Sickness

Emesis is the Greek term for vomiting. An *anti-emetic*, of course, blocks this action. Many effective anti-emetics require a doctor's prescription. Others are available over-the-counter. Both the Panel and the FDA believe that these preparations should be used only to quell the nausea and vomiting associated with motion sickness. If these symptoms are not related to motion sickness, medical help should be sought if they do not rapidly subside.

Non-medicinal Help for Motion Sickness

Popular folk remedies for motion sickness, such as "soda crackers and 7 Up®" and "cola syrup over ice," have not been shown—scientifically—to work, say medical specialists who treat motion sickness and other forms of dizziness (the American Academy of Otolaryngology/Head and Neck Surgery). But these ear, nose, and throat doctors do have some suggestions:

1. Sit in the front seat of the car and watch the distant scenery, or, aboard ship, go up on deck and watch the horizon. In planes, choose a window seat over the wings where there is less motion. Always ride facing forward.

2. Don't read.

3. Don't watch or talk to another traveler who is suffering motion sickness.

4. Avoid strong odors and spicy or greasy foods.

APPROVED ACTIVE INGREDIENTS

• *BENHYDRYL PIPERAZINES: MECLIZINE HYDROCHLORIDE AND CYCLIZINE HYDROCHLORIDE:* These antihistamines are both evaluated as safe and effective for the prevention and treatment of motion sickness. They are especially useful if taken a half-hour to an hour *before* setting out on a journey. There is no explanation of exactly why or how they work to quell motion sickness, although they are thought to reduce the excitability of balance centers within the inner ear.

Meclizine hydrochloride is a well-studied and widely used drug that had been available by prescription for more than a quarter of a century. The evaluators decided that it is safe and effective when sold and used as an over-the-counter product. Cyclizine hydrochloride appears to have been used and studied less extensively. But it is chemically similar to meclizine, and the Panel and the FDA rate it as safe and effective.

Fears were raised in the 1960s that these drugs could cause birth defects if used by pregnant women. However, a study of more than 1000 women who used meclizine during their first trimester indicates that this is not true. So the FDA canceled its required label warning that suggests that these drugs not be used during pregnancy unless urgently needed.

Both meclizine and cyclizine cause drowsiness in some users. Neither should be taken by a person who is driving a car or other vehicle, piloting a boat or plane, or operating heavy machinery. Neither should they be taken by a person who is drinking; alcohol and antihistamines have an additive, sleep-inducing effect.

Meclizine hydrochloride has the advantage that a single 25-to 50-mg dose remains effective up to 24 hours. It should not be given to children under 12 years of age except as directed by a doctor.

The adult dosage for cyclizine hydrochloride is 50 mg every 4 to 6 hours, up to 4 times in 24 hours. For children 6 to 12 years old, 25 mg per dose, up to 3 times in 24 hours is allowed. Do not give to children under 6 years of age except as directed by a doctor.

WARNING:

 These drugs may cause *marked drowsiness.*

- *AMINO ALKYL ETHERS: DIPHENHYDRAMINE HYDROCHLORIDE, DIMENHYDRINATE:* The safety and effectiveness of these drugs against seasickness and airsickness have been shown repeatedly in the 40 years since diphenhydramine first was introduced, the evaluators noted. These drugs are relatively free of side effects in the recommended doses, although some users do become very drowsy. So passengers can use them, but not drivers, pilots, or nautical captains. Drinking liquor may make a person drowsier still, which some seasickish passengers may find welcome!

Antihistamines have a drying effect on some glands and tissues. These drugs should not be used by sufferers of asthma, glaucoma, or enlarged prostate (disorders already marked by glandular problems) except under a doctor's supervision.

The adult dosage of diphenhydramine hydrochloride is 25 to 50 mg every 4 to 6 hours, not to exceed 300 mg in 24 hours, or as directed by a doctor. For children 6 to 12 years old, it is 12.5 to 25 mg every 4 to 6 hours, not to exceed 150 mg in 24 hours, or as directed by a doctor. Do not give to children under 6 years old unless directed by a doctor.

The dosage of dimenhydrinate required to prevent or relieve motion sickness in adults is 50 to 100 mg every 4 to 6 hours, not to exceed 400 mg in 24 hours, or as directed by a doctor. For children 6 to 12 yars of age, it is 25 to 50 mg every 6 to 8 hours, not to exceed 150 mg in 24 hours, or as directed by a doctor. For youngsters 2 to 6 years of age, the dosage is 12.5 to 25 mg every 6 to 8 hours, not to exceed 75 mg in 24 hours, or as directed by a doctor. Dimenhydrinate is the only anti-emetic approved for young children. But do not give it to children under 2 years of age unless directed by a doctor.

WARNING:

 These drugs may cause *marked drowsiness*.

CONDITIONALLY APPROVED ACTIVE INGREDIENTS
None.

DISAPPROVED ACTIVE INGREDIENTS
None.

When Greater Relief Is Needed

Several drugs, including tranquilizers and nervous systems depressants, are available on prescription. Some *anticholinergic agents*, which depress the involuntary (autonomic) nervous system previously were available without prescription. But OTC drug reviewers decided that they are not safe when used without medical supervision, and the FDA agreed. These drugs now are available only on prescription (℞). One of the trendiest of them is a new scopolamine adhesive patch that can be stuck under a person's ear a few hours before traveling. It provides protection from motion sickness for up to 3 days.

Safety and Effectiveness: Active Ingredients in Over-the-Counter Motion-Sickness Medicines

Active Ingredient	Assessment
cyclizine hydrochloride	safe and effective
dimenhydrinate	safe and effective
diphenhydramine hydrochloride	safe and effective
meclizine hydrochloride	safe and effective

Motion-Sickness Medicines: Product Ratings

Product and Distributor	Dosage of Active Ingredients	Rating*	Comment
cyclizine hydrochloride			
Marezine (Burroughs-Wellcome)	tablets: 50 mg	A	
dimenhydrinate			
Dimenhydrinate (generic)	liquid: 15 mg per teaspoonful tablets: 50 mg	A A	
Dramamine (Upjohn)	tablets: 50 mg liquid: 12.5 mg per teaspoonful	A A	
Tega-Vert (Ortega)	capsules: 50 mg	A	
diphenhydramine hydrochloride			
Benadryl 25 (Parke-Davis Consumer)	capsules, tablets: 25 mg	A	Ŗ to OTC switch
Benylin Cough Syrup (Parke-Davis Consumer)	syrup: 12.5 mg per tsp.	A	Ŗ to OTC switch
Diphenhydramine hydrochloride (generic)	capsules: 25 mg, 50 mg liquid, syrup: 12.5 mg per tsp.	A A	Ŗ to OTC switch Ŗ to OTC switch

Motion-Sickness Medicines: Product Ratings (contd)

Product and Distributor	Dosage of Active Ingredients	Rating*	Comment
meclizine hydrochloride			
Bonine (Pfizer)	**chewable tablets:** 25 mg	A	
Dizmiss (JMI Canton)	**chewable tablets:** 25 mg	A	
Meclizine hydrochloride (generic)	**tablets:** 12.5 mg	A	
	tablets: 25 mg	A	
	chewable tablets: 25 mg	A	

*Author's interpretation of FDA criteria. Based on contents, not claims.

Mouthwash for Oral Hygiene

Bad breath *is* unpleasant. If you go by mouthwash commercials, it is the ultimate social sin! It is no wonder that Americans spend a million dollars a day on mouthwashes, gargles, and other breath fresheners.

These products are promoted to encourage daily use by persons with no symptoms or evidence of disease. However, manufacturers claim these products prevent dental decay and gum and mouth diseases; these of course are *medicinal* claims. Many mouthwashes contain pharmacologically active ingredients—principally antimicrobials (germicides), which kill or inhibit the growth of bacteria, viruses, funguses, and other microorganisms. Both the medicinal claims and the pharmacological ingredients define these products legally as drugs as opposed to cosmetics, and, therefore, they were assessed as part of the OTC Drug Review.

The Panel took a dim view of medicated mouthwashes. It rated many of the claims made for them as sheer hogwash. Aside from questionable benefits, there may be significant risk in the daily use of

MOUTHWASH FOR ORAL HYGIENE is based on the report of the FDA's Advisory Review Panel on OTC Oral-Cavity Drug Products.

antimicrobials by healthy people. This cautionary view is shared by the FDA, the National Academy of Science, and researchers at the National Cancer Institute. The Panel said: "The absurd notion that antimicrobial agents in gargles, mouthwashes, and mouth rinses are necessary for daily cleansing of the mouth and throat is based on tradition, promotional appeal by manufacturers, and misunderstandings concerning their effectiveness and safety, rather than on well-documented facts . . . . There are few, if any, indications justifying the use of [these products] for self-medication or for oral health care by lay consumers."

None of the antimicrobials used in these products has been demonstrated to be safe and effective for routine use by healthy people. Some of these preparations also are marketed for brief use in treating sore throat, sore mouth, and other minor oral-cavity irritation. (*See* MEDICAMENTS FOR SORE GUMS, MOUTHS, AND THROATS.) Thus far, none of the antimicrobial agents has been found to be safe and effective for these purposes.

Of much greater import—since promotional efforts and sales both are booming—is the claim that some of these same antimicrobial agents in mouthwashes, rinses, and toothpastes will prevent or reduce the buildup of dental plaque. Since bacteria in the mouth *do* play a key role in plaque formation, and since these germicides *do* kill bacteria, these claims have some credence. However, despite huge sales, the evidence that these products kill sufficient numbers of the right bacteria to control plaque, and can do so safely, simply does not exist at this time (1992) insofar as the FDA is concerned. These important anti-plaque claims, and the ingredients and products for which they are made, are treated separately in TEETH: ANTI-PLAQUE PRODUCTS. This Unit, then, focuses on the use of these and some other ingredients in mouthwashes, for which other health claims may be made.

 Claims

Accurate

None. The Panel could not discern any accurate claim for the safe and effective use of antimicrobial active ingredients in mouthwash products intended for routine daily use by healthy people.

False or Misleading

• "Inhibits odor-forming bacteria"

- "Deodorizing mouthwash and gargle"
- "Oral antiseptic cleanser"
- "For oral hygiene, bad breath"
- "Management of mouth odors, bad breath"
- "An aid to daily care of the mouth"
- "For causing the mouth to feel clean"

The Healthy Mouth

Millions of microorganisms enter the nose and mouth each day in the air we breathe, the food we eat, and the water we drink. Many come to rest in the gastrointestinal tract or respiratory system. These "germs" normally do not cause disease because the body has a potent defense system to kill or remove them. *Saliva* is one key element in this system.

A third of a liter of saliva is secreted into the mouth each day. It cleans the inside of the mouth and the teeth and also inhibits bacterial growth. The body's immunological defense mechanisms also are constantly at work in the mouth destroying invading microorganisms. What is more, bacteria that normally are present in the mouth appear to help resist colonization by their invading, disease-producing relatives.

These defense mechanisms sometimes fail, and infections and other disorders may result. But a healthy mouth requires no ongoing help in the form of medicated mouthwash to stay fresh and clean. And there is no evidence, the Panel says, that using these products will prevent infections and diseases.

Mouthwash and Cancer

In 1983, just as the first edition of this Guide (*The Essential Guide to Nonprescription Drugs*, New York: Harper & Row, 1983) was published, the National Cancer Institute (NCI) issued an advisory notice to the public that said: "An apparent association between mouthwash use and increased risk of cancers of the mouth and throat has been found among a small group of women who are usually considered at low risk for these cancers, according to an NCI study." The study was conducted by biostatistician William J. Blot, Ph.D., and several associates.

Almost a decade later, Blot and his NCI associates published a larger, follow-up study that shows that people who use mouthwash containing 25 percent alcohol or more for a period of 20 years or longer have a significantly higher rate of mouth and throat cancers: 1.5 times higher for men, and almost twice as high for women, compared with matched groups of men and women who do not use these products (D.M. Winn *et al., Cancer Research*, vol. 51, pp. 30044-30047, June 1, 1991).

Mouthwash manufacturers (particularly Warner-Lambert, which makes *Listerine*—alcohol content: 26.9 percent) say the Blot study does not stand up to scrutiny. Warner-Lambert says no evidence exists to support an association between alcohol-containing mouthwashes and cancer, the *"Pink Sheet"* reports (Jan. 29, 1992).

But the FDA, which collected a couple of other, confirmatory reports on the putative link between alcoholic mouthwash and cancer has told nonprescription drug makers and manufacturers of other mouthwash products that it is concerned about the "potential health risk for consumers who use oral health care drug products that contain high concentrations of alcohol." The FDA said that although the scientific findings by Blot and others "do not firmly establish the risk relationship between alcohol-containing mouthwash use and these cancers, they show a need to look further at this relationship."

Oral Malodor

Whether it is called *bad breath, halitosis, foul breath*, or, as the Panel preferred, *oral malodor*, this is an age-old problem. Remedies employed against it have ranged from chewing pleasant-smelling berries like teaberry to taking enemas, scraping the tongue, using perfumes, and smoking flavored cigarettes. Today, the principal remedy is the scented mouthwash. Scented mouthwashes are cleansing and freshening preparations—that is, *cosmetics*—unless they contain an antimicrobial or other drug or carry medicinal claims on their labels, as many do. Any substance that is promoted as a germ killer is being promoted as a drug.

Some diseases cause unusual—and in some instances quite unpleasant—odors on the breath. But the Panel said that most oral malodor is not associated with sore throat, sore mouth, or any particular systemic or local oral-cavity disease. Bad breath, the Panel said, is not a disease.

Oddly, bad breath usually is not detected by the person who has it. Putting into more delicate language the scripts of many a mouthwash commercial, the Panel declared: "Unless a social contact informs an individual that he or she has malodor, the individual may be unaware of its presence."

Bad breath can be associated with medical conditions: Diabetes, for example, creates a sweetish smell on the breath. Persons whose kidneys are failing and who no longer can get rid of body wastes in their urine may have a urine-like smell on their breath. Upper-respiratory infections, not surprisingly, can produce a purulent smell. These malodors, of course, do not occur in healthy people.

Having studied the medical literature, the Panel concluded that only about 10 percent of all oral malodors are due to outside causes like food and drink, or disease. The rest represent local oral conditions in people who are healthy.

Researchers long quarreled about what *kind* of chemicals produce bad breath. In recent years, an analytic method called *gas chromatography*—which can detect airborne molecules in parts-per-billion concentrations—has demonstrated that a halitosis-affected mouth has minute traces of sulfur compounds. These volatile and foul-smelling gases include hydrogen sulfide, methylmercaptan, and, to a lesser extent dimethylsulfides.

These sulfurous gases cannot be made by cells of the human body. But they can be made by bacteria that are normally present in the mouth. Two species, Fusobacterium and Peptostreptococcus, are principal culprits. These microbes thrive in nooks and crannies in the mouth where there is little or no oxygen. This means they are principally found in crevices in the gums, between the teeth, in small folds in the tonsils, and in tiny intercellular spaces in the tongue. (This last location has long been believed to be one of their principal places of concealment.) Neither the volatile sulfurs nor the bacteria that produce them appear to be dangerous.

Eating candy and other sweets does not lead to bad breath—contrary to what some parents tell their children. Rather, according to the experts, the offensive bacteria consume sulfur-containing proteins and amino acids that are most abundant in meat, fish, and dairy products.

Methods for Eliminating Bad Breath

The Panel had several suggestions for eliminating bad breath. These suggestions refer specifically to malodor that arises from within the throat and mouth—*not* to "garlic breath" and other such situations that can be avoided simply by not eating or drinking the offending substance before a date or other social function.

Purging

It is often possible to temporarily rid yourself of bad breath by rinsing out your mouth with water, brushing your teeth, using dental floss, or eating a meal. These methods sometimes work and sometimes do not. The improvement results from the physical removal or dilution of volatile sulfur compounds, the bacteria that produce them, and the food debris they consume. This dilution is part of the beneficial effect of most liquid preparations and products sold to relieve mouth odor—but water will serve as well.

Masking

Bad odors sometimes can be covered up with good odors. Many mouthwashes contain anise, cinnamon, peppermint, spearmint, or sage oils to provide this coverup. These masking agents are effective only until the saliva dilutes them and carries them away—usually in about 15 to 20 minutes.

Chemical Neutralization

Some substances react chemically with bad-smelling airborne compounds to form nonodorous substances, usually nonvolatile sulfides. The effect they produce depends on how long the neutralizing agent remains in the mouth and how much of the malodorous compounds needs to be neutralized. This method provides longer-lasting protection than purging or masking substances. Unfortunately, the Panel failed to identify what these neutralizing substances are.

Bacterial Inhibition

An antimicrobial that kills or slows the growth and reproduction of the bacteria that cause mouth malodor *will* freshen the breath for longer periods than purging or masking methods. But after a meal or during sleep, the Panel said, the bacteria will usually return to their original numbers, bringing back the odor.

Theoretically, the best results should be obtained by using germicides that specifically and selectively attack the relatively few bacteria that appear to be responsible for bad breath. But the Panel said it does not know whether antimicrobials really work this way. What *is* known is that the bacteria rarely if ever are completely destroyed, and they will quickly repopulate the mouth once the antimicrobial is gone.

Evaluators estimate that to obtain long-lasting protection the antimicrobial dose would have to be repeated every 3 or 4 hours, as long as the malodor persisted. This heavy use of antimicrobials, which can upset the normal, healthy balance of microorganisms in the mouth, cannot be justified. So the Panel stressed its objection to the routine, self-prescribed use of medicated oral-health preparations, particularly those with antimicrobial agents.

This hard stance against over-the-counter sales and self-treatment with antimicrobial mouthwashes does not mean that the reviewers wholly oppose efforts to use drugs to eliminate odor-forming bacteria in the mouth. Rather, they feel that drug-research progress—which has produced far more effective germ-killing agents than the ones found in over-the-counter preparations—requires that such treatment be supervised by a doctor or a dentist. The professional may be able to identify the responsible microorganisms and then prescribe a potent prescription antimicrobial prescription that will fairly specifically and selectively reduce or eliminate them. These drugs for the most part are administered systemically, not topically in mouthwashes.

Active Ingredients in Over-the-Counter Mouthwash

A glance at mouthwash labels in any drugstore will reveal that most contain antimicrobials. A few also contain astringents, anesthetics, or other types of drugs. The Panel assessed all ingredients in the preparations submitted for its evaluation and automatically disapproved any that were not submitted for review. (For assessment of these active ingredients in oral-health-care products intended for short-term use, *see* MEDICAMENTS FOR SORE GUMS, MOUTHS, AND THROATS.)

Among the astringents that may be found in mouthwashes, the FDA says alum and zinc chloride are safe and effective, but tincture of myrrh is neither safe nor effective. Among the many antimicrobials that are the principal medicinal ingredients in these washes, the Panel could not find even one that it felt was safe and effective for self-treatment under any circumstances.

APPROVED ANTIMICROBIAL ACTIVE INGREDIENTS

None.

CONDITIONALLY APPROVED ANTIMICROBIAL ACTIVE INGREDIENTS

• BENZALKONIUM CHLORIDE: The safety of this antimicrobial, which is described on p. 678, has not been well researched: "The Panel finds no data from controlled studies on the cumulative side effects resulting from absorption from the mucous membranes of benzalkonium chloride when used on a day-to-day basis in mouthwashes or rinses for years." Surprisingly, nonetheless, it rated this compound safe. The Panel went on to say that benzalkonium chloride is an effective germ killer. But the evidence indicating its efficacy in mouthwashes and oral rinse products is deficient, the Panel said, and it does not endorse the use of benzalkonium chloride for this purpose. The Panel's assessment thus was: safe, but not proved effective.

• BENZETHONIUM CHLORIDE: The Panel said that this antimicrobial, which is described more fully on p. 678, is relatively nontoxic and probably safe for short-term use. But its safety for continuing use in daily-use mouthwashes and similar products has not been established. The Panel could find "no substantial evidence to establish the rationale for healthy people to use benzethonium chloride on a continuing day-to-day basis as an antimicrobial agent in mouthwashes or rinses." In short, both safety and effectiveness remain to be proved.

• CETALKONIUM CHLORIDE: This is a quaternary ammonium compound, or "quat," that is quite similar to benzalkonium chloride and benzethonium chloride, described previously. (*See* also pp. 679-680.) Although this compound is safe, generally speaking, for short-term use, the Panel said the available data did not convince it that cetalkonium chloride will not cause cancer, birth defects, or hidden genetic damage when used on a long-term basis in mouthwashes, rinses, and gargles. The Panel found the testing methods used to demonstrate cetalkonium chloride's effectiveness in mouthwashes inadequate. It concluded, surprisingly, that the compound is safe. It said that cetalkonium chloride's effectiveness in mouthwash products has yet to be proved.

• CETYLPYRIDINIUM CHLORIDE: This "quat," like the ones described above, is of dubious value when used on a short-term basis for minor infections and inflammations of the throat and mouth (*see* p. 680). What is worse, the Panel said, is that data on its cumulative effects after long-term use simply are not known. Cetylpyridinium chloride acts against only a narrow spectrum of bacteria and may be quickly neutralized by chemicals naturally present in the mouth and by food debris. The Panel said "there are no data to justify the use of cetypyridinium chloride in oral health products on a continuing day-to-day basis for protracted periods of time . . ." Its decision was that both the safety and the effectiveness of cetypridinium chloride need to be proved.

Cetylpyridinium chloride's anti-plaque potential is described on page 934.

- *CHLOROPHYLL:* Since this is the natural green substance in broccoli, spinach, and all other green plants, it obviously is safe. Commercial chlorophyll products in fact are made from broccoli leaves and also from alfalfa, the Panel said. Chlorophyll inhibits the growth of some bacteria, but the Panel said: "It has not been demonstrated that it is an effective deodorant." So, while safe, chlorophyll's efficacy remains to be proved.

- *DOMIPHEN BROMIDE:* This antimicrobial (*see* pp. 680-681) is unlikely to cause an immediate toxic reaction. But insufficient data were presented to the Panel to rule out the possibility that long-term use could cause cancer, genetic damage, or birth defects in the children of women who used the compound during pregnancy. Much evidence shows that domiphen bromide kills bacteria. But the Panel did not believe its effectiveness as an active ingredient in mouthwash was established by the available data. Safety and effectiveness need to be established.

Domiphen bromide's anti-plaque potential is described on page 935.

- *ETHYL ALCOHOL:* This is ordinary grain alcohol (*see* p. 681). It is used in mouthwash preparations in part because of its intrinsic antimicrobial effect and in part because it acts as a solvent for other germ-killing ingredients. The Panel declared it safe. It should be noted, however, that high-alcohol mouthwashes recently have been implicated by the National Cancer Institute researchers as a risk factor for cancers of the mouth and throat in people who used these products habitually on a daily basis for 20 years or longer. Men had a 1.6-fold increased risk, and women a 1.9-fold increased risk, the study by biostatistician William J. Blot, Ph.D., and his associates showed, according to a summary in the *Journal of the National Cancer Institute* (vol. 83, No.

11, p. 751, June 5, 1991).

Mouthwashes with less than 25 percent alcohol did not increase the cancer risk, the study found. According to the *Journal of the National Cancer Institute*, the product singled out by the press as falling into the risk category was *Listerine* (Warner-Lambert), which contains 26.9 percent alcohol. Only one other mouthwash product listed in the *Handbook of Nonprescription Drugs*, 9th ed. (Washington: American Pharmaceutical Association, 1990) contains a higher alcohol concentration.

Warner-Lambert disputes the findings of the NCI study by biostatistician Blot and his associates. It says that it intends to continue to market *Listerine*. In June 1992, Warner-Lambert introduced a new mouthwash, called *Cool Mint Listerine*, that has a lower, 21.6 percent alcohol content.

In terms of efficacy, the FDA says ethyl alcohol is ineffective in concentrations under 48 percent. So a 20 or 25 percent alcohol mouthwash is unlikely to be effective, according to the Panel's evaluation. However, lower concentrations of alcohol in combination with other antimicrobials may indeed be germicidal. But this efficacy, if it exists, remains to be proved. The Panel's conclusion, pre-dating the NCI study, is that ethyl alcohol is safe but its effectiveness remains to be proved.

• *EUCALYPTOL:* As described on p. 681, the Panel decided that eucalyptol is safe for use in the mouth and throat. But the evidence submitted to establish its short-term efficacy was inadequate, in the Panel's view. It can be inferred that while it may be safe, its effectiveness when used on a daily basis by healthy people remains to be proved. Verdict: safe but not proved effective.

• *MENTHOL:* The Panel ruled this peppermint-oil extract safe. But it found that the data submitted to demonstrate its effectiveness in sore-throat-and-mouth preparations, and particularly mouthwash, was inadequate. So, while safe, menthol's effectiveness is yet to be proved.

• *METHYL SALICYLATE:* Like menthol, with which it frequently is combined, methyl salicylate is rated as safe by the Panel. But the evidence to show that it is effective was not convincing. So safety and efficacy both remain to be proved.

• *PHENOL:* The Panel did not assess any data on the safety and effectiveness of phenol as an antimicrobial for long-term use in mouthwash, mouthrinse, or gargle preparations. But while phenol in concentrations of 0.5 to 1.5 percent appears safe at least for short-term use in the mouth and throat, its effectiveness remains to be proved. From this it can be inferred that effectiveness will have to be proved before a phenol-based mouthwash could be ruled safe and effective for long-term use in healthy people. In sum: safe but not proved effective.

- **THYMOL:** This aromatic alcohol is widely used in products used for treating sore mouth and throat, for which the Panel rated it safe but not proved effective. (*See* p. 685.) It kills germs and has a pleasant, clean taste. But its effectiveness for relieving sore mouth and sore throat is unproved, and the Panel apparently did not receive significant data on its effectiveness over the long term when used as a mouthwash in healthy men and women. Verdict: safe, not proved effective.

DISAPPROVED ANTIMICROBIAL ACTIVE INGREDIENTS

It is not clear whether any disapproved active ingredients currently are being formulated into mouthwash, mouthrinse and gargle products for long-term use by healthy teenagers and men and women. The following ingredients have been declared to be not safe and effective by the FDA in products used for treating sore mouth and throat. They would also be unsafe for chronic use:

- **BORIC ACID:** This drug is derived from the non-metallic element *boron*, a potent nerve poison. Skin can block the absorption of boric acid but mucous membrane cannot. The early signs of boron poisoning or boric-acid poisoning are nausea, vomiting, diarrhea, and stomach pain.

   Boric acid is only weakly effective, at best, in killing microorganisms in the mouth and throat. The Oral Cavity Panel therefore classifies boric acid (and the related compounds sodium borate and borax) as both unsafe and ineffective.

- **BOROGYLCERIN GLYCERITE:** As its name suggests, this is a compound of boric acid and glycerin. No convincing scientific evidence is available on its worth in the case of sore throat and sore mouth, and it also shares the toxic risk of boric acid (*see* immediately preceding). The Panel's verdict: not safe and effective.

- **CAMPHOR:** Despite its long use, concern persists about the toxicity of this substance. Lacking data showing that camphor is effective on the mucous membranes of the throat and mouth, evaluators judged it both not safe and not effective.

- **CRESOL:** This is a phenol derivative that may be more irritating to body surfaces than phenol itself is. Cresol is readily and rapidly absorbed into the body through mucous membranes and produces local damage to tissues even in dilute solutions. For these reasons, it was declared not safe. It is more active against some bacteria than is phenol, but the Panel did not rule on cresol's effectiveness: It disapproved cresol wholly on grounds of safety.

• *FERRIC CHLORIDE:* An iron salt that is reddish or brownish in color, ferric chloride is irritating to the mucosal lining of the gastrointestinal tract. It is fairly toxic, and large doses, accidentally swallowed, could cause death. The Panel ruled it unsafe. Also, since they were provided no data indicating that ferric chloride effectively combats the microorganisms that cause sore throat and mouth, the Oral Cavity Panel declared ferric chloride not effective as well as unsafe.

• *METHYL SALICYLATE:* The pleasant wintergreen aroma and taste of this aspirin-like drug tend to conceal its high toxicity. It is also extremely irritating to the gums. The Dental Panel says it is both not safe and not effective.

When Greater Relief Is Needed

Persistent bad breath or bad taste in the mouth should be evaluated and often can be successfully treated. Start with your dentist. If he or she cannot help resolve or reduce the problem, ask for a referral to an infectious disease specialist, otolaryngologist, or other specialist whom the dentist feels may help with the problem.

Safety and Effectiveness: Antimicrobial Active Ingredients in Over-the-Counter Mouthwash, Rinse, and Gargle Products For Chronic Use by Healthy People

Active Ingredient	Assessment
benzalkonium chloride	safe, but not proved effective
benzethonium chloride	not proved safe or effective
boric acid	not safe and effective
boroglycerin glycerite	not safe and effective
camphor	not safe and effective
cetalkonium chloride	safe, but not proved effective
cetylpyridinium chloride	not proved safe or effective
chlorophyll	safe, but not proved effective
cresol	not safe and effective
domiphen bromide	not proved safe or effective
ethyl alcohol	safe, but not proved effective
eucalyptol	safe, but not proved effective
ferric acid	not safe and effective
menthol	safe, but not proved effective
methyl salicylate	not proved safe or effective
phenol	safe, but not proved effective
thymol	safe, but not proved effective
tincture of myrrh	not safe and effective

Mouthwash for Oral Hygiene: Product Ratings*

Product and Distributor	Dosage of Active Ingredients	Rating†	Comment
Cepacol (Marion Merrell Dow)	**mouthwash:** 0.05% cetylpyridinium chloride + 14% alcohol	B	not proved safe or effective
Chloraseptic (Richardson-Vicks)	**mouthwash, spray, gargle:** 1.4% phenol as phenol and sodium phenolate	B	not proved effective
Laryglan (Ayerst)	**spray:** 0.3% antipyrine + 0.05% pyrilamine maleate + 0.5% sodium caprylate	C	antipyrine not approved for this purpose
Listerine Antiseptic (Warner-Lambert)	**liquid:** 0.06% thymol + 0.09% eucalyptol + 0.06% methyl salicylate + 0.04% menthol + 26.9% alcohol	C	most ingredients not proved effective; methyl salicylate and alcohol not proved safe at these concentrations
Cool Mint Listerine (Warner-Lambert)	**liquid:** essentially the same ingredients as previous product, but with 21.6% alcohol	C	all 4 active ingredients are doubtfully effective, and methyl salicylate has not been proved safe; this is not an approved combination

| Scope (Procter & Gamble) | 0.45% cetylpyridinium xhloride + 0.005% domiphen bromide | C | neither ingredient proved safe and effective; combination is not approved |

*The FDA and Panel do not approve regular daily use of any mouthwash product that contains active medicinal ingredients.

†Author's interpretation of FDA criteria. Based on contents, not claims.

Nail-Biting and Thumb-Sucking Deterrents

Drugs used to discourage children from biting their fingernails or sucking their thumbs rely on a very basic principle: Make things taste bad enough, and people will not put them in their mouths!

This approach may work, according to the Panel that assessed these deterrent products. These bitter drugs are considered safe. But the reviewers say that the evidence that the one FDA-approved ingredient has value in breaking nail-biting and thumb-sucking habits remains inconclusive. They suggest caution in using preparations made with this substance.

A common parental error is to worry too much and too early about thumb-sucking. It is a natural act that may continue normally until about age 4 years. To forestall parental efforts to stop it prematurely, the reviewers stipulate that these drugs should *not* be used on children under age 4 years.

NAIL-BITING AND THUMB-SUCKING DETERRENTS is based on the report on nail-biting and thumb-sucking deterrent drug products by the FDA's Advisory Review Panel on OTC Miscellaneous External Drug Products and FDA's Tentative Final Monograph on these products.

Fingernails and Their Biters

Nail-biters are quite numerous. One study reported that 43 percent of children bite their nails, as do 25 percent of college students and 10 percent of other adults.

Hard-bitten nails, surprisingly, grow back faster than nails that are not bitten. The normal growth rate for fingernails is about 0.1 mm per day—which means 36 mm (just under 1 inch) per year. Nail-biters can expect almost 3 inches of annual growth.

The horny *keratin*, or hard material of the nail, is produced continuously by the *matrix*, which is the white, half-moon-shaped material visible at the base of the exposed part of the nail. It extends back under the skin.

Nail-biting goes by the technical name *onychophagia*. People who do it may nip and pull the ends off the nails until they are past the normal attachment point of nail and bed. The bed then may bulge upward where the nail should be. The sharp and rough edges left by biting can cause inflammation, and excessive biting can cause open wounds that are apt to become infected.

Why people bite their nails is not fully known. Biting is sometimes thought to express discontent, stress, or emotional maladjustment. In most cases, it is an unconscious habit that seems to provide oral gratification. The consequences nevertheless can be quite distressing not only to parents, grandparents, and friends but also to nail-biters themselves, who often try available nail-biting drug products in the hope of breaking the habit.

Less distasteful approaches may, however, be more effective. Reviewers cite one study of a behavioral modification method called The Habit Reversal procedure. First, children are reminded by their parents and therapist that they are biting their nails; then they are helped to understand why this is a bad habit; and finally they are offered alternative self-gratifying behavioral choices. In a study of 14 chronic nail-biters, all stopped biting their nails after a month of this treatment. Pediatricians, dentists, psychologists, and psychiatrists may be able to provide this kind of therapy.

In one recent study in chronic nail-biters, investigators at the National Institute of Mental Health, near Washington, D.C., found that the antidepressant drug clomipramine hydrochloride reduced or stopped nail-biting in about half of the patients who completed the 10-week clinical trial.

The drugs used to discourage nail-biting are the same ones used to deter thumb-sucking and will be described later in this unit.

Thumb-Suckers

Many children suck their thumbs: studies indicate that between 16 and 40 percent of kids of various ages do. Thumb-sucking is so natural that it starts before birth—as has been shown in X-rays of unborn babies. It usually stops at about 4 years of age. Why it continues longer in some children than others is not known, but the Panel said that professionals believe thumb-sucking in older children is an "empty or simple habit, a result of [previously] learned behavior," and does *not* signify that a child is emotionally disturbed.

Thumb-sucking may, however, be damaging—more so for the mouth that sucks than to the thumbs that are sucked. Sucking may delay or disrupt the eruption of a child's incisor teeth. It can distort the development of muscles in the lips, affecting a child's ability to swallow. The dental arch and palate of the mouth may become deformed, causing difficulties in breathing, chewing, and speaking.

Deterrent Drug

The active ingredient in drugs intended to keep fingers out of mouths tastes extremely bitter. It is meant to be painted onto the fingertips or nails. It is *not* to be swallowed. This ingredient has not been demonstrated to be effective. But if it should be approved, the claim that could be made for it is

- "For use as a nail-biting and thumb-sucking deterrent in persons aged 4 years and older"

APPROVED ACTIVE INGREDIENTS

None.

CONDITIONALLY APPROVED ACTIVE INGREDIENT

• *SUCROSE OCTAACETATE:* This ingredient is so bitter that wildlife biologists have tried to use it to keep nuisance species of wild birds from eating food crops. In one test to establish its safety, a researcher was unable to feed or force-feed animals enough of the chemical to kill them. When he did manage to get it into their stomachs, he could not detect toxic changes after dosing the animals with sucrose octaacetate for 90 days. Two other researchers believe that stomach irritation or vomiting would occur long before a dangerous dose could be ingested.

On the basis of such findings, evaluators concluded that sucrose octaacetate is safe. But they believe there is insufficient data from controlled scientific studies to adequately judge how well it works. In fact, the only study of this substance in humans that the Panel cited is one in which it is combined with another, now-banned bitter substance, denatonium benzoate. Verdict: safe but not proved effective.

DISAPPROVED ACTIVE INGREDIENTS

None.

Safety and Effectiveness: Active Ingredient in Over-the-Counter Nail-Biting and Thumb-Sucking Remedies

Active Ingredient	Assessment
sucrose octaacetate	safe, but not proved effective

Nail-Biting Deterrents: Product Ratings

Product and Distributor	Dosage of Active Ingredients	Rating*	Comment
Thum (Numark)	Liquid: cayenne pepper extract + citric acid	C	ingredients not submitted to or assessed for this use in over-the-counter drug review

No OTC retail product containing conditionally-approved sucrose octaacetate is listed in 1992 *Drug Topics Red Book*. Such a product may be available from local distributors.

*Author's interpretation of FDA criteria. Based on contents, not claims.

Pain, Fever, and Anti-Inflammatory Drugs Taken Internally

Pain is the most common problem for which people use medicines, and pain relief is the most common reason why people take nonprescription drugs. The pain relievers that are applied to the skin, and work externally, are described elsewhere in the book. (*See* ITCH AND PAIN REMEDIES APPLIED TO THE SKIN.) This Unit is concerned with pain relievers taken internally—usually by mouth.

Americans spend about $2.5 billion annually on over-the-counter pain-relievers, according to FDA and market researchers. This should relieve much pain, given that a safe and effective dose of aspirin—two 325 mg tablets—can be purchased in quantity for about two cents. (Gussied up into capsule-shaped tablets, the same dose can cost half a dollar when purchased a dose at a time.)

Many internal analgesic drugs also relieve fever; that is, they

PAIN, FEVER, AND ANTI-INFLAMMATORY DRUGS TAKEN INTERNALLY is based on the report of the FDA's Advisory Review Panel on OTC Internal Analgesic and Antirheumatic Drug Products; and on the FDA Tentative Final Monograph, Notice of Proposed Rulemaking on Internal Analgesic, Antipyretic, and Antirheumatic Drug Products for OTC Human Use.

have an *antipyretic* (antifever) effect. Many, too, soothe the inflammatory distress of arthritis and so are said to have an antirheumatic effect. All three symptoms—pain, fever, and inflammation—were treated together by the Panel because most safe and effective drugs in the group are advertised and used to relieve two or even all three symptoms. So, for convenience, drugs that provide these several benefits are referred to collectively as *pain-relievers*, or *analgesics*, or *analgesic-antipyretics*. They also may be called *pain-fever relievers*.

Drugs that thus far have been proved to be safe and effective for self-medication include aspirin and several chemically related salicylates, ibuprofen, and acetaminophen (although the latter is not effective against inflammation). Evaluations of effectiveness were based on published and unpublished studies that the Panel and the FDA believed to be scientifically valid. Criteria for judging safety included the incidence and risk of adverse reactions and significant side effects when the drug is used correctly, the potential for misuse or abuse when the drug is easily available without prescription, and the benefit-to-risk ratio.

More money is spent advertising internal analgesics than any other category of nonprescription drugs. Ad campaigns have attained high levels of sophistication, with advertisers' referring to wholly new—and medically unrecognized—ailments like "file-cabinet backache" and "camper-noise tension." The Panel said that more effective government regulation of such promotions, particularly on television commercials that are seen by children, is needed. But the FDA and other regulatory agencies have been quite permissive with regard to manufacturers' promotional activities in recent years.

 Claims

Accurate

• "For the temporary relief of minor aches and pains including those associated with the common cold, sore throat, headache, toothache, muscular aches, backache, premenstrual or menstrual periods (dysmenorrhea); for the minor pain from arthritis; and to reduce fever"

• For acetaminophen only, "for flu"

False or Misleading

• The product is especially effective against certain types of pain; for example, "postpartum pain," "pain due to cancer," "tooth extraction pain"

• Confusing terms like "jumpy nerves," "fretfulness," "night-time pain and its tension," and "under the weather"

• "Fast pain relief," "special pain-relieving formula," "so strong and so gentle," "so gentle can be taken on an empty stomach," "acts 5 times faster than aspirin," "reaches peak action 12 times faster than aspirin," "long-lasting pain reliever," "enhanced relief of pain"

• References to "depression" and "nervous tension" (over-the-counter pain relievers are clearly ineffective against them)

Pain

It is usually best to have a doctor determine the cause of pain. On the other hand, minor pain, of mild to moderate intensity, often can be successfully treated with over-the-counter drugs used at home. Minor pain is sometimes referred to as self-limited pain. That means it can be expected to go away by itself, without a doctor's diagnosis or treatment.

Persons who must work or maintain other normal daily activities while suffering a toothache, headache, or sore muscles may find over-the-counter analgesics particularly useful. The several active ingredients and many products that are safe and effective work predominantly by blocking the transmission of pain impulses to the brain.

These nonprescription drugs should not be taken to relieve pain for more than 10 days by adults or more than 5 days by children. And, if pain persists, you should see a doctor. These drugs should not be taken for more than 3 days to relieve fever except under a doctor's direction.

Common Cold

The use of pain-fever relievers for colds is described in COLD AND COUGH MEDICINES.

Headache

In the Panel's view, headache is in a class by itself because it is so common—almost everyone suffers from one from time to time—and also because nonprescription analgesics are widely used and vigorously promoted to treat it. While self-medication most often is both appropriate and successful, experts caution that headaches vary greatly in intensity, feeling, persistence, and cause—as well as in the part of the head where the pain is felt. So in some instances prescription medication or medical supervision is needed, as outlined in the following paragraphs.

Vascular Headache

This pain usually occurs when blood vessels inside the brain and adjacent areas dilate or distend, so that their walls do not adapt well to blood-pressure changes. As a result, pressure variations are more keenly felt by sensory receptors in the blood-vessel walls. These sensations are experienced as pain.

One common vascular headache, hypertensive headache, is caused by a sudden rise in blood pressure. It is a dull, generalized pain, usually in the forehead, that characteristically is worse in the morning, then lessens as the day progresses.

Migraine headache, a recurrent, throbbing headache often on one side of the head, is another common form of vascular headache. Millions of people are afflicted by migraine.

Headache experts say that *neither hypertensive nor migraine headache should be treated with nonprescription analgesics. Both require medical diagnosis and, usually, prescription drugs.* However, the same experts note that headaches from fever, hangover, and caffeine withdrawal—all of which involve the vascular system—can be successfully treated with nonprescription drugs.

Tension Headache

This is an extremely common plight that accounts for up to 9 out of 10 headache complaints for which sufferers see doctors. Causes include apprehension, anxiety, depression, and other emotional states. Job, social, or marital stress can also induce these headaches. Tension headaches are more common after 30 years of age. The pain usually is diffuse and difficult to describe; it is rarely confined to one side of the head. Some people experience these emotionally induced headaches as "pressure" rather than pain; this sensation may be accompanied by persistent contractions of the head, neck, and facial muscles.

There has been considerable difference of opinion as to whether these headaches can be treated successfully with nonprescription drugs.

The Panel felt they could not. But recent studies have shown that the pain of occasional and non-persisting tension headaches can be treated successfully with aspirin, acetaminophen, ibuprofen, and similar over-the-counter drugs. The National Headache Foundation, in Chicago, endorses this view. But, as the FDA stresses, these drugs do not relieve the underlying anxiety or tension.

Traction and Inflammatory Headaches

These headaches, much rarer than vascular headache and tension headache, are caused by organic disease. For example, inflammation of the sinuses (sinusitis, or allergic rhinitis) may cause a deep, dull, non-pulsating pain in the front of the head. But the pain of sinusitis can be relieved temporarily by over-the-counter pain relievers. Traction headaches may also result from pressure from brain tumors or from inflammation of the membranes surrounding the brain. Clearly, medical care is required for these headaches.

Menstrual and Premenstrual Cramps

The use of pain and fever relievers for menstrual and premenstrual pain (dysmenorrhea) is described in MENSTRUAL DISTRESS PREPARATIONS.)

Muscular Aches

This pain may be treated with either internal pain-fever relievers taken by mouth or with preparations applied externally to the skin. (*See* LINIMENTS AND POULTICES FOR ACHES AND PAINS.)

Sore Throat

The use of pain-fever relievers to calm sore-throat pain is described in MEDICAMENTS FOR SORE GUMS, MOUTH, AND THROAT.

Fever

Normal body temperature is about 98.6° F (37° C). There is a slight variation in baseline temperatures between individuals, and most people's temperature rises and falls slightly throughout the day. Fever is defined medically as temperature above 98.6° F.

The body's balance between heat production and heat loss is controlled by the hypothalamic nuclei, tiny areas in the brain stem. In fever, this "thermostat" is set too high. Fever-lowering drugs, it is believed, act to reset this regulator so that the temperature falls back toward normal. The hypothalamus accomplishes this by increasing blood flow to vessels near the body surface and by inducing sweating, both of which serve to carry off heat.

Fever is a signal that something is wrong in the body. Current medical practice focuses on finding and treating what has caused the rise in temperature; treating the fever itself is of secondary importance. Antibiotics can be used, with good result, to treat many infections that cause fever. In general, fever is a less common and less persistent problem than it once was. Many pain relievers—such as acetaminophen, aspirin, and ibuprofen—do relieve fever, and they can be safely used for this purpose. Since high or persistent fever may indicate a serious illness, call or see a doctor whenever an individual's temperature goes above 103° F (39.5° C) or if fever persists for more than 3 days (72 hours).

'Normal' Temperature Is Not Quite Exact

The number 98.6° F—"normal" human body temperature—should not be cast in stone. This mixed number on the fahrenheit scale is equal to a whole number—37°—on the centigrade scale.

These "normal" values are obtained by taking many peoples' temperatures and averaging them. The range, however, is quite wide. Physiologist Andrew Ivy, M.D., recorded the oral temperature of 276 medical students seated in classes between 8 A.M. and 9 A.M. A few temperatures were under 97° F; a few were over 99° F. The average in this group was 98.1° F.

In addition, if the students had taken their temperatures through a different orifice, the results would have been different—and higher: A person's *rectal* temperature, other experts have shown, is almost 1° F higher, on average, than the same person's *oral* temperature taken at the same time.

Arthritis

A major use of aspirin and other nonprescription analgesics is to combat the pain and inflammation of red, swollen, sore joints that are the hallmark of osteoarthritis, rheumatoid arthritis, gout, and other rheumatic disorders. Between 20 and 50 million Americans are estimated to suffer from these conditions, which together are called *arthritis*. Arthritis usually comes on with age, so that most people will have some arthritic aches and pains by the time they are 65. Yet some forms of arthritis strike very young children; so no age group is exempt.

Aspirin and related drugs, called *salicylates*, and the drug *ibuprofen* are effective ingredients for relieving this distress; acetaminophen is not. The exact way in which salicylates relieve arthritic tenderness and swelling is still not known, even though these medications have been widely used for this purpose for many decades. One current theory is that aspirin and similar drugs inhibit the body's production of substances called *prostaglandins*, which are believed to contribute to the inflammatory process.

Despite the wide use of salicylates to relieve rheumatic symptoms and related muscular discomfort, the Panel urged the FDA not to let nonprescription drugs be labeled for this purpose. It recommended that claims such as "for temporary relief of minor arthritic and rheumatic aches and pains" be forbidden because salicylates act on 2 levels, depending on dosage. Lower doses—up to 4000 mg (4 grams) of aspirin daily—can be taken safely as self-medication for temporary relief of pain, and perhaps with some limited effect on the inflammation and underlying symptoms. But the larger doses—5300 mg (5.3 grams) daily—that actually appear to stop the underlying disease process may be toxic for some people. So these amounts should be taken only on prescription and under close medical supervision. Ibuprofen, by the same token, is safe and effective at low doses approved for self-medication, of up to 1200 mg daily, for relieving arthritic pain. The higher doses, up to 3200 mg daily, that are effective in relieving inflammation *should be taken only at a doctor's direction*.

Reviewers also saw danger in self-medication at the safer, lower dosage level that may relieve the immediate pain but allow the underlying disease to smolder on. To protect people from this risk, the FDA has added, and consumers should heed, this warning:

WARNING:

 If new symptoms occur, or if redness or swelling—which often occur in arthritis—is present, then you should consult a doctor, since these could be signs of a serious condition.

Dosage

Aspirin is the most widely used and widely studied of the effective over-the-counter pain relievers, so it is used as the baseline for dosage recommendations that also apply to sodium salicylate and to acetaminophen. The Panel believes they are roughly equivalent in potency. Acetaminophen has somewhat different side effects than the salicylates, and it is not effective against inflammation and some other arthritic symptoms. It also has been used and studied far less than aspirin; so until there are more data, dosages for acetaminophen should not exceed those for aspirin.

The most commonly used dosage unit for these drugs—that is, the amount contained in many, perhaps most tablets, pills, or other dosage forms is 325 mg. This amount, 325 mg, is also considered the minimum effective dose. The comparable dose of ibuprofen is 200 mg.

Equivalent Dosage

Dosage for over-the-counter pain relievers is sometimes given in *grains* (an apothecary measure) instead of in *milligrams* or *grams*, which are part of the now-preferred metric system. A 325-mg tablet contains 5 grains. Here are some common equivalences:

    1 grain = 65 mg

    1.25 grains = 80 or 81 mg (child's usual dosage unit)

    5 grains = 325 mg (adult's usual dosage unit)

    10 grains = 650 mg (adult's usual dosage)

    61.54 grains = 4000 mg (maximum 24 hours' dosage of aspirin and acetaminophen for adults)

Of the other approved over-the-counter pain relievers, magnesium salicylate, while less well-studied than aspirin, is believed to be a little less potent in the form that is currently marketed in some products. Thus its minimum effective dose is 377 mg. The other two approved salicylates are weaker. The minimum effective dose of carbaspirin calcium is 414 mg; that of choline salicylate is 435 mg. The approved dose of ibuprofen is 200 mg, or 400 mg if necessary.

These drugs all would be far safer and easier to use if they were sold only in a standard 325-mg dosage unit (or the equivalent for the weaker ones), as the Panel recommended. But at present products are sold in dosage units that may deliver as little as 452 mg of aspirin in two tablets. This amount is less than the 650 mg dose usually recommended for an adult.

The Panel wished to create *standard dosage units*—fixed amounts for tablets, pills, and so on—and ban all others. For aspirin and acetaminophen, for example, the standard dosage unit would have been 325 mg, which is the minimal effective dose. Two tablets, 650 mg, would always be the standard and usual dose. This regulatory step, the Panel said, would help ensure that users obtained effective doses of medication if they took one or two tablets. It also would prevent manufacturers from confusing consumers with ads saying things like "higher levels of pain reliever," which means that the product contains a little more aspirin or acetaminophen than some other product.

To the detriment of the consumer, the FDA disagrees with the Panel's scheme. The FDA plans not to establish "standard" dosage units but to stipulate only the approved doses—the amount of the drug in however many tablets or other dosage units—that should be taken. The Panel's plan would serve consumers better, so in the Product Table for these drugs, a plus sign—"+"—has been added to the ratings for products that meet both the FDA's requirements and the Panel's recommendation for standard dosage units.

Dosage for Adults

Two tablets every 4 hours is the most common dosage recommendation for nonprescription pain relievers for adults. This is the correct dosage for aspirin, sodium salicylate, and acetaminophen, provided that tablets or other dosage units each contain 325 mg (5 grains) of one of the active ingredients. Translated into total quantities, this dosage means 650 mg (10 grains) of an active ingredient every 4 hours. For ibuprofen, the recommended dose is 200 or 400 mg, which is 1 or 2 tablets of 200 mg each every 4 to 6 hours.

An initial dose of 975 mg of aspirin, sodium salicylate, or acetaminophen—or 3 tablets—provides increased benefit for some people, the Panel said. But only one such dose is safe; a repeat could cause bad reactions such as (with aspirin) ringing in the ears. The FDA does not approve of this stronger initial, or *loading dose*, in part because it is too difficult to describe on small-print product labels.

Just as there is a recommended adult dose for these drugs, so there also is a maximum daily amount—except for arthritics under a doctor's supervision.

No one should take over 4000 mg of aspirin, sodium salicylate, or acetaminophen (or their equivalents in other nonprescription pain relievers) in 24 hours. This limit comes to about 167 mg per hour. What this means is that no more than 12 of the 325-mg tablets or caplets of acetaminophen, aspirin, or sodium salicylate should be taken during a 24-hour period. The limit for ibuprofen is 6 tablets, or 1200 mg in 24 hours.

Beyond these limits, there is a dramatic, rapidly rising risk of toxic side effects, with little if any added pain relief.

Dosage for Children

The standard dosage unit for children is 80 or 81 mg (about 1.23 grains) of aspirin or acetaminophen. Children under age 2 years should not be medicated with these drugs except when recommended by a doctor, who should determine the dose. For older children, the dose rises with age from 160 mg (2 tablets) for 2- to 4-year-olds, up to 480 mg (6 tablets) for 11- to 12-year-olds. Older children can use adult doses in the recommended schedule of one dose every 4 hours.

There is no FDA-approved dosage of ibuprofen for children under 12.

APPROVED PAIN-RELIEVING ACTIVE INGREDIENTS

Seven drugs are approved as active ingredients for nonprescription pain relievers: acetaminophen, aspirin, calcium carbaspirin, choline salicylate, ibuprofen, magnesium salicylate, and sodium salicylate. They are safe and effective for allaying mild to moderate pain.

Acetaminophen

Acetaminophen is a safe, effective over-the-counter pain reliever when taken in the recommended dosage of 325 to 650 mg every 4 hours with limits of 4000 mg per 24-hour period and use of no longer than 3 days

Recommended Adult Dosage Schedule for Aspirin, Acetaminophen, and Sodium Salicylate

Dose*	Interval	24-hour Maximum Dosage
325 to 650 mg	every 4 hr	4000 mg (4 gm)
325 to 500 mg	every 3 hr	4000 mg (4 gm)
650 to 1000 mg (1 gram)	every 6 hr	4000 mg (4 gm)

Recommended Adult Dosage Schedule for Ibuprofen

Dose	Interval	24-hour Maximum Dosage
200 to 400 mg	every 4 to 6 hr	1200 mg (1.2 gm)

* A dose may be tablet, caplet, packet of powder, or measure of liquid containing the same amount of the drug.

Recommended Children's Dosage Schedule for Aspirin or Acetaminophen

Age in Years	Dose and Frequency Standard Dosage: 80 or 81 mg*	Equivalent Dose in 325-mg (adult) tablets	24-hour Maximum Dosage
Under 2	No recommended dosage except with advice and supervision of doctor		
2 to under 4	2 tablets every 4 hr (or a total of 160 mg)	1½ (162 mg)	800 mg
4 to under 6	3 tablets every 4 hr (or a total of 240 mg)	(244 mg)	1200 mg
6 to under 9	4 tablets every 4 hr (or a total of 320 mg)	1 (325 mg)	1600 mg
9 to under 11	4 to 5 tablets every 4 hr (or a total of 320 to 400 mg)	1 to 1¼ (325 to 406 mg)	2000 mg
11 to under 12	4 to 6 tablets every 4 hr (or a total of 320 to 480 mg)	1 to 1¼ (325 to 487 mg)	2400 mg
Over 12	See Recommended Adult Dosage Schedule, p. 769		

* Dosage units are listed here as tablets but may be chewable tablets, syrups, or other products containing the same amount of drug. If children-strength products are unavailable, the second column can be used to reckon appropriate amounts of 325-mg aspirin or acetaminophen tablets. Examples: for a 2-year-old, 160 mg recommended dosage is one-half of a 325-mg adult aspirin tablet; for an 11-year-old, 480 mg is one-and-a-half adult tablets.

for fever or 10 days for pain. (If fever or pain lasts longer, seek a doctor's help.) It is also available in suppositories in strengths of 120 mg to 650 mg.

Acetaminophen is safe and effective for relieving flu symptoms and fever and pain for chicken pox and measles in children. Aspirin and other salicylates are not safe for this use.

Acetaminophen was introduced before aspirin, in 1893. Milligram for milligram, it has been shown to be about as effective as aspirin—except against inflammatory conditions like arthritis, for which it is not effective.

Numerous clinical studies have shown that in recommended doses, the drug is relatively free of adverse effects in most age groups—even in persons suffering a variety of illnesses. Unlike aspirin, for example, it does not cause gastrointestinal bleeding and it does not interfere with drugs used to treat gout. However, it may minimally affect blood-clotting, and some people are allergic to it (and so should not use it).

Some advertisements claim that acetaminophen is safer and less toxic than aspirin. Actually, the drug is metabolized by the liver, and overdoses can cause severe liver damage, even death. Alcoholics and other persons whose livers are damaged or diseased may be more vulnerable to acetaminophen toxicity—even at lower doses—than normal people with healthy livers. In case of overdosage, seek medical care *at once*, even if you are not feeling ill or upset.

 Claims for Acetaminophen

Accurate

- "For the temporary relief of minor aches and pains associated with the common cold, flu, sore throat, headache, toothache, muscular aches, backache, premenstrual or menstrual periods (dysmenorrhea); for the minor pain from arthritis; and to reduce fever"

False or Misleading

- For "nervous tension headache," "simple exertion," "simple pain of teething," "simple pain of immunization," "simple pain of tonsillectomy," "fretfulness," "pain of neuralgia," "pain of neuritis," "pain following dental procedures," "overexertion," "bursitis," "sprains"

Aspirin

When taken in the recommended dosage of 325 to 650 mg every 4 hours, aspirin is a safe and effective nonprescription pain reliever. Self-medication with aspirin should not go beyond 10 days for pain or 3 days for fever (after which you should consult a doctor if the symptoms persist), nor should you take more than 4000 mg in a 24-hour period.

Aspirin's technical name is acetylsalicylic acid; it is one of a group of compounds that are called salicylates. Aspirin is the active medicinal ingredient in birch bark, and in other traditional plant remedies that long have been used by people around the globe. It is a very powerful drug for which important new uses continue to be found. (*See* p. 790).

Aspirin is effective against mild to moderate pain that is localized or widespread, including some cancer pain. But it is not effective against severe pain. The lowest effective dose of aspirin is a little over 300 mg; increments of around 200 to 300 mg—up to somewhat over 900 mg—produce noticeable increases in pain relief. But different people respond differently to any pain reliever, so a dose of aspirin that quells one person's pain may not help another's. Interestingly, two standard aspirin tablets (a total of 650 mg) have been found to be more effective that the standard (60 mg) dose of the narcotic pain killer codeine in calming the pain of some types of advanced cancer.

Because aspirin has been widely used for such a long time, and has produced comparatively few side effects, its safety has been well established for the majority of people; the risk-benefit ratio is low. But aspirin can have adverse effects:

- Effects on Blood: Aspirin interferes with blood-clotting (coagulation). So persons who have blood-coagulation defects, who are receiving anticoagulant drugs, or who suffer severe anemia should avoid it. Constant use may also cause persistent iron-deficiency anemia.

- Effects on gastrointestinal tract: Aspirin can trigger or aggravate peptic ulcer and may cause stomach upset or heartburn. It can cause imperceptible bleeding from the stomach lining, and in some individuals can trigger massive bleeding into the stomach.

- Allergic effects: Aspirin produces allergic reactions in an estimated 2 persons per 1000 who are hypersensitive to the drug, and, more commonly, in some asthma sufferers. These reactions range from rash, hives, and swelling to asthmatic attacks that may be life-threatening.

• Effects in pregnancy: Aspirin interferes with blood-clotting in both mother and fetus; it can lengthen pregnancy and the process of delivery. It produces birth defects in animals and increases the incidences of stillbirths and of deaths of newborn babies. It should not be taken in the last 3 months of pregnancy except under the advice and supervision of a physician.

• Effects on central nervous system: Aspirin overdose may stimulate the brain and spinal cord, producing ringing in the ears—a warning sign. Subsequently there is a depression in central nervous system functioning that may appear as respiratory failure, circulatory collapse, coma, and then death.

• Effect on kidneys: In rare instances, aspirin can make a severe existing kidney disorder worse. If you have a kidney problem, do not take aspirin except under a doctor's direction.

• Effects of taking aspirin with other drugs: Aspirin interferes with the action of some anticlotting and antidiabetic drugs, as well as some drugs used to treat gout. It may also enhance the ulcer-producing risk of medications taken for arthritis.

Ringing in the ears (*tinnitus*) is the most common and reliable sign that you are taking too much aspirin or too much of another salicylate. Hearing loss is also a fairly common early warning sign. If either occurs, the drug must be discontinued or the dose drastically reduced. These symptoms will vanish—hearing will return to normal—within hours to days, and at most a month after the medication is stopped.

Other early signs of aspirin toxicity include headache, dizziness, vomiting, rapid breathing, extreme irritability, and even bizarre behavior. The danger signs of aspirin toxicity in children may be different from those in adults. For example, nausea or rapid breathing may occur before ringing in the ears.

As noted in the list of adverse reactions, above, aspirin interferes with the blood's ability to clot. Therefore, persons who are scheduled for surgery or dental work should tell their doctors ahead of time if they are taking aspirin.

Never use aspirin to treat youngsters who have chicken pox, flu, or late-winter flu-like symptoms. The danger is this: a very high percentage of children who suffer or who die from a rare liver disorder called Reye's syndrome turn out to have been treated with aspirin to relieve chicken pox or flu symptoms. How aspirin enhances their risk is not known. Treatment with acetaminophen appears not to carry this risk.

 Claims for Aspirin

Accurate

- For "the temporary relief of minor aches and pains associated with the common cold, sore throat, headache, toothache, muscular aches, backache, premenstrual or menstrual periods (dysmenorrhea); for the minor pain from arthritis; and to reduce fever

False or Misleading

- For "comforting relief of aches," "pains caused by: colds and flu, inoculations, minor ailments, tonsillectomy," "pains caused by teething," "under the weather," "pains of neuralgia," "pains of neuritis," "pains of mild migraine," "pains of minor injuries," "pains of sciatica," "swollen tissues," "jumpy nerves," "sleeplessness caused by minor painful distress," "the blues," "nervous tension headache," "feeling of depression," "muscular fatigue," "muscle tension," "low back pain," "bursitis," "lumbago," "low body ache due to fatigue," "body aches"

Aspirin, far more than any other approved pain reliever, has been formulated into a wide variety of special products intended to enhance its effectiveness, safety, and appeal. Some of these formulations— chewable aspirin for children and buffered aspirin, to name just two— make the medication easier to take for persons who tolerate ordinary aspirin tablets poorly.

Forms of Aspirin

- *BUFFERED ASPIRIN:* Buffering agents, principally antacid compounds—are alkaline, as opposed to acidic. Aspirin is an acid, and the stomach is naturally acidic. When the stomach contents are neutralized, briefly, by the alkaline buffering, the aspirin supposedly can dissolve and will be absorbed into the bloodstream more rapidly, which supposedly speeds up pain relief. The buffering also is intended to relieve gastric irritation by the aspirin.

There is more alkaline in highly buffered effervescent powders, which must be mixed with water before being swallowed, than in the buffered tablets. Both kinds of preparations—which usually are identified as "buffered" in the product name or on the label—may speed up the absorption of aspirin from the stomach. Also, some highly buffered aspirins have been shown to significantly decrease mild, unnoticed bleeding in the stomach. Because they facilitate absorption, highly buffered preparations are an ideal way to take aspirin. There is, however, little scientifically meaningful difference in the absorption rates between many buffered and nonbuffered aspirin products. Moreover, few if any data exist satisfactorily demonstrating that buffered aspirin provides pain relief with a more rapid onset, a greater peak intensity, or prolonged duration.

Buffered and highly buffered aspirins may diminish the stomach distress that a relatively small number of people experience when they take aspirin. But they do not necessarily reduce the rare-but-real risk of massive gastrointestinal bleeding, so they cannot be considered safer in that regard. Some buffering ingredients are more effective than others, and some poorly formulated preparations may dissolve no more rapidly than ordinary aspirin. Also, some unbuffered calcium salts of aspirin dissolve more rapidly than buffered aspirin.

 ### Claims for Buffered Aspirin

Accurate
- "Contains buffering ingredients"

Unproved
- "Faster to the bloodstream than plain aspirin," "provides ingredients that may prevent the stomach distress that plain aspirin causes…"

- *CHEWABLE ASPIRIN TABLETS:* Flavored, chewable tablets are convenient for children or for grown-ups who cannot or will not swallow whole tablets; they are an acceptable way to formulate aspirin. Children should be told to drink water after they take chewable aspirin.

• *FILM-COATED TABLETS:* At least one major manufacturer (Glenbrook) coats aspirin tablets with a thin, smooth, transparent film that briefly retards dissolution. This facilitates swallowing and shields users from aspirin's bitter taste.

• *DELAYED-RELEASE TABLETS AND CAPLETS:* Aspirin tablets can be given special coatings to keep them from dissolving in the stomach, as a way to prevent gastric irritation and possible bleeding. The aim is to delay dissolution of the tablets until they leave the stomach, and so are absorbed from the small intestine instead. But there are problems: The tablets may take several hours to reach the intestine, so that pain relief may be delayed, and some tablets may fail to dissolve at all. For these reasons, these products were given only conditional approval by the Panel. Based on a manufacturer's data, the FDA now has approved *8-Hour Bayer Timed-Release Caplets* (Glenbrook) as safe and effective.

• *MICRONIZED ASPIRIN:* There is no convincing scientific evidence that formulating aspirin in tinier-than-ordinary particles improves it in any way, the Panel said.

• *ASPIRIN POWDERS:* While not commonly used, aspirin powders may be absorbed and reach effective blood levels faster than tablets. They may be easier to give to children than tablets or capsules are, once the powder is dissolved in a full glass of sweetened fruit juice or water.

 Claims for Aspirin Powders

Unproved
• "faster to the bloodstream than plain aspirin"

• *CHEWING-GUM ASPIRIN:* Aspirin in a gum base is safe and effective. It should not be used for a week after oral surgery or tonsillectomy, as it may reopen the surgical wounds.

• *RECTAL SUPPOSITORIES:* Aspirin-impregnated rectal suppositories are a good way of giving the drug to people who are vomiting, unconscious, or otherwise unable to take it by mouth. But absorption is slow and the suppositories can slip out—thus the value of rectal suppositories as nonprescription medications remains to be proved outside of use in these special circumstances. These products are much more expensive than most aspirin tablets.

Carbaspirin Calcium

This nonprescription pain reliever is safe and effective nonprescription pain reliever when you take the recommended dosage of 414 to 828 mg every 4 hours, 414 to 637 mg every 3 hours, or 828 to 1274 mg every 6 hours. You should take no more than 4970 mg during 24 hours and use it for no longer than 3 days for fever or 10 days for pain. (After that length of time, see a doctor if the fever or pain persists.)

Carbaspirin calcium is often called soluble calcium aspirin. It is similar to ordinary aspirin, but it contains calcium and urea (which aspirin does not). It is only four-fifths as strong on a milligram-for-milligram basis, so more must be taken to get the same result.

The usual dosage unit of calcium carbaspirin is 414 mg (roughly one and a quarter times the 325-mg usual dose for aspirin), so the usual adult dose is 828 mg. (For children, multiply the dosages in the Recommended Children's Dosage Schedule on page 770 by 1.24 to obtain the right equivalences.)

Carbaspirin calcium dissolves in the stomach more rapidly than ordinary aspirin, but one team of researchers found that it offers no significant advantage over aspirin in the rate at which it gives relief from pain. It may produce slightly less gastrointestinal bleeding than aspirin, but this has not been scientifically demonstrated. Beyond the possibility that carbaspirin calcium might be slightly less irritating to the stomach and intestines, the drug's effectiveness and safety are quite like aspirin's—given the difference in dosage requirements.

 Claims for Carbaspirin Calcium

Accurate
• For "the temporary relief of minor aches and pains associated with the common cold, sore throat, headache, toothache, muscular aches, backache, premenstrual or menstrual periods (dysmenorrhea); for the minor pain from arthritis; and to reduce fever

Unproved
• "Faster to the bloodstream than plain aspirin," "provides

ingredients that may prevent the stomach distress plain aspirin occasionally causes..." (for buffered carbaspirin)

Choline Salicylate

Choline salicylate is a safe and effective nonprescription product for relief of pain as long as it is taken as recommended: 435 to 870 mg every 4 hours, or 435 to 669 mg every 3 hours, or 870 to 1338 mg every 6 hours while symptoms persist. Take no more than 5220 mg in a 24-hour period. If fever persists after 3 days, or pain persists after 10 days, seek medical care.

Medicinally, choline salicylate is similar to aspirin. But unlike aspirin it is highly soluble. Because of this, it may be sold and stored as a stable, palatable liquid. One of its particular advantages is that it is the only aspirin-like drug available over-the-counter in liquid form. This can be an advantage when a child, or an older person who has trouble swallowing tablets needs to take aspirin.

Choline salicylate is absorbed from the stomach rapidly, which may forestall the stomachaches and cramps that sometimes follow ingestion of ordinary aspirin. But there is no evidence that this faster absorption brings quicker relief of pain; one investigator noted that even if this were so, it would be absurd to claim advantages for any compound that may hasten relief by no more than a few minutes.

Milligram for milligram, choline salicylate is weaker than aspirin, so that a larger dose is needed to produce the equivalent pain relief. The standard dosage unit of the drug, 435 mg, is 1.3 times greater than the standard dosage of aspirin. The choline salicylate standard dosage for adults is 870 mg (the equivalent of 650 mg of aspirin) every 4 hours. For children, multiply by 1.3 the aspirin doses in the Recommended Children's Dosage Schedule on p. 770.

Choline salicylate is less well studied than aspirin, but the comparisons that have been made suggest that its actions and risks appear comparable to those of aspirin.

 Claims for Choline Salicylate

Accurate

For "the temporary relief of minor arches and pains, associated with the common cold, sore throat, headache, toothache, muscular aches, backache, premenstrual or menstrual periods (dysmenorrhea); for the minor pain from arthritis; and to reduce fever

False or Misleading
"Five times faster than aspirin," "reaches peak action 12 times faster than aspirin," "does not cause the gastrointestinal bleeding associated with . . . aspirin . . ."

Unproved
"Faster to the bloodstream than plain aspirin," "causes less gastric irritation"

Ibuprofen

This is a safe and effective pain-reducer and fever-reliever for adults when used in the recommended dosage of 200 to 400 mg every 4 to 6 hours but no more than 1200 mg (1.2 grams) in 24 hours. Do not use longer than 3 days for fever, or 10 days for pain without consulting a doctor. Ibuprofen is not approved for use as a nonprescription drug for children under 12 years of age.

This is the first new safe and effective pain-reliever to become available to consumers without a prescription in half a century. It is a synthetic compound, of the class called *nonsteroidal anti-inflammatory drugs* (NSAIDs).

Ibuprofen was not assessed in the OTC Review. Rather, it was a prescription product that was switched to OTC status, at low dosages, on the basis of manufacturers' petitions. The prescription to over-the-counter switch became effective in 1984.

Ibuprofen is stronger than aspirin or acetaminophen, so the usual nonprescription doses—either 200 mg or 400 mg every 4 to 6 hours—are lower than comparable doses of these other fever-reducing, pain-relieving over-the-counter compounds. The conservative *Medical Letter on Drugs and Therapeutics* (7/6/84) said, at the time ibuprofen was approved for nonprescription sales: "For treatment of mild to moderate pain, 200 mg ibuprofen appears to be at least as effective as 650 mg of aspirin, and 400 mg of ibuprofen appears to be more effective."

Ibuprofen is effective against fever as well as pain and is considered by drug analysts at the American Medical Association (*Drug Evaluations* 1991) to be particularly effective against menstrual cramps and other forms of menstrual distress (*see* MENSTRUAL DISTRESS PREPARATIONS), and also particularly effective against the minor pains of arthritis. (At far-higher prescription (℞) dosages, ibuprofen is a safe, effective and well-regarded drug for treating the inflammation that characterizes arthritis and other inflammatory disorders.)

Side effects are uncommon, and the AMA and other medical authorities say they are less severe than with aspirin. However, there have been some reports of persons who have mild and chronic kidney failure—which they may not even be aware of—suffering acute kidney failure after taking ibuprofen at approved OTC dosages for brief periods of time. So, while almost a decade has passed since ibuprofen was approved for OTC sales and self-treatment of aches, pains, and fever, the last word has not been written on the risks of this usage.

Generally speaking, however, the consensus is that ibuprofen is safe, probably safer than aspirin.

People who are intolerant of aspirin may have similar problems with ibuprofen, since they are somewhat similar, chemically. Ibuprofen side effects include nausea, vomiting, diarrhea, constipation and upset stomach. Taking ibuprofen with a glass of milk can reduce these gastrointestinal side effects.

 Claim for Ibuprofen

Accurate
- "For the temporary relief of minor aches and pains associated with the common cold, headache, toothache, muscular aches, backache, for the minor pain of arthritis, for the pain of menstrual cramps, and for the reduction of fever."

WARNINGS:

 Do not take for pain for more than 10 days or fever for more than 3 days, unless directed by a doctor. If pain or fever persists or gets worse, or if the painful area is red or swollen, consult a doctor.

If you are under a doctor's care for any serious condition, consult a doctor before taking ibuprofen.

If you experience any symptoms which are unusual or seem unrelated to the condition for which you took ibuprofen, consult a doctor before taking any more of it.

It is especially important not to use ibuprofen during the last 3 months of pregnancy unless specifically directed to do so by a doctor because it may cause problems in the unborn child or complications during delivery.

Magnesium Salicylate

This magnesium-aspirin compound is a safe and effective nonprescription analgesic when taken as recommended. It is slightly less potent than aspirin, and the approved dosages are: 377 to 754 mg every 4 hours, or 377 to 580 mg every 3 hours, or 754 mg every 6 hours, not to exceed 4640 mg in 24 hours. It should be used no longer than 3 days for fever or 10 days for pain without consulting a doctor. (Note: different chemical forms of magnesium salicylate have somewhat different strengths. Currently marketed products appear to be based on the more potent of these forms, for which 325 mg of magnesium salicylate is equal to 325 mg of aspirin; they are sold in 325-mg tablets.)

Magnesium salicylate has been studied far less extensively than ordinary aspirin, but it seems essentially equivalent. Claims that it may be the drug to use when aspirin is not tolerated in the stomach remain to be proved. It may not cause asthmatic attacks in susceptible persons, which can happen with aspirin and some other salicylates. Thus, this compound may be particularly useful for the few asthmatic individuals who are sensitive to aspirin. In general, the warnings that apply to aspirin apply to this compound as well.

 Claims for Magnesium Salicylate

Accurate
- For "the temporary relief of minor aches and pains including those associated with the common cold, sore throat, headache, toothache, muscular aches, backache, premenstrual or menstrual periods (dysmenorrhea); for the minor pain from arthritis; and to reduce fever"

False or Misleading
- For "pains of sciatica," "overexertion," "fatigue," "aches and pains due to fatigue"

Unproved
- "Has less potential for gastrointestinal bleeding than aspirin"

Sodium Salicylate

When used in the recommended dosage—325 to 650 mg every 4 hours, or 325 to 500 mg every 3 hours, or 650 to 1000 mg every 6 hours—this drug is safe and effective. Use no more than 4000 mg in a 24-hour period, and use it for no longer than 3 days for fever or 10 days for pain without a doctor's consultation. One pharmacology source, *drug facts and comparisons*, says sodium salicylate is less effective than aspirin.

Originally, aspirin was introduced to the market because it was believed to be more palatable and cause less stomach distress than sodium salicylate. But the two ingredients are essentially similar in these and all other matters of safety, save that sodium salicylate appears not to provoke asthmatic attacks in susceptible persons, as ordinary aspirin does. However, if you are on sodium-restricted diets because of high blood pressure or other disorders, use other over-the-counter pain relievers that do not contain sodium.

 Claims for Sodium Salicylate

Accurate
- For "the temporary relief of occasional aches and pains, including those associated with the common cold, sore throat, headache, toothache, muscular aches, backache, premenstrual or menstrual periods (dysmenorrhea); for the minor pain from arthritis; and to reduce fever"

CONDITIONALLY APPROVED PAIN-RELIEVING ACTIVE INGREDIENTS

There are several pain-relieving nonprescription drugs for which there still is too little evidence for evaluators to decide if they are safe and effective.

• *ALUMINUM ASPIRIN:* This salicylate, very similar to ordinary aspirin, is safe. But it may not be wholly effective in the dosage reviewed by the Panel of 365 to 730 mg every 4 hours. No more than 4380 mg should be taken in a 24-hour period; if fever continues beyond 3 days, or if pain continues beyond 10 days, consult a doctor.

     The problem with aluminum aspirin is that it dissolves very slowly in the stomach, and may be absorbed far less rapidly than ordinary aspirin. There are some indications in unpublished reports that this slow dissolution and absorption may prolong the pain relief it provides. However, this claim remains to be proved.

• *ANTIPYRINE:* While widely used in Europe, antipyrine has seen limited use in the United States. It is in a wholly different class of drugs from aspirin and acetaminophen. In terms of safety, it is said not to interfere with blood-clotting, as aspirin does, nor is it believed to damage the liver—even when taken in large doses—as acetaminophen can do. But more studies are needed to confirm these tentative findings. The major block to full approval is that a small number of persons, apparently many of them black Americans, are highly allergic to antipyrine. Before 1950, 394 poisoning cases and 23 deaths were reported; since 1950 there have been no reported fatalities. Severe skin eruptions are one of the principal allergic reactions; anyone who notices a rash while taking antipyrine should stop using the drug and see a doctor.

     Antipyrine has a long-lasting effect against pain: a single dose of 975 mg provides relief for 24 hours. So the majority of Panel members believed it should be carefully studied, as it has not yet been, to see if antipyrine can be recommended for persons who cannot tolerate other analgesics. However, a minority of the evaluators—in an unusual division of opinion—felt that the drug's side effects can be so severe in the small percentage of people who appear to be highly allergic to it that it is too dangerous to study in human subjects. These members argued that antipyrine should be banned at once as a nonprescription drug. There are few if any antipyrine products on the OTC market in the U.S.

Antipyrine is not recommended for children under 12 years of age.

• **POTASSIUM SALICYLATE:** This is an aspirin-like drug appears in some nonprescription pain-relief products. It was not submitted to the FDA for the OTC Review, and so the agency has no scientific evidence to assess its safety and effectiveness in this context. It has not been proved safe and effective according to current standards, the FDA says.

• **SALICYLAMIDE:** Chemically less closely related to aspirin than its name would suggest, salicylamide became widely used in the last 30 years in combination products; that is, in pain relievers combined with cold preparations, in quantities between 100 and 400 mg per dosage unit. There are too few data to determine whether it is either safe or effective in these doses.

Much larger amounts—up to 1000 mg or even 2000 mg every 4 to 6 hours—appear to be effective, but studies that would establish the safety of these larger doses have not been completed as yet. Reviewers' skepticism about the lower doses that are currently used reflects the findings that small amounts of salicylamide are almost completely broken down—extremely quickly—in the body. Most of the substance is gone before it ever gets into the bloodstream, where it could be carried throughout the body to relieve pain. It appears that the only way to get an effective amount of this drug into the bloodstream is to give a dose of 1000 mg or more—enough to overwhelm the enzyme system that controls its breakdown. On the other hand, in doses under 600 mg, salicylamide has been shown to provide no more pain relief than dummy medication (placebo). Salicylamide also lacks aspirin's anti-inflammatory property, so it is far less effective against arthritic symptoms.

The drug's safety has been inadequately studied. It does not cause the gastrointestinal irritation and bleeding that aspirin can and ought to be safer in this respect, although large doses can produce stomachaches. Very large doses have also produced toxic effects in other organs, particularly in children, for whom it is not recommended for use without prescription.

• **SALSALATE:** Also called salicylsalicylic acid, salsalate has not been shown to be safe or effective in the recommended dosage of 5000 to 1000 mg every 4 hours. Little research has been done on the substance. It is known to dissolve rather slowly, so it might be expected to be absorbed slowly or incompletely. Because of the slow absorption, salsalate is at best only two-thirds as potent as aspirin, despite claims that it may approach aspirin in its ability to relieve pain and fever.

Because salsalate is composed of 2 molecules of salicylic acid, the active ingredient in ordinary aspirin, it has been assumed that its safety is like aspirin's. This simplistic view is not justified, and studies to establish the agent's safety remain to be done. Claims that it is safer than aspirin particularly need to be proved. In the meantime, the drug seems comparable to aspirin in the severity and incidence of its side effects, so warnings applicable to aspirin are appropriate for salsalate too. Few if any nonprescription products containing this ingredient are currently marketed in the United States.

DISAPPROVED PAIN-RELIEVING ACTIVE INGREDIENTS

Many over-the-counter pain relievers still marketed contain active ingredients that are ineffective, unsafe, or mislabeled. The Panel has recommended that they be banned from nonprescription products sold in the United States.

• *ACETANILIDE:* Though marketed for many years for the relief of pain and fever, this drug is currently not readily found in over-the-counter products because the effective dose is very close to the toxic dose. There are many reports of poisoning; a number of these incidents resulted in death. The toxic compound is the breakdown product *aniline*, which has no beneficial effect. The pain-relieving property of acetanilide comes from another breakdown product, acetaminophen, which does not have aniline's poisonous properties. But acetaminophen is available as such (*see* Acetaminophen, p. 771), so it makes no sense to take acetanilide to obtain acetaminophen's benefits.

• *CODEINE:* This narcotic agent, derived from opium, is a very effective pain killer in the dosages used in prescription drugs. But in the small amounts—from 10 to 20 mg codeine per dose—that the federal government now allows in nonprescription products, it is ineffective against pain. Moreover, because it is a narcotic, codeine has the potential for abuse; it may cause narcotic dependence when taken in large amounts over a period of time.

Because of its addictive properties codeine is not sold over-the-counter as a single-ingredient product in the United States. It is available in combination products for treating coughs, for which it is recognized as safe and very effective. (*See* Codeine in COLD AND COUGH MEDICINES.)

- *IODOANTIPYRINE:* There is no scientific evidence to show that this compound—more widely used in Europe than in the United States—is actually effective. As for safety concerns, it liberates free iodide in the body. This can cause iodine poisoning, so the risks outweigh any possible benefits from its use.
- *QUININE:* The ground-up bark of the cinchona tree has long been known to relieve fever. It also relieves pain. However, reviewers concluded that the high dosage required for this kind of relief should be prescribed by a doctor. But: *see* QUININE FOR LEG CRAMPS.

    Quinine is quite toxic, causing ringing in the ears, headache, nausea, visual disturbances, and other symptoms. The drug is poisonous to the cardiovascular system and can cause death. Such risks heavily outweigh any value it might have as an over-the-counter drug for relieving common kinds of pain and fever.

OTHER INGREDIENTS

A number of substances besides active ingredients are put into over-the-counter pain relievers. Some are believed by manufacturers to be active ingredients, contrary to the Panel's judgment. Others are included for different reasons, and reviewers classify them as described here.

Adjuvants

In the amounts used, *adjuvants* or "helpers," have no significant pain-relieving ability, but they may contribute (directly or indirectly) to the effectiveness of an active ingredient. Some adjuvants enhance a drug's response by increasing its effect at the sites where it acts in the body. Others act elsewhere to modify the drug's absorption, breakdown, distribution, or excretion from the body.

Caffeine

This substance is one of the best known of those believed to act as an adjuvant for pain relief. It is safe in amounts up to 75 mg per dose. Caffeine is mildly habit-forming and mildly toxic. It has been said to have pain-relieving properties in its own right, but because this has not been demonstrated scientifically, caffeine cannot be claimed to be an active ingredient in over-the-counter pain medication. However, growing evidence suggests that relatively small amounts—75 mg per dosage unit—may enhance the effects of active pain-relieving drugs such as aspirin or acetaminophen with which it is combined. In these circumstances the caffeine may be acting as a mood elevator. Another possibility is that caffeine helps to relieve pain from headaches by tightening the distended blood vessels that are causing the pain. Exactly how this ingredient works remains to be established.

Antihistamines

Small amounts of antihistamines are sometimes added to over-the-counter pain relievers.

Although these substances are useful for other purposes (*see* COLD AND COUGH MEDICINES and ALLERGY DRUGS), they are not effective against pain. They may have adjuvant value in boosting the pain relief provided by aspirin and other active ingredients, but this use has not been proved. They are safe for this purpose. Compounds in this category include pheniramine maleate, phenyltoloxamine, and pyrilamine maleate.

Salicylamide

Despite some questions regarding safety, this compound, already discussed as an active ingredient on p. 784, is known to be effective in doses of 1000 mg every 4 hours. But because it is so rapidly broken down before it reaches the general circulation, lower doses are unlikely to have any direct pain-killing activity. Yet salicylamide is marketed in a variety of over-the-counter pain-killing combination products—usually with aspirin or acetaminophen—in amounts of about 200 mg per dose. There is some evidence that in these lower doses it enhances the analgesic effect of the other compounds. But this remains to be demonstrated conclusively, and if true, knowledge of how it actually works and what doses are appropriate must be more clearly defined.

Benzoic Acid Compounds

Some over-the-counter antirheumatic medications contain benzoic acid and related compounds. They include aminobenzoic acid, which is also called para-aminobenzoic acid (or PABA), and sodium para-aminobenzoate. These compounds have not been proved effective, and they are not safe.

Correctives (side-effect reducers)

These ingredients are intended to reduce one or more undesirable side effects of an active agent. Their principal role in over-the-counter analgesics is to act as antacid and buffering agents; for example, speeding aspirin's dissolution and buffering the stomach lining against its acidity. These compounds include

- AMINOACETIC ACID (GLYCINE, GLYCOCOLL)
- CALCIUM CARBONATE
- CALCIUM PHOSPHATE DIBASIC (MONOCALCIUM PHOSPHATE)
- CITRIC ACID (SODIUM CITRATE)
- DIHYDROXYALUMINUM AMINOACETATE (ALUMINUM GLYCINIATE)
- DIHYDROXYALUMINUM SODIUM CARBONATE
- DRIED ALUMINUM HYDROXIDE GEL
- MAGNESIUM CARBONATE
- MAGNESIUM HYDROXIDE
- SODIUM BICARBONATE
- SODIUM CARBONATE

Descriptions and evaluations of these compounds can be found in the Unit ANTACIDS.

Combination Products

The nonprescription pain-relieving active ingredients are formulated into a large number of combination products. The medicinal advantage of buffering aspirin and aspirin-like ingredients has been established. But the advantage of most other combined products—which may be much more expensive than single-ingredient products—is less clearcut, since the user is tied to the properties of each ingredient in the combination. In general, the Panel ruled that an over-the-counter product with fewer ingredients provides greater safety. The FDA currently has these views of combination products:

Combinations of Two Pain Relievers

The FDA, for now, approves pain-fever relieving combination products that include 325 to 500 mg acetaminophen per dose with a comparable dose of a salicylate (325 to 500 mg of aspirin or sodium salicylate; 414 to 637 mg of carbaspirin calcium; 436 to 669 mg of choline salicylate; or 377 to 580 mg of magnesium salicylate). Combinations that contain 2 salicylates are *not* approved.

The FDA says that a conference on analgesic-associated kidney disease, held by the National Institutes of Health in 1984, issued a statement saying there was "considerable evidence" that analgesic combination products taken in large doses over a long period of time can cause "a specific form of kidney disease and chronic kidney failure," as well as tumors. "The Conference also concluded that, in contrast, there is little evidence that preparations containing a single analgesic ingredient have been similarly abused and similarly harmful. The Conference recommended that serious consideration should be given to limiting OTC drug products to those containing a single antipyretic-analgesic agent."

The FDA says it has this recommendation under advisement. Meanwhile, people who frequently use pain-fever relievers may wish to take heed—and limit themselves to single-ingredient products.

Combination products that contain conditionally approved or disapproved ingredients are not approved by the FDA as safe and effective.

Combinations of Pain Relievers + Other Active Ingredients

One or 2 safe and effective pain relievers, in effective amounts, may be combined with other approved active ingredients intended to achieve a different purpose. But all active ingredients must help relieve at least one of the symptoms for which the combination is intended. Further, the whole must be as safe and as effective as any of its parts.

Mixes that FDA approves include those in which acetaminophen or aspirin is combined with one or more safe and effective antitussive agents, expectorants, nasal decongestants, or antihistamines. See COLD AND COUGH MEDICINES and also *see* ALLERGY DRUGS.

Acetaminophen may be combined with antacids. Aspirin and other salicylates, in solid form, may be combined with small amounts of antacids that act to buffer acidity. Aspirin may be combined with one or more antacids to treat pain and fever, in combination with acid indigestion or related gastric symptoms. (*See* ANTACIDS.) Pain-fever relievers may be combined with a diuretic to relieve menstrual distress. (*See* MENSTRUAL DISTRESS PREPARATIONS.)

Combinations of aspirin + a bronchodilator (bronchial muscle relaxer) are unsafe because a small percentage of asthmatic persons who may have urgent need for bronchodilators are also fatally allergic to aspirin. Another disapproved combination is analgesics that are mixed with laxatives or vitamins; despite wide availability, their use makes no sense because the need for the amount of each ingredient should be determined individually. Premixed combinations may not meet these individual needs.

All combinations that contain adjuvant caffeine are only conditionally approved. Caffeine is not in itself an effective pain reliever and it remains to be determined whether relatively small amounts of it will boost the pain relief provided by other ingredients.

When Greater Relief Is Needed

Over-the-counter pain-fever relievers can be very effective for the mild, even moderate pain they are intended to treat. If they fail in the relatively low doses approved by the FDA for self-medication, they may prove effective in the significantly higher doses a doctor can prescribe.

A wide variety of other, stronger single-ingredient and combination products are available by prescription to treat sudden, strong pain, or other pain that will not go away. Besides non-narcotic and narcotic drugs, doctors use biofeedback, electrostimulation, and nerve ablation surgery to help people cope with significant pain.

Some kinds of pain can be wholly relieved. Others cannot. But specialists working in hospitals and in special pain clinics should be able to provide most sufferers with significant relief.

Aspirin's Other—Life-Saving—Uses

The salicylates, and particularly aspirin, are extremely powerful drugs. So much so, in fact, that experts say that if aspirin were to be brought to market for the first time today, it would be restricted to prescription use rather than being made available without prescription. Important new uses for aspirin continue to emerge.

Two of these uses should be of keen interest to middle-aged and older Americans. These uses are described in the professional labeling for aspirin products that is available to doctors but are not detailed on the package of the drug product that you buy in the drug or variety store.

Heart Attack Prevention

Aspirin has a powerful effect of thinning the blood: It melts, or prevents, the formation of fibrous blood clots, which may enter and block the delicate coronary arteries that nourish the heart, causing a heart attack (myocardial infarction). In one study, daily aspirin reduced the risk of death or subsequent heart attack in patients who had suffered an initial heart attack by about 20 percent. Chest pain (unstable angina) was significantly reduced as well.

Other studies have shown that aspirin prevents *initial* heart attacks in middle-aged men. This benefit recently has been shown to apply to women, too. The FDA suggests that one ordinary 325-mg aspirin tablet, plain or buffered, each day may be "a reasonable, routine dose" for preventing heart attacks. This dose is large enough to be effective but small enough to spare users some of the gastrointestinal side effects that may accompany aspirin's use. Evidence from another major study suggests that half this amount, namely 160 mg per day, may be the optimal dosage. This dosage can be obtained by taking, each day, two baby aspirins (80 mg); or by breaking an ordinary 325 mg aspirin tablet in half; or by taking one of the new, half-strength, enteric-coated 160 mg aspirin tablets marketed specifically to prevent heart disease. Liquid aspirin (choline salicylate) preparations also may be used. The FDA has not yet announced its final recommendations for this heart-protecting use of aspirin.

Because aspirin has side effects—it can bring on or worsen gout, for example, this daily preventive regime should not be undertaken without your doctor's approval.

Strokes in Men

When the blood supply to small vessels in the brain is cut off by "blood clots" composed of fibrin and platelet cells from the bloodstream, brief, mild strokes, called TIAs, for *transient ischemic attacks*, often result. A TIA may cause a person to black out briefly, temporarily lose function in a limb or other body part, or experience sudden difficulty in thinking, speaking, or moving. These tiny strokes may be harbingers of more serious strokes, where large parts of the brain are deprived of oxygenated blood. Paralysis and death may result.

Studies have shown that men who have had TIAs, and who are at risk of more serious strokes, can be protected with aspirin, in doses of 1300 mg daily, in divided doses of 650 mg twice daily, or 325 mg four times each day. The risk of a major stroke or death can be cut by one-third. Women, too, may benefit, but as of 1988, when the FDA published its current document on these drugs, this effect had not been proved.

If you have had TIAs, you should speak to your doctor about preventive use of aspirin, if he or she has not already recommended it, along with other drugs he or she may have prescribed. Using buffered aspirin rather than ordinary aspirin may make this therapy easier to tolerate.

Safety and Effectiveness: Active Ingredients in Over-the-Counter Drugs for Pain, Fever, and Arthritic Symptoms

Active Ingredient	Pain Relief †	Fever Reduction	Arthritic (Rheumatic) Symptom Relief
acetaminophen	safe and effective	safe and effective	safe, but not effective
acetanilide	not safe	not safe	not safe or effective
aluminum aspirin*	safe, but not proved effective	safe, but not proved effective	safe, but not proved effective
antipyrine	not proved safe or effective	not proved safe or effective	not proved safe or effective
aspirin (acetylsalicylic acid)*	safe and effective	safe and effective	safe and effective
carbaspirin calcium*	safe and effective	safe and effective	safe and effective
choline salicylate*	safe and effective	safe and effective	safe and effective
codeine	not safe or effective	not safe or effective	not safe or effective
ibuprofen	safe and effective	safe and effective	safe and effective
iodoantipyrine	not safe	not safe	not safe
magnesium salicylate*	safe and effective	safe and effective	safe and effective
potassium salicylate*	not proved safe or effective	not proved safe or effective	not proved safe or effective
quinine	not safe	not safe	not safe or effective
salicylamide*	not proved safe or effective	not proved safe or effective	not effective

salsalate*	not proved safe or effective	not proved safe or effective	not proved safe or effective
	safe and effective	safe and effective	safe and effective
sodium salicylate*	safe and effective	safe and effective	safe and effective

* These ingredients belong to the aspirin family (salicylates).

† Pain may include headache, minor aches and pain associated with colds, sore throat, toothache, muscular aches, backache, premenstrual and menstrual periods, and minor pain of arthritis.

Safety and Effectiveness: Adjuvant ("Helper") Ingredients in Over-the-Counter Drugs for Pain, Fever, and Arthritic Symptoms

Adjuvant	Evaluation
aminobenzoic acid (PABA)	not safe
sodium para-aminobenzoate	not safe
caffeine	safe, but not proved effective
pheniramine maleate	safe, but not proved effective
phenyltoloxamine citrate	safe, but not proved effective
pyrilamine maleate	safe, but not proved effective
salicylamide	not proved safe or effective

Pain, Fever, and Anti-Inflammatory Drugs Taken Internally: Product Ratings

SINGLE-INGREDIENT PRODUCTS

Product and Distributor	Dosage of Active Ingredients	Rating*†	Comment
acetaminophen[§§]			
Acetaminophen or APAP (generic)	tablets, capsules: 325 mg	A+	adult dosage
Anacin-3 (Whitehall)		A+	
Panex (Hauck)		A+	
Tylenol Caplets (McNeil-CPC)		A+	
Tylenol Regular Strength (McNeil-CPC)		A+	
Acetaminophen (generic)	tablets, capsules: 500 mg	A	
Datril Extra Strength (Bristol-Myers)		A	
Acetaminophen (Philips Roxane)	tablets: 650 mg	A+	
Acetaminophen or APAP (generic)	elixir: 120 mg per teaspoonful (5 ml)	A	
Oraphen PD (Great Southern)		A	
Dolanex (Lannett)	elixir: 325 mg per teaspoonful (5 ml)	A+	
Acetaminophen (generic)	suppositories: 120 mg	A	
	325 mg	A+	
	650 mg	A+	

Pain, Fever, and Anti-Inflammatory Drugs Taken Internally: Product Ratings (contd)

Product and Distributor	Dosage of Active Ingredients	Rating*†	Comment
Children's Tylenol (McNeil-CPC)	chewable tablets: 80 mg	A+	children's dosage
Tylenol Infant Drops (McNeil-CPC)	liquid: 100 mg per ml	A	for young children
St. Joseph Aspirin-Free Infant Drops (Schering-Plough)		A	for young children
Tylenol Extra Strength (McNeil-CPC)	liquid: 500 mg per teaspoonful (5 ml) capsules: 500 mg	A	
aspirin (acetylsalicylic acid)			
Aspirin (generic)	tablets: 325 mg	A+	
Genuine Bayer Aspirin (Glenbrook)		A+	
Empirin (Burroughs-Wellcome)		A+	
Ecotrin Tablets and Caplets (SmithKline Beecham)	tablets, enteric coated: 325 mg	A+	
Aspirin (generic)		A	
Aspirin (URL)	tablets: 500 mg	A	
Aspirin (generic)	tablets, enteric coated: 650 mg suppositories: 60 mg through 600 mg	A+ A	
Aspergum (Schering-Plough)	chewable gum tablets: 227.5 mg	A	

8-Hour Bayer Timed-Release Aspirin (Glenbrook)	**timed-release tablets:** 650 mg	A+
Bayer Children's Aspirin (Glenbrook)	**tablets:** 81 mg	A+ children's dosage unit
aspirin, buffered		
Arthritis Pain Formula (Whitehall)	**tablets:** 500 mg + 100 mg magnesium hydroxide + 27 mg aluminum hydroxide	A
Ascriptin Regular Strength (Rhone-Poulenc Rorer)	**enteric coated tablets:** 325 mg + 50 mg aluminum hydroxide + 50 mg magnesium hydroxide + calcium carbonate	A+
Buffered aspirin (generic)	**tablets:** 325 mg + buffers	A+
Bufferin (Bristol-Myers)	**tablets:** 325 mg + 34 mg magnesium carbonate + 63 mg magnesium oxide +158 mg calcium carbonate	A+
Cama Arthritis Pain Reliever (Sandoz)	**tablets:** 500 mg + 150 mg magnesium hydroxide + 150 mg aluminum hydroxide	A
Halfprin (Kramer)	**enteric coated tablets:** 81 mg, 165 mg	A dosages for heart attack prevention; when recommended by a doctor

Pain, Fever, and Anti-Inflammatory Drugs Taken Internally: Product Ratings (contd)

Product and Distributor	Dosage of Active Ingredients	Rating*†	Comment
choline salicylate			
Arthropan (Purdue-Frederick)	liquid: 870 mg per teaspoonful (5 ml)	A	
ibuprofen			
Advil Tablets and Caplets (Whitehall)	tablets, caplets: 200 mg	A	℞ to OTC switch
Ibuprofen (generic)	tablets: 200 mg	A	℞ to OTC switch
Motrin IB Tablets and Caplets (Upjohn)	tablets, caplets: 200 mg	A	℞ to OTC switch
magnesium salicylate			
Original Doan's Pills (Ciba)	tablets: 325 mg	A+	
quinine sulfate			
Quinine sulfate (generic)	tablets: 325 mg	C	not safe
sodium salicylate			
Sodium salicylate (generic)	tablets, enteric coated: 325 mg	A+	
	650 mg	A+	

EFFERVESCENT PRODUCTS

Product and Distributor	Dosage of Active Ingredients	Rating*†	Comment
Alka-Seltzer with Aspirin (Miles)	**effervescent tablets:** 325 mg aspirin + 1.9 g sodium bicarbonate + 1 g citric acid	A+	
Bromo Seltzer (Warner-Lambert)	**effervescent granules:** 325 mg acetaminophen + 2.781 g sodium bicarbonate + 2.224 g citric acid per capful measure	A+	

NARCOTIC LIQUID COMBINATION PRODUCTS‖

Product and Distributor	Narcotic	Acetaminophen	Rating*	Comment
Acetaminophen with codeine elixir (generic)	12 mg codeine phosphate	12 mg per teaspoonful	C	codeine not safe or effective
Tylenol with Codeine Elixir (McNeil-CPC)			C	codeine not safe or effective

NON-NARCOTIC COMBINATION PRODUCTS

Product and Distributor	Aspirin	Acetaminophen	Other Analgesic	Other	Rating*	Comment
Anacin Caplets (Whitehall)	400 mg			32 mg caffeine	B	caffeine not proved effective
Anacin Maximum Strength Tablets (Whitehall)		500 mg		32 mg caffeine	B	

Pain, Fever, and Anti-Inflammatory Drugs Taken Internally: Product Ratings (contd)

NON-NARCOTIC COMBINATION PRODUCTS

Product and Distributor	Aspirin	Acetaminophen	Other Analgesic	Other	Rating*	Comment
Aspirin Free Excedrin Caplets (Bristol-Myers)		500 mg		65 mg caffeine	B	caffeine not proved effective
BC Powder (Block)	650 mg			195 mg salicylamide + 32 mg caffeine	B	salicylamide and caffeine not proved effective
BC Tablets (Block)	325 mg			95 mg salicylamide + 16 mg caffeine	B	salicylamide and caffeine not proved effective
Cope (Glenbrook)	421 mg			32 mg caffeine + 50 mg magnesium hydroxide + 25 mg aluminum hydroxide	B	caffeine not proved effective

Excedrin Extra Strength Caplets and Tablets (Bristol-Myers)	250 mg	250 mg	65 mg caffeine	B	caffeine not proved effective
Gemnisyn Tablets (Kremers-Urban)	325 mg	325 mg		A+	
Momentum Tablets (Whitehall)	500 mg		15 mg phenyltoloxamine citrate	B	the antihistamine not proved effective
Vanquish Caplets (Glenbrook)	227 mg	194 mg	33 mg caffeine + 50 mg magnesium hydroxide + 25 mg aluminum hydroxide	B	caffeine not proved effective

*Author's interpretation of FDA criteria. Based on contents, not claims.

†A "+" indicates uniform dosage; proposed by Panel, but rejected by FDA, that acetaminophen and aspirin and other equally potent salicylates be formulated in simple fractions or multiples of 325 mg—the standard dose—including 81 mg, 162 mg, 325 mg, and 650 mg.

‡The acetaminophen ratings are for pain and fever relief. Acetaminophen is not effective against *inflammation* due to arthritis and other conditions and injuries.

§Products are arranged by dosage form and strength of active ingredient(s).

||Not available in all states, and if available may not be displayed on open shelves.

Pancreatic Enzyme Supplements

The pancreas—which is a fish-shaped organ between the stomach and kidneys—produces digestive enzymes that play a key role in breaking down food so that it can be absorbed from the intestinal tract and used by the body for energy. When these enzymes are unavailable because the pancreas is diseased or has been removed surgically because of illness or injury, a person's digestion may be seriously impaired. Foodstuffs, and particularly fats, may pass through the gut and be excreted basically unchanged. As a result, diarrhea and malnutrition may occur. The feces may smell foul.

The normal human pancreas has the capacity to produce far greater amounts of these enzymes than the body actually needs. Some 90 percent of the organ—and thus, its enzymes—must be gone before digestive function is threatened. Short of serious pancreatic insufficiency, therefore, these supplements are not needed.

The lack of pancreatic enzymes can be overcome with replacements sold to fulfill this purpose. These supplements come from hog

PANCREATIC ENZYME SUPPLEMENTS is based on the report "Exocrine Pancreatic Insufficiency Drug Products" by the FDA's Advisory Review Panel on Miscellaneous Internal Drug Products; FDA's Tentative Final Monograph on these products; and a follow-up policy document.

pancreases. However, the Panel cautions that the need for these preparations cannot be self-diagnosed, and the serious illnesses that cause pancreatic insufficiency cannot be self-treated. Children with cystic fibrosis, for example, are particularly dependent on these enzymes. So while some of these products are available over-the-counter, both the diagnosis and the treatment of pancreatic insufficiency must be supervised by a doctor.

Normally the pancreas produces 3 digestive enzymes, each with a different function:

- *Lipase* digests fat.

- *Protease* digests protein.

- *Amylase* digests starch.

Supplements of these enzymes together are called *pancreatin*. A similar drug product, which contains a higher proportion of lipase, is called *pancrelipase*.

The FDA asked for public comment on the rules that it planned to issue to regulate over-the-counter sales of pancreatic enzymes. In doing so, the agency discovered a number of serious problems with these preparations. Many of these problems were called to the agency's attention by cystic fibrosis patients and their doctors:

- There is extreme variation in the amount of biologically active enzymes in the assortment of products on the market. This indicates that each batch of finished products must be individually assayed, which can be done only through prescription (℞) registration of products. Such testing cannot be done for products marketed over-the-counter.

- Individual patients have different and varying needs for these supplements, through time. Hence, they need to see their doctors regularly to adjust their dosages, and this adjustment can be achieved more effectively with prescription rather than with nonprescription dispensing.

- Many patients rely on insurance to pay for their drugs. Insurers are more likely to reimburse prescription medications than nonprescription ones.

Based on these reasons, and several others, the FDA decided in 1991 to ban nonprescription dispensing of the pancreatic enzyme supplement *pancreatin*, and said it would retain pancrelipase's prescription status. Barring a bureaucratic change of heart, the agency said, these supplements would be banned from the over-the-counter marketplace, and sometime in the next several years, will be available only on a doctor's prescription.

Subsequently, just such a change of bureaucratic heart did occur: Prompted by fears of cystic fibrosis sufferers that a change to prescription status would raise the cost and limit the availability of pancreatin—which they sometimes need *urgently*—the FDA switched gears: It declared that "currently marketed exocrine pancreative insufficiency drug products may be considered safe and effective."

What is needed, the agency added, is a way to ensure that batches of these products meet the standards printed on their labels. The FDA has set in motion technical and regulatory initiatives to see if pancreatin can be kept up to standard if it continues to be sold without prescription.

 Claims

Accurate

"For the treatment of exocrine pancreatic insufficiency when conducted under the care of the physician"

APPROVED ACTIVE INGREDIENTS

• **PANCREATIN:** This preparation is obtained from hog pancreases. It is described earlier in this Unit.

CONDITIONALLY APPROVED ACTIVE INGREDIENTS

None.

DISAPPROVED ACTIVE INGREDIENTS

None.

Safety and Effectiveness: Active Ingredients in Over-the-Counter Pancreatic Supplements

Active Ingredient	Assessment
Pancreatin (lipase + protease + amylase)	safe and effective

Pancreatic Enzyme Supplements: Product Ratings

Product and Distributor	Dosage of Active Ingredients	Rating*	Comment
Dizymes Tablets (Recsei Labs)	250 mg pancreatin (6,750 units lipase + 41,250 units protease + 43,750 units amylase)	A	enteric coated
Hi-Vegi-Lip Tablets (Freeda)	2400 mg pancreatin (12,000 units lipase + 60,000 units protease + 60,000 units amylase)	A	
Pancreatin (Lilly)	tablets: 325 mg pancreatin USP (8125 amylase + 650 units lipase + 8125 units protease)	A	
Pancreatin Enseals (Lilly)	enteric-coated tablets: 1000 mg pancreatin USP (25,000 units amylase + 2000 units lipase + 25,000 units protease)	A	

*Author's interpretation of FDA criteria. Based on contents, not claims.

Phenol: Special Note

The phenol story is one of the classics in pharmacology. This drug, of lowly origins, rose quickly to world fame a century ago. Then, it was pushed from center stage by new and better performers, and also by a growing awareness of its inherently destructive nature. Yet, phenol's popular appeal remains strong to this day. Nevertheless, as signaled by decisions about it in the Over-the-Counter (OTC) Drug Review, phenol's medicinal use may be waning.

Phenol is an alcohol. It was discovered in 1834, as a constituent of coal tar, which is why it also is called *carbolic acid*. Later, it was discovered that phenol can be distilled from hardwood and also can be made synthetically from benzene. In 1867, phenol became critically important to the practice of medicine when the English surgeon Joseph Lister showed that the high death toll from post-operative infections could be greatly reduced by spraying phenol in the operating room, cleansing a patient's skin with it before surgery, and applying phenol-soaked dressings to the surgical wound after the operation. The drug

PHENOL: SPECIAL NOTE is based on the report "OTC Topical Antimicrobial Products" by the FDA's Advisory Review Panel on OTC Topical Antimicrobial Drug Products for Repeated Daily Human Use (Antimicrobial I Panel); the FDA's Tentative Final Monograph on OTC Topical Antimicrobial Products; and reports by other OTC Review Panels.

quickly gained wide acceptance among doctors and lay people as a disinfectant for sanitary, medical, and surgical purposes. There is no denying phenol's ability to kill or inhibit disease-causing bacteria and other microorganisms; its characteristic, easily recognized pungent odor has come to be the olfactory symbol of "medicine."

Even today, in medical facilities, phenol continues to be widely used as a *disinfectant*; that is, as a chemical used to cleanse and degerm equipment, floors, and other surfaces. People continue to think of phenol as the germ-killing solution with the "medicinal smell."

For many years, phenol was the principal odoriferous ingredient in a popular soap that was widely and successfully promoted for its ability to kill the bacteria that supposedly cause body odor. It is a clear sign of phenol's decline that—in the United States at least—this soap no longer contains phenol or its engaging smell.

Through the years phenol was discovered to have useful pharmacological properties other than killing germs. It can, for example, penetrate the sensory nerve endings in the skin and temporarily inactivate them, providing an *anesthetic*, or numbing, effect. Phenol has therefore been widely used in topical drugs for relieving pain and itching. The drug has been used as an acne remedy, as an antifungal against athlete's foot, and for many other purposes. It is one of the most widely represented active ingredients in over-the-counter drugs, and was assessed— for different purposes—by 7 of the 17 review Panels.

The Dangers of Phenol

The fates began to change for phenol early in this century, when more-effective germicidal and anesthetic drugs came on the market. Phenol, meanwhile, was found to be extremely toxic. It is dangerous, whether swallowed, applied to the skin or mucous membranes, or even when inhaled from the air.

Taken orally, just a half an ounce of concentrated phenol is lethal; death occurs within minutes. Smaller amounts or weaker concentrations produce nausea, vomiting, physical collapse, pallor, cold sweats, and a feeble pulse rate. The victim may sink into a stupor. For these reasons, it is not safe to keep phenol around the house if there are children in the family.

When phenol is applied to the skin, concentrations of over 2 percent in water are irritating and may cause the skin to peel and die. The drug is readily absorbed through both normal and injured skin or mucous membranes, so systemic poisoning can result from its use on external body surfaces.

It is particularly dangerous to use phenol to treat diaper rash—a practice that may still continue. The drug is more readily absorbed through a rash than it would be through normal skin, and a large area of the baby's body is involved. Diapering over the phenol retards its evaporation and increases its absorption. Worst of all, an infant's ability to break down and neutralize the drug may not be fully developed, so toxic amounts can accumulate quickly in the liver and other organs.

Many chemical injuries in people of all age groups have now been attributed to phenol. Recent studies suggest the drug also may cause cancer.

Similar risks are being found or are suspected for a number of other compounds that are related to phenol. They include:

chlorothymol

chloroxylenol

cresols (including m-*cresol and secondary amyltricresols)*

dichlorophen

phenolate sodium (also called *sodium phenolate)*

resorcinol

Few of these drugs were assessed as safe and effective, except when they are used on very tiny body areas (such as the gums) or in extremely weak solutions.

WARNING:

 Do not use for diaper rash, or use over large areas of the body, or cover the treated area with a bandage or dressings.

Specific Phenol Concentrations

After a careful study of phenol drugs (phenolates), the Antimicrobial I Panel proposed a formulation standard for phenol that was then endorsed by the FDA. This standard is now being applied to most nonprescription uses of these drugs:

• *PHENOL 1.5 PERCENT OR GREATER IN AQUEOUS OR ALCOHOLIC SOLUTIONS:* Concentrations above 1.5 percent are too dangerous for use without prescription, according to the Antimicrobial I Panel and the FDA. The FDA plans to ban their use unless manufacturers present satisfactory evidence on safety and effectiveness.

• *PHENOL 5 PERCENT OR LESS IN GLYCERIN OR OIL BASE:* Phenol is released onto and absorbed into the skin less rapidly when it is formulated with glycerin or in an oil-based preparation with camphor. The FDA has set a 5 percent upper limit for safety for these formulations.

• *PHENOL 1.5 PERCENT OR LESS IN AQUEOUS OR ALCOHOLIC SOLUTIONS:* Low concentrations of 1.5 percent phenol or less in aqueous or alcoholic solutions do not present a known hazard to the consumer. But they may be too weak to be effective. Whether manufacturers will try to prove that weak phenol preparations are effective remains to be seen. At present, however, only these uses are approved as both safe and effective by OTC Review Panels and the FDA:

> • For relieving itching and pain on the skin at concentrations of 0.5 to 1.5 percent or, combined with camphor, in light mineral oil, at a ratio of 1 part phenol to 2 or 3 parts camphor, up to 5 percent phenol and 11 percent camphor.
>
> • As a first-aid antiseptic at concentrations of 0.5 to 1.5 percent, or in the higher concentrations combined with camphor and light mineral oil (as just indicated).
>
> • For the relief of anal itching and pain in the same amounts as were described for the relief of itching and pain on the skin.
>
> • For relieving fever, pain, and itching of cold sores (fever blisters) at the aforementioned concentrations.
>
> • For relieving poison ivy-oak-sumac and insect-bite welts at the same concentrations.
>
> • For the relief of soreness and irritation of the gums and mucous membranes of the mouth and throat at concentrations of 0.5 to 1.5 percent.

None of these judgments is final.

Conditional approval—pending proof of safety, effectiveness, or both—has been granted to phenol by Panels for several other uses. (*See* Index.)

• *PHENOL UNDER 0.5 PERCENT, AS AN INACTIVE INGREDIENT:* At very low concentrations—under 0.5 percent, or one-half of 1 percent—phenol is safe, the FDA says, and may continue to be used as "an inactive ingredient for its aromatic characteristics." In other words, the FDA is willing to allow manufacturers to practice a small smell deception on over-the-counter drug users, since the "medicinal odor" will come from an ingredient that no longer is present in concentrations high enough to be of medicinal value.

Among the other phenol-like drugs, phenolate sodium and resorcinol have a few uses. (*See* Index.)

Safety and Effectiveness: Phenol

Active Ingredient	*Assessment*
phenol over 1.5% in aqueous or alcoholic solutions	not safe
phenol over 5% in anhydrous glycerin, or formulated in oil preparation with camphor	not safe
phenol 0.5 to 1.5% in aqueous or alcoholic solutions	safe, or may be safe—and may or may not be effective
phenol up to 5% in anhydrous glycerin or in oily preparations with camphor up to 11%	safe, or may be safe—and may or may not be effective
phenol under 0.5%	safe but inactive as a drug

Phenol: Product Ratings—Rated for Safety Only

Product and Distributor	Dosage of Active Ingredients	Rating*	Comment
Anbesol (Whitehall)	0.5%	A	
Campho-Phenique (Winthrop)	4.7%	A	
Cheracol Sore Throat Spray Liquid (Richardson-Vicks)	1.4%	A	
Chloraseptic Mouthwash and Spray (Richardson-Vicks)	1.4%	A	
Skeeter Stik (Triton)	2%	C	
Unguentine Plus (Norwich-Eaton)	0.5%	A	

*Author's interpretation of FDA criteria. Based on contents, not claims.

Poison Ivy-Oak-Sumac Preventives and Palliatives

The plant poisons—poison ivy, poison oak, and poison sumac—are the scourge of many a fishing trip, golf game, and gardening day. Children playing in the backyard or nearby woods may encounter these plants, too. It would be nice if there were a preventive medicine that could be swallowed or rubbed onto the skin before exposure; but no drug is available that safely and effectively fulfills this need. It would be nice, too, if there were drugs that could be used safely and effectively after exposure to prevent the rashes from erupting on the skin, but there are none.

Once the rash has erupted, more can be done about it: Safe and effective drugs *are* available to relieve the itching and pain. Some are marketed specifically for plant poisoning, others as general remedies for skin rashes. This Unit focuses on safe and effective itch-pain relievers and skin protectants to quell these plant rashes' distress. Many of these ingredients and many additional products can be found

POISON IVY-OAK-SUMAC PREVENTIVES AND PALLIATIVES is based on the report "OTC Poison-Ivy, -Oak, and -Sumac Prevention Drug Products" by the FDA's Advisory Review Panel on OTC Miscellaneous External Drug Products and the FDA's Tentative Final Monographs on Skin Protectant Drug Products and on External Analgesic Drug Products used for poison ivy-oak-sumac and insect bites.

in the Units ITCH AND PAIN REMEDIES APPLIED TO THE SKIN, and UNGUENTS AND POWDERS TO PROTECT THE SKIN.

Preventive Measures

The best way to avoid poison ivy-oak-sumac is to learn to recognize these poisonous plants and stay away from them. Remember, too, that direct contact with the plant is not required for trouble to erupt. A dog that runs through patches of the plant, or a boat or other equipment that is dragged through them, will pick up enough toxin to cause a serious rash if you pet the dog or handle the boat or equipment. Even airborne

What To Do

If you have touched the leaves, stems or creepers of a poison ivy, poison oak, or poison sumac plant, here are some self-care steps recommended by experts at the Mayo Clinic, in Rochester, Minn.:

1. Wash with ordinary soap and water—within ten minutes or less if possible. This may prevent or reduce the reaction. Be sure to scrub under your fingernails so that you do not spread the poisons by scratching.

2. If a rash begins to arise, soak it in cool tap water or use a nonprescription aluminum acetate solution. These methods may provide partial relief.

3. Use a hydrocortisone cream, spray or ointment, for which 1 percent concentrations are readily available without prescription. Stronger steroid skin preparations require a prescription.

4. An oral antihistamine, such as chlorpheniramine maleate or diphenhydramine, may help. (See ALLERGY DRUGS.)

5. If these measures (combined with use of other nonprescription products described in this Guide) do not avail, the Mayo Clinic doctors advise: See your physician promptly. Earlier treatment is more effective.

material from the plants can be poisonous to highly sensitive persons, particularly when the plants are burned in brush-clearing efforts.

Persons seriously afflicted with poison ivy should discuss their problem with an allergist. Some helpful medical measures are available, including oral desensitizing doses of ivy toxin.

Preventive Drugs

At least one nonprescription oral drug is marketed with the claim that it prevents plant poisoning. The Panel concerned with miscellaneous internal drugs was supposed to assess such compounds, but it was disbanded before it could do so.

Several currently available preparations are *claimed* to help prevent ivy poisoning when applied to the skin. No data were submitted— or were assessed by the Panel on these active ingredients. The FDA has now performed a preliminary analysis on them.

APPROVED PREVENTIVE ACTIVE INGREDIENTS

None.

CONDITIONALLY APPROVED PREVENTIVE ACTIVE INGREDIENTS

None.

DISAPPROVED PREVENTIVE ACTIVE INGREDIENTS

• **FERRIC CHLORIDE:** This iron salt is formulated into a couple of long-selling products to prevent poison ivy-oak-sumac eruptions. The manufacturer said that consumers like these products and have registered few complaints. But the FDA, reiterating some notational material left by the Panel, found no substantial data on the safety or effectiveness of ferric chloride. For now the verdict is: not safe or effective.

• **POLYVINYLPYRROLIDONE-VINYL ACETATE:** A long name but the FDA said, no data: not safe or effective. The FDA lists this ingredient by the shorthand name *povidone* (*see* p. 821).

Drugs to Relieve the Sting

Many products are available to treat bumps, blisters, rashes, and other eruptions from poison ivy and related plant poisons. Because of fiscal and governmental policy constraints, the present Panel was disbanded by the FDA before it could specifically evaluate active ingredients in these preparations with one exception: the Panel approved an astringent, *aluminum acetate solution*, as safe and effective for treating poison ivy-oak-sumac (*see* Aluminum Acetate, in STYPTIC PENCILS AND OTHER ASTRINGENTS).

The FDA now has rectified the Panel's shortcoming, in part by recognizing poison ivy-oak-sumac symptom relievers under two additional classes: *itch-pain relievers applied to the skin,* and *skin protectants.* These ingredients are described in, respectively, the Units ITCH AND PAIN REMEDIES APPLIED TO THE SKIN and UNGUENTS AND POWDERS TO PROTECT THE SKIN. These two groups also will be treated cursorily in this Unit with cross references to the pages in which they are described in the other two Units. A few ingredients, such as *sodium bicarbonate* and *tannic acid,* that are particularly labeled or possibly useful for the relief of poison ivy-oak-sumac will be described briefly here. This information will be summarized in the Safety and Effectiveness table at the end of the Unit. Some products that are labeled specifically for the relief of poison ivy will be listed in the Poison Ivy-Oak-Sumac Product Ratings table that concludes this Unit. Many other safe and effective (and other) products to relieve itching, and to dry and protect the skin in sufferers of poison ivy-oak-sumac, as well as for sufferers of other itchy or painful skin conditions, are listed in the Product Tables in ITCH AND PAIN REMEDIES APPLIED TO THE SKIN and UNGUENTS AND POWDERS TO PROTECT THE SKIN.

External Pain-Relieving Active Ingredients

 Claims

Accurate
- "For the temporary relief of itching and pain associated

with poison ivy, poison oak, poison sumac"
- "For the temporary relief of rashes due to poison ivy, poison oak, poison sumac"

APPROVED PAIN-RELIEVING ACTIVE INGREDIENTS

- BENZOCAINE (5 TO 20 PERCENT): *See* pp. 557-558.
- BENZYL ALCOHOL: *See* p. 558.
- BUTAMBEN PICRATE: *See* pp. 558-559.
- CAMPHOR: *See* p. 559 and CAMPHOR: SPECIAL NOTE pp. 124-129.
- CAMPHORATED METACRESOL: *See* p. 559.
- DIBUCAINE: *See* pp. 559-560.
- DIBUCAINE HYDROCHLORIDE: *See* p. 560.
- DIMETHISOQUIN HYDROCHLORIDE: *See* p. 560.
- DIPHENHYDRAMINE HYDROCHLORIDE: *See* p. 560.
- DYCLONINE HYDROCHLORIDE: *See* pp. 560-561.
- HYDROCORTISONE: *See* pp. 561-562.
- HYDROCORTISONE ACETATE: *See* pp. 561-562.
- JUNIPER TAR: *See* p. 562.
- LIDOCAINE: *See* p. 562.
- LIDOCAINE HYDROCHLORIDE: *See* p. 562.
- MENTHOL: *See* pp. 562-563.
- PHENOL: *See* p. 563 and PHENOL: SPECIAL NOTE pp. 807-812.
- PHENOLATE SODIUM: *See* p. 563.
- PRAMOXINE HYDROCHLORIDE: *See* pp. 563-564.
- RESORCINOL: *See* p. 564.
- TETRACAINE: *See* p. 564.
- TETRACAINE HYDROCHLORIDE: *See* p. 565.
- TRIPELENNAMINE HYDROCHLORIDE: *See* p. 565.

CONDITIONALLY APPROVED PAIN-RELIEVING ACTIVE INGREDIENTS

- BENZOCAINE UNDER 5 PERCENT: *See* pp. 557-558.
- DEXPANTHENOL: Only one study on the safety of dexpanthenol—when fed to rats—was submitted to the FDA, and the agency said it was a

poor and unconvincing piece of work. Several clinical studies showed no skin reactions to dexpanthenol. The FDA says its safety has not been established. No well-controlled data on the efficacy of dexpanthenol were submitted. The FDA's current judgment is: not proved safe or effective. This compound is virtually identical to *panthenol* , for which the same judgments pertain.

- GLYCOL SALICYLATE: *See* p. 565.
- PANTHENOL: *See Dexpanthenol.*
- TANNIC ACID: This is the substance that hardens and toughens cow hide into leather in *tanneries.* It is extracted from tree bark. Tannic acid was once widely used in nonprescription medications. However, it is quite toxic and can cause side effects even at fairly low concentrations. The OTC Drug Review has weeded it out of many types of products.

   One manufacturer has sold combination products containing 8 to 10 percent tannic acid for the relief of minor itching and pain of poison ivy-oak-sumac, as well as other causes, for half a century, with—he says—few problems or complaints. At least two Panels looked at this manufacturer's data and were not impressed by it. Nevertheless, the FDA is willing to give this maker a pass on the safety issue, based on the product's long and seemingly innocent use. What the FDA will not let pass are the data submitted to demonstrate the substance's efficacy in relieving poison ivy-oak-sumac discomfort. Temporary ruling: Tannic acid is safe but not proved effective for relieving these rashes.

- TROLAMINE: *See* pp. 532-533.
- TROLAMINE SALICYLATE: *See* p. 566.

DISAPPROVED PAIN-RELIEVING ACTIVE INGREDIENTS

None.

Drying and Skin Protecting Medications

The FDA has made the following judgments on skin protectant active ingredients for the relief of itching, pain, and discomfort from poison ivy-oak-sumac.

Claims for Drying and Skin-Protecting Medications

Accurate

• "Poison ivy-oak-sumac drying cream [or "lotion" or "powder"] (excludes colloidal oatmeal and sodium bicarbonate)"

• "Poison ivy-oak-sumac treatment"

For colloidal oatmeal and sodium bicarbonate used as soak, or for sodium bicarbonate as wet dressing or paste:

• "Provides temporary skin protection and relieves minor irritation and itching due to poison ivy-oak-sumac."

Unproved

For sodium bicarbonate:

• "For drying oozing and weeping"

APPROVED DRYING AND SKIN-PROTECTING ACTIVE INGREDIENTS

• ALUMINUM HYDROXIDE GEL: *See* p. 973.

• CALAMINE: *See* p. 973.

• COLLOIDAL OATMEAL: *See* pp. 281-282. This substance may be particularly appropriate for treating widespread rashes and welts from poison ivy-oak-sumac and the wheals left by insect bites. The colloidal oatmeal soothes the skin and leaves a protective layer of the material on it after treatment. The treatment can be given as a soak in a tepid bath (about a cupful of colloidal oatmeal per tubful of water). This can be repeated twice daily. For children under 2 years of age, consult a doctor.

• KAOLIN: *See* p. 974.

• SODIUM BICARBONATE (BAKING SODA): This is a standard household remedy. *See* p. 975. It can be used as a soak—one or two cupfuls to a tub of warm water—or can be made up at home and applied as a paste or a wet dressing. Repeat application as needed. For children under 2 years of age, consult a doctor.

• ZINC ACETATE: *See* p. 976.

• ZINC CARBONATE: *See* p. 976.

• ZINC OXIDE: *See* p. 977.

CONDITIONALLY APPROVED DRYING AND SKIN-PROTECTING ACTIVE INGREDIENTS

- **BUFFERED MIXTURE OF CATION + ANION EXCHANGE RESINS:** This preparation, which appears not to be sold in the United States at this time, contains resins that are said to pick up both acid and base plant proteins (*antigens*) that provoke reactions to plant poisons. The resins are then washed off, carrying the toxins away.

  A few safety tests were submitted for review. They indicate that the mixture produces little skin irritation during the first two weeks of use but later can provoke severe sores in the skin and underlying tissues. So the mixture was judged safe when used briefly.

  Evaluators were not impressed by the evidence on how well this drug works. In an uncontrolled study, 13 doctors reported on 32 instances in which they used the resins. All claimed the mixture was effective. Another doctor said the rashes dried up quickly in the 40 patients he treated with the resins. But in a controlled study of 20 men who were sensitive to poison ivy, the mixture was not clearly superior to dummy medication. The Panel concluded that, while safe, a buffered mixture of anion and cation exchange resins has not been proved effective. The FDA agreed.

  There now appear to be one or more additional experimental products that may protect the skin from poison ivy-oak-sumac toxins in much the same way. None as yet has passed the FDA's tests for safety and effectiveness.

- **TOPICAL STARCH (CORN STARCH):** This is an inert drying powder that is safe and effective for many uses (*see* p. 976). But the FDA is concerned that it will cause poison ivy-oak-sumac eruptions to crust over rather than to weep freely—and so may hinder rather than hasten healing. Few data are available on the effectiveness of topical starch in treating plant poison rashes. So the agency says: safe, but not proved effective.

DISAPPROVED DRYING AND SKIN-PROTECTING ACTIVE INGREDIENT

- **FERRIC CHLORIDE:** A manufacturer claims this chemical will prevent poison ivy-oak-sumac poisoning. No data were submitted. The FDA's ruling: not safe and effective.

When Further Relief Is Needed

If you have inhaled smoke from burning poison ivy-oak-sumac plants, or note eruptions from them in your mouth and throat, go to the emergency room or see your doctor at once. If nonprescription drug products do not adequately relieve the itching from these plant poisons, see your family doctor or a dermatologist. Much more powerful drugs— particularly steroids—are available on prescription to quell the itching, pain, and inflammation.

For many other products that are safe and effective for relieving itching, pain, and discomfort of poison ivy-oak-sumac poisoning, see the Product Table in ITCH AND PAIN REMEDIES APPLIED TO THE SKIN. For drying and skin-protecting products to treat and dry welts and rashes of poison ivy-oak-sumac, see the Product Table in UNGUENTS AND POWDERS TO PROTECT THE SKIN.

Safety and Effectiveness: Active Ingredients in Over-the-Counter Medications Used to Treat Poison Ivy, Oak, and Sumac

Active Ingredient	Function	Assessment
aluminum acetate solution (modified Burow's solution)	astringent	safe and effective
benzocaine	itch-pain reliever	safe and effective
benzyl alcohol	itch-pain reliever	safe and effective
buffered mixture of cation and anion exchange resins	preventive	safe, but not proved effective
Burow's solution (see aluminum acetate solution)		
butamben picrate	itch-pain reliever	safe and effective
calamine	skin protectant	safe and effective
camphor	itch-pain reliever	safe and effective
camphorated metacresol	itch-pain reliever	safe and effective
colloidal oatmeal	skin protectant drying agent	safe and effective
dexpanthenol	itch-pain reliever	safe, not proved effective
dibucaine	itch-pain reliever	safe and effective
dibucaine hydrochloride	itch-pain reliever	safe and effective

dimethisoquin hydrochloride	itch-pain reliever	safe and effective
diphenhydramine hydrochloride	antihistamine	safe and effective
dyclonine hydrochloride	itch-pain reliever	safe and effective
ferric chloride	preventive	not safe and effective
hydrocortisone preparations (hydro-cortisone, hydrocortisone acetate)	itch relievers	safe and effective
juniper tar	itch-pain reliever	safe and effective
lidocaine	itch-pain reliever	safe and effective
lidocaine hydrochloride	itch-pain reliever	safe and effective
menthol (0.1 to 1%)	itch-pain reliever	safe and effective
panthenol (see dexpanthenol)		
phenol (0.5 to 1.5% in aqueous or alcoholic solution)	itch-pain reliever	safe and effective
phenolate sodium (0.5 to 1.5% phenol)	itch-pain reliever	safe and effective
pramoxine hydrochloride	itch-pain reliever	safe and effective
polyvinylpyrrolidone-vinyl acetate copolymers (povidone)	preventive	not safe and effective
resorcinol	itch-pain reliever	safe and effective

Safety and Effectiveness: Active Ingredients in Over-the-Counter Medications
Used to Treat Poison Ivy, Oak, and Sumac (contd)

Active Ingredient	Function	Assessment
sodium bicarbonate (baking soda)	skin protectant	safe and effective
tannic acid	itch-pain reliever	safe, not proved effective
tetracaine	itch-pain reliever	safe and effective
tetracaine hydrochloride	itch-pain reliever	safe and effective
topical starch	skin protectant	safe, not proved effective
tripelennamine hydrochloride	antihistamine	safe and effective
trolamine*	skin protectant	safe, not proved effective
trolamine salicylate*	itch-pain reliever	safe, not proved effective
zinc acetate	skin protectant	safe and effective
zinc carbonate	skin protectant	safe and effective
zinc oxide	skin protectant	safe and effective

* FDA documents not in accord on these ingredients.

Poison-Ivy Palliatives and Preventives: Product Ratings

SINGLE-INGREDIENT PRODUCTS

Product and Distributor	Dosage of Active Ingredients	Rating *	Comment
aluminum acetate solution (Modified Burow's solution)			
Domeboro Powder and Tablets (Miles)	**powder:** 2.36 g packet produces 1 pint 1:40 modified Burow's solution	A	
Modified Burow's Solution (generic)	**liquid:** aluminum acetate solution	A	
benzocaine	*See p. 571, Product Ratings in ITCH AND PAIN REMEDIES APPLIED TO THE SKIN*		
calamine			
Calamine (generic)	**lotion:** 8% calamine + 8% zinc oxide + 2% glycerin	A	
colloidal oatmeal			
Aveeno Shower and Bath Oil (Rydelle)	**bath oil:** 5%	A	
dexpanthenol			
Panthoderm (Jones)	**cream:** 2%	B	not proved safe or effective

Poison-Ivy Palliatives and Preventives: Product Ratings (contd)

Product and Distributor	Dosage of Active Ingredients	Rating *	Comment
diphenhydramine hydrochloride			
Benadryl (Parke-Davis)	spray, cream: 1%	A	
Maximum Strength Benadryl (Parke-Davis)	spray, cream: 2%	A	
hydrocortisone and hydrocortisone acetate			
See pp. 571-572, Product Ratings in ITCH AND PAIN REMEDIES APPLIED TO THE SKIN			
sodium bicarbonate			
Arm & Hammer Baking Soda (Church & Dwight)	powder	A	
Sodium Bicarbonate (generic)	powder	A	

COMBINATION PRODUCTS

Product and Distributor	Dosage of Active Ingredients	Rating *	Comment
Caladryl (Parke-Davis)	**cream:** 1% diphenhydramine hydrochloride + 8% calamine **lotion:** 1% diphenhydramine hydrochloride + calamine + camphor	A	

Product and Distributor	Dosage of Active Ingredients	Rating*	Comment
Dermarest Plus (Commerce)	**gel, spray:** 2% diphenhydramine hydrochloride + 1% menthol	A	
Ivarest (Blistex)	**cream, lotion:** 14% calamine + 5% benzocaine	A	
Phenolated Calamine (Humco)	**lotion:** 8% calamine + 8% zinc oxide + 1% phenol	A	
Rhuli Cream (Rydelle)	**cream:** 3% calamine + 5% benzocaine + 0.3% camphor	A	
Rhuli Gel (Rydelle)	**gel:** 2% benzyl alcohol + 0.3% menthol + 0.3% camphor	B	inadequate dosage of benzyl alcohol
Rhuli Spray (Rydelle)	**spray:** 13.8% calamine + 5% benzocaine + 0.7% camphor	A	
Ziradryl (Parke-Davis)	**lotion:** 1% diphenhydramine hydrochloride + 2% zinc oxide	A	
PREVENTIVES			
Ivy-Rid (Hauck)	**spray:** povidone + other ingredients	C	not safe and effective
Ivy-Check (JMI)		C	not safe and effective

*Author's interpretation of FDA criteria. Based on contents, not claims.

Poisoning Antidotes

Most poisonings occur in children and are accidental. Adults must be prepared to provide first aid, with the help—if available—of poison control operators or other emergency health-care professionals. Teenagers and adults who overdose on licit or illicit drugs or who have taken poison deliberately are a different matter; they are likely to be uncooperative. Police help should be sought *immediately*.

Steps to Take Right Now

Find the phone number of two nearby poison-control centers by asking your telephone information operator, calling your local or state health department, or family doctor, or contacting your local hospital, police or fire department. It is best to have two poison-center numbers because one center may be closed at the time you need it or may not

POISONING ANTIDOTES is based on the report of the FDA's Advisory Review Panel on OTC Laxative, Antidiarrheal, Emetic, and Antiemetic Drug Products; the FDA's Tentative Final Order on Emetic Drug Products for OTC Human Use; the report "Drug Products for OTC Use for the Treatment of Acute Toxic Ingestion," by the Advisory Review Panel on OTC Miscellaneous Internal Drugs; the FDA's Tentative Final Monograph on these products; and material on first aid provided by the director of the now disbanded National Poison Center Network.

answer for some other reason. Write the phone numbers of these centers, and the other phone numbers indicated, in the spaces provided:

Poison Control Center #1 _____

Poison Control Center #2 _____

Doctor _____

Police _____

Emergency Medical Facility _____

      Purchase over-the-counter antidotes from your druggist. Buy syrup of ipecac. Also buy activated charcoal. These ingredients are available in kits that contain pre-measured doses of each antidote, plus instructions. Keep kit where it is in clear sight—in a bathroom, kitchen, or bedroom—and from time to time remind all adults in the house where it is.

Steps to Take in Case of Poisoning

In case of poisoning or suspected poisoning, follow these steps in order. Do not panic.

General First Aid

1. Call a poison control center, a doctor, or an emergency health facility *immediately*. If possible, begin first-aid treatment at once while another person does the phoning.
2. Loosen tight clothing—be sure the airway is clear from nose and mouth to lungs. You may have to remove or reposition false teeth in older persons.
3. Apply artificial ventilation—mouth-to-mouth resuscitation—if breathing has stopped. Keep the airway open if the victim is unconscious.
4. Keep the victim warm (not hot) with blankets.
5. Do not give the victim liquor, soft drinks, or drugs in any form.

Treating the Poisoning

Take these steps next. Stay calm.

1. If you can, tell the expert at the poison control center or the emergency medical facility the victim's condition, the type of poison involved, and the amount taken. Decide with the medical authority whether to bring the victim to an emergency room, wait for an ambulance, or begin additional treatment on the spot.

2. If the victim is transported for help, take along the poison container. If the victim has vomited, take a sample of the vomited matter.

3. If a petroleum distillate or similar hydrocarbon product has been swallowed—for example, *cleaning fluid, furniture polish, gasoline, turpentine* or other *paint-thinner, lighter fluid,* or *kerosene*—first-aid instruction must come from poison center staff, your physician, hospital emergency room personnel, or another health professional. You may be able to smell a petroleum distillate on the victim's breath if no container can be found.

4. Do *not* induce vomiting if the victim

   • is unconscious

   • is having convulsions

   • complains of pain or a burning sensation in the mouth or throat and

   • has swallowed a *corrosive acid* or *corrosive alkali*

   corrosive acids include:
       toilet-bowl cleaner (sodium bisulfate)
       sulfuric, nitric, oxalic, hydrochloric, or phosphoric acids

   corrosive alkalis include:
       chlorine bleach (sodium hypochlorite)
       lye or drain cleaner (sodium or potassium hydroxide)
       washing soda (sodium carbonate)
       ammonia
       bleaching powder (sodium perborate)
       dishwashing detergent

   a. If the victim of corrosive poisoning is conscious, is alert, and can swallow, give him or her water or milk: For babies up to age 5 years, 1 to 2 cups of fluid; for older persons, 2 to 3 cups of fluid.

b. Do *not* give activated charcoal and do *not* induce vomiting.

5. If the poison is not a corrosive substance, first give 1 to 2 cups of *water* or other clear fluid—not milk—to dilute the poison in the stomach.

6. Induce vomiting if directed to do so by a medical authority. If no emergency medical source can be reached, take the responsibility yourself.

a. You can usually induce vomiting by irritating the back of the victim's throat with back end of a spoon or with your finger. This stimulates the gag reflect. When retching and vomiting begins, help victim stand or sit, leaning forward, with head lower than hips. This prevents poisoned vomitus from being sucked into the lungs where it could cause further damage.

b. If this mechanical method does not work—and it often does not—attempt to induce vomiting with *syrup of ipecac*. Dosages are as follows: For babies 6 months to 1 year of age, 1 teaspoon (5 ml) followed by ½ to 1 glass of water. For children ages 1 to 12 years, 1 tablespoon (15 ml) followed by 1 to 2 glasses of water or other clear liquid—*not* milk. For older persons, 2 tablespoons (30 ml) followed by 1 to 2 glasses of water. Do not give ipecac to babies under six months of age except on a health professional's advice.

c. Keep the patient active and moving.

d. If vomiting has not occurred within 30 minutes, repeat the dose of ipecac and water.

e. If vomiting *still* has not occurred, seek emergency medical help.

f. After vomiting has occurred—*not before*—give activated charcoal. This is an adsorbent which will grab onto, bind, and so neutralize many poisons. If you know how much of the toxic substance was swallowed, give 8 to 10 times that amount of activated charcoal. Otherwise, give 4 to 6 tablespoons (20 to 30 grams). Each dose should be mixed in 1 glass of water (8 ounces) to facilitate swallowing. Do not give activated charcoal if the poison is a *corrosive acid* or *corrosive alkali*, as described previously.

7. Keep victim active and moving.

8. Bring the victim to a medical facility as quickly as possible.

Understanding the Poisoning Problem

The need to know about and be able to deliver first-aid treatment for poisoning is clear from the statistics: Over two million poisonings occur in the United States each year. The National Safety Council says 5700 of these episodes are fatal. Most accidental poisonings occur in youngsters. According to one estimate, children account for 70 percent of accidental poisonings. Sixty children 14 years or younger died of accidental poisoning by solids or liquids in 1990, according to the National Safety Council.

Many of these poisonings could be prevented by what some parents call "child-proofing" the house, as soon as an infant is able to crawl:

Preventing Poisoning

- *IN THE KITCHEN:* Put household chemicals and cleaners in a locked cabinet or on high shelves out of reach. A bicycle padlock with a long hasp can be used to secure kitchen cabinet-door handles.
- *IN THE BATHROOM:* Lock the medicine cabinet if possible, and keep all drugs and medicines on a high shelf. Do not trust safety caps. Get "Mr. Yuck" stickers from your poison control center or druggist for all medicine bottles.
- *IN THE BEDROOM:* Take perfumes and other cosmetics and medicine off the night stand or dresser, and store them in a secure place children cannot reach.
- *IN THE BASEMENT AND GARAGE:* Do not put paint-thinner, solvents, fuels, or other toxic substances in milk or soft-drink bottles. Store weed killers and pesticides as manufacturers recommend: out of children's reach. Be sure that laundry detergents are out of reach, too.

At the grocery, hardware, paint or utility store, and at the gas station: Select products that have been laced with tiny amounts of denatonium benzoate (*Bitrex*, Henley Chemicals): It is claimed to be the world's most bitter substance. The denatonium benzoate is not harmful, but it will cause a child to stop, and spit out any poisonous household chemical that contains it after the first taste. Look for products that carry the *Bitrex* trademark.

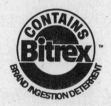

Drugs Used to Counteract Poisoning

A number of chemicals and mixtures have been used as antidotes. Most are ineffective and hence dangerous. Contrary to what some people believe, there is no universal antidote. Preparations recommended for this purpose in the past have consisted of activated charcoal, tannic acid, and magnesium oxide. While activated charcoal can be helpful, tannic acid and magnesium oxide are worthless and may interfere with the activated charcoal's action.

The only two useful antidotes to keep in the house are syrup of ipecac and activated charcoal.

Activated Charcoal Alone, Might Be Better

Several scientific studies suggest that activated charcoal by itself may be better than syrup of ipecac followed by the charcoal. In one clinical study in young children, emergency-room pediatricians at Children's Hospital of Buffalo, N.Y., found that mild-to-moderately poisoned youngsters given only the charcoal received this remedy an hour and a half sooner than children who were started on ipecac (*Annals of Emergency Medicine*, vol. 20, pp. 648-51, 1991). The charcoal-only children had an easier time in the emergency room and were sent home sooner. So the pediatricians say young, awake patients treated in emergency rooms should be given activated charcoal *first*, without prior syrup of ipecac.

Claims

Accurate for Syrup of Ipecac
• "For emergency use to cause vomiting of swallowed poisons"

Accurate for Activated Charcoal
• "For emergency use to adsorb swallowed poisons"

WARNING:

 Before using, call a physician, poison control center or other emergency medical facility or health professional for advice, if you can reach them. Do not give either of these preparations to a person who is not fully conscious.

APPROVED ANTIDOTES

• *IPECAC SYRUP:* This is the *first* antidote to use (*see* previously, under Steps To Take in Case of Poisoning). Ipecac is prepared from a powder obtained from the plant *Cephaelis ipecacuanha*, where it gets its unusual name. Its only recommended use is as an antidote in poisoning, and it has been shown to be safe and effective for this purpose. Ipecac acts on the vomiting center in the brain and also by directly irritating the lining of the gastrointestinal tract, according to FDA.

   The recommended dose for children 6 months to 1 year of age is 1 teaspoon (5 ml), followed by ½ to 1 glass of water. For children ages 1 to 12, the dose is 1 tablespoon (15 ml) followed by 1 to 2 glasses of water or other clear liquid—but *not* milk. If vomiting does not occur within 30 minutes, repeat the dosage *once*. Do not give a third dose: Seek emergency medical help.

   For older children and for adults, the FDA recommends a dose of 2 tablespoons (30 ml) followed by 1 to 2 glasses of water (8 to 16 ounces). If vomiting does not occur within 30 minutes, the initial dose can be repeated *once*. Do not give a third dose.

• *CHARCOAL, ACTIVATED:* This substance should only be taken *after* ipecac has been given and *after* vomiting has occurred. Otherwise, it will interfere with the ipecac's ability to stimulate vomiting. Strictly speaking, activated charcoal is not an antidote; that is, it does not act specifically against any poison or group of poisons. Rather, it acts by binding to, holding, and thus neutralizing many poisons—a pharmacological and chemical property called *adsorption.*

Activated charcoal's enormous adsorptive capacity comes in large part from its highly porous, honeycomb-like internal structure. It is here that poisonous particles become stuck and entrapped. Unbelievable as it may seem, the internal surface area of a standard 1-ounce (30 gram) dose of activated charcoal is 300,000 square feet—the equivalent of a square that is 500 feet on a side.

Many tests in animals and long clinical use in humans have demonstrated that activated charcoal is safe. Its binding and neutralizing functions have been demonstrated in the laboratory, in hospital emergency rooms, and through the follow-up of poisoning victims who were treated at home. It will not adsorb all poisons, however, and should be used as advised by your poison control center or other health-care professionals.

Although activated charcoal should not be given in advance of ipecac syrup, except when recommended by a health professional, it works best when it is given within the first half-hour after poisoning, before the poison leaves the stomach and enters the small intestine. Luckily the charcoal *can* catch up with the poisons, and so it can be given later if necessary.

Activated charcoal is a black powder and is unpleasant to take. The Panel recommended that drug makers find an inactive base like carboxymethylcellulose that would make it more palatable. Meanwhile, each 4 to 6 tablespoon (20 to 30 gram) dose should be mixed in a glass of water (8 ounces). This is the usual dose, but the more that the victim can be made to take, the better, so give another full dose immediately if the poisoning victim can and will take it.

CONDITIONALLY APPROVED ANTIDOTES

None.

DISAPPROVED ANTIDOTES

None.

Safety and Effectiveness: Active Ingredients in Over-the-Counter Antidotes for Poisons

Active Ingredient	Assessment
charcoal, activated	safe and effective
ipecac syrup	safe and effective

Ipecac Syrup—Fast Dosage Information

Bottles of syrup of ipecac sold without prescription should contain 30 ml or 2 tablespoons of the drug.

For persons over 12 years of age, 1 dose = 1 bottle

For children aged 1 to 12, 1 dose = ½ bottle

For children 6 months to 1 year, 1 dose = 1 teaspoon of ipecac

For children under 6 months of age, consult a health professional

Poisoning Antidotes: Product Ratings

SINGLE-INGREDIENT PRODUCTS

Product and Distributor	Dosage of Active Ingredients	Rating*	Comment
ipecac syrup			
Ipecac syrup (generic)	**syrup:** 1.5%	A	
charcoal, activated			
Activated charcoal (generic)	**powder:** 15 and 30 g single-dose containers and in larger quantities	A	
Activated charcoal liquid (generic)	**liquid:** 12.5 g in propylene glycol per 60 ml bottle	A	
	liquid: 25 g in propylene glycol per 120 ml bottle	A	
Charcoaid (Requa)	**liquid:** 30 g in 150 ml sweetened suspension	A	

Poisoning Antidotes: Product Ratings (contd)

COMBINATION PRODUCTS

Product and Distributor	Dosage of Active Ingredients	Rating*	Comment
Res-Q (Boyle)	**powder:** 50% activated charcoal + 25% magnesium hydroxide + tannic acid in 15 packets	C	magnesium hydroxide and tannic acid not safe or effective; combination not approved

EMERGENCY ANTIDOTE KITS

Product and Distributor	Dosage of Active Ingredients	Rating*	Comment
Poison Antidote Kit (Bowman)	**package includes:** 1 bottle syrup of ipecac (30 ml) + 4 bottles charcoal suspension (60 ml)	A	

*Author's interpretation of FDA criteria. Based on contents, not claims.

Premature Ejaculation Retardants

Many men reach sexual climax too soon—when the penis first enters the vagina, or even before. This is embarrassing for the man and frustrating for his partner.

Premature ejaculation is caused by a variety of problems, some of which require medical or psychiatric correction. But the Panel that evaluated miscellaneous external self-treatment products believes that their use can be beneficial to many men. These preparations may carry labels that describe them as "cream for relief of premature ejaculation," "desensitizing lubricant for men," "world-famous delay spray for men," or "climax-control spray for men." The active ingredients are topical anesthetics, which act by temporarily diminishing penile sensations. Although some claims made for these products are judged misleading or inappropriate, the Panel decided that the drugs themselves are safe and effective.

PREMATURE EJACULATION RETARDANTS is based on the report "OTC Male Genital Desensitizing Drug Products" by the FDA's Advisory Review Panel on OTC Miscellaneous External Drug Products and on FDA's Tentative Final Monograph on these products.

Claims

Accurate

- "Aids in the prevention of premature ejaculation"
- "For temporary male genital desensitization helping to slow the onset of ejaculation"
- "Aids in temporarily retarding the onset of ejaculation"
- "Aids in temporarily slowing the onset of ejaculation"
- "Aids in temporarily prolonging time until ejaculation"
- "For reducing oversensitivity in the male in advance of intercourse"

False or Misleading

- "Aids in temporarily retarding rapidity of ejaculation or slowing the speed of ejaculation" (the preparation can *delay* ejaculation but not slow it once it has started)
- "To strengthen sexual confidence"
- "Original and unchallenged throughout the world for quality, effectiveness, and satisfaction"

WARNING:

 Premature ejaculation may be due to a condition requiring medical care. If a product, used as directed, does not provide relief, discontinue using it and consult a doctor. If you or your partner develops a rash or irritation, such as burning or itching, discontinue use. If symptoms persist, consult a doctor.

In about 75 percent of men, orgasm occurs about two minutes after entry of the penis into the vagina. But in what the Panel says is a "considerable number" of others, climax is reached in under a minute, or even within 10 or 20 seconds or less. The Panel obtained these statistics from a urological specialist, who pointed out that the condition can usually be attributed to one of three basic causes:

- The penis may be so highly sensitive to sexual stimulation that it starts the ejaculatory response too soon.

- Inflammation of the urethral tissues can serve as an ejaculatory trigger mechanism.

- Psychoneurotic problems can interfere with the individual's sex life.

The same report notes that a man's orgasm may occur within a normal span of time but that his partner may require a much longer time to reach climax — if she does so at all. Pondering this problem, the urologist hit on the idea of delaying the male partner's ejaculation by temporarily desensitizing the penis, using a numbing (anesthetic) drug. He tried this method with his patients, and reported (in 1963) that anesthetic preparations in fact raised the level of resistance to sexual excitation, thereby delaying a man's orgasm.

In a study of 13 men—aged 22 to 39—who complained that they ejaculated prior to or upon insertion of the penis into the vagina, the researcher found that treating the head and shaft of the penis with 3 percent benzocaine cream corrected premature ejaculation in all 13 men. The average time from insertion to orgasm lengthened to a minute and a half. Other studies, described below, have confirmed this initial finding. According to other inconclusive evidence related by the Panel in its report, this use of the anesthetic drug does not desensitize the clitoris or diminish the woman's pleasure.

Drugs Used to Treat Premature Ejaculation

Products marketed to retard ejaculation all contain an anesthetic. They may also contain passion fruit; the Panel lists it as an inactive ingredient.

APPROVED ACTIVE INGREDIENTS

- *BENZOCAINE:* This is a widely used topical anesthetic. Because of its excellent safety record, reviewers assess it as safe for use as a penile anesthetic. Benzocaine's effectiveness was initially suggested by the study described previously. In a larger study with 120 men who had premature ejaculation problems, another investigator reported that 108 benefited: They were able to maintain control over the ejaculatory reflex for 2 minutes or longer when they used a 7.5 percent benzocaine ointment before intercourse; 72 men were able to delay orgasm for 3 minutes or more. Only 8 of the 120 men benefited from using a dummy preparation.

Use of the active drug was reported to please their partners, too; 72 percent of them achieved orgasm when the man used the active drug, compared with only 2.5 percent when the man used an ointment without the benzocaine.

The Panel concluded that benzocaine is safe and effective in concentrations of 3 to 7.5 percent when applied in small amounts to the head and shaft of the penis before intercourse. It should be washed off afterward.

• LIDOCAINE: Another widely used local anesthetic, lidocaine, has a good safety record when used in small amounts. The Panel says it is safe for use on the penis. The studies submitted to demonstrate lidocaine's effectiveness as a penile anesthetic showed that the drug significantly prolonged the time required for men to masturbate to orgasm. Another study showed that it reduced the penis's sensitivity to a variety of stimuli, including pressure, pain, warmth, cold, and mechanical vibrations. The Panel said that these results show lidocaine's ability to retard the onset of ejaculation, and they assessed it safe and effective for that purpose. The approved concentration is 9.6 percent lidocaine in an aerosol spray dispensed from a dose-metered container that delivers measured amounts of about 10 milligrams of lidocaine. The Panel said that a nonmetered spray container is unsafe because the amount of anesthetic applied is not measured.

CONDITIONALLY APPROVED ACTIVE INGREDIENTS
None.

DISAPPROVED ACTIVE INGREDIENTS
None.

Safety and Effectiveness: Active Ingredients in Over-the-Counter Premature Ejaculation Retardants

Active Ingredient	Assessment
benzocaine	safe and effective
lidocaine	safe and effective

Premature Ejaculation Retardants: Product Ratings

Product and Distributor	Dosage of Active Ingredients	Rating*	Comment
Benzocaine Topical (generic)	cream: 5%	A	
Detane (Commerce)	gel: 7.5% benzocaine	A	
Stud 100 (Pound)	spray: lidocaine 9.6%	A	this is a sex shop item; it may also be available in drug stores

*Author's interpretation of FDA criteria. Based on contents, not claims.

Psoriasis Lotions

Sufferers of psoriasis usually are well aware of their problem *and* its name. This intensely itchy and often unsightly skin disorder may wax and wane, but once present it usually remains for a lifetime.

Severe psoriasis is a demoralizing, occasionally life-threatening ailment that requires medical management. Mild cases may fall more into the nuisance category. It is this latter group that may be appropriate for self-treatment with nonprescription drugs. The Panel that evaluated nonprescription products used for psoriasis finds that only two types of drugs—coal-tar preparations and salicylic acid—are safe and effective for relieving the itching, inflammation, and scaling that occur in these mild cases. The FDA concurs with this judgment and tentatively lists hydrocortisone and hydrocortisone acetate as safe and effective as well.

PSORIASIS LOTIONS is based on the report "Dandruff, Seborrheic Dermatitis, Psoriasis Control Drug Products," by the FDA's Advisory Review Panel on OTC Miscellaneous External Drug Products and on FDA's Tentative Final and Final Monographs on these products.

Claims

Accurate

• "For the relief of psoriasis"

• "Controls the itching, redness, irritation and scaling associated with the symptoms of psoriasis on the skin"

WARNING:

 If psoriasis covers a large area of the body, consult your doctor before attempting self-treatment. If the condition worsens or fails to improve after several days, a physician should be seen. These drugs should not be used in or around the rectum or in the genital area or the groin except on the advice of a physician.

Pink Patches and Silvery Scales

Psoriasis is a chronic inflammatory disease that afflicts several million Americans. The cause is unknown. The disease is characterized by sharply demarcated pink or dull red splotches on the skin that are covered with tiny silvery scales. These lesions may come and go or they may be continually present.

In persons with psoriasis, the outer layer of the skin (the epidermis) turns over extremely rapidly. Skin cells may take only three or four days to grow, mature, and die. This is 10 to 20 times faster than the normal turnover rate, which is 25 to 30 days.

The plaques of psoriasis may appear on the scalp or on virtually any other body surface; common sites are the elbows and knees. These plaques are particularly likely to develop at the site of a cut, burn, sunburn, or pre-existing rash. Emotional stress can also bring on these distressing eruptions. Pregnancy, on the other hand, may bring dramatic remissions.

Nonprescription Drugs Used for Psoriasis

The drugs that have been formulated into body lotions, shampoos, and other over-the-counter preparations for treating psoriasis fall into several classes. They include *cytostatic agents*, which retard skin-cell growth; *keratolytic agents*, which loosen and dissolve scales; *tar preparations*, whose mode of action is uncertain; *hydrocortisone preparations*, which reduce itching and inflammation; and others (*See* DANDRUFF AND SEBORRHEIC-SCALE SHAMPOOS to learn more about these various kinds of drugs.) The FDA still is mulling over hydrocortisone's suitability as a nonprescription drug for treating psoriasis—but for the moment lists it as safe and effective. The FDA has rejected—and banned—all other over-the-counter drugs sold for this purpose save the three described here.

APPROVED ACTIVE INGREDIENTS

• COAL-TAR LOTIONS AND SHAMPOOS: These tar preparations, derived from coal and petroleum products, are assessed as safe when formulated as shampoos for twice-weekly application to the scalp or as lotions, creams, and ointments that are intended to leave a residue of tar on the skin. Tars have been used for a long time to treat psoriasis and other skin conditions. But there have been few double-blind studies in which coal tar by itself was tested against the base in which it was formulated (the kind of testing the Panel preferred).

In one such study, however, 7.5 percent coal-tar solution with 1.5 percent menthol, formulated as a shampoo, proved to be superior to the shampoo alone after a month of regular use. The redness, itching, and scaling were measurably reduced in participants who used the medicated product. Basing their judgment on this and a few other studies, the reviewers list coal-tar shampoos as safe and effective for twice-weekly use to relieve scalp psoriasis.

Coal-tar lotions are intended to be applied to the body once or twice daily to relieve itching and other distress of psoriasis.

While several fairly convincing scientific studies suggest that these lotions effectively relieve psoriatic itching and inflammation, there was a lingering fear among Panel members that continued use of coal-tar products might eventually lead to skin cancer. The FDA therefore studied the world scientific literature on coal tar and cancer and as a result discounted this risk. Its verdict: 0.5 to 5 percent coal tar is safe and effective when used as directed.

The approved dosages are: 0.5 to 5 percent coal tar or its equivalent in other coal-tar preparations.

The Panel warns that coal-tar products may make the skin

hypersensitive to sunlight. Try to stay out of bright, direct sun for a day following its application.

• *HYDROCORTISONE PREPARATIONS: HYDROCORTISONE AND HYDROCORTISONE ACETATE:* These potent anti-inflammatory agents have excellent safety records, and are widely used to relieve itching and discomfort of psoriasis. The FDA has not said its final word on the preparations' suitability in concentrations up to 1 percent for this purpose. But the agency's interim ruling is: safe and effective.

• *SALICYLIC ACID:* This is a keratolytic (skin-peeling) agent that is widely used to treat skin disorders. The Panel has assessed it as safe. Evaluators were not presented with results from any scientifically controlled, double-blind study of salicylic acid used by itself as a psoriasis treatment. (It may have seen—but does not describe any—studies in which the drug was used in combination with other ingredients to treat this condition.) Nevertheless, salicylic acid in concentrations of 1.8 to 3 percent was judged safe and effective for controlling psoriasis of the body and scalp.

CONDITIONALLY APPROVED ACTIVE INGREDIENTS
None.

DISAPPROVED ACTIVE INGREDIENTS
None.

When Further Relief Is Needed

Dermatologists do not know how to cure psoriasis. But they have developed several effective methods to control its symptoms. One method is exposure of the skin to a light-sensitizing agent, *methoxsalen*, followed by long-wave ultraviolet light. A wide variety of other (R) drugs, including corticosteroids and methotrexate also can be quite helpful.

Safety and Effectiveness: Active Ingredients in Over-the-Counter Psoriasis Drugs

Active Ingredient	Assessment
coal tar (0.5-5%)	safe and effective
hydrocortisone (0.25 to 1%)	safe and effective
salicylic acid (1.8-3%)	safe and effective

Psoriasis Lotions: Product Ratings*

Product and Distributor	Dosage of Active Ingredients	Rating†	Comment
coal-tar shampoos			
See pp. 264-267, Product Ratings in DANDRUFF AND SEBORRHEIC-SCALE SHAMPOOS			
coal-tar body lotions and bath preparations			
Aqua Tar (Allergan Herbert)	**gel:** 2.5% coal tar extract	A	
Balnetar (Westwood)	**bath additive:** 2.5% coal tar	A	
Coal tar or carbonis detergens (generic)	**solution:** 20% coal tar	A	safe if diluted in bath water
Neutrogena T/Derm Tar Emollient (Neutrogena)	**ointment:** 5% coal tar extract	A	
PsoriGel (Owen/Galderma)	**gel:** 7.5% coal tar solution	A	
Tarlene (Medco Labs.)	**lotion:** 2% refined coal tar + 2.5% salicylic acid	C	combination of coal tar and salicylic acid not approved
Tegrin for Psoriasis (Reedco)	**cream, soap, lotion:** 5% coal tar solution	A	
salicylic acid			
P & S (Baker Cummins)	**shampoo:** 2%	A	

Salicylic Acid (Stiefel)   soap: 3.5%   A

---

*For hydrocortisone preparations, *see* ratings on pages 571-572 . But note: hydrocortisone preparations are not proved safe and effective for nonprescription use to relieve psoriasis. The FDA is studying this use of these drugs.
†Author's interpretation of FDA criteria. Based on contents, not claims.

Quinine for Leg Cramps

As people get older they sometimes are awakened during the night by *cramps*—pain—in the legs. These nocturnal leg cramps may occur only rarely, or quite frequently, and they may vary, too, in severity. They can be quite distressing.

The cause can be difficult to find. In some people, poor blood flow in the legs may deprive muscles of the oxygen they need to function. This oxygen reduction will cause painful muscle spasm—cramps. In other people, the breakdown products of muscle metabolism, particularly lactic acid, can build up in the muscles and adjacent tissues. This also is painful. (Runners' cramps, too, may be due to lactic acid buildup.)

Another possible cause of cramps, when you are lying down trying to sleep at night, is the expansion of veins in the legs. These veins may fill with blood from the capillary circulation more rapidly than they can return the blood to the heart. The pressure in the over-filled veins causes the crampy pain.

QUININE FOR LEG CRAMPS is based on the report "Quinine for the Treatment of Nocturnal Leg Muscle Cramps for OTC Human Use" by the FDA's Advisory Review Panel on Miscellaneous Internal Drugs and on the FDA's Tentative Final Monograph on these products.

There are other causes for leg cramps as well. If you continue to be bothered by them, your best recourse is to see a doctor.

Youngsters often suffer cramps at night during growth spurts; these are commonly called "growing pains." Warm soaks in the tub will relieve them temporarily, and eventually they should go away.

WARNING:

 The discussion here is restricted to cramps in middle-aged and older persons; the drugs used to relieve them may be *dangerous* for children and should not be used to treat their leg pains.

One drug, quinine, has been used successfully by doctors for many years to prevent and relieve leg cramps. A second drug, vitamin E, also is used sometimes, albeit the FDA says there is virtually no scientific evidence to support this use. Both drugs have only qualified approval, pending scientific studies that persuade the FDA that they are safe and effective.

APPROVED ACTIVE INGREDIENTS
None.

CONDITIONALLY APPROVED ACTIVE INGREDIENTS
There are two conditionally approved drugs for the prevention and relief of nocturnal leg muscle cramps.
* QUININE SULFATE: This is the legendary bitter drug, derived from the bark of the tropical cinchona tree. It made its fame in the Far East where it was—and still is—taken to kill malarial parasites and so relieve the debilitating fever-and-chills disease *malaria*.

But note: Malaria should never be self-treated. The disease requires the medical care of a tropical medicine specialist, who may or may not recommend quinine.

British colonial officers mixed their daily quinine ration with gin to improve its taste and, of course, their own dispositions. Eventually, they came to enjoy the bitter taste—from whence came the mixed drink *gin and tonic*, the tonic being quinine water. A can of the carbonated quinine-water tonic sold in the United States today in grocery stores for mixed drinks contains a fraction of the dose—perhaps 5 to 10 percent— of the amount used to treat malaria and nocturnal leg cramps. Quinine reduces pain and relaxes muscles, which may be why it relieves leg cramps. But nobody knows for sure.

Many doctors think quinine is effective, based on reports from their patients. But the scientific evidence to back this belief is extremely thin. Unless manufacturers, or others, produce such evidence soon, the FDA says it will ban quinine as an OTC drug for leg cramps.

Quinine has a high incidence of side effects. It can cause ringing in the ears, headache, nausea, vomiting, and disturbances in vision. Even tiny amounts of quinine—the quantity in a gin and tonic—can cause life-threatening symptoms in highly susceptible individuals; the heart, kidneys, optic nerves, and other organs may be significantly damaged. Quinine can also induce abortions, and damage the fetus, and so should never be used by pregnant women.

• **VITAMIN E:** People taking this vitamin for other purposes noticed a reduction in the incidence and severity of nocturnal leg muscle cramps. Some began taking it for this reason—and reported good results. But there is absolutely no scientific evidence to support this use of vitamin E as a drug for leg cramps.

DISAPPROVED ACTIVE INGREDIENTS
None.

Combination Products

Some leg-cramp remedies contain both quinine sulfate and vitamin E. The FDA demands stringent proof that these combinations are more effective than either single ingredient. So far, it is not in evidence.

When Greater Relief Is Needed

Quinine can be administered as a prescription drug, under a doctor's supervision, in higher doses than would be safe for self-treatment. But persistent and severe leg cramps should not be treated symptomatically. A medical workup may identify a specific, treatable cause for the problem, for example, narrowing of blood vessels in the legs that can be treated effectively with a vasodilating drug.

Safety and Effectiveness: Active Ingredients in Over-the-Counter Drugs to Prevent and Relieve Nocturnal Leg Muscle Cramps

Active Ingredient	Assessment
quinine sulfate	not proved safe or effective
vitamin E	not proved safe or effective

Nighttime Leg Muscle Cramp Relief and Prevention: Product Ratings

SINGLE-INGREDIENT PRODUCTS

Product and Distributor	Dosage of Active Ingredient	Rating*	Comment
quinine sulfate			
Quinine sulfate (generic)	capsules: 200 mg	B	not proved safe or effective
	tablets: 260 mg	B	not proved safe or effective
	capsules: 325 mg	B	not proved safe or effective
Quinine sulfate (Major)	capsules: 300 mg	B	not proved safe or effective

COMBINATION PRODUCTS

Product and Distributor	Dosage of Active Ingredients	Rating*	Comment
Formula Q (Major)	capsules: 65 mg quinine sulfate + 400 IU vitamin E	C	quinine not proved safe and effective; vitamin is of doubtful value
M-KYA (Nature's Bounty)	capsules: 64.8 mg quinine sulfate + 400 IU vitamin E + lecithin	C	FDA dismisses lecithin out of hand
Q-vel Soft Caplets (Ciba)		C	FDA dismisses lecithin out of hand

*Author's interpretation of FDA criteria. Based on contents, not claims.

Reducing Aids

The 17 Review Panels made tens of thousands of decisions about the safety and effectiveness of ingredients in the quarter-million over-the-counter drug products sold in the United States. But of all these decisions, the most controversial is the vote to list the drug phenyl-propanolamine hydrochloride (PPA) as safe and effective as a reducing aid.

This endorsement of PPA triggered a major marketing effort that quickly helped boost sales to $141 million last year, according to industry sources. The Panel's approval also set off a sharp backlash among medical colleagues and other health authorities, who charge that PPA is a fad and a fraud—and dangerous to boot.

Officials at the FDA were disquieted by the Panel's decision on PPA. The agency has demanded further safety testing and has already cut back the Panel's recommended dosages.

The reasons for the Panel's approval of PPA are not altogether clear. Members perhaps felt that the wide public constituency for

---

REDUCING AIDS is based on the report "Weight-Control Drug Products for OTC Human Use" by the FDA's Advisory Review Panel on OTC Miscellaneous Internal Drug Products and on the FDA's Final Rule on most of the active ingredients used in these products.

agents to combat overweight was entitled to *some* help in the over-the-counter marketplace. But the reviewers conceded that the studies upon which they based their approval were flawed as well as unpublished. It certainly seems reasonable to want far better evidence to support a drug that is taken for weeks at a time by millions of people, many of them women of childbearing age.

 Claims

Accurate
- "For appetite control to aid weight reduction"
- "Helps curb appetite"
- "Appetite depressant in the treatment of obesity"
- "An aid in the control of appetite"
- "For use as an adjunct to diet control"

Unproved
- "Provides bulk to add to low caloric intake and helps to satisfy the feeling of hunger caused by emptiness"
- "Contains one of the most powerful diet aids available without prescription"
- "Easy-to-follow reducing plan built around food you love to eat. You will eat well but less and lose weight without going hungry"
- "The modern aid to appetite control"
- "Now enjoy a slim, trim figure. Lose pounds. Reduce inches"
- "Lose weight starting today . . . . Look your best, feel your best!"
- "The delightful aid to appetite control"
- "Delightfully delicious, scientifically formulated to help you control your appetite quickly, pleasantly"
- "Trim pounds and inches without crash diets or strenuous exercise"
- "Get rid of unsightly bulges"

WARNING:

 These products should not be used for longer than 3 months. They should not be given to children under 12 years old, since there is no evidence to show they are safe and effective for youngsters.

Appetite Suppressants

Many Americans *are* fat and many others *fear* that they are. And we all face a world in which thinness is prized. Little wonder then that there is tremendous demand for new and better ways to lose weight—for a miracle drug that has yet to be developed!

The Panel said that over-the-counter reducing aids (anorexiants) have a real—if brief—therapeutic role to play in helping people lose weight. These drugs can help you eat less and may contribute to the development of a long-standing self-commitment to staying in negative caloric balance: that is, to burn more calories than you consume. However, the experts stress that these preparations must be used only temporarily, and never longer than 3 months, which may be time enough to develop spare, new eating habits.

An enormous range of drugs and other substances claimed by manufacturers to have medicinal benefit has been formulated into weight-loss products. Some have no pharmacological activity at all, and many others were dismissed out-of-hand by the Panel for want of any shred of evidence that suggests they may be helpful. Of the multitude, reviewers winnowed out a dozen drugs that have at least promise of benefit. They further decided that two of them, PPA and benzocaine, are safe and effective. FDA has now banned all but these two, upon which its judgment is pending.

Combination Products

The evaluators took a dim view of combination diet products. None were approved.

Guar Gum Can Be Deadly

One ingredient the FDA may have waited too long to ban is *guar gum*. This is a soluble fiber, like cellulose, that is used—safely—in low concentrations as an additive to thicken food products. In more concentrated doses, it long was sold as a weight-loss ingredient. Guar gum was claimed to create a full feeling in the stomach and so allegedly reduced hunger so that users consumed less food.

The FDA never was convinced that guar gum is effective. But it delayed acting on it for years, while the OTC Review ground slowly forward. Then, in the late 1980s, reports began to be published of consumers suffering obstruction of the esophagus (food pipe) after taking over-the-counter weight-control products containing the gum. The FDA then said "Ten of the cases of esophageal obstruction required hospitalization, and one person eventually died as an indirect result of the obstruction. [This person developed] massive [blood clots in the lungs] one week after open-chest surgery to repair an esophageal tear sustained during the removal of the guar gum obstruction."

The FDA *still* was procrastinating when problems with a guar gum product were described at a hearing held by the House Subcommittee on Regulation, Business Opportunity, and Energy, chaired by Rep. Ron Wyden (Dem.-Ore.). CBS-TV ran an expose on its *Inside Edition*. Meanwhile, the U.S. Postal Service and some local governmental agencies acted to restrict promotion and distribution of the product.

Finally, in 1990, the FDA ruled that guar gum is not safe and not effective as a nonprescription weight-loss medication. The agency banned it in 1991. Nevertheless, it may still be sold.

Whether they find it being sold as a medication, or as health food, or under some other guise, consumers should carefully avoid products containing guar gum in concentrations greater than the 2 to 3 percent permitted in food products.

Weight-Reducing Ingredients

Only two ingredients were evaluated as safe and effective for nonprescription sales and self-medication for weight loss. These drugs both have problems, and could still be ruled off the market.

APPROVED ACTIVE INGREDIENTS

• **BENZOCAINE:** This is a widely used anesthetic with an excellent safety record. The Panel lists it as safe. We eat partly because we like the taste of our food. Benzocaine acts as an appetite suppressant by temporarily deadening the taste receptors in the mouth, dulling our pleasure. It particularly interferes with our ability to detect varying degrees of sweetness. The Panel reviewed several studies that suggest that benzocaine can help a person lose weight, but did not indicate if the studies were controlled or not controlled nor how they were conducted. The Panel also neglected to say how quickly appetite returns when the benzocaine wears off. Nevertheless, in a conclusion based on this seemingly meager record, the Panel said 3 to 15 mg of benzocaine in chewing gum or candy, used just before eating, is safe and effective for weight control.

• **PHENYLPROPANOLAMINE HYDROCHLORIDE (PPA):** This drug's therapeutic activity is similar to that of the *amphetamines*, a class of prescription drugs that have long been used as dieting aids, but which have a high potential for abuse and dependence because of the "highs" they produce. Although PPA may be free of this addictive risk, the Panel does say that even low doses can be expected to tighten blood vessels and speed up the heart rate, which will elevate blood pressure. Large doses may cause anxiety, excitement, sleeplessness, headache, irregular heartbeat, convulsions, and circulatory distress.

Despite these hazards, the Panel said that in manufacturers' recommended doses of 25 to 50 mg before meals, PPA has low toxicity and can be safely used without professional supervision. Of course, because of PPA's stimulating effect on the body, persons with high blood pressure, heart disease, diabetes, or thyroid disease should ask their doctor's advice before they use the drug.

The question of how PPA acts to reduce appetite remains unanswered. But work it does, the Panel said, at least temporarily. The Panel cited double-blind, placebo-controlled investigations show the drug's effectiveness, but it concedes that these studies were flawed and may be criticized for improper study design that has resulted in "confusing or contradictory findings." Some studies are inconclusive. Nonetheless, the evaluators said that they adequately establish PPA's ability to facilitate weight loss over short periods, of 4 to 6 weeks. One study shows that the active drug is better than dummy medication for up to 16 weeks. So the Panel considered the available data adequate to establish PPA's effectiveness for periods of up to 12 weeks, in dosages up to 150 mg daily, divided into 25 to 50 mg doses before meals.

The reviewers did not say how many people were studied, what percentage lost weight, or how much was lost. All these questions seem highly relevant when one considers the virtually simultaneous assessment by the American Medical Association's Department of Drugs. This professional group maintained that products containing PPA—with or without caffeine—"are only minimally effective" (AMA Drug Evaluations, 4th ed., 1980).

In a more recent (1991) edition, the AMA said that if someone is participating in a comprehensive weight management program that includes diet, exercise, and behavioral modification, then adding PPA to the regimen can add an additional half pound a week to the weight that is lost. But, the AMA evaluators noted, PPA's "effectiveness for longer than three months has not been studied."

The Panel's approval of PPA proved to be a fast-acting stimulant to the diet-aid business. The leading U.S. manufacturer, Thompson Medical Company, promised druggists $21 million in advertising to launch what it called a "gigantic growth in diet-aid sales" that aimed at exceeding $300 million dollars per year. As sales rose, so did adverse-reaction reports. Particularly worrisome to the FDA was a report from Australia, published in The Lancet (January 12, 1980), about tests in which a single 85-mg dose of PPA was given to normal, healthy medical students in their twenties. The capsule pushed the blood pressure up in one-third of them; 3 of the 37 subjects required anti-hypertensive medication. The Australian investigators concluded that the high-dose PPA capsules are potentially hazardous.

The FDA reacted by noting that, based on the Panel's recommendations, U.S. drug companies were selling higher-dosage units of PPA than it had formally approved. The agency said the maximum dosage it would sanction is 75 mg daily, not the 150 mg that the Panel had recommended. It set a limit of 37.5 mg for ordinary, immediate-release tablets or capsules and 75 mg for sustained-release PPA capsules.

Reporter Joseph Carey meanwhile searched out the studies upon which the Panel based its approval of PPA. He noted in New York's *Daily News* (February 2, 1981) that one study, conducted by a Philadelphia internist, was funded by Thompson Medical (which, in fact, is how most drug studies are done). In the test, 35 subjects were given PPA plus caffeine, and 35 were given dummy drugs. Of the participants who took the active drug, 50 percent lost 6 or more pounds; only 22 percent of those who took the dummy drug lost this much. Of those who took the active drug, 35 percent lost 8 or more pounds while only 9 percent of those on the dummy drug achieved this result.

But after considering all the published evidence on PPA, a number of medical authorities came to conclusions quite at odds with the Panel's. The well-regarded *Medical Letter on Drugs and Therapeutics* (vol. 21, no. 16) declared: "There is no good evidence that PPA . . . can help obese patients achieve long-term weight reduction." An editorial in the *Journal of the American Medical Association* (vol. 245, no. 13) said: "Clearly, the use of PPA poses a danger to the public."

When the FDA published the Panel's report approving PPA, it expressed strong doubts about the drug's safety but did not override the Panel's decision that it is safe and effective. The agency did insist, however, that "further studies" be conducted "to resolve the safety questions" and promised to monitor dieters' use of the drug with the eye to "immediate...regulatory action" if new evidence of risk were to warrant it. The agency noted, too, that sustained-release capsules and tablets that contain more PPA than immediate-action capsules must be proved safe and effective under the stringent guidelines that apply to all new drugs.

Ten years have passed since the Panel made its decision approving PPA as safe and effective. The FDA, having spoken its doubts, seems to be taking an inordinately long time to make up its regulatory mind about a drug that continues to be used by millions of Americans. Prodded by Congressman Ron Wyden (Dem.-Ore.), drug analyst Carl Peck, M.D., who is director of FDA's Center for Drug Evaluation and Research, promised an agency decision on phenylpropanolamine hydrochloride as a reducing aid by the end of 1992.

The approved daily dosage for phenylpropanolamine now is 75 mg, divided into 2 or 3 smaller doses or as a single sustained release capsule.

WARNING:

 For phenylpropanolamine hydrochloride (PPA): Do not exceed the recommended dosage. If nervousness, dizziness, or sleeplessness occurs, stop the medication and consult your physician. If you are being treated for high blood pressure or depression, or have heart disease, diabetes, or thyroid disease, do not take this product except under the supervision of a physician.

CONDITIONALLY APPROVED ACTIVE INGREDIENTS
None.

DISAPPROVED ACTIVE INGREDIENTS
None.

When Further Help Is Needed

Tens of millions of American men and women want desperately to lose weight. There are no easy ways, and the value of drugs—whether nonprescription or prescription (R)—is extremely limited: They are not very helpful, and the more potent they are, as a rule, the more dangerous they can be.

The two keystones for people who are moderately overweight, and wish to lose weight, are to burn more calories through exercise and to consume fewer calories through dieting. A person can be helped along this difficult path by Weight Watchers and similar self-help groups.

A person who is significantly overweight ought to see a reputable endocrinologist or other internist at a teaching hospital associated with a medical school. Flashy "fat doctors" who make grandiose promises (which are likely to be costly, and which they probably cannot fulfill) should be avoided. In some cases reputable and conservative physicians can diagnose a hormonal dysfunction or other factor, which may be correctable, to explain why a person is overweight. In some cases, they may be able to recommend effective medical or even surgical treatment to relieve the problem.

There are, however, few magic bullets. A careful and conservative diet program and an enjoyable exercise program that you can sustain through months and years are two of the best measures for controlling weight—and helping you *feel* better.

Safety and Effectiveness: Ingredients in Over-the-Counter Reducing Aids

Active Ingredient	Assessment
benzocaine	safe and effective
phenylpropanolamine hydrochloride (PPA)	safe and effective

Safety and Effectiveness: Combination Products Sold Over-the-Counter as Reducing Aids

Safe and Effective
  None

Conditionally Safe and Effective
  None

Not Safe or Effective
  contains active ingredient at more or less than approved dosage(s)
  contains any active ingredient disapproved as unsafe or ineffective

Reducing Aids: Product Ratings

SINGLE-INGREDIENT PRODUCTS

Product and Distributor	Dosage of Active Ingredients	Rating*	Comment
benzocaine			
Diet Ayds (DEP Corp.)	candy: 6 mg	A	
Slim Mint Gum (Thompson)	chewing gum: 6 mg	A	
phenylpropanolamine hydrochloride (PPA)			
Acutrim 16 Hour (Ciba)	steady-release tablet: 75 mg	A	
Acutrim II, Maximum Strength (Ciba)	timed-release tablets: 75 mg	A	
Control (Thompson)	timed-release capsules: 75 mg	A	
Dexatrim Pre-Meal (Thompson)	timed-release capsules: 25 mg	A	
Maximum Strength Dex-A-Diet Caplets (O'Connor)	timed-release tablets: 75 mg	A	
Maximum Strength Dexatrim (Thompson)	timed-release tablets: 75 mg	A	
Phenoxine (Lannett)	tablets: 25 mg	A	

COMBINATION PRODUCTS

Product and Distributor	Dosage of Active Ingredients	Rating*	Comment
Dieutrim T.D. (Legere)	**timed release capsules:** 75 mg phenylpropanolamine hydrochloride + 9 mg benzocaine + 75 mg sodium carboxymethylcellulose	C	the first two ingredients are okay, but this is not an approved, or even conditionally approved, combination
Pretts Diet-Aid (MiLance)	**chewable tablets:** 200 mg alginic acid + 100 mg sodium carboxymethylcellulose + 70 mg sodium bicarbonate	C	none of these is approved as a diet aid; the combination is not approved

Note: Phenylpropanolamine is often combined with citrus extract, fiber, vitamins and other nutrients. The FDA does not recognize any of these add-ons as adding anything to the medicinal value of the phenylpropanolamine.

---

*Author's interpretation of FDA criteria. Based on contents, not claims.

Salt Supplements and Substitutes: Preliminary Report

People who sweat a lot, either because they are working (or playing) very hard or because they are exposed to heat, often take salt tablets to counteract the loss of body salt.

These salt supplements and salt substitutes were to have been evaluated by the Advisory Review Panel on OTC Miscellaneous Internal Drugs, but the group was disbanded before the review could be completed. The FDA or a supplemental panel may someday complete this task, but a decade has passed since the Panel disbanded. Meanwhile, persons on sodium-restricted diets should ask their doctors whether they can use salt substitutes and how much they can use. Many older persons, particularly those who have kidney or heart ailments, must shun table salt (sodium chloride) and they may be advised to use potassium chloride or potassium iodide instead.

Your family doctor or a sports-medicine specialist may be able

---

SALT SUPPLEMENTS AND SUBSTITUTES: PRELIMINARY REPORT is based on an FDA study report on the OTC Drug Review.

to enlighten you on the value of taking salt pills when you are hot and sweating. *Drinking a lot of water* and other fluids may be at least as important as replacing the salt.

Sleep Aids

From time to time, many people have difficulty falling asleep or staying asleep. Therefore, both the FDA and the Panel see a valid need for safe and effective nonprescription medication to induce and sustain sleep.

 Claims

Accurate
For adults only, the FDA says the only claims that can legitimately be made for a safe and effective over-the-counter sleep aid are:

- "Helps [you] fall asleep if you have difficulty falling asleep"

- "For relief of occasional sleeplessness"

SLEEP AIDS is based on the report of the FDA's Advisory Review Panel on OTC Sedative, Tranquilizer, and Sleep-Aid Drug Products; the FDA's Tentative Final and Final Orders for OTC Nighttime Sleep-Aid and Stimulant Products; the Final Order on OTC Daytime Sedatives; and official addenda in the OTC Drug Review.

- "Reduces [the] time to fall asleep if you have difficulty falling asleep"

Benefits and Risks

The principal active ingredients in sleep aids have been drugs of the class called *antihistamines*. They make many people drowsy. How they achieve this is not clear. It *is* known that antihistamines depress the activity of the central nervous system; this may in part explain how they act.

A nonprescription drug that induces drowsiness and sleep can be useful and convenient. Unfortunately, however, the Panel's assessment is that most active ingredients that had been used in sleep aids were unsafe, ineffective, or both and that many of the claims made for these products were false and misleading. The FDA, by and large, agreed and proposed severe restrictions in the ingredients and in the claims that could be made for such preparations. However, the FDA subsequently granted its approval to three antihistamines as sleep-aid active ingredients. The approved ingredients are doxylamine succinate, diphenhydramine hydrochloride, and diphenhydramine citrate.

When to Consider Sleep Aids

Brain-wave recordings made while subjects are asleep in a sleep laboratory have become the principal means that scientists use to study normal sleep and its disturbances. The recordings show the exact moment that a subject falls asleep and then the minute-by-minute progression through now well-recognized sleep stages. Most people go through essentially the same sequences, although there is considerable variation in sleep patterns from person to person.

The effectiveness of over-the-counter sleep aids can be determined in part by users' subjective reports or by trained observers who watch them sleep. But all-night sleep recordings made in sleep laboratories are preferable: They are the most objective method for assessing the action of these drugs. Such action should not seriously interfere with the behavioral and brain-wave patterns of normal sleep, the Panel warns. Neither should the drug's effects persist into the following day to interfere with normal daytime tasks.

A person's normal sleep patterns tend to be similar night after night. An occasional sleep disturbance is valid reason for buying and using an over-the-counter sleep aid, the Panel says. The medication can be expected to help one fall asleep, or remain sleeping, if the problem is untimely awakenings at night or early in the morning. But a sleep-aid should not be used longer than 2 weeks. Persons with severe or continuing insomnia should consult a doctor, who can offer more potent remedies.

Sleep aids specifically depress brain activity. So the FDA warns that they may act additively, and prove to be particularly hazardous for persons drinking alcoholic beverages, which have a similar depressant effect.

Antihistamines used in sleep aids also have the effect of reducing fluid secretions throughout the body. This can be particularly dangerous to persons with asthma or glaucoma and to men with enlarged prostate glands. Such individuals therefore should avoid taking sleep aids except under the advice and supervision of a physician. These preparations are also inappropriate for children under 12 years of age, whom they may *stimulate* rather than sedate!

Antihistamines

Antihistamines, as their name implies, block the action of the body protein *histamine*, which triggers runny nose, watery eyes, and a variety of other allergic symptoms. These drugs were introduced in the 1940s and are widely used for allergic relief. (*See* ALLERGY DRUGS.)

It soon was discovered that sedation is one of the principal side effects of antihistamines. Antihistamines may produce an inability to concentrate, dizziness, loss of coordination, and drowsiness.

This sedative effect was soon recognized as a hazard: Antihistamine users are routinely warned not to drive, operate heavy machinery, or do other jobs that require mental alertness while they are taking these drugs. On the other hand, pharmacologists recognized that this soporific side effect might also be used to advantage. Antihistamines began to be formulated into sleep-aid products, which quickly became quite popular. Now, more than 10 million Americans use antihistamine-based sleep aids.

Different chemical groups of antihistamines have different sedative effects; the most pronounced are in a group of potent antihistamines called *ethanolamines*. This group includes diphenhydramine hydrochloride, diphenhydramine citrate, and doxylamine succinate—the three antihistamines recently approved by the FDA as safe and effective.

Common side effects of antihistamines include:

> dizziness
>
> ringing in the ears
>
> lassitude
>
> fatigue
>
> blurred or double vision
>
> mood changes (e.g., euphoria, anxiety, disorientation, confusion, and even delirium)

Some other side effects are:

> loss of appetite
>
> nausea
>
> vomiting
>
> both constipation and diarrhea
>
> dry mouth
>
> heart palpitations and irregularities in heart rate or rhythm
>
> frequency or difficulty in urination
>
> skin rashes
>
> rare but serious events (e.g., convulsions, coma, even death)

APPROVED ACTIVE INGREDIENTS

The FDA, acting on the basis of new data submitted by manufacturers, has approved two kinds of antihistamines for this purpose.

• DIPHENHYDRAMINE: DIPHENHYDRAMINE HYDROCHLORIDE AND DIPHENHYDRAMINE CITRATE: The antihistamine diphenhydramine has a pronounced tendency to induce drowsiness. The Panel granted it conditional approval, and then the FDA approved it as safe and effective in 1981.

This decision was reached because of two studies conducted by a manufacturer in which healthy people who occasionally had trouble sleeping alternated in the use of diphenhydramine hydrochloride and a dummy medication to fall asleep. Neither the subjects nor the researchers dispensing the drugs knew which tablets contained the active drug and which did not. The diphenhydramine turned out to be "significantly better" than did the dummy drug in terms of shortening the time it took users to fall asleep, the depth of sleep they obtained, and their assessments of how well they slept.

A dozen manufacturers' studies that then were submitted to the agency resolved outstanding issues on diphenhydramine's safety and effectiveness. The FDA's analysis of the studies showed the side effects to be minimal and mild, so the drug was judged safe when used to induce sleep. The FDA approved dosages of 50 mg of diphenhydramine hydrochloride and 76 mg of diphenhydramine monocitrate, which is rapidly converted to the hydrochloride in the stomach. The citrate is weaker than the hydrochloride, thus the two dosages are equivalent.

• *DOXYLAMINE SUCCINATE:* This antihistamine, like diphenhydramine, has a marked tendency to induce drowsiness. Although it has a long record of use as a prescription drug for a variety of purposes, doxylamine succinate had not previously been marketed as an over-the-counter sleep aid. Following the Panel and the FDA's decision that none of the existing nonprescription sleep aids was safe and effective, a manufacturer submitted a New Drug Application and supporting data requesting the FDA's permission to market doxylamine succinate as a nonprescription sleep aid. This application was studied and approved under the rigorous scientific standards applicable to all new drugs examined in the late 1970s. The drug quickly became the top-selling over-the-counter sleep aid.

The approved dosage is 25 mg. While it has not yet been proved dangerous to pregnant women, neither has it been proved to be safe for them or for their babies. For this reason, the label warns that pregnant or nursing women should not use this sleep aid.

CONDITIONALLY APPROVED ACTIVE INGREDIENTS
None.

DISAPPROVED ACTIVE INGREDIENTS
None.

Combination Products

No combination sleep-aid products are approved at present. Manufacturers are trying to show that there is a need and a market for a sleep aid and a pain reliever for people who have arthritis. The FDA wants to see some convincing data.

When Greater Relief Is Needed

Several types of prescription drugs will help insomniac people fall asleep. But most are effective only for a few days. What is more, some of these drugs, like phenobarbital, can be dangerously addictive.

The consensus among doctors is that the safest prescription sleeping aids are benzodiazepines. The most widely used for sleep has been triazolam (*Halcion*, Upjohn). But questions have been raised in the early 1990s about its safety. Other benzodiazepine soporifics also are available.

Sleeplessness may be a sign of depression (which is not a surprising feeling in hard times) or of some other emotional or physical disorder. Medical help should be sought. You may wish to ask your doctor for referral to a sleep specialist or a sleep clinic if ordinary and obvious measures do not restore restful sleep.

Safety and Effectiveness: Active Ingredients in Over-the-Counter Sleep Aids

Active Ingredient	Assessment
diphenhydramine hydrochloride	safe and effective
diphenhydramine monocitrate	safe and effective
doxylamine succinate	safe and effective

Sleep Aids: Product Ratings

SINGLE-INGREDIENT PRODUCTS

Product and Distributor	Dosage of Active Ingredients	Rating*	Comment
diphenhydramine hydrochloride			
Compoz Nighttime Sleep Aid (Med-Tech)	**tablets:** 50 mg	A	R̸ to OTC switch
Nytol (Block)	**tablets:** 25 mg	A	R̸ to OTC switch
Sominex2 Tablets (SmithKline Beecham)	**tablets:** 25 mg	A	R̸ to OTC switch
doxylamine succinate			
Unisom Nighttime Sleep Aid (Pfizer)	**tablets:** 25 mg	A	R̸ to OTC switch
COMBINATION PRODUCTS			
Sominex 2 Pain Relief Formula (SmithKline Beecham)	**tablets:** 25 mg diphenhydramine hydrochloride + 500 mg acetaminophen	B	FDA not convinced of merit of sleep aid + pain reliever; R̸ to OTC switch (diphenhydramine)

| Unisom with Pain Relief (Pfizer) | tablets: 50 mg diphenhydramine hydrochloride + 650 mg acetaminophen | B | FDA not convinced of merit of sleep aid + pain reliever; Rx to OTC switch (diphenhydramine) |

*Author's interpretation of FDA criteria. Based on contents, not claims.

Smelling Salts: Preliminary Report

Fainting—if you believe the classically romantic English novelists—was once a fashionable method of responding to emotional distress. Individuals who were subject to fainting spells carried bottles of smelling salts, which, when opened and waved under their noses, appear to have successfully revived them.

Fainting can signal the presence of a serious underlying illness. It also can be dangerous in and of itself, if a person falls or passes out in an unsafe place. People who find themselves feeling faint, or fainting from time to time, should see a doctor.

These days smelling salts are sold over-the-counter in convenient, single-use ampules. Their principal active ingredient is ammonia, so they are called *ammonium inhalants*. A few drops of household ammonia sprinkled on a handkerchief or other cloth that is then passed back and forth under the nose of a person who has fainted, or who feels faint, may serve the same purpose.

The FDA's Advisory Review Panel on OTC Miscellaneous

SMELLING SALTS: PRELIMINARY REPORT is based on an FDA status report on the OTC Drug Review.

Internal Drugs was scheduled to assess ammonium inhalants, but it was disbanded before the task could be done. Over a decade later, no further review work appears to have been done by the FDA on these drugs. The agency formerly listed the two active ingredients in ammonium inhalants as *ammonium carbonate* and strong ammonium solution. They also are called *aromatic ammonia spirits*.

Smoking Deterrents

Many people want to stop smoking, and more than 50 million Americans have succeeded in this effort since 1964, when the Surgeon General of the United States Public Health Service first confirmed cigarette smoking's high risk of causing lung cancer. Since then, cigarette smoking has also been documented to be a major contributing factor in heart and artery disease and a variety of breathing disorders. Every day, more than 1000 Americans die of smoking related illnesses!

Most Americans know these facts. Many who have not yet stopped smoking, and would like to, ask whether the readily available over-the-counter drugs that are promoted as smoking deterrents actually work. The Panel's answer: Maybe, for brief periods of time, and only if you *really* want to stop and are willing to mobilize the self-discipline that may be needed to free yourself from the habit. In fact, it is will power, or fear, or at least a desire to stop smoking, that is the ingredient that is necessary for success. To make this clear, the Panel thought that each smoking-deterrent product should carry this notice:

SMOKING DETERRENTS is based on the report "Smoking Deterrent Drug Products for OTC Human Use" by the FDA's Advisory Review Panel on OTC Miscellaneous Internal Drug Products, and FDA's Tentative Final Monograph on these products.

"This product's effectiveness is directly related to the user's motivation to stop smoking cigarettes."

At present, nonprescription drugs are not a very useful route to stopping smoking. They all may be worthless.

 ### Claims

Accurate (if one were shown to be safe and effective, which none has)
- "A temporary aid to those who want to stop smoking cigarettes"
- "A temporary aid to breaking the cigarette habit"

Misleading or Unproved
- "A temporary aid to cut down on smoking"
- "An aid to those who want to reduce the smoking habit"
- "Curbs the tobacco urge"
- "Helps to stop smoking without requiring will power"

The Allure of Smoking

In 1623, Sir Francis Bacon noted that "the use of tobacco is growing greatly; it conquers men with a certain secret pleasure so that those who have once become accustomed thereto can hardly be restrained therefrom." The FDA's expert advisers, writing 357 years later, found no reason to dispute Bacon's account.

Rolling up corn silk, coffee grounds, or dried lettuce leaves in cigarette paper and smoking it—as some persons have done—simply will not deliver pleasure comparable to tobacco's. This led the Panel to conclude that tobacco contains some element that causes drug-like behavioral changes—one of which, of course, is difficulty in stopping. The dependency-producing element almost certainly is *nicotine*, a substance that strongly stimulates the central nervous system.

Products

How then to stop, once the smoker comes to accept that the habit is detrimental to health? Many professionally guided and self-help methods have been developed in the last two decades. But, as judged by the medical literature, long-term success rates are low, and many people slip back into the habit.

For the smoker seeking the way to go, the Surgeon General's recent findings may offer a useful clue. He estimates that of the 50 million persons who have successfully stopped smoking since 1964, the large majority have done so *without counseling or using a structured program.* In other words, the do-it-yourself method has proved to be the most successful.

How much the use of nonprescription drugs can contribute to this effort remains unclear. Reviewers were unable to approve any of the over-the-counter smoking deterrents they examined. But a few nonprescription drugs have shown some promise in clinical tests, so they might provide a margin of success for the smoker who has seriously set himself or herself to the hard, but certainly not impossible, task of stopping.

All over-the-counter smoking deterrents claim one of two possible mechanisms: Either they change the taste of tobacco smoke so that smoking is no longer pleasurable, or they substitute a nicotine-like drug in an oral form such as candy or gum. This latter method creates an alternative habit that is claimed to be pleasurable enough to help the smoker forsake cigarettes.

These drugs may also be promoted to help a person "cut down" on smoking. The Panel strongly disapproved of this goal. They felt that this use of the drugs is a waste of time and money, since most such efforts are doomed to fail. The only meaningful role for a smoking deterrent is to help a smoker *stop.*

The hardest time will be the first few weeks, so this is when smoking deterrents will be of most value. Because of this time element the evaluators assessed the effectiveness of these drugs in terms of how they work during the three weeks after a person throws away his or her last pack of cigarettes.

Ingredients in Smoking Deterrents

A variety of active ingredients are sold in smoking deterrents.

APPROVED ACTIVE INGREDIENTS

None.

CONDITIONALLY APPROVED ACTIVE INGREDIENTS

• LOBELINE PREPARATIONS: LOBELINE SULFATE, NATURAL LOBELINE ALKALOIDS, LOBELIA INFLATA
HERB: Lobeline preparations are plant products and extracts whose active substance, lobeline, is similar to though weaker than nicotine. *How* they help is not altogether clear from the Panel's description, but it appears that lobeline may provide a temporary and alternative oral gratification for the smoker who is trying to lessen the craving for inhaling nicotine.

Large doses of lobeline can cause belching, heartburn, stomach ache, and other symptoms, but in the small 2-mg recommended doses, few such symptoms result. Based on these findings in the handful of studies available, the Panel declared lobeline safe.

In one double-blind, scientifically controlled study, over 80 percent of smokers who used lobeline had stopped smoking after 5 or 6 days, compared with fewer than 10 percent who stopped smoking among the group taking dummy medication. But of 10 other controlled studies assessed, only 2 studies confirmed these results; the other 8 did not. So the Panel and the FDA believe further testing is in order. Conclusion: lobeline preparations are safe but not proved effective.

• SILVER ACETATE: A silver compound, this drug has one minor adverse effect—it can discolor the skin, turning it bluish. The Panel therefore calls it safe.

Silver acetate is usually formulated into a chewing gum, to prolong its presence in the mouth. It reputedly affects the mucous membranes of the mouth so that cigarette smoke has a nasty, metallic sweet taste, which smokers find discouragingly unpleasant. This aversive effect may last up to 4 hours.

Three double-blind placebo-controlled studies were submitted as evidence that silver acetate gum is effective; none of them were considered to be objective enough. In the first study, 11 of 30 smokers who used the medicated gum said they had stopped smoking by the end of 2 weeks, a significantly greater percentage than was recorded among members of a control group who chewed a dummy, nonmedicated gum. But the investigators relied on mail-in answer forms and telephone interviews to obtain these results, and evaluators say self-reports of this kind are highly suspect. So the Panel and the FDA concluded that while silver acetate is safe, it has not been proved effective.

DISAPPROVED ACTIVE INGREDIENTS

None.

When Further Help Is Needed

The major new element in smoking cessation, as of 1992, is the nicotine patch. This is a prescription drug product, formulated as a removable patch that can be placed on one or another skin surface.

Nicotine leaches slowly out of the patch, through the skin, and into the bloodstream, which carries it rapidly to the brain. This reduces nicotine craving, and so may help a smoker overcome the urge to smoke. After a person wearing a patch has had time to develop other coping mechanisms for tension, stress, and other triggers for smoking, he or she graduates to a smaller patch that delivers less nicotine—and after several more weeks the person is weaned off nicotine altogether.

Initial quit rates have been as high as 50 percent among smokers who were strongly motivated to quit. But some back-sliding occurs. Nevertheless, abstinence rates of 10 to 20 percent after one to two years have been reported in the medical literature. For a smoker who is intent on quitting, and finds that he or she cannot stop cold turkey—which is what most successful quitters do—more medicinal help may be found from the nicotine patch than from any other available ℞ or OTC drug.

Safety and Effectiveness: Active Ingredients in Over-the-Counter Smoking Deterrents

Active Ingredient	Assessment
lobeline preparations: lobeline sulfate, natural lobeline alkaloids, and *Lobelia inflata* herb	safe, but not proved effective
silver acetate	safe, but not proved effective

Smoking Deterrents: Product Ratings

Product and Distributor	Dosage of Active Ingredients	Rating*	Comment
BanSmoke (Thompson)	**gum:** 6 mg benzocaine	C	not an approved drug for this purpose
Bantron (Dep Corp.)	**tablets:** 2 mg lobeline sulfate	B	not proved effective

*Author's interpretation of FDA criteria. Based on contents, not claims.

Stimulants

Everybody seems to have an idea of what stimulants are. The Panel defined them as drugs that keep a person awake and alert. It decided that occasional use of safe and effective nonprescription stimulant preparations is not harmful to adults. These mild nonprescription stimulants may be useful in counteracting the boredom and fatigue of long, tedious work that requires continuous vigilance. The Panel singled out the "highway hypnosis" that long-distance truck and auto drivers sometimes experience as one of these cases. When greater stimulation is required, prescription drugs—including amphetamines and desoxyephedrine—are available through a doctor.

To qualify as safe and effective, the Panel declared, an over-the-counter stimulant should

- enable the user to perform whatever tasks are necessary even if he or she is drowsy or fatigued
- last long enough for the task to be completed

STIMULANTS is based on the report of the FDA's Advisory Review Panel on OTC Sedative, Tranquilizer, and Sleep-Aid Drug Products and the FDA's Tentative Final and Final Monographs on stimulants.

- provide a very wide margin of safety between a helpful dose and a dangerous one
- not unduly excite the heart
- not make the user restless or irritable
- not interfere with normal sleep
- not interact in an unpleasant or a dangerous way with ordinary food or beverages

 Claims

Accurate
- "Helps restore mental alertness or wakefulness during fatigue or drowsiness"

Nonprescription Stimulants

APPROVED ACTIVE INGREDIENT

- *CAFFEINE:* The only over-the-counter stimulant that meets the Panel's standards is caffeine. The FDA concurred that caffeine is both safe and effective. The recommended dosage is 100 to 200 mg, not more often than every 3 or 4 hours. Medicinal caffeine preparations should not be used for longer than a week or two at a time, and they should not be used by children under 12 years of age.

Caffeine stimulates both the heart and the brain. This effect is greater when you are tired than when you are rested and alert. But the claim that caffeine "enhances performance" when a person is not fatigued has *not* been proved. One scientific review concludes, however, that caffeine can increase precision in a "wide range of behavior ... from putting the shot to monitoring a clock face."

The Panel noted: "In contrast to the irritating qualities of many coffee extracts, caffeine itself does not seem to cause irritation of the gastrointestinal tract in the usual doses. This is an advantage when the drug is used for its stimulant properties."

Taking large amounts of caffeine at one time—more than about

Caffeine Content of Beverages and Foods

Item	Average mg	Range of mg
coffee (5-oz cup) brewed, drip method	115	60-180
brewed, percolator	80	40-170
instant	65	30-120
decaffeinated, brewed	3	2-5
decaffeinated, instant	2	1-5
tea (5-oz cup) Brewed, major U.S.brands	40	20-90
brewed, imported brands	60	25-110
instant	30	25-50
iced (12-oz glass)	70	67-76
cocoa beverage (5-oz cup)	4	2-20
chocolate milk beverage (8 oz)	5	2-7
milk chocolate (1 oz)	6	1-15
dark chocolate, semi-sweet (1 oz)	20	5-35
baker's chocolate (1 oz)	26	26
chocolate-flavored syrup (1 oz)	4	4

Source: FDA

240 mg—can cause nervousness, headache, and irritability, however. Anxiety may develop. Since caffeine also is in coffee, tea, and cola drinks, medicinal supplements of this drug should be used cautiously when you are drinking large amounts of these beverages. The recommended medicinal dose of 100 to 200 mg is comparable to the caffeine in a cup of coffee (roughly 125 mg) or strong tea (roughly 100 to 115 mg) or in four 8-ounce glasses of cola drinks (25 to 30 mg per glass).

The FDA says the evidence shows that caffeine *restores* alertness when a person is drowsy or fatigued. But it will *not* prevent drowsiness or fatigue if taken on a preventive basis beforehand. This means that coffee will perk you up when you get to the truck stop but will not help you once you are back on the road, unless you continue sipping it from a take-out container when you get back on the road.

Caffeine can be habit-forming. But severe problems of addiction appear to be rare. Sudden withdrawal, however, can produce severe headache.

Dependency on caffeine was explored in an interesting set of experiments several years ago. Researchers found that chronic coffee drinkers became sleepy and irritable when given de-caffeinated coffee. They felt alert and contented when given coffee that contained caffeine. These regular coffee drinkers did not miss much sleep at night. But non-coffee drinkers who took coffee during the experiment could not sleep. Moreover, they became jittery and suffered stomach aches, while the habituated users reported only "contentment." The conclusion seems to be that coffee does not adversely affect regular coffee drinkers but may cause problems in other people.

There has been concern that coffee drinking—and by implication other uses of caffeine—may cause genetic or developmental defects in unborn babies or may cause heart ailments in older persons. The FDA believes these fears to be unfounded. The FDA also notes that no fatal caffeine poisonings have ever been reported as the result of oral overdosage; it is calculated that an adult male would have to swallow the equivalent of 100 cups of coffee—or more—at one time to kill himself with caffeine.

WARNING:

 Limit the use of caffeine-containing medications, food, or beverages while taking a nonprescription stimulant product, because too much caffeine may cause nervousness, irritability, sleeplessness, and occasionally, rapid heart beat. For occasional use only...

CONDITIONALLY APPROVED ACTIVE INGREDIENTS

None.

DISAPPROVED ACTIVE INGREDIENTS

None.

Safety and Effectiveness: Active Ingredients in Over-the-Counter Stimulants

Active Ingredient	Assessment
caffeine	safe and effective

891

Stimulants: Product Ratings

Product and Distributor	Dosage of Active Ingredients	Rating*	Comment
caffeine			
Caffeine (generic)	tablets: 125 mg	A	
NoDoz (Bristol-Myers)		A	
Caffedrine (Thompson)	tablets, capsules, timed-release: 200 mg	A	
Enerjets (Chilton)	lozenges	B	no dosage given on label
Vivarin (SmithKline Beecham)	tablets: 200 mg	A	

*Author's interpretation of FDA criteria. Based on contents, not claims.

Styptic Pencils and Other Astringents

When a man nicks himself shaving, touching the cut with the moistened end of a styptic pencil will produce a stinging sensation and then usually will coagulate the blood so that the bleeding stops. This is an *astringent effect*, as are other effects of drugs in this class that slow or stop oozing, discharge, or bleeding from the skin or mucous membranes.

When astringents are defined in this way, the drugs' benefits seem clearcut. But the Panel that grappled with evaluating them concedes that they appear to act in several interrelated ways. They confer benefits that are partly *medicinal* and also perhaps partly *cosmetic*, in the sense that they create clean, puckery, refreshed feelings.

The principal astringent chemicals are compounds of aluminum, zinc, manganese, iron, and bismuth, and other chemical groups that contain these metals (such as permanganates). The tannins, like tannic acid, are also astringents. Some acids, alcohols, and phenols will sepa-

STYPTIC PENCILS AND OTHER ASTRINGENTS is based on the report "OTC Astringent Drug Products" by the FDA's Advisory Review Panel on OTC Miscellaneous External Drug Products and on the FDA's Tentative Final Monograph on these products.

rate out proteins, but they also readily penetrate cell surfaces and may damage cells and tissues. Therefore, according to the Panel's standards they are not technically astringents.

How They Work

Although some astringent substances are potent chemicals, they do not enter human body cells—which is their virtue. Rather, all their activity occurs at the cell surface—where they may block noxious substances from entering the cell or the space between cells. They *coagulate* body chemicals, which means that they pull the proteins out of blood, serum, sweat, and other body fluids so that they form clots, crusts, or other solid deposits. If the serum is carrying an irritating body substance (histamine, for example), the astringent appears to trap and remove it. Thus, the irritant can no longer enter its target cells, where it would provoke inflammation and itching.

Some astringent benefit may result from direct action on the protein-type surface molecules of body cells. Astringents are said to draw these molecules, and thus cells, together, reducing their surface area. This may account for the puckering sensations that astringents produce. Certain foods, like lemon or unripe persimmon, cause what appear to be comparable sensations when they pucker the inside of the mouth.

In drawing together and shrinking cells or cell-membrane surfaces, astringents block the passage of blood, serum, and other fluids from one body compartment to another. To go back to the original example of the man who cuts himself while shaving, an astringent styptic pencil not only precipitates the solids out of the blood so that they dry and block further flow, but it also shrinks and tightens cells of the injured capillary vessels, which helps to staunch the flow.

Combination Products

The Panel says it is unaware of any products that combine 2 or more astringent substances, but it does know of combinations with other classes of active ingredients. These combinations are safe and effective only if they meet the over-the-counter review standards, which require that both active ingredients contribute to the claimed effect or effects of the combination product and do not counteract or diminish each other's effectiveness or safety. The combination must provide concurrent therapeutic benefit for a significant number of people who require the action of *both* active ingredients.

The FDA approves these combinations as safe and effective:

- 1 approved astringent + 1 approved itch-pain reliever for external use
- 1 approved astringent + 1 approved skin protectant for treating itchiness and discomfort around the anus

The following combinations are only conditionally approved:

- 1 approved astringent + 1 approved skin protectant for treating areas other than the perianal skin
- 1 approved astringent + 1 approved itch-pain reliever + 1 skin protectant

 Claims

Accurate for Styptic Pencils

- "Stops bleeding caused by minor surface cuts and abrasions as may occur during shaving"

Accurate for Aluminum Acetate (modified Burow's solution)

- "For relief of inflammatory conditions of the skin such as poison ivy"
- "For the temporary relief of minor skin irritations due to poison ivy, poison oak, poison sumac, insect bites, athlete's foot, [and] rashes caused by soaps, detergents, cosmetics or jewelry"

Accurate for Products Containing Hamamelis Water, NF XI (witch hazel)

- "For relief of minor skin irritations due to insect bites, minor cuts [or] minor scrapes"

WARNING:

 For external use only. Avoid contact with the eyes.

Astringent Active Ingredients

Dozens of putative astringent active ingredients were surveyed. Only a tiny few met the test of treatment success.

APPROVED ASTRINGENT ACTIVE INGREDIENTS

• *ALUMINUM ACETATE (MODIFIED BUROW'S SOLUTION):* This aluminum compound is used medicinally in an aqueous solution. When it is applied to the skin, as it should be, the Panel says complications are rare or nonexistent. However, drinking aluminum acetate solution can result in poisoning.

The medical record on aluminum acetate is more anecdotal than scientific. In the one study cited by the reviewers, a researcher induced poison ivy in six persons who were highly sensitive to this plant poison. Two days later, he treated the blisters with compresses containing either tap water, salt water, aluminum acetate 2.5 percent, or aluminum acetate 5 percent. The latter, stronger aluminum acetate solution was the only one that significantly reduced the inflammation and itching. Basing its conclusion on that study, and on doctors' wide clinical experience with this preparation, the Panel says aluminum acetate is safe and effective for relieving poison ivy and other irritating skin conditions. The solution should contain 0.13 to 0.5% aluminum acetate—which are the concentrations that result when 2.5 to 5 percent concentrations of modified Burow's solution are properly diluted. It can be used as a soak or applied to a larger skin area as a wet dressing.

• *ALUMINUM SULFATE:* This ingredient, also known as *cake alum* or simply *alum*, is used to make styptic pencils. It stings when applied to the cut, but this Panel, in contrast to the Antiperspirant Panel, said it does not irritate the skin. In the 75 years styptic pencils have been marketed, reviewers say, there are no reports of side effects from their use. So aluminum sulfate is judged safe for this purpose. There is only sparse scientific data on aluminum sulfate's effectiveness. But its long history of consumer and medical acceptance and use persuaded the FDA to stamp it "effective." The approved dosage is 46 to 63 percent aluminum sulfate. To use, moisten the top of the styptic pencil with water and apply the pencil to the cut, nick, or other small lesion.

• *HAMAMELIS WATER NF XI:* This fragrant plant extract, also called *witch hazel* is a popular aftershave lotion. *Hamamelis* is the Latin name for the shrub whence the astringent is extracted; *NF XI* means simply that it is described in the *National Formulary*, 11th edition.

So little witch hazel is left in the final product that the Panel did not quibble about its safety. As for effectiveness, these reviewers at first felt that the 14 percent alcohol that is typically present in witch hazel preparations may be responsible for whatever astringent benefit they possess. However, a witch-hazel manufacturing company presented a study demonstrating that hamamelis water in 14 percent alcohol speeds up the clotting of human plasma while plain 14 percent alcohol does not. This indicates, the company said, that hamamelis water is "superior" to its alcohol base.

The Panel concurred and assessed witch hazel as safe and effective. The dosage? Apply to the affected area as often as needed.

CONDITIONALLY APPROVED ASTRINGENT ACTIVE INGREDIENTS

• ALUMINUM CHLORIDE HEXAHYDRATE: This astringent, which is chemically similar to the two approved aluminum salts astringents (*see* under previous headings), got lost in the shuffle in the Over-the-Counter drug review, and was not evaluated by the Panel. So the FDA took up the task.

Aluminum chloride hexahydrate is usually applied to irritated skin in a wet dressing, and one scientific study indicates that it will effectively pull proteins out of solution (coagulation), which is what it is claimed to do. But the FDA analysts felt that the studies submitted were inadequate to establish this astringent's efficacy. So the agency rates it only conditionally approved—for now.

• TANNIC ACID: A tanning agent, this drug will harden the skin and form a protective coating over mucous membranes, curtailing the oozing of blood and other body fluids.

When used over large areas of damaged skin, tannic acid can be dangerous because it is absorbed into the body and acts as a liver poison. But it has little if any action on unbroken skin, and the Panel believes it is safe when applied to small painful areas such as an ingrown toenail. (*See* INGROWN-TOENAIL RELIEVERS.)

The only studies submitted to the evaluators were on the use of tannic acid for treating ingrown toenails. But the panelists believe it may also be useful in treating cold sores and fever blisters, and they would like to see it tested for such use. Meanwhile, they granted it only conditional approval: safe but not proved effective as an astringent.

The FDA seems to concur, but the agency's position is not wholly clear. In its Proposed Rule on Astringent Drug Products, it lists tannic acid as not safe and effective. But in a later summary of the ingredients in the OTC Review, it concurs with the Panel that this is a safe ingredient whose effectiveness remains to be demonstrated.

DISAPPROVED ASTRINGENT ACTIVE INGREDIENTS

A variety of compounds were summarily rejected by the Panel because no information was submitted or otherwise made available concerning safety and effectiveness. (*See* the Safety and Effectiveness table.)

Safety and Effectiveness: Active Ingredients in Over-the-Counter Astringents

Active Ingredient	Assessment
acetone	summarily disapproved
alcohol	summarily disapproved
alcohol 14%	summarily disapproved
aluminum acetate (modified Burow's solution)	safe and effective
aluminum chlorhydroxy complex	summarily disapproved
aluminum chloride hexahydrate	safe, but not proved effective
aluminum sulfate	safe and effective
ammonium alum	summarily disapproved
aromatics	summarily disapproved
benzalkonium chloride	summarily disapproved
benzethonium chloride	summarily disapproved
benzocaine	summarily disapproved
benzoic acid	summarily disapproved
borax	summarily disapproved

Safety and Effectiveness: Active Ingredients in Over-the-Counter Astringents (contd)

Active Ingredient	Assessment
boric acid over 0.6%	summarily disapproved
Burow's solution, modified (See aluminum acetate)	
calcium acetate	summarily disapproved
camphor (gum camphor)	summarily disapproved
colloidal oatmeal	summarily disapproved
cresol	summarily disapproved
cupric sulfate	summarily disapproved
eugenol	summarily disapproved
ferric subsulfate	summarily disapproved
hamamelis water, NF XI	safe and effective
honey	summarily disapproved
isopropyl alcohol	summarily disapproved
menthol	summarily disapproved
oil of cloves	summarily disapproved
oil of eucalyptus	summarily disapproved
oil of peppermint	summarily disapproved
oil of sage	summarily disapproved
oil of wintergreen	summarily disapproved
oxyquinoline sulfate	summarily disapproved
para-tertiary-butyl-meta-cresol	summarily disapproved
phenol (carbolic acid)	summarily disapproved
polyoxyethylene monolaurate	summarily disapproved
potassium alum	summarily disapproved
potassium ferrocyanide	summarily disapproved
silver nitrate	summarily disapproved

Safety and Effectiveness: Active Ingredients in Over-the-Counter Astringents (contd)

Active Ingredient	Assessment
sodium diacetate	summarily disapproved
starch	summarily disapproved
talc	summarily disapproved
tannic acid	safe, but not proved effective
tannic acid glycerite	summarily disapproved
thymol	summarily disapproved
witch hazel (*See* hamamelis water NF XI)	
zinc chloride	summarily disapproved
zinc oxide	summarily disapproved
zinc phenolsulfonate	summarily disapproved
zinc stearate	summarily disapproved
zinc sulfate	summarily disapproved

Astringents: Product Ratings

Product and Distributor	Dosage of Active Ingredients	Rating*	Comment
aluminum acetate			
Modified Burow's solution (generic)	**solution:** aluminum acetate solution	A	makes modified Burow's solution when diluted in water
aluminum sulfate			
Bluboro Powder (Allergen)	**powder:** aluminum sulfate + calcium acetate	A	
Mammoth Styptic Pencil (Woltra)	**styptic pencil**	B	concentration of active ingredient not listed on label
tannic acid			
Tannic acid (generic)	**powder**	B	not proved effective
witch hazel			
Tucks (Parke-Davis)	**cream:** 50%	A	

Witch hazel (generic)

solution

A

Sunscreens

Judged by their active ingredients, most sunscreen products sold in the United States are safe—and remarkably effective. Some products can block 99 percent of the ultraviolet B (UVB) light rays, which cause sunburn, in the billionth of a second before these rays strike the skin.

Sunscreens have only one direct role: They prevent sunburn. Sunbathers who use them can spend more hours of more days in the sun, pursuing a tan if they so choose.

 Claims

Accurate

- "Filters out the sun's burning rays to prevent sunburn"
- "Screens out the sun's harsh and often harmful rays to prevent sunburn"

For avobenzone only:

SUNSCREENS is based on the report "Sunscreen Drug Products for OTC Human Use," prepared by the FDA's Advisory Review Panel on OTC Topical Analgesic, Antirheumatic, Otic, Burn and Sunburn Prevention and Treatment Drug Products.

- "Absorbs throughout the UVA spectrum"

False or Misleading
- "Promotes suntanning"
- "Facilitates rapid, deeper, darker, or longer-lasting tans"

The tan-seeker in a sense tempts fate, the Panel said. With or without a sunscreen, the fastest way to tan is to expose the skin to the sun daily up to the point that it becomes vividly red, *before* covering up or going indoors. It takes about twice as long to get a painful, blistering burn as it does to achieve the initial non-painful reddening; therefore, if, after an hour of sunning, your skin is bright red but not sore, then you can anticipate that after just one more hour of such exposure you will be badly burned. Using a sunscreen slows this process. Unlike most over-the-counter drugs, using too little of a sunscreen is more dangerous than using too much. Apply the product liberally to cover the skin, and reapply after swimming, sweating or other activities that may wash or rub it away.

Note: For sun*burn* product ingredients, *see* pp. 967-968

Skin Protection Factor (SPF)

Most manufacturers—following the Panel's recommendation—provide guide numbers on product labels to help a consumer pick an appropriately graded product to fulfill his or her need for protection. To use this guide number, you first must determine your sensitivity to sunlight. This estimate, based on past sunbathing and sunburning experience will in turn indicate how strong a sunscreen you will need. (*See* the table Skin Types and Recommended Sunscreen Product.) This measure of a product's effectiveness is called its *skin protection factor*, or *SPF*. The SPFs range from a low of SPF 2, which is appropriate for a dark and insensitive skin that needs little or no sunscreen protection, to SPF 15 or above, which is for supersensitive skins that must be heavily shielded almost all the time to prevent painful, blistering sunburn. The average white-skinned American requires a product that has an SPF 4 for most fairly casual outdoor exposures.

The SPFs have been correlated by the Panel with the descriptive words *minimal, moderate, extra, maximal,* and *ultra.* A product that provides *minimal* product will permit tanning but will also allow burning. A *maximal* product will protect against sunburn but also will prevent tanning, even in very sun-sensitive persons.

Using the table given here, you can keep track of sunscreen needs for yourself and each family member.

Family Member	Skin Sensitivity	Skin Protection Factor (SPF)	Product Category
Self	_____	_____	_____
Spouse	_____	_____	_____
Child ____	_____	_____	_____
Child ____	_____	_____	_____
Child ____	_____	_____	_____

SPFs do more than tell you which product to buy. They indicate how long it is safe to stay out in the sun with use of the recommended sunscreen. They also show which product to use if you need or want to stay out *longer.*

Cover up on Mauna Loa

The most intense and burning UVB sunlight thus far discovered on the face of the earth is atop the Mauna Loa volcano on the island of Hawaii. An average white-skinned person who spent the day there would be exposed to *five times* the UVB light needed to produce painful sunburn.

Skin Types and Recommended Sunscreen Products

Skin Sensitivity on First 30- to 45-Minute Exposure (e.g., after winter)	Skin Protection Factor (SPF)	Recommended Sun Product
highly sensitive: always burns very easily, never tans	SPF 15 or above	ultra
sensitive: always burns easily, never tans	SPF 8 to under 15	maximal
sensitive: always burns easily, tans minimally	SPF 6 to under 8	extra
normal: burns moderately, tans gradually to light brown	SPF 4 to under 6	moderate
normal: burns minimally, always tans well to moderate brown	SPF 2 to under 4	minimal
insensitive: rarely burns, tans profusely to dark brown	SPF 2	minimal
very insensitive: never burns, skin is deeply pigmented	under SPF 2	(none needed)

Using no sunscreen, an average light-skinned person—who usually uses products that are SPF 4—will get red, but not painfully burned, after about 40 minutes of sun on his or her first beach outing of the season without any sunscreen protection. However, by using a *moderate* sunscreen, labeled SPF 4, this individual can extend his or her safe exposure time by a factor of 4: that is, to 160 minutes (4 x 40 = 160), or 2 hours and 40 minutes.

If, however, this person uses a *maximal* product, SPF 8, he or she can extend his or her safe time to 320 minutes (8 x 40 = 320), or more than 5 hours.

Thus a person will be protected in this way throughout the entire dangerous midday period (from 10:00 A.M. to 2:00 P.M.), when the sun is high in the sky. But a fisherman who normally uses SPF 4 products, but who now plans a day in an open unshaded boat on the ocean, should select a maximal or an ultra protective product (SPF 8 or above) if he hopes to eat his fish dinner in comfort.

Using like calculations, a fair-skinned woman who usually burns after 20 minutes by the pool can extend her protected period to 2 hours by using an extra protective sunscreen with SPF 6 (6 x 20 = 120). If however, she uses a darker-skinned friend's sunscreen, SPF 4, to avoid burning, she must cover up with clothing after only 1 hour and 20 minutes (4 x 20 = 80) or risk a burn.

A sun-tanned skin, like an inherently dark one, provides protection against burning. So as the season advances, and skin darkens, it is safe to stay longer in the sun each day. Alternatively, you can switch to a less-protective sunscreen—one with a lower SPF—which in turn will enhance tanning. Most white people, nevertheless, will require repeated daily exposure to the sun for about two weeks to appreciably darken their skins.

"Tanning," the Panel cautioned, "cannot be rushed!"

Armed with this knowledge, a person taking a long summer vacation may decide to limit his or her daily sun exposure at the start, in order to slowly build a satisfying tan. But on a 5-day winter jaunt to a tropical island, a wise person might renounce *tanning* as largely unattainable, and instead use a *maximal-* or *ultra*-protective product in order to play safely all day in the hot sunshine.

Sunlight and the Skin

Sunburns and Suntans

Sunburn and suntan are both caused by UVB light rays, which cannot be seen with the naked eye. They are not caused by the sun's visible light rays. Ultraviolet rays that are between 290 and 320 nanometers (nm)— or about one ten-millionth of an inch in length—are the most immediately dangerous. Burning occurs because this solar radiation is transformed into heat as it strikes the skin. Tanning occurs (much more slowly) because these same UVB rays stimulate pigment-producing cells called *melanocytes* to produce the dark pigment (melanin) in the skin. It is melanin that makes black people's skin black. It is melanin that white sunbathers must induce in order to enhance their appearance as *tanned*.

Melanin blocks UVB rays from reaching and burning the deep inner layers of the skin. White people who have achieved good tans can, like black people, stay in the sun longer without burning. But the Panel warned that untanned, light-complexioned white persons—particularly redheads and blondes of Northern European descent—are about 33 times more susceptible to sunburn than dark-skinned persons of African descent. Thus both vulnerability to sunburn and the ability to tan are to a large extent inherited traits.

The closer you go to the Equator, by and large, the more intense the sun's UVB light. A fair-skinned person who will be vividly red after 40 minutes of June sun in New Jersey (which is 40° N) will reach the same vivid redness after only 25 minutes of sun exposure in the Florida Keys (25° N).

The UVB light rays are filtered by the earth's atmosphere. So the higher upward you go, the more intense they become—a fact that persons skiing in high mountains should keep in mind. Ice, snow, water, and desert sands that reflect a lot of UVB light also decrease the safe interval before sunburn.

The New Worry: Ultraviolet A (UVA)

The sunscreens assessed by the Panel, more than 15 years ago, were—and still are—designed primarily to stop UV rays in the spectrum of 280 to 320 nm, which are called ultraviolet B, or *UVB*, sun rays.

But the recent discovery that the ozone layer, which protects against longer, lower-energy sun rays of roughly 320 to 400 nanometers, is thinning in spots and may be threatened has changed the demand for sunscreen products. Reason: These longer rays, designated ultraviolet A, or *UVA*, have been shown to cause slower and more subtle, but also more damaging, injury to the skin. The UVA light specifically causes skin cancers, including, possibly, the dangerous but ever-more-common cancers called *malignant melanoma*. It also causes most "sun allergies" and other photosensitive reactions to sunlight, experts say.

The "ozone hole" and the risk of skin cancer attributed to it is blamed on the destructive effects of compounds called *chlorofluorocarbons* that are used in aerosol propellants and other products, which now are being phased out. Whether this international conservation effort will stop the erosion of ozone in the upper atmosphere remains to be seen.

The ozone hole usually appears in Antarctica, or in the high Arctic, in winter—where there are likely to be few sun-bathers. Whether this ozone thinning and loss of UVA protection also occurs at lower, temperate, and tropical zones in summer, when and where sunbathers are baring their skins, is still uncertain. But many people feel they need UVA protection at least as much as UVB. They now can have it, but the price is dear: about $2.50 an ounce according to *Consumer Reports* (June, 1991).

The FDA has approved, as a new drug, the first specific UVA blocker, *avobenzone*, also known as Parsol 1789. It effectively blocks UVA, but is only mildly effective against UVB and so is combined with another ingredient, padimate O, that blocks UVB. Some other, long-standing ingredients, such as benzophenone-3, are moderately effective in blocking both UVA and UVB. But these claims are *not* FDA approved.

In sunscreens, unlike many other over-the-counter drug products, the FDA allows and even encourages combinations of two or more active ingredients. Some combination products now being marketed that do not contain avobenzone *may* be effective against *both* dangerous ultraviolet light sources. Perhaps when the FDA publishes its Tentative Final Monograph on these products it will provide a yardstick on the value of these ingredients in blocking both UVB and UVA light rays.

A number of products are now promoted as "broad spectrum" sun-blockers because the UVB blockers they contain provide some protection against UVA. But one expert, dermatologist Vincent A. DeLeo, M.D., who is director of environmental dermatology at the Columbia

Presbyterian Medical Center in New York City, warns that these standard UVB blockers provide "relatively little protection against UVA" (*The Skin Cancer Foundation Journal*, vol. IX, 1991, pp. 11, 65-66). He says these ingredients provide UVA protection analogous to a UVB SPF 1 to SPF 5. The ingredients that provide this protection are indicated in the description of the individual ingredients further on, and in the Ingredients table at the end of this Unit.

Harmful Effects of Sunlight

The most immediate effect of overexposure to sunlight is sunburn, which can be an excruciatingly painful and even dangerous condition. Sunburned skin is reddest some 6 to 20 hours after sunning. The long-term risks are more insidious.

Skin Cancer

Exposure to sunlight is a major causative factor in the 630,000 cases of skin cancer diagnosed in the United States each year, according to the U.S. Centers for Disease Control (CDC) in Atlanta. The CDC estimates that there are 8500 skin-cancer deaths each year. These cancers may take several decades to develop. White people have a higher risk of skin cancer than black people, and men a higher rate than women— perhaps because they have traditionally spent more time working out-of-doors. Farmers, sailors, and construction workers are at greatest risk. The incidence of skin cancer doubles for every 3 or 4 degrees you travel south toward the Equator.

The Panel found it ironic that sunscreens for the most part are promoted toward and used by women, who are engaged in recreational pursuits. Yet it is working men outdoors who need them most. The experts had few suggestions on how to persuade hard hats to use these products.

Premature Aging of the Skin

The sun exposure that produces tanning also thins, dries, and wrinkles the skin. This condition is called *premature aging of the skin*, although at the cellular level these skin changes are different from normal aging. The UV sunlight appears to stimulate the growth of elastic fibers in the skin. These fibers eventually disintegrate into an amorphous mass that deprives the skin of its elasticity, and gives it an aged appearance.

A majority of the Panel members, in a close vote, proposed that all sunscreen products carry a statement that says in effect: "Overexposure to the sun may lead to premature aging of the skin and skin cancer. The liberal and regular use over the years of this product may help reduce the chance of these harmful effects." A minority of the Panel (three of its seven members) disagreed. "Sunlight can cause premature aging and cancer," they said, "but because [the] data are not yet conclusive that skin cancers are preventable by these over-the-counter products...a claim of...preventing cancer is unwarranted at this time."

Which view is more accurate still is unknown.

A Cautionary Word About Caution

Skin doctors, sunscreen manufacturers, and the media have whipped up a hysteria about the hazards of sun exposure. They point, rightly, to a significant increase in skin cancers, particularly of the dangerous type, *malignant melanoma*, in the United States in recent decades. But few of their scary charts and projections are correlated either with the nation's population increase or with the migration into the Sun Belt during and following World War II: More people live in places where there is more sunshine, so more skin cancers of course can be expected.

As the result of the fear that has been engendered, some people now hide from the sun or only venture out when lathered with high SPF sunscreens. At one level, they may be denying themselves healthy fun. At a more serious level, people need sunlight to produce vitamin D, and some sun exposure is required for them to do it. In several surveys many Americans in northern areas have been shown to have marginal vitamin D levels; this is particularly true for older people. Vitamin D, it should be noted, is important for *preventing* several cancers.

This vitamin can be supplied with supplements. (*See* VITAMINS AND MINERALS. But the healthier way may be to walk, rest, or play in the sunshine for a while each day. (For a report on possible overreaction to skin cancer warnings, *see Medical Tribune*, December 14, 1989, pp. 1, 17.)

Sun-Blocking Agents and Sunburn Preventives

If sunburn is bad news, the good news is that a remarkably large number of drugs will effectively protect the skin from the sun.

Opaque Sunblock Agents

Often used to cover the nose, ears, toes, or other vulnerable small areas of the body, opaque sunblocks reflect or scatter *all* light that strikes them from both the visible and UV spectra. The life guard with a sunblock-covered nose is a classic example of the use of these agents.

Sunscreens

Two types of sunscreen admit some UV light. A *sunscreen-sunburn* preventive agent contains an active ingredient that absorbs 95 percent or more of UVB light in the immediately dangerous 290- to 320-nm range. A *sunscreen-suntanning* agent absorbs between 85 percent and 95 percent of these rays, and hence lets more UVB light get through to the skin. Clearly the protective agent permits faster tanning and burning than does a preventive product.

Avobenzone blocks UVA in the range of 320 to 400 nm; these rays produce photosensitivity and may lead to skin cancer or other conditions over a long period of time. These rays do not cause sunburn or even tanning in ordinary out-of-doors doses.

The safety and effectiveness of a sunscreen depend in part on the concentration, or dosage, of active ingredients that it contains. The Panel's decisions on the safe and effective dosage for each approved active ingredient is presented in the Safety and Effectiveness table at the end of this Unit.

The evaluators said that the majority of sunscreen products they assessed contained only 1 or 2 sunscreen active ingredients. More may be contained if each is present in a safe and effective concentration and contributes to the product's effectiveness without interacting with or compromising any other ingredient's effectiveness or safety. A combination of a safe and effective sunscreen with a safe and effective ingredient from another drug category (for example, a skin protectant) is also safe and effective if it meets these requirements.

Sunless Tanners

The current rage in the sun product world is a group of products, sometimes called "bronzers," that temporarily dye the skin a tannish color *indoors*, without the need for you ever to set foot outside in the sun. It appears that some of these products are marketed as drugs, some as cosmetics. Most, if not all contain as an active ingredient the skin dye *DHA*, or *dihydroxyacetone*, which is being assessed as a drug in the OTC Drug Review. *See* lawsone + DHA, p. 919, below. It is not clear whether the current products also contain lawsone.

The self-tanning creams, lotions, and gels now are estimated to account for 20 percent of the $500 million annual sun products market. They cost between a dollar and about six dollars an ounce.

These dyes will color only the outer layer of skin, so they last only a few days, until that layer is naturally and normally sloughed off. The self-tanner then must be reapplied. The application itself is tricky—and needs to be done slowly and carefully—in order to obtain a smooth, even, ersatz tan.

Dihydroxacetone *does not* screen out the sun's UVA or UVB rays. Some self-tanners are combined with safe and effective sunscreens, albeit usually at low SPFs. So if you use one of these products, and then plan a day in the sun, you also may have to use ordinary sunscreens, of about your usual SPF, and observe your customary exposure limit in order not to sunburn through your "tan."

Dosage

Many people suffer serious sunburns each summer. Yet most sunscreen products sold in the United States contain effective protective ingredients. So it must be concluded that many people use either too little of these products or none at all.

One remedy, the Panel said, is to apply these products liberally before sunning and again after swimming or performing sweat-inducing exercises. The preparations must be spread over and must *cover* body surfaces in order to protect them.

Because sunscreens are believed to be quite safe, the Panel proposed no upper limits to the amounts adults and older children can use. Youngsters' skin is more sensitive to the sun than is adults'. So products that provide only minimal protection (SPF less than 4) should not be used on children under 2 years of age, except with medical supervision. Products that offer more protection (SPF 4 and above) may be used for babies 6 months to 2 years old. Except with the advice and supervision of a doctor, sunscreens should not be used on younger babies, who should be kept out of the sun. Their tender skin and eyes can be badly injured by bright sunlight.

A Word About 'Tanning Pills'

Can you get a tan without going out into the sunlight? Many people try to. Some use so-called tanning pills, which turn out to be food colors. They are synthetic analogues of the natural food coloring substances *beta carotene* and *canthaxanthin*, which belong to a class of compounds called *carotenoids*. It is the carotenoids that account for the yellowish-orange color in carrots, peaches, and melons.

Tanning pills *do* color the skin, but the FDA says the tan often has a distinctive orange tinge, particularly on the palms of the hands and the soles of the feet, and so does not look quite right. The agency also points out that a dye tan, unlike a natural one, does not protect against sunburn when you venture out with it onto a beach. The "tan" takes several weeks to develop and fades slowly when the pills are stopped.

A few individuals have suffered gastrointestinal distress and skin eruptions from taking tanning pills. Of far more serious concern, a recent report in the medical literature describes an apparently healthy young woman from Nashville, Tenn., who went to a tanning studio and was given canthaxanthin tanning pills. She took them. They turned her skin deep orange.

A few months later she became very ill—and soon died of the blood disorder *aplastic anemia*. (Because she was a Jehovah's Witness, she had refused treatment with human blood products.) Aplastic anemia is very often fatal. The woman's doctors say her death was "associated with" use of the tanning substance, but they could not prove cause and effect (*Journal of the American Medical Association*, vol. 264, pp. 1141-42, Sept. 5, 1990).

The FDA says that selling these tablets in interstate commerce is illegal until the agency has been presented with—and accepts—scientific evidence that they are safe and effective. These steps have not been taken. Verdict: Not safe and effective as a non-prescription drug. Products containing these ingredients usually are sold as cosmetics.

The way that a sun product is formulated can strongly influence its effectiveness and durability, including the preparation's resistance to sweating and washing off during swimming. A person who becomes sunburned while using a particular product should consider switching to another product that is prepared in a different way (lotion, cream, ointment, or solution), or one that has a higher, more protective SPF.

Ingredient Names in
Over-the-Counter Sunscreen Products

Standard Name	Alternate Names and Abbreviations
the combination of allantoin + aminobenzoic acid	allantoin-*p*-aminobenzoic acid (ALPABA)
aminobenzoic acid	*p*-aminobenzoic acid (PABA)
avobenzone	Parsol 1789 methoxydibenzoyl-methane 4-tert-butyl-4'-methoxydibenzoylmethane
cinoxate	2-ethoxyethyl-*p*-methoxycinnamate
diethanolamine p-methox-cinnamate	*p*-methoxycinnamic acid diethanolamine salt
dioxybenzone	2,2'-dihydroxy-4-methoxyben-zophenone
ethyl 4-[bis(hydroxypropyl)] aminobenzoate	2-mole propoxylate of aminoethyl-benzoate ethylhydroxypropyl PABA
2-ethylhexyl 2-cyano-3,3-diphenylacrylate	2-ethylhexyl-alpha-cyano-beta-phenylcinnamate
ethylhexyl *p*-methoxycinnamate	2-methoxycinnamic acid 2-ethyl-hexyl ester
2-ethylhexyl salicylate	octyl salicylate
glyceryl aminobenzoate	glyceryl *p*-aminobenzoate
homosalate	3,3,5-trimethylcyclohexyl salicylate homomenthyl salicylate

Ingredient Names in
Over-the-Counter Sunscreen Products (contd)

Standard Name	Alternate Names and Abbreviations
the combination of lawsone + dihydroxyacetone lawsone dihydroxyacetone	2-hydroxyl-1, 4-naphthoquinone 1,3-dihydroxy-2-propanone DHA
oxybenzone	2-hydroxy-4-methoxybenzophenone benzophenone-3
padimate A	amyl-dimethyl-p-aminobenzoate isoamyl-p-dimethylaminobenzoate pentyl 4-(dimethylamino) benzoate
padimate O	2-ethylhexyl p-demethylaminobenzoate 2-ethylhexyl 4-(dimethylamino) benzoate octyl dimethyl PABA 2-ethylhexyl PABA
red petrolatum	red veterinary petrolatum
sulisobenzone	2-hydroxy-4-methoxybenzophenone-5-sulfonic acid

APPROVED ACTIVE INGREDIENTS

• **AMINOBENZOIC ACID (PABA):** While this substance, commonly known as PABA, was not widely used in commercial sunscreen preparations until the 1970s, careful and exhaustive tests have shown that aminobenzoic acid is very effective—and also very safe—as a sunscreen. It has become the standard against which other sunscreens are judged. One study revealed aminobenzoic acid to be more effective than 100 other sunscreen formulations; another found it superior to 24 commercially available sunscreen products.

This ingredient provides day-long protection if the user does not swim or sweat heavily. Accounts vary on its retention after swimming, and the Panel recommends that it be reapplied when you emerge from the water.

Aminobenzoic acid appears to be more effective when applied two hours *before* sunning. This gives it time to diffuse into the outer layer of the skin, where it is retained.

Considerable data show that aminobenzoic acid is safe. But rashes and other skin eruptions may result from its use, and it may not be as popular now as it once was. As to effectiveness, aminobenzoic acid can protect the skin against sunburn in cases of extremely strong UV irradiation such as is found on glaciers or on the ocean. The Panel's approval is based predominantly on its ability to block UVB rays. In sum: safe and effective.

- **AVOBENZONE:** This compound has been judged by the FDA to safely and effectively block the full spectrum of UVA light rays (*see* previously under The New Worry: Ultraviolet A). It is the only active ingredient specifically approved for this purpose. It may be listed on containers as *Parsol 1789* or as methoxydibenzoyl-methane. It is particularly effective in the high UVA range of 340 to 380 nm, where other sunscreens are ineffective. The hope is that avobenzone will help prevent photosensitivity reactions as well as long-term damage, although it is not yet clear that it will. This ingredient is sold in combination with a UVB sun screen, padimate O, and the FDA approves the claim that these combinations are "broad-spectrum" sunscreen products. Avobenzone is safe and effective.

- **CINOXATE:** A 1 percent preparation of this substance totally absorbs UVB light rays in the immediately dangerous 290- to 320-nm range. Several studies have shown that most users get good to excellent tans when they use cinoxate. Its effectiveness depends in part on the vehicle in which it is formulated; one study showed that a lotion provided much better protection against exposure to fluorescent sunlamps than did a slightly weaker liquid solution.

Extensive tests in animals and in humans have failed to turn up serious toxic or allergic reactions. One manufacturer reported no complaints from the sale of 400,000 units of a 2 percent cinoxate sunscreen lotion and only 9 complaints (of which 8 were minor) from the sale of 2 million units of a 1.7 percent cinoxate solution. The Panel's verdict: safe and effective.

- **DIETHANOLAMINE P-METHOXY-CINNAMATE:** This tannish substance, also known as *p*-methoxycinnamic acid diethanolamine salt, is highly water-soluble; therefore, it may wash off when you swim or perspire. Studies in animals show that it is not irritating to the eyes or skin, and does not trigger allergic sensitization. These studies, plus wide use without reports of adverse effects, persuade the Panel that it is safe. Several tests on human subjects indicate that this sunscreen provides significant protection against the burning UVB rays of the sun; it is most effective against rays that are 290 nm in length. The Panel judges it safe and effective at dosages of 8 to 10 percent for adults and children over 6 months of age.

- *DIGALLOYL TRIOLEATE:* A derivative of tannic acid, this substance has been used as a sunscreen for 40 years. No scientifically controlled experiments were submitted to demonstrate its effectiveness. But a number of less-rigorous studies have shown that it blocks sunburn, even in people with extremely sun-sensitive skins. Digalloyl trioleate has been an "approved" sunscreen agent under United States Army specifications.

  Safety tests have uncovered no major risks. One company that sold 2 million units of a digalloyl trioleate sunscreen product over 20 years reported only six consumer complaints, only one of which may have been serious. The Panel evaluates digalloyl trioleate as safe and effective.

- *DIOXYBENZONE:* Dioxybenzone has been widely marketed in a combination product with padimate A (*see* p. 920), over which it has a wider spectrum of UV wavelength coverage. Several double-blind studies—conducted in real-life situations in which participants sat, played, or went swimming in the sun—indicate that this combination is an effective sunscreen, comparable with combinations of padimate A and aminobenzoic acid. A wide variety of safety tests failed to identify any significant risk with its use, so the Panel concluded that dioxybenzone is both safe and effective. It absorbs some radiation in the UVA spectrum over 360 nm.

- *ETHYL 4-[BIS(HYDROXYPROPYL)] AMINOBENZOATE:* This formulation of aminobenzoic acid in a waxy ointment remains on the skin and will block UVB light effectively after immersion and vigorous activity in the water. So it may be preferable to other aminobenzoic acid preparations for sunbathers who go in and out of the water frequently or sweat profusely. Animal and human tests, doctors' clinical experience with the substance in sun-sensitive patients, and manufacturers' marketing experiences all indicate that it effectively blocks UVB light rays. Yet it causes little irritation or other untoward effects, even when used in liberal amounts and for several days at a time. The Panel calls the compound safe and effective.

- **2-ETHYLHEXYL 2-CYANO-3,3-DIPHENYLACRYLATE:** A water-soluble sunscreen ingredient, this compound is formulated into a variety of oil-, alcohol-, and cream-based products. Tests in animals show that it is not an allergic sensitizer, and one manufacturer said he had received no complaints about sensitivity or intolerance to it after he marketed 15,000 product units. Studies show that it is very effective in absorbing UVB light and in protecting the skin, albeit less effectively than aminobenzoic acid. It absorbs some radiation in the UVA spectrum over 360 nm. The Panel's judgment: safe and effective.

- **ETHYLHEXYL P-METHOXYCINNAMATE:** This is an almost odorless, pale-yellow liquid with a slightly oily feeling. Diluted in alcohol, a 2 percent solution absorbs 84 percent of UVB light rays; a 5 percent solution absorbs 98.8 percent of these rays before they reach the skin.

  Extensive tests show that it is non-irritating and does not cause allergic sensitization; the Panel could find no reports of adverse effects in the medical literature. In comparative tests, products containing ethylhexyl p-methoxycinnamate "performed well" against aminobenzoic acid. So the Panel evaluated this substance as safe and effective as a sunscreen active ingredient.

- **2-ETHYLHEXYL SALICYLATE:** A clear, pale, odorless liquid, 2-ethylhexyl salicylate meets the technical requirements (light absorption) for an effective sunscreen. It is widely used; one company sells 55,000 pounds of it in sunscreens each year.

  Although 2-ethylhexyl salicylate was introduced long ago, in 1938, when safety testing requirements were less rigid than they are now, there have been no reports of adverse effects in the medical literature. Continuing consumer demand confirms the theoretical and experimental data that show that it effectively absorbs UV light rays. So the Panel pronounced it safe and effective.

- **GLYCERYL AMINOBENZOATE:** The virtue of this substance is that, unlike the related aminobenzoic acid, it is not soluble in water. Tests show that in some product formulations, although not in all of them, glyceryl aminobenzoate remains present and protective even after an ocean swim. It commonly is combined with a chemically related substance, p-dimethylaminobenzoate, but one study submitted to the Panel indicates that 3 percent glyceryl aminobenzoate by itself is as protective as 3 percent of each of these 2 aminobenzoates together.

  Tests in animals and in humans, as well as sunbathers' reports, suggest that some people will experience very mild itching in the eyes and minor skin irritation from glyceryl aminobenzoate preparations.

But no serious or long-lasting problems have been reported. The Panel said that this is a safe and effective sunscreen active ingredient—one that could be particularly useful for swimmers.

• HOMOSALATE: This oily, faintly yellow liquid blocks out less UVB light than aminobenzoic acid. Therefore it may be more appropriate for persons who are actively seeking a suntan than for people with extremely sensitive skin who are trying to avoid sunburn at all cost. Sweating and washing with water decrease homosalate's protective value so that it then needs to be reapplied.

The way that homosalate products are formulated will influence their effectiveness. In one test, a cream that contained 4 percent homosalate provided greater protection than a lotion that contained an 8 percent concentration.

In safety tests, homosalate has been shown to be nonirritating and nonsensitizing. One manufacturer reported that, over a decade of marketing experience, homosalate-containing products prompted about one letter of complaint for every quarter-million units sold. No serious ill effects were reported, so homosalate was judged by the Panel to be safe as well as effective.

• COMBINATION OF LAWSONE + DIHYDROXYACETONE (DHA): These chemicals are dyes. Lawsone is the principal dye component of henna, the red hair-dye. When the two substances are used in sequence—first the DHA, then the lawsone—they bind to the skin and effectively protect it from the sun's UVB rays. People whose skin is so sensitive that they can tolerate very little sunlight at all use this combination. It allows some—though not all of them—to go outside, travel, and even swim and play out-of-doors in daylight without danger. This combination is effective even for people who are not adequately protected by aminobenzoic acid. It absorbs some radiation in the UVA spectrum over 360 nm.

The exact way this double-dye method works to block UV light is not known. The two ingredients are effective sunscreens *only* when used together. They do not cause allergic sensitization, and serious complications are quite rare; accordingly the Panel found the combination of lawsone with DHA to be safe and effective.

It is claimed that this combination also acts to tan the skin even *without* exposure to sunlight. The DHA does, in fact, interact with the horny substance keratin in the outer layer of skin and dye the skin reddish brown. *No sun exposure is needed.* Repeated DHA applications progressively darken the skin. This "coloration" persists for some time, the Panel said. But it may be uneven because thicker skin (on the palms of the hands, for example) contains more keratin than thinner skin and so becomes darker. Coloring the skin with DHA is a cosmetic and not a medical activity, the Panel decided, and so is outside the purview of the OTC Drug Review. These cosmetics became quite faddish—and expensive—in the early 1990s.

DHA also may have a delayed effect on sun exposure. A person who has "pre-tanned" with it on one day will burn less-readily the next day. However, this protection is no greater than might be obtained with a single safe and effective sunscreen active ingredient by itself and the cost may be an artificial and uneven DHA "dye job" rather than a sun-induced natural tan. Nevertheless, DHA does darken the skin more quickly than sunlight, without risk of sunburn.

• *MENTHYL ANTHRANILATE:* Although its name does not immediately suggest it, this compound is an aminobenzoate. It is much less effective in blocking UV light rays than aminobenzoic acid, the standard against which other sunscreens are judged. But it has the advantage that it is less likely to irritate or sensitize the skin than some other aminobenzoates, so the Panel assessed it as safe and effective.

• *OXYBENZONE:* This compound is virtually insoluble in water. It is often combined with a second active ingredient. The evidence relating to its effectiveness is sparse and less convincing than the evidence for some other sunscreen active ingredients. But its safety has been better studied, and on the basis of available evidence, the Panel judged oxybenzone to be both safe and effective.

• *PADIMATE A:* While chemically related to aminobenzoic acid, padimate A is insoluble in water; thus it is more resistant to the effects of swimming and sweating. One researcher finds it comparable to aminobenzoic acid in effectiveness. (The two compounds are combined in some sunscreen products.) In a test, a 1 percent preparation of padimate A blocked 90 percent of dangerous UVB rays; a 2 percent preparation was a total sunblock. On the negative side, padimate A has been shown to irritate some people's skin. However, these reactions have not proved serious, so the Panel considered the ingredient safe and effective.

• *PADIMATE O:* Like padimate A (*see* immediately preceding), padimate O is a chemical relative of aminobenzoic acid. But it is not soluble in water. It is, in fact, more water-resistant than most sunscreen agents that have been tested. For example, more than half the padimate O remained on test subjects' arms after they swirled them around in tap water for half an hour. The Panel cites one researcher who says that a combination of padimate A + padimate O + oxybenzone should provide at least a half-day's protection against sunburn, even after swimming. Like padimate A, padimate O will irritate the skin of some users. But since these reactions tend to be mild, the Panel says padimate O is safe and effective.

- **2-PHENYLBENZIMIDAZOLE-5-SULFONIC ACID:** This fine, white, crystalline powder has been used for a long time as a sunscreen, usually in combination with other active ingredients. Controlled tests show that these combination products tend to provide effective protection against sunburn. The compound's safety has been established in many tests in animals and humans. One manufacturer told the Panel that in a recent 10-year period 50 tons were marketed around the world, with no adverse effects reported. So the ingredient was judged both safe and effective.

- **RED PETROLATUM:** As the name suggests, this is a petroleum product: one of the residues that remain after gasoline and home heating oil are removed from crude oil. The red color, an intrinsic pigment, is what blocks the UV sun rays. Long-term successful use confirms that it is effective. During World War II the United States Army Air Corps chose red petrolatum as the most effective protective substance for men marooned on life rafts or in the desert after plane crashes, because of its effectiveness and because a little bit covers a lot of skin. Red petrolatum absorbs some radiation in the UVA spectrum over 360 nm. It also holds in moisture. Surprisingly, while red petrolatum contains some paraffin wax and other petroleum byproducts, it spreads to a smooth, almost invisible film on the skin and leaves no visible greasy film as other forms of petrolatum may do.

  Red petrolatum is considered to be inert, and so safe that it is used as the vehicle for a number of other drug and cosmetic products. The manufacturer reports fewer than one complaint per 100,000 product units sold. As a sunscreen active ingredient, red petrolatum is safe and effective, according to the Panel.

- **SULISORBENZONE:** This is a chemical derivative of oxybenzone that has been shown in tests to be safe and effective as a sunscreen active ingredient. It absorbs some radiation in the UVA spectrum over 360 nm. But sulisorbenzone appears to be less protective against UVB than the aminobenzoates, and it is highly soluble in water. So it provides virtually no continuing protection after swimming, although the Panel evaluates it as safe and effective.

- **TITANIUM DIOXIDE:** This brilliant white powder reflects and scatters UVB light, much as whitewash will; it is an opaque sun block. It also reflects some UVA light rays above 360 nm. Titanium dioxide is used in face powders and beauty creams, as well as in sunscreen ointments, lotions, and protective powders. One skin specialist says it is "perhaps the most suitable and widely-used" light-scattering ingredient employed to protect people from the sun.

Titanium dioxide is chemically inert, and its wide use confirms that it is safe. Some 3.5 million units of a sunscreen containing titanium dioxide were sold between 1949 and 1972, and the manufacturer says no complaints were received that were attributable to the substance. The Panel's view: Titanium dioxide is safe and effective.

• TROLAMINE SALICYLATE: This substance has been studied less rigorously than some other active ingredients in sunscreens, but the tests that have been done indicate that it is effective. The available data show that while it may irritate the skin of some users, these reactions tend to be rare and mild. So the preparation was assessed as both safe and effective.

CONDITIONALLY APPROVED ACTIVE INGREDIENTS

• COMBINATION OF ALLANTOIN + AMINOBENZOIC ACID: A manufacturer claims he has combined these two substances in a single molecular complex. The Panel was not convinced that such is the case; neither was it convinced that there is any additional protective benefit to be gained from such a combination. The available data indicate that the combination is safe; they simply do not establish that allantoin—a tannic acid derivative—enhances the already great protective power of aminobenzoic acid. Pending such proof, the Panel rates this combination as conditionally approved.

• 5-(3,3-DIMETHYL-2-NORBORNYLIDEN)-3-PENTEN-2-ONE: The Panel received no studies documenting the effectiveness of this agent as a sunscreen active ingredient, even though it has been marketed for this purpose since 1973 and seems safe.

• DIPROPYLENE GLYCOL SALICYLATE: While animal tests indicate that this substance is not highly toxic, no data were submitted to the Panel on its safety or its effectiveness as a sunscreen. So it is given only conditional approval: not proved safe or effective.

DISAPPROVED ACTIVE INGREDIENTS

The Panel found three sunscreen active ingredients that it said were neither safe nor effective. While none of them is used in sun products marketed in the United States, travelers abroad should be aware of the disapprovals.

- **2-ETHYLHEXYL 4-PHENYLBENZOPHENONE-2-CARBOXYLIC ACID:** No experimental or marketing data were submitted on the safety of this compound when used by humans. Neither were studies concerning its effectiveness. The Panel concluded that it is not safe and not effective, and recommended that it not be marketed in the United States until adequate studies are submitted to the FDA. Subsequently, however, this ingredient has been listed in an FDA summary document as safe and effective. Its status, for now, seems unclear.

- **3-(4-METHYLBENZYLIDENE)-CAMPHOR:** The safety of this compound has been studied in mice, rats, and rabbits but not in humans. There is no data to show that it is effective as a sunscreen. The Panel judged it as neither safe nor effective.

- **SODIUM 3,4-DIMETHYLPHENYL-GLYOXYLATE:** There are no data on the safety and effectiveness of this substance when used as a sunscreen agent. The Panel says: not safe and not effective.

INACTIVE INGREDIENTS

There is more to most sunscreen products than their active ingredients. The sun-blocking chemical is usually dissolved or suspended in a vehicle—an ointment, a lotion, a cream, or a solution—so that the sunscreen can be applied to the skin. Perfumes, skin-softening compounds, and other inactive components may also be added.

Some of these inactive ingredients have complex chemical names, just as the active ingredients do. It can be difficult to decide which is which by reading the label. To help the consumer differentiate, some of these inactive components are

alcohol
allantoin
beeswax
benzyl alcohol
BHA

BHT
2-bromo-2-nitropropane-1, 3-diol
camphor
carbomer 934
carboset
cellulose gum
cetyl alcohol
cetyl palmitate
cetyl stearyl glycol
citric acid
clove oil
cocoa butter
color
dimethicone
dimethyl polysiloxane
ethyl alcohol
FD&C yellow No. 5
FD&C red No. 4
fragrances
glycerin
glyceryl stearate
isopropyl myristate
isopropyl palmitate
lanolin
lanolin alcohol
lanolin derivatives
lanolin oil
menthol
methylparaben
microcrystalline titanium-coated mica platelets
microcrystalline wax
mineral oil
oleth-3-phosphate
parabens
paraffin
PEG 2 stearate
petrolatum
polyoxyl-40-stearate
polysorbate 60
propellant 46

propellant 12/114
propylparaben
propylene glycol
propylene glycol stearate
quaternium 15
SD alcohol 40
sesame oil
silica
sodium carbomer
sorbitan oleate
sorbitan stearate
stabilized aloe vera gel
stearyl alcohol
synthetic spermaceti
wax
zinc oxide

When Further Relief Is Needed

If prevention fails, and a sunburn results, *see* ITCH AND PAIN REMEDIES APPLIED TO THE SKIN, and particularly, the Product Ratings on pp. 571-575, for anesthetics and other preparations to relieve the burning and pain. *See* also UNGUENTS AND POWDERS TO PROTECT THE SKIN to find soothing and protective ingredients and products to protect mildly burned, chapped, or chafed skin.

If sunburn is very red, and particularly if it is painful or the sun-burned person is feverish, faint, or feels ill, call your physician or visit a hospital emergency room without delay. While taking these steps, be sure that the sun-burned person is drinking sufficient quantities of water.

Safety and Effectiveness: Active Ingredients in Over-the-Counter Sunscreens

Ingredient	Panel's Assessment	Concentration (%)
allantoin + aminobenzoic acid	safe, but not proved effective	
aminobenzoic acid (PABA)	safe and effective	5-15
avobenzone	safe and effective* against UVA (but not UVB)	3
avobenzone + padimate O	safe and effective against UVA and UVB*	3% avobenzone, 7% padimate O
beta carotene (taken internally)	not safe or effective*	
canthaxanthin (taken internally)	not safe or effective*	
cinoxate	safe and effective	1-3
diethanolamine p-methoxycinnamate	safe and effective	8-10
digalloyl trioleate	safe and effective	2-5
5-(3,3-dimethyl-2- norbornyliden)-3-penten- 2-one	not proved effective	
dioxybenzone	safe and effective (absorbs some UVA)	3
dipropylene glycol salicylate	not proved safe or effective	

ethyl 4-[bis(hydroxypropyl)] aminobenzoate	safe and effective	1-5
2-ethylhexyl 2-cyano-3, 3-diphenylacrylate	safe and effective (absorbs some UVA)	7-10
ethylhexyl p-methoxycinnamate	safe and effective	2-7.5
ethylhexyl salicylate	safe and effective	3-5
2-ethylhexyl 4-phenylbenzophenone-2'-carboxylic acid	status not clear	
2-ethylhexyl salicylate	safe and effective	3-5
glyceryl aminobenzoate	safe and effective	2-3
homosalate	safe and effective	4-15
lawsone + dihydroxyacetone lawsone dihydroxyacetate	safe and effective (absorbs some UVA)	0.25 3
menthyl anthranilate	safe and effective	3.5-5
3-(4-methylbenzylidene)-camphor	not safe or effective	
oxybenzone	safe and effective	2-6
PABA (see aminobenzoic acid)		
padimate A	safe and effective	1-5
padimate O	safe and effective	1.4-8

Safety and Effectiveness: Active Ingredients in Over-the-Counter Sunscreens (contd)

Ingredient	Panel's Assessment	Concentration (%)
2-phenylbenzimidazole-5-sulfonic acid	safe and effective	1-4
red petrolatum	safe and effective (absorbs some UVA)	30-100
sodium 3,4-dimethylphenylglyoxylate	not safe or effective	
sulisobenzone	safe and effective (absorbs some UVA)	5-10
titanium dioxide	safe and effective (blocks some UVA)	2-25
trolamine salicylate	safe and effective	5-12

* FDA assessment.

Sunscreens: Product Ratings

Product and Distributor	Dosage of Active Ingredients	Rating*	Comment

Because of the long (15-year) lapse since the most recent OTC Drug Review publication on sunscreens (the panel report), it is not possible to provide a meaningful analysis of these products. One problem is that the nomenclature on the labels has become extremely confusing, with ingredients listed by names that differ from those used in the panel report. More important, many manufacturers are not yet supplying dosages on labels and in product information. Matters should become clearer when—finally—the FDA Tentative Final Monograph on these products is published.

*Author's interpretation of FDA criteria. Based on contents, not claims.

Teeth: Anti-Plaque Products

Dental plaque—and claims that mouthwashes, rinses, toothpastes and powders will reduce or control it—have become a central focus of oral health interest and marketing in the 1990s. Mouthwashes, which are now promoted and sold at least as much as anti-plaque agents as they are as breath-fresheners, are a $750 million annual market in the United States, according to industry sources. (*See* MOUTHWASH FOR ORAL HYGIENE.) What remains unclear is whether these products, re-dressed as plaque attackers, are safe or effective for routine use, according to FDA standards. Serious doubts exist that they are.

The fault in large part lies with the FDA, which has been extraordinarily slow in forcing manufacturers to back up claims for their products' safety and effectiveness, as anti-plaque claims became a font of promotional effort in the early 1980s. Both the Dental and the Oral Cavity Panels evaluated some ingredients—most of them *antimicrobials*, or germ-killers—that are now claimed to control plaque. But for a series of bureaucratic and administrative reasons, including the lack

TEETH: ANTI-PLAQUE PRODUCTS is based on the reports of the FDA's Advisory Review Panels on OTC Oral Cavity Drugs and on OTC Dentifrice and Dental-Care Products; on FDA's request for data and information on OTC Dental and Health Care Drug Products for Antiplaque Use, Safety and Efficacy Review; and on other sources cited in the text.

of forceful anti-plaque claims for some of these ingredients and products, neither of these original sets of evaluators in the Over-the-Counter (OTC) Drug Review definitively assessed such claims. But they did express some doubts about them.

Later, starting in the mid-1980s, the FDA began to talk about convening a new panel to assess anti-plaque claims. In 1988, it established this supplemental consultant group, called the Dental Products Panel. Two years later, it called for manufacturers and others to present scientific and dental evidence on the safety and effectiveness of products marketed with anti-plaque claims. This new information was due at the FDA in 1991. Since the agency process to evaluate, seek comment on, and regulate anti-plaque preparations may take several more years, consumers will have spent billions on these products before the verdict is in on their worth.

The FDA is allowing manufacturers who previously marketed active ingredients and products for which they now are making anti-plaque claims to continue to do so, provided they do not change the dosage or dosage forms. The agency also has acted to temper some manufacturers' outrageously inflated claims, and to exclude as new drugs some purported plaque-fighting substances that have not previously been sold in the United States to any significant degree.

For now, however, the consumer is largely on his or her own. *Caveat emptor!* (Let the buyer beware!)

 ## Claims

Approved
None.

Pending
There are no approved claims for anti-plaque products. The claims that the FDA's new Dental Products Panel and the agency itself are evaluating include

• "Anti-plaque"

• "For the reduction or prevention of plaque, tartar, calculus, film, sticky deposits, bacterial build-up and gingivitis"

What Is Plaque?

The original Dental Panel described plaque as a gel-like mat that has become firmly stuck to natural or artificial tooth surfaces. It is made up of masses of microbes and their secretions and detritus, and some non-bacterial cellular matter as well. The Oral Cavity Panel added that plaque is a soft and tenacious material found on the surface of teeth. Its composition varies, depending on where in the mouth it develops, diet, and other factors. Dental plaque leads to sore gums (gingivitis) and other diseases, the latter Panel said, a view reiterated in the standard *Dorland's Illustrated Medical Dictionary*, 27th ed. (Philadelphia: W.B. Saunders Company, 1988); it says plaque plays an "important" causative role in the development of dental cavities and diseases of the soft tissues, or *periodontal tissues*, that surround and support the teeth.

Cleaning the teeth has previously been treated as a cosmetic effort by the FDA; ordinary toothpastes, for example, are regulated under relatively unrestrictive rules that pertain to cosmetics. (Fluoride toothpastes and other fluoride products, however, are claimed to prevent disease—dental cavities—and so are regulated more stringently, as drugs. (*See* FLUORIDE TOOTHPASTES AND RINSES FOR CAVITY PREVENTION.)

The FDA now has made an important regulatory decision: Anti-plaque claims and the products for which they are made will be regulated under the stricter drug sections of the federal Food, Drug and Cosmetic Act. Plaque is usually not visible on the surface of the teeth, unless a stain or other disclosant substance is first applied to the teeth. Removing plaque cannot be a cosmetic activity that makes teeth look better, since there is no visible sign that in fact it has. More important perhaps, the agency says, anti-plaque active ingredients are intended to prevent cavities, calculus, and other forms of periodontal disease, so anti-plaque claims *are* medicinal claims and should be regulated as such.

The agency identifies two classes of anti-plaque products:

• Mouthwashes, gels, toothpastes, or other products that contain antimicrobial or chemical agents that are claimed to reduce or remove plaque.

• Toothpastes and powders and other products that contain abrasive substances that will scour away plaque when brushed onto the teeth with a toothbrush or other implement.

In assessing claims made for these ingredients and products, consumers should bear in mind that they may have been over-sold to the public. "Recently, products with anti-plaque claims have been heavily promoted," FDA says. In its *FDA Consumer* (May, 1990, pp. 9-13), public health specialist Steven Shepherd, M.P.H., adds: "The good news is that most of us have less to fear than we may have been led to believe. Periodontal disease is often described as almost universal—a disease that can or will affect almost everyone, and that can have 'devastating' results. But . . . recent studies suggest that only about 10 percent of adults have periodontitis severe enough to possibly cause tooth loss. The percentage is lower in younger people . . ."

Anti-microbial Active Ingredients

One combination of active ingredients and several individual ingredients are claimed to prevent or reduce plaque by killing the microbes of which it is largely composed. The list that follows probably is not complete; but it covers the major market share of these products.

• ALCOHOL *26.9* PERCENT + EUCALYPTOL *0.09* PERCENT + MENTHOL *0.04* PERCENT + METHYL SALICYLATE *0.06* PERCENT + THYMOL *0.06* PERCENT: This is an important combination drug product: First, because the formulation (*Listerine Antiseptic*, Warner-Lambert) was the first mouthwash to receive the American Dental Association (ADA) Seal of Acceptance for anti-plaque efficacy; second, because *Listerine* and the related *Listermint* have been market leaders, accounting for 35 to 40 percent of the mouthwash market; third, because researchers at the National Cancer Institute and elsewhere have reported an association between regular, long-time use of high-alcohol content mouthwashes, containing greater than 25 percent alcohol, and cancer of the throat and mouth (*see* MOUTHWASH FOR ORAL HYGIENE for a discussion of the possible cancer risk for high-alcohol content mouthwash.) Warner-Lambert says that the alcohol in *Listerine* is not an active ingredient (the concentration of which must be listed on the label). It says the alcohol is only a solvent for the antimicrobial ingredients. The company also has introduced a new product, *Cool Mint Listerine*, which contains 5 percent less alcohol: 21.6 percent.

The ADA standard that *Listerine* met requires two well-designed clinical studies showing that a product has significant effect against plaque and gingivitis. The *Listerine* studies, according to *Consumer Reports* (August 1989, pp. 504-509) reduced plaque scores 20 to 35 percent. The product-rating magazine's dental consultants said that the test results showed a "meaningful" reduction in plaque and gingivitis, so the product "could help many people."

Whether the FDA will agree, and whether the agency's concerns about the potential cancer risk of high-alcohol content mouthwashes will lead it to a different conclusion remain to be seen. *Consumer Reports* concurs with Warner-Lambert that *Listerine's* efficacy is based on its four phenol-like essential oils—eucalyptol, menthol, methyl salicylate and thymol—which are described elsewhere in this Guide. (*See* Index.)

• CETYLPYRIDINIUM CHLORIDE (CPC): This antimicrobial agent is a half-century-old quaternary ammonium compound, or "quat." (*See* p. 422.) It is a common ingredient in mouthwashes, some of which do, and some of which do not, make anti-plaque claims for it. *Consumer Reports* said several years ago that the one six-month study that it was aware of yielded only a 14 percent reduction in plaque—far less than *Listerine*. Side effects of cetylpyridinium chloride include tooth staining, a burning sensation in the mouth, and increased tartar formation, the product-rating periodical said.

• CHLORHEXIDINE GLUCONATE: This compound is an antimicrobial (antiseptic). The FDA and its panelists have dragged their feet in assessing its anti-plaque value for more than a decade. Although chlorhexidine is very effective at killing a wide range of microorganisms, its safety and effectiveness in over-the-counter products have not been demonstrated to the agency's satisfaction. Chlorhexidine *is* FDA-approved in the prescription mouthrinse *Peridex* (Procter & Gamble) which also has the ADA anti-plaque seal of approval.

Chlorhexidine sticks to the teeth, which may be one reason why it stays in the mouth long enough to effectively kill significant numbers of bacteria: It reduces plaque scores by 40 to 50 percent, and gingivitis by 30 to 50 percent, according to *Consumer Reports*. The beneficial effects have been shown to continue for two years, while the product continues to be used. Chlorhexidine stains the teeth, but the stain can be removed by a dentist. Chlorhexidine also has an unpleasant bitter taste.

While *Peridex* (which contains 0.12 percent chlorhexidine) remains a prescription drug, a toothpaste called *Elgydium* from France—where this antimicrobial substance is available without prescription—is sold in some stores in the United States. But it contains "only a small fraction" of the chlorhexidine dosage that has been shown to be effective in *Peridex*.

The effectiveness of this lower dosage has not been ratified either by the ADA or the FDA. *Consumer Reports* doubts its efficacy. Chlorhexidine has one other disadvantage: It can *promote* a slight buildup of *tartar*, which is calcified plaque, according to *Consumer Reports*.

• **DOMIPHEN BROMIDE:** This compound kills germs. But its safety and effectiveness as an anti-plaque active ingredient were in doubt when the Oral Cavity Drug Panel evaluated it a decade ago, and they remain in doubt today. (*See* p. 747.)

• **SANGUINARIA:** Sanguinaria is an extract from the bloodroot plant, for which plaque reduction of up to 68 percent has been claimed by a manufacturer. *Consumer Reports* noted that this was based on only a four-week study; other studies that showed only a 20 percent reduction required twice daily use of both a toothpaste *and* a mouthwash containing sanguinaria. The ADA has rejected a plaque-fighter claim for a sanguinaria product, according to *Consumer Reports*; the FDA's consultants have not had their say yet.

• **SODIUM BENZOATE:** The *Handbook of Nonprescription Drugs*, 9th ed. (1990) identifies sodium benzoate as the active ingredient in a high-selling pre-brushing mouthrinse (*Plax*, Pfizer), for which some extraordinary anti-plaque claims have been made. The *Handbook* says that, "upon further investigation, use of *Plax* yielded results comparative to placebo [dummy medication.]"

Abrasive Substances

• **CALCIUM PHOSPHATE:** This is a polishing and whitening agent that one maker says also acts to improve fluoride's penetration into the tooth enamel—a reputed anti-cavity action. This manufacturer also claims that the calcium helps "remove plaque."

• **SODIUM BICARBONATE (BAKING SODA):** This is a mild antimicrobial as well as an abrasive that is formulated into a tooth powder. The maker has claimed that sodium bicarbonate "fights plaque all the way to the gumline." FDA's dental consultants have not yet said if they concur. But a report in the agency's publication *FDA Consumer* (May 1990) describes a four-year study at the University of Minnesota School of Dentistry, in which baking soda was compared with ordinary toothpaste: Over all, according to the researchers quoted in the FDA magazine, there was no evidence that a baking soda brushing regimen "will contribute more toward periodontal health than use of a commercial toothpaste, a toothbrush, and dental floss."

- **ZINC CHLORIDE:** This astringent, a long-standing mouthwash ingredient (*see* p. 689), is formulated into some plaque-fighting products.

When Greater Relief Is Needed

Regular tooth-brushing and flossing are recommended methods to control plaque, and its hardened, calcified late stage, called *tartar*, or *calculus*. Your dentist can prescribe *Peridex*. Hardened deposits and softer plaque as well can be removed by a dentist or a dental hygienist in about ten minutes. Given the high price for some anti-plaque self-treatment products, plaque removal in the dental chair, along with brushing and flossing, may be a more effective and economical way to manage dental plaque.

Safety and Effectiveness: The FDA's Evaluation of Active Ingredients in Over-the-Counter Anti-Plaque Products Assessment

Active Ingredient	In Mouthwash or Rinse	In Toothpaste or Powder
alcohol 26.9% + eucalyptol 0.09% + menthol 0.04% + methyl salicylate 0.06% + thymol 0.06%	pending	
calcium phosphate		pending
cetylpyridinium chloride	pending	
chlorhexidine gluconate	safe and effective in dosage in Rx mouthrinse	pending
domiphen bromide	pending	
sodium bicarbonate (baking soda)		pending
zinc chloride	pending	pending

Anti-Plaque Preparations: Product Ratings

Product and Distributor	Dosage of Active Ingredients	Rating*	Comment

The FDA has not announced even its preliminary assessment of plaque-prevention claims for mouthwashes, toothpastes, and other products. So a meaningful rating of these products is not yet possible. It is worth noting, however, that most, if not all of these products contain antimicrobial (germ-killing) ingredients, and that the FDA has not approved *any* antimicrobial ingredient for routine daily use in the mouth.

*Author's interpretation of FDA criteria. Based on contents, not claims.

Teeth Desensitizers

Pain can arise and persist in a tooth without a cavity being present and without the pulp being exposed. Some teeth, in some people, simply seem to be more sensitive—indeed, painfully hypersensitive—to quite minor stimuli such as heat, cold, and pressure that others would not even notice.

Hypersensitive teeth are a common problem. One estimate presented to the FDA by a dentifrice manufacturer is that 12 percent of the adult population in the United States, about 19 million people, have sensitive teeth. A hypersensitive tooth may feel as painful as one with a cavity. This means the consumer cannot self-diagnose hypersensitivity; the dentist must do so, by ruling out cavities and all other causes of pain. Once the diagnosis has been made, however, nonprescription medications are available to treat dentin hypersensitivity.

The *dentin*—the calcified matter that makes up the bulk of the tooth between the crown enamel and the root cementum—appears to be capable of conveying sensations inward toward the sensitive pulp that lies at the tooth's center. Whether the dentin is laced with microscopic

TEETH DESENSITIZERS is based on the report "Drug Products for the Relief of Oral Discomfort for OTC Human Use," by the FDA's Advisory Panel on OTC Dentifrice and Dental-Care Drug Products and the FDA's Tentative Final Monographs on these products.

nerve fibers, or conveys sensations in some other way remains unclear. What *is* certain, the Panel says, is that even tiny nicks, scratches, or malformations in the enamel or cementus can expose the dentin, making it vulnerable to these unpleasant sensations.

The way that drugs act to relieve this discomfort is not really clear. Some drugs may alter the tiny nerve endings in the dentin so that they are less sensitive. Some may temporarily cover and block these sensitive endings. Others are claimed to form a new, hard outer layer of tooth that re-covers the exposed dentin.

One combination of active ingredients is approved by the FDA: 5 pecent potassium nitrate + 1 approved fluoride in a toothpaste or gel for treating hypersensitive teeth and preventing cavities.

 ### Claims for Desensitizers

Accurate
- "Helps reduce painful sensitivity of the teeth to cold, heat, acids, sweets, or contact"
- "Builds increasing protection against painful sensitivity of the teeth to cold, heat, acids, sweets, or contact"

WARNING:

 Sensitive teeth may indicate a serious problem that may need prompt care by a dentist. See your dentist if this condition persists or worsens. Do not use desensitizers for longer than 4 weeks unless recommended by a dentist or a doctor.

APPROVED TEETH-DESENSITIZING ACTIVE INGREDIENTS

- POTASSIUM NITRATE 5 PERCENT: Dentists have long used potassium nitrate, often in higher, 8.5 to 10 percent concentrations, as an office treatment for dental hypersensitivity. Since large amounts of nitrates are also consumed daily in food—principally from lettuce, beets, celery, radishes, and spinach—the reviewers decided that the relatively small amounts that might be ingested from a medicated toothpaste are safe.

Dentifrice makers recently have sponsored careful tests, using several hundred subjects, in which toothpastes containing 5 percent potassium nitrate were compared with identical toothpastes without potassium nitrate. As weeks and months went by, the medicated products proved consistently better than the unmedicated ones: The potassium nitrate reduced sensitivity to heat, cold, or pressure from a dental probe by about twice as much at each time as the non-medicated toothpastes. What is more, the teeth became less and less sensitive with time.

The FDA therefore approves two brushings daily with 5 percent potassium nitrate toothpaste. Brush at least one minute each time, using a soft tooth brush. For children under 12 years of age, consult a dentist or doctor.

CONDITIONALLY APPROVED TEETH-DESENSITIZING ACTIVE INGREDIENTS

- CITRIC ACID + SODIUM CITRATE IN POLOXAMER 407 (PLURONIC F-127 GEL): The individual ingredients in this preparation, which is marketed abroad as a tooth desensitizer, are widely used in foods and drugs. So the Panel accepts them, together, as safe. But the reviewers received only scant and inadequate data to show that the combination quells discomfort inside sensitive teeth. Verdict: effectiveness remains to be proved.

- FLUORIDE PREPARATIONS: SODIUM FLUORIDE, SODIUM MONOFLUOROPHOSPHATE, AND STANNOUS FLUORIDE: These ingredients are the fluoride preparations used in cavity preventive dentifrices; in the concentrations used in these products they are safe. (See FLUORIDE TOOTHPASTES AND RINSES FOR CAVITY PREVENTION.)

Fluorides act by hardening the enamel and perhaps by helping to re-enamel worn areas. It makes sense, then, that they would cover up exposed dentin, thereby reducing sensitivity to heat, cold, pressure, and other stimuli. Several controlled studies submitted to the Panel suggested that fluorides are beneficial in this way. But more recent research, evaluated by the FDA, failed to confirm this.

The FDA *does* agree, however, with manufacturers' claims that fluorides and teeth desensitizers serve a *complementary* role in hardening and armoring the teeth against injury and discomfort. So it approves a combination of potassium nitrate, the one safe and effective desensitizer, and any of the fluoride preparations approved for preventing cavities by hardening and strengthening the outer layer of tooth enamel.

- **FORMALDEHYDE SOLUTION:** This solution is a weak preparation, usually about 1.4 percent formaldehyde by weight in water, of the pungent gas that is also a principal ingredient in embalming fluid. It can be formulated as a toothpaste for treating hypersensitive teeth, and the Panel judged it safe after one manufacturer reported only 27 complaints of mouth reactions or gum injuries following the sale of 3,681,000 tubes of his product.

    However, formaldehyde's effectiveness in soothing hypersensitive teeth is less clearcut. Some controlled scientific studies indicate that a small percentage of users experience reduced sensitivity, compared with subjects who used a dummy medication. But reviewers found defects in the design of these experiments and commented on their lack of statistical significance. In short, while safe, formaldehyde's effectiveness as a teeth desensitizer remains to be proved.

- **STRONTIUM CHLORIDE:** This mineral compound has been shown to be extremely nontoxic. Over a twelve-year period, published reports on a 10 percent strontium chloride hexahydrate toothpaste showed no adverse effects. So reviewers concluded that strontium chloride is safe.

    The studies that are purported to demonstrate this mineral salt's effectiveness in relieving tooth hypersensitivity are far less convincing. Of these studies, the best was double-blind, meaning that neither the patients nor the dentist knew who were using the medicated toothpaste and who was using a dummy preparation. Both the test group and the controls showed measurable reductions in hypersensitivity at 4, 8, and 12 weeks. But users of the strontium chloride toothpaste did not improve much more than those using the dummy preparation.

    In another, comparable study, the investigator obtained similarly inconclusive results after subjects had used medicated and dummy toothpastes for 3 months. Only after 6 months was there a statistically significant advantage—in reduced sensitivity—among those who used the strontium chloride preparation. The lack of early and consistently significant improvement led the Panel to doubt the drug's effectiveness. The FDA concurs. Conclusion: safe but not proved effective.

DISAPPROVED TEETH-DESENSITIZING ACTIVE INGREDIENTS

- **COMBINATION OF EDETATE DISODIUM + SODIUM FLUORIDE (0.44 PERCENT) + STRONTIUM**

CHLORIDE: The sodium fluoride level in this preparation is 0.44 percent, which is double the level that the Panel has approved as safe for daily use against cavities. (*See* Fluoride in FLUORIDE TOOTHPASTES AND RINSES FOR CAVITY PREVENTION.) Along with the added risk of doubling the fluoride concentration, edetate disodium is unsafe because it can soften the teeth. Furthermore, no evidence has shown that the latter drug alone or in this combination of compounds is effective. In sum: not safe and not effective.

When Greater Relief Is Needed

More potent potassium nitrate toothpastes are available by prescription. Ask your dentist.

Safety and Effectiveness:
Over-the-Counter Teeth Desensitizers

Active Ingredient	Assessment
citric acid + sodium citrate in poloxamer 407 (Pluronic F-127) gel	safe, but not proved effective
edetate disodium + sodium fluoride + strontium chloride	not safe or effective
fluoride preparations: sodium fluoride, sodium monofluorophosphate (0.44%), and stannous fluoride	safe, but not proved effective
formaldehyde solution	safe, but not proved effective
potassium nitrate (5%)	safe and effective
potassium nitrate (5%) + one approved fluoride preparation, if labeled both for tooth desensitization and cavity prevention	safe and effective
strontium chloride	safe, but not proved effective

Teeth Desensitizers: Product Ratings

Product and Distributor	Dosage of Active Ingredients	Rating*	Comment
Denquel Sensitive Teeth (Procter & Gamble)	**toothpaste:** 5% potassium nitrate	A	
Mint Sensodyne (Block)	**toothpaste:** 5% potassium nitrate	A	
Original Sensodyne (Block)	**toothpaste:** 10% strontium chloride hexahydrate	B	not proved effective

*Author's interpretation of FDA criteria. Based on contents, not claims.

Teething Easers

When a several-months-old baby suddenly becomes fussier than usual, it is a good bet that he or she is cutting a tooth. Teething babies need to "work" their gums, and do so by chewing on crib edges, teething rings, bottle nipples, parents' fingers—or their own. They also may need occasional relief from the pain, which can be provided by cooling the gums with a bit of crushed ice or giving the infant a baby bottle containing a few ounces of cool water. An *anesthetic*, or numbing teething medication also may help.

 Claim

Approved
"For the temporary relief of sore gums due to teething in infants and children 4 months of age and older"

No combination products are approved for the relief of teething pain.

TEETHING EASERS is based on the report "Drug Products for the Relief of Oral Discomfort for OTC Human Use" by the FDA's Advisory Review Panel on OTC Dentifrice and Dental-Care Drug Products and the FDA's Tentative Final Monograph on these products.

Anesthetics for Pain of Teething

APPROVED ACTIVE INGREDIENTS

Two anesthetics are approved for use—without consulting a doctor—to relieve teething distress in infants from 4 months to 2 years of age. For younger infants with sore gums, or who appear to be teething, consult a doctor or dentist.

- BENZOCAINE (5 TO 20 PERCENT): This drug acts within seconds when applied to the gums and it provides pain relief that may last 5 to 10 minutes or longer. Benzocaine is widely used as an anesthetic and is considered very safe (see p. 671) and also effective for the relief of teething distress. However, it should not be used on infants younger than 4 months without first checking with the baby's doctor.

  The safe and effective dosage is 5 to 20 percent benzocaine, applied with a swab or small piece of cotton, up to 4 times daily.

- PHENOL (0.5 PERCENT): This alcohol is regarded as safe and effective when applied in small amounts to the gums. It blocks nerve conduction of pain impulses. Use up to six times daily, or as directed by a doctor or dentist.

CONDITIONALLY APPROVED ACTIVE INGREDIENTS
None.

DISAPPROVED ACTIVE INGREDIENTS
None.

Safety and Effectiveness: Active Ingredients in Over-the-Counter Teething Easers

Active Ingredient	Assessment
benzocaine (5-20%)	safe and effective
phenol (0.5%)	safe and effective

Teething Easers: Product Ratings

Product and Distributor	Dosage of Active Ingredients	Rating*	Comment
Babee Teething (Pfeiffer)	lotion: 2.5% benzocaine	B	inadequate concentration of benzocaine
Baby Anbesol (Whitehall)	gel: 7.5% benzocaine	A	
Baby Orajel (Commerce Drug)	gel: 7.5% benzocaine	A	

*Author's interpretation of FDA criteria. Based on contents, not claims.

Thyroid Protectors for Nuclear Emergencies

Escape of radioactive gases and liquids from atomic power plants and other nuclear facilities can occur suddenly and without warning—as was demonstrated by the 1979 Three Mile Island mishap near Harrisburg, and the 1986 nuclear reactor explosion at Chernobyl, in what is now the Ukraine. The Chernobyl explosion carried a variety of dangerous materials into the surrounding environment.

A self-treatment drug, potassium iodide, which once was a standard ingredient in over-the-counter cough remedies, can provide significant protection from one important form of radiation damage. *But it should be taken before or immediately after exposure to be of maximal value.* Taking it later, however, also may be helpful.

THYROID PROTECTORS FOR NUCLEAR EMERGENCIES is based on the FDA Summary of Basis for Approval for New Drug Applications 18-307 and 18-308, and on final recommendations for the use of potassium iodide as a thyroid-blocking agent in a radiation emergency, prepared by the FDA's Center for Devices and Radiological Health, and its Bureau of Drugs; it also is based on related federal documents.

Vulnerability of the Thyroid Gland

In nuclear accidents, some of the released material is almost certain to be radioactive iodines, particularly the nuclide called *iodine-131*, or I-131. After these iodines—which may be gases, liquids, or solid particles—are inhaled from the air, or ingested with foods or drink, they are picked up by the blood. The bloodstream carries them to the thyroid gland which normally regulates food intake and digestive metabolism. This gland quickly takes up and holds radioactive iodine. It does this because it normally takes up and holds other, non-radioactive iodines, which it uses, in tiny amounts, to regulate metabolism and other body functions.

Thyroid uptake of radioactive iodine is particularly dangerous because this gland is highly sensitive to radiation damage. Radiation can cause thyroid cancer, which, however, may not become evident for a decade or more after exposure. It also can cause non-cancerous growths, called *thyroid nodules*, and can inhibit thyroid function. Children are more vulnerable to this injury than adults.

Protective Preparations

Despite its great vulnerability, the thyroid can be treated with a nonprescription drug to forestall damage from radiation fallout.

To protect itself from overload of ordinary, non-radioactive iodine, the gland will stop taking up iodine once it has as much as it needs. So thyroid specialists and the FDA proposed a way of taking advantage of this protective mechanism: Supply the thyroid with enough *non*-radioactive iodine to make it stop taking this element up *before* the radioactive iodine arrives and is absorbed by the body. To be most effective, the blocking dose should be taken very quickly.

A protective dose of potassium iodide (KI), taken before or at the time that radioactive fallout or other leaked material reaches the body, will provide 90 to 100 percent protection. A substantial benefit—a block of 50 percent—is attainable during the first 3 to 4 hours after exposure, the FDA says. Longer delay will further diminish benefits.

The need to act quickly means that persons who live close to nuclear facilities probably should have KI close at hand in the home.

The efficacy of this public health measure, even when delayed, was demonstrated in the Chernobyl disaster: While there apparently is little solid data available from what formerly was the Soviet Union, some very useful information has been collected from nearby Poland, according to health physicist Donald Thompson, Ph.D., of the FDA's Center for Devices and Radiological Health. He cites information provided by University of Warsaw endocrinologist Janusz Nauman, M.D., on the results of emergency KI distribution. This did not begin in Poland until about twenty seven hours *after* I-131 from Chernobyl was first detected falling from the sky.

The KI had been stockpiled at government-run pharmacies. The druggists that worked in them were ordered to stop all other business on the second day after the explosion, and only dispense KI tablets, which they did. Ironically, a comparable emergency effort could no longer be undertaken, Dr. Janusz said in 1992, in a talk at the National Institutes of Health (NIH), in Bethesda, Maryland, because Poland's pharmacies no longer are state run. At that time, the pharmacists and Polish citizens diligently followed government instructions: about 85 percent of the public received at least one KI dose.

Those who took it had a five- to sixfold *lower* uptake of I-131 than other Poles who did not, Dr Nauman said. This is statistically a "very significant" benefit, according to Thompson, who heard Janusz's NIH talk. Side effects were infrequent, and mostly mild, Thompson related, confirming the FDA's earlier prediction that the method is safe as well as effective.

If a comparable disaster were to occur in the United States, or close by in Canada, would Americans be similarly or perhaps even *better* protected? Incredibly, the answer is a resounding no!

Federal officials talked for several years of stockpiling KI for emergency public distribution, or of providing it ahead of time to people living near nuclear facilities to keep in their homes. But they did neither.

A pre-Chernobyl (1985) federal policy document, still operative, acknowledges that "the use of KI is effective as a thyroid blocking agent in reducing accumulations by the thyroid gland of radioiodine..."

But people might be confused, the fed says, and might wrongly assume that KI protected against *all* forms of radiation, and so might not protect themselves by evacuating the area or staying in shelters. So—amazingly—the present policy says: "The federal position with regard to the pre-distribution or stockpiling of potassium iodide for use by the general public is that it should not be required."

Since it is not federally required, few if any of the states, which are directly responsible for citizens' well-being in a nuclear emergency, have stockpiled KI for the public. What they *have* done is make small stockpiles, of a few thousand doses, for the exclusive use of rescue workers and institutionalized persons (prisoners and hospitalized patients) who could not flee. The general public, however, will not be served.

To make matters worse, the FDA has licensed three companies to produce nonprescription KI tablets and liquid for nuclear emergencies. But the two larger ones, Wallace Laboratories in New Jersey, and Roxane Laboratories in Ohio, do not make it for retail distribution, and, according to news accounts, refused to supply it to people who phoned for it during the Three Mile Island mishap (*New York Times*, Aug. 31, 1983). One of the makers said the federal government had asked it *not* to provide KI to the public!

One frightened citizen who could not buy KI was a New York marketing specialist, Alan Morris. He thereupon quit his job, and started a company, called Anbex, Inc., to make and distribute KI supplements for use in nuclear emergencies; the FDA licensed his company for this purpose. A decade later, Morris apparently is the only source of brand-name nonprescription KI tablets, which he sells by mail. (For specific information, *see* the table Thyroid Protectors: Product Ratings at the end of this Unit.)

One other nonprescription KI source exists: According to FDA physicist Thompson, local pharmacies legally can (and should be willing to) prepare it, without prescription, when asked, provided the label stipulates: For thyroid blocking in a radiation emergency.

KI has a long shelf life. Thompson says ongoing tests show that it remains stable in the bottle at least five years. Given the small governmental stockpiles and absence of a plan to distribute KI to the public, the only way consumers can be assured of it, if they need it, is to obtain it from one of the sources mentioned here and keep it on hand. The declaration of a nuclear emergency (the cue to start taking the drug) is a state or local decision, not a federal one, U.S. officials say. Given the confusion that might occur in a nuclear emergency, some people might choose not to wait for the governor to make an announcement.

Some other iodine compounds as well as some other drugs will block thyroid uptake of radioactive iodine. In an emergency, if you do not have KI on hand, phone your doctor or pharmacist for advice, and listen to health advisory warnings on the radio or television.

Claims

Accurate
• "For thyroid blocking in a radiation emergency only"

WARNING:

 Potassium iodide should not be used by people allergic to iodine. In case of overdose or allergic reaction, contact a physician or public health authority.

Thyroid-Blocking Agents

While a variety of iodines may provide protection against radioactive iodine, only one is well studied and approved.

APPROVED ACTIVE INGREDIENT

• **POTASSIUM IODIDE (KI):** This iodine compound is present in small amounts in ordinary food, and in iodized table salt. It has been widely used medicinally as a salt substitute and is available by prescription as an expectorant for persons with bronchial asthma.

The doses used to treat bronchial asthma and other respiratory diseases are from 300 to 1200 mg daily for adults. This is far higher than the dosage recommended for use in the brief period following a nuclear emergency. So the FDA says potassium iodide is safe as well as effective in recommended dosages. For persons who are allergic to iodine, the risk probably outweighs the potential benefit.

The approved dosage for adults, including pregnant women, and for children over one year of age is 130 mg once daily. The approved dosage for babies up to a year old is 65 mg once daily. Treatment should continue for 10 days unless public health officials say stop.

CONDITIONALLY APPROVED ACTIVE INGREDIENTS

None.

DISAPPROVED ACTIVE INGREDIENTS

None.

When Greater Relief Is Needed

If you are unable to obtain KI without a prescription, via the routes suggested in this Unit, you can ask your physician to write a prescription for it. The druggist almost certainly will fill it.

Safety and Effectiveness: Active Ingredients in
Over-the-Counter Thyroid-Protecting Agents for Nuclear Emergencies

Active Ingredient	RECOMMENDED DAILY DOSAGE		Assessment
	Infants Under Age 1 year	*Adults and Children Over Age 1 year*	
potassium iodide	65 mg	130 mg	safe and effective

Thyroid Protectors: Product Ratings

Product and Distributor	Dosage of Active Ingredients	Rating*	Comment
			The two major companies that have been licensed by the FDA to sell potassium iodide over the counter as a thyroid blocker for nuclear emergencies (*Thyro-Block*, Wallace; *Oral Potassium Iodide*, Roxane), appear not to be marketing it retail through drug stores. Your pharmacist, however, stocks or can easily obtain this substance. If he or she has doubts about the propriety of dispensing it without prescription, a phone call to FDA's Center for Devices and Radiological Health (301-443-2850) should dispel these concerns. The third licensed supplier, listed below, is a mail order company.
Iosat (Anbex)	**tablets:** 130 mg	A	send $6† per treatment packet (10-day supply) to Anbex, POB 863, Radio City Station, NYC 10019

*Author's interpretation of FDA criteria. Based on contents, not claims.
†Price is subject to change.

Toothache Relievers

Quick relief is what everybody wants when a tooth suddenly starts aching. A number of drugs are sold for this purpose. Their instructions say to apply the drug to the cavity or crack in the tooth or to temporarily use it to plug the hole until a dentist can be seen.

Most of these drugs are unsafe, ineffective, or both, according to Panel reviewers and the FDA. So, from the evaluators' findings, it seems that anyone who hopes for the repair and saving of an aching tooth ought to avoid over-the-counter drugs that are applied to the teeth. Instead, a toothache sufferer should make an emergency dental appointment, and, in the meantime, use a hot water bottle, ice pack, aspirin, or prescription pain killers to relieve pain.

The only tooth that the Panel believed is a candidate for treatment with topical nonprescription toothache relievers is the one that is so badly damaged that the dentist is going to have to extract it anyway. How do you decide? If the pain is intermittent (coming and going) the tooth is probably still alive and salvageable. If the pain is throbbing

TOOTHACHE RELIEVERS is based on the report "Drug Products for the Relief of Oral Discomfort for OTC Human Use" by the FDA's Advisory Panel on OTC Dentrifice and Dental-Care Drug Products and the FDA's Tentative Final Monograph on these products.

and relentless, the tooth is likely to be irreversibly damaged.

One way of treating tooth pain is by *counterirritation*: By setting up what is presumably a more tolerable irritation or pain in the nearby gum, you are supposed to forget the pain in the tooth. But the reviewers have strong reservations about using counterirritants in treating toothaches as well as about the drug—essence of red pepper—that is used for this purpose. (*See* further on.)

Claims for Toothache Relievers

Accurate

None.

False or Misleading

• "For temporary relief of cavity toothache"

• "Eases pain due to cavities fast"

• "Quickly forms temporary filling"

• "Fast relief from toothache due to cavities"

WARNING:

Do not use for intermittent pain. Toothaches and open cavities indicate serious problems that need prompt attention by a dentist. A dentist must be seen as soon as possible, whether or not the pain has been temporarily relieved.

The Panel adds an additional warning for toothache relievers that are marketed in small, porous bags (poultices) designed to be held in the mouth so that the drug will be released slowly onto the sore tooth and surrounding gum: To avoid choking, do not leave a poultice in the mouth when you may fall asleep.

Types of Toothache Relievers

Some toothache remedies are intended to act as "temporary fillings," which allegedly protect the tooth pulp by shielding it against saliva, food particles, and other items that can provoke pain. The serious problem with this approach is that the dental pulp easily becomes inflamed when exposed to any foreign matter—including the temporary filling. The dental pulp swells and may secrete fluids and gases that must be drained. Without proper drainage, pressure within the tooth can cause further, perhaps uncorrectable, damage. Putting beeswax, sandarac, or other semi-solid temporary fillings into the tooth prevents necessary drainage and decompression. The Panel says such temporary fillings are unsafe and are also unlikely to be effective in relieving pain.

WARNING:

 The FDA specifically concurs that beeswax should *never* be used as a temporary filling, as it may cause festering—and further pain—inside a damaged tooth.

Many toothache relievers are alcohols, which dry out the calcified hard material (the dentin) that forms the bulk of the tooth. Some of these drugs are also irritants. The drugs have a medicinal taste and smell and, as irritants, cause a new and perhaps helpful sensation of pain. "These properties distract the patient and may provide some psychological feelings of benefit," the Panel said, "but the major problems of deep cavities, pulp inflammation, and infection remain untreated."

Combination Products

The Panel listed no safe and effective combinations, and granted conditional approval to only three:

- A combination of 2 approved or conditionally approved toothache relievers that act by different mechanisms
- 1 approved or conditionally approved toothache reliever + 1 gingival (gum) anesthetic (specifically: eugenol + benzocaine)
- 1 approved or conditionally approved gingival anesthetic + 1 approved or conditionally approved counterirritant

All other combinations that include toothache-relief drugs are disapproved.

Toothache Pain Relievers

APPROVED PAIN-RELIEVING ACTIVE INGREDIENTS
None.

CONDITIONALLY APPROVED PAIN-RELIEVING ACTIVE INGREDIENTS

- **BENZOCAINE:** Generally speaking, this is a safe anesthetic and also a highly effective one. But there are few data on its value when applied directly to dental nerve tissue in the cavity of a tooth. Verdict: safe but not proved effective.

- **BENZYL ALCOHOL:** This drug irritates soft tissues, so that its safety—even in the low concentrations of 1 to 3 percent in which it is formulated into toothache remedies—remains to be proved. No scientific evidence is available to show that it effectively relieves toothache when applied directly to a decayed or broken tooth. In sum, benzyl alcohol is not proved safe or effective for this purpose.

- **BUTACAINE SULFATE:** An anesthetic, this substance is safe and effective when applied to the gums, as is benzocaine. But there is insufficient documentation to show that it is either safe or effective when put directly onto sensitive nerve tissue inside a diseased or injured tooth. Conclusion: not proved safe or effective.

- **CREOSOTE:** This is a distillate of wood tar. Because it paralyzes sensitive nerves, and so acts anesthetically, it has been reported to provide temporary relief from toothache. But it is an irritant to the tooth pulp, and a safe dosage has never been established. Creosote is usually formulated into toothache remedies as dilute solutions, and evidence is lacking to show it is effective in these concentrations. So the Panel and the FDA say: not proved safe or effective.

- **CRESOL:** This is a phenol-like alcohol that is fairly irritating to tissues, so the Panel cannot vouch for its safety. The Panel searched widely for a scientific study demonstrating cresol's effectiveness as a dental anesthetic, but it could find none. Therefore cresol is listed as not proved safe or effective as a toothache remedy.

- *EUGENOL PREPARATIONS 85 TO 87 PERCENT EUGENOL IN CLOVE OIL OR OTHER BLAND OIL:* These pungent, spicy-tasting preparations are obtained from cloves, although eugenol now also is extracted from other sources, according to the *United States Pharmacopeia XIX*. Clove oil contains 85 to 87 percent eugenol; the Panel felt that only full-strength (85 to 87 percent) preparations contain enough eugenol to be effective.

    Eugenol's pain-deadening property has been known for 300 years. Dentists long have used it as a local anesthetic. Eugenol was previously available only as a prescription drug. The reviewers decided, with some misgivings, that it should be made available without prescription. A major argument in favor of this step was the evaluators' lack of confidence in the safety and effectiveness of existing nonprescription toothache drugs. A major argument against it was that eugenol acts as an extreme irritant to the nerve tissue of the tooth pulp.

    The decision to approve eugenol was made despite a lack of well-controlled contemporary studies on its use as a self-treatment drug. Approval was based largely on the clinical experience of Panel members and the views of consultants. While the Panel approved it, the FDA demurred and said it needed to see proof of eugenol's safety and effectiveness.

WARNING:

 Because of this tooth-destroying trait, the Panel warned strongly that eugenol preparations should be used only on teeth that already are irreparably damaged.

- *EUGENOL PREPARATIONS 1 TO 84 PERCENT EUGENOL:* There is no evidence that lower concentrations of eugenol will relieve toothache or are safe for that purpose. Conclusion: not proved safe or effective.
- *PHENOL PREPARATIONS PHENOL AND PHENOLATE SODIUM:* Phenol is safe and effective for use on the gums. But it has never been established through acceptable scientific studies that it is either safe or effective when instilled into a rotten or broken tooth. Conclusion: not safe or effective.
- *THYMOL PREPARATIONS THYMOL AND THYMOL IODIDE:* These medicinal extracts of thyme are aromatic, like clove oil and eugenol. In dentistry they are used after a cavity is drilled clean to form a protective layer between the dentin and the inlay (filling) that will be packed in. They are also used as deodorant ingredients in antiseptic mouthwash and gargles. So, despite a paucity of scientific evidence, reviewers judged the

drugs safe. But the Panel could not find sufficient evidence to demonstrate thymol's effectiveness as a toothache remedy. The FDA concurred: These preparations are listed as not proved effective.

DISAPPROVED PAIN-RELIEVING ACTIVE INGREDIENTS

- **CAPSICUM:** This red-pepper extract is highly irritating to the tooth pulp, the gums, and other tissues. The Panel says the substance will injure viable tooth pulp and is unsafe. Also, no studies could be found to show that currently marketed capsicum toothache drops or gum effectively relieve pain. Verdict: neither safe nor effective.
- **MENTHOL:** This pepperminty substance is extremely irritating to living tissues, so it is not safe for the temporary relief of toothaches. Evidence shows that it is also ineffective. Verdict: menthol is not safe and not effective.
- **METHYL SALICYLATE:** This minty alcohol is extremely irritating to soft tissues and should not be put into a tooth cavity. What is more, there is no evidence whatsoever that the drug acts as a pain killer. In sum: methyl salicylate is not safe and not effective.

Counterirritants

Given the general ineffectiveness of over-the-counter toothache pain relievers, it is little wonder that some people desperately try to defeat the pain by deliberately irritating the gums that surround a sore tooth. The rationale is that the sufferer's attention is shifted from the toothache, or perhaps the tolerable irritation from the counterirritant blocks the intolerable tooth pain. Another theory is that the counterirritant draws additional blood into the area, hastening the removal of poisonous products from the injured tooth. None of these theories has been proved.

 Claims for Counterirritants

Accurate
None.

APPROVED COUNTERIRRITANT ACTIVE INGREDIENTS

None.

CONDITIONALLY APPROVED COUNTERIRRITANT ACTIVE INGREDIENTS

None.

DISAPPROVED COUNTERIRRITANT ACTIVE INGREDIENTS

• CAPSICUM: This red-pepper extract is sold in poultices that may also contain a pain-relieving ingredient. It also comes in the form of drops and gums. The capsicum dose is very weak: about 2 parts per 10,000 in the base in which the drug is formulated. So the Panel judged it safe. Several small studies have been done to try to establish whether capsicum relieves toothache pain; the Panel judged the results to be inconclusive. The FDA says: Not safe or effective.

When Further Relief Is Needed

See a dentist at once. If you cannot make an emergency appointment, or cannot wait for relief, go to the nearest hospital emergency room. They can provide enough of a potent prescription (R) pain-killer to get you comfortably to a dental appointment or a dental clinic.

Safety and Effectiveness: Over-the-Counter Toothache Pain Relievers and Counterirritants

Active Ingredient	Assessment
beeswax (inactive ingredient)	not safe
benzocaine	safe, but not proved effective
benzyl alcohol	not proved safe or effective

Safety and Effectiveness: Over-the-Counter
Toothache Pain Relievers and Counterirritants (contd)

Active Ingredient	Assessment
butacaine sulfate	not proved safe or effective
capsicum (as pain reliever)	not safe or effective
capsicum (as counterirritant)	not safe or effective
creosote	not proved safe or effective
cresol	not proved safe or effective
eugenol preparations with 85 to 87% eugenol	not proved safe or effective
eugenol preparations with 1 to 84% eugenol	not proved safe or effective
menthol	not safe or effective
methyl salicylate	not safe or effective
phenol preparations: phenol and phenolate sodium	not proved safe or effective
thymol preparations: thymol and thymol iodide	safe, but not proved effective

Toothache Relievers: Product Ratings

Product and Distributor	Dosage of Active Ingredients	Rating*	Comment
Anbesol (Whitehall)	**liquid:** 6.3% benzocaine + 0.5% phenol	B	benzocaine not proved effective; phenol not proved safe or effective
Num-zit jel (Purepac)	**gel:** benzocaine + menthol	C	menthol not safe or effective
Orajel (Commerce)	**gel:** 10% benzocaine	B	benzocaine not proved effective for relieving toothache
Orajel-d (Commerce)	**gel:** 10% benzocaine + eugenol	B	neither ingredient proved effective
Poloris Dental Poultice (Block)	**poultice:** 7.5 mg benzocaine + 4.6 mg capsicum	C	capsicum not safe or effective

*Author's interpretation of FDA criteria. Based on contents, not claims.

Unguents and Powders to Protect the Skin

For centuries certain substances have been used as dusting powders, lotions, ointments and creams for temporary coverage, protection, and relief of burned, chafed, chapped, scraped, or otherwise irritated and injured skin. These substances, technically called *skin protectants*, differ from most of the medications described in this book. Most medications *act* in some way. For example, they may have a biochemical effect on the body's cells and fluids or on bacteria or other "germs." Skin protectants, however, tend to be *inert*. They form a physical barrier that protects injured, vulnerable skin from dryness, wetness, or irritating chemicals, or from external pressure or frictional contact with clothing, bandages, or even other body surfaces. Some skin protectants grab, hold, dilute, or dissolve irritants. In a paradoxical sense, some of these substances are inactive active ingredients. Yet, as the reviewers noted, they can produce dramatic relief—for example, when a lubricant

---

UNGUENTS AND POWDERS TO PROTECT THE SKIN is based on the report on "Skin Protectant Drug Products for OTC Human Use" prepared by the FDA's Advisory Review Panel on OTC Topical Analgesic, Antirheumatic, Otic, Burn and Sunburn Prevention and Treatment Drug Products, and on FDA's Tentative Final Monograph on these products.

and anti-drying agent is applied to sunburn; when moisture retainers are used for chapped lips; and when lubricants soften the skin and increase its pliability. Technically, for the purposes of the OTC Drug Review, skin protectants are categorized as *active ingredients*.

 Claims

Accurate

- "For the temporary protection of minor cuts, scrapes, burns and sunburn"
- "Helps prevent and temporarily protects chafed, chapped, cracked, or wind-burned skin and lips"
- "Dries the oozing and weeping of poison ivy, poison oak and poison sumac"

False or Misleading

- Any reference to the "cure" of anything
- "Aids healing" (this has yet to be proved)

WARNING:

 If the condition worsens or does not improve within 7 days, consult a doctor.

Uses for Skin Protectants

Depending on their physical traits, skin protectant ingredients can serve three different purposes. Some fulfill only one of these purposes; others serve two. The Uses for Approved Skin Protectants table defines these uses.

The skin protectants described in this Unit also have other specific uses. *See* POISON IVY-OAK-SUMAC PREVENTIVES AND PALLIATIVES. Other uses are described in the Units COLD-SORE BALMS, DIAPER-RASH RELIEVERS, INSECT REPELLENTS AND BITE AND STING TREATMENTS, and ITCH AND PAIN REMEDIES APPLIED TO THE SKIN.

Uses for Approved Skin Protectants

Ingredients	USES		
	For the temporary protection of minor cuts, scrapes, burns, and sunburn	Helps prevent and temporarily protects chafed, cracked, or windburned skin and lips	Dries the oozing of poison ivy, oak, and sumac
allantoin	yes	yes	
cocoa butter	yes	yes	
petrolatum	yes	yes	
white petrolatum	yes	yes	
shark-liver oil	yes	yes	
dimethicone	yes	yes	
sodium bicarbonate (bicarbonate of sodium, baking soda)	yes		
glycerin		yes	
aluminum hydroxide gel			yes
calamine			yes
kaolin			yes

Uses for Approved Skin Protectants (contd)

Ingredients	USES		
	For the temporary protection of minor cuts, scrapes, burns, and sunburn	Helps prevent and temporarily protects chafed, cracked, or windburned skin and lips	Dries the oozing of poison ivy, oak, and sumac
topical starch			yes
zinc acetate			yes
zinc carbonate			yes
zinc oxide			yes

Burns

Many of the ingredients used to treat minor burns are skin protectants. Serious burns, in which one or more layers of skin have been destroyed, require medical attention. Only first-degree burns, in which the skin is reddened but initially not broken, and mild second-degree burns, where small areas of the outer layer of skin have been damaged, should be self-treated.

When a person is seriously burned, medical help should be quickly sought. Covering a wide or deep burn with a first-aid product or skin protectant can complicate later treatment, since the temporary material may have to be removed by the emergency room doctor or nurse—a procedure that can make the pain worse.

Fast action is the key to first aid for minor burns. The burned surface should be immediately immersed in a basin of still, cool, or even cold water, or covered *gently* with cold-water compresses (cloths soaked in cold water and wrung out). Do *not* use running water: The pressure and friction of the water stream may increase the pain. Do *not* use ice cubes or ice water: They are too cold and can cause further injury and pain.

Cold-water treatment of a mild burn should continue for 20 minutes to half an hour. If the burn pain subsides, little further treatment (other than possible use of a skin protectant) will be needed.

A number of household remedies have been used to treat burned skin. These include application of butter, lard, goose grease, and other oily substances. Although they may offer some initial relief, these substances are *not* recommended. They are likely to be unsterile and so may promote infection. They may contain salt, which can increase the pain. The nonirritating skin protectants described in this Unit are the better choice.

Wound Healing

Three active ingredients that are claimed to promote wound healing are being assessed in the Over-the-Counter (OTC) Review. Two of them—*allantoin* and *zinc acetate*—have been found to be safe and effective as skin protectants but *not* as wound healers. The other, *live-yeast-cell derivative*, was evaluated only as an agent to promote healing, and it is still being considered by the FDA. The Hemorrhoid Panel said it has not been proved safe and effective. (*See* p. 506, in the unit HEMORRHOID MEDICATIONS AND OTHER ANORECTAL APPLICATIONS.)

The present Panel was extremely skeptical of all wound-healing claims. Similar doubts were raised by two other Panels, which evaluated antibiotics and other antimicrobial agents. Manufacturers will have to substantiate the wound-healing claims by scientific studies or drop them from their product labels.

Standards of Approval for Skin Protectants

The evaluators appear to have been more tolerant in granting approval to skin-protectant ingredients than they (or other over-the-counter reviewers) were with any other class of ingredients. One reason is that these protectants traditionally have been popular because they are soothing and non-irritating. Their safety and effectiveness are attested to by druggists and by doctors' medical experience—and by the long-time use of satisfied consumers.

Because these agents are inert, or neutral (and so appear safe), several of them are used as *vehicles*. This means that manufacturers and druggists use them for mixing other pharmacologically active ingredients to make products that are applied to the skin or mucous membranes. The Panel therefore recommended that the FDA waive its usual test requirements because of (1) wide use, (2) the protectants' inclusion in standard drug compendiums, and (3) their established effectiveness in providing a mechanical barrier that protects the skin. The FDA accepted this proposal.

A Possible Hitch?

It can be argued, of course, that occasionally a drug that is universally regarded as safe turns out to be a hazard. One noteworthy example is boric acid, which for a long time was used as a skin protectant in diapering powders for babies as well as in lotions, ointments, and pastes to prevent irritation and infection, speed healing, and relieve the pain of burns. Only after a half-century of widespread use was boric acid found to be potentially lethal. The danger arises because of the ease with which boron—its principal base, which is now known to be very poisonous—is absorbed through the skin. Moreover, on careful reexamination, boric acid has now been found to have little or no protective value! Accordingly, it has been assessed in the OTC Drug Review as both unsafe and ineffective for nonprescription use. It is being banned for most if not all nonprescription drug products.

Conceivably, other skin-protectant ingredients that now are considered safe and effective, despite the lack of definitive scientific proof, will one day be discarded as boric acid has been.

Combination Products

In the liberal spirit with which they assessed skin-protectant active

Cow Balm Relieves Chapped Human Hands

This Guide is about over-the-counter drugs legally sold for *human* uses. But there is one product, once made and marketed in huge tubs exclusively to relieve milk cows' chafed, chapped udders, that now enjoys widening sales in small containers as a human skin-care product. As dairy herds dwindle around the town of Lyndonville, Vermont, where it originates, *Bag Balm* (Dairy Association Co., Inc.) is selling nicely in local drug stores, and elsewhere as well.

Bag Balm is labeled as an antiseptic and contains 8-hydroxyquinoline sulfate 0.3 percent in a base of petrolatum and lanolin.

The FDA has not been persuaded that 8-hydroxyquinoline sulfate (also called *oxyquinoline sulfate*) is safe and effective for human use. But it certainly would have no problem with petrolatum and lanolin as skin protectants.

Bag Balm is sold in colorful green and red tins, at up to $3 an ounce, and is promoted by retailers and mail-order companies to gardeners, fishermen, and others who spend much time out-of-doors. As one garden catalogue puts it, "The same properties which soothed and healed cows provide wonderful relief for hands which have been exposed to cold and wet."

The label carries the mandatory warning "for veterinary use only," and provides these special directions: "Massage thoroughly, and allow ointment to remain for full antiseptic and softening effect on the udder."

ingredients, the evaluators imposed no limit on the number of these substances that can be formulated into a product, provided that each ingredient makes a contribution to the whole.

But ingredients in combination products cannot interact with each other or act in an opposing way to each other. Thus an ingredient like cocoa butter, which is moisture-retaining, cannot be combined, say, with calamine lotion, which has the opposite (drying) effect.

The approved combinations are any 2 or more ingredients in each list in approved concentrations:

- allantoin + cocoa butter + petrolatum + shark liver oil + white petrolatum
- allantoin + cocoa butter + dimethicone + glycerin + petrolatum + shark liver oil + white petrolatum
- aluminum hydroxide gel + calamine + kaolin + zinc acetate + zinc carbonate + zinc oxide

Combinations with safe and effective itch-pain relievers are also approved but not those that include hydrocortisone. See p. 567.

Skin Protectants

APPROVED SKIN-PROTECTING ACTIVE INGREDIENTS

- **ALLANTOIN:** Allantoin is a compound for which few, if any, adverse reactions have ever been reported in the medical literature. It appears to be non-toxic, non-allergenic, and non-irritating when applied to the skin. It has the ability to protect even very young and tender bottoms against the moisture and irritation of diaper rash. Allantoin also is a skin softener.

In one series of controlled experiments, with an emulsion that contained allantoin, silicones, and the now-banned germicidal agent hexachlorophene, only 5 percent of several hundred babies developed diaper rash. In a control group of babies who were not so treated, the incidence of diaper rash was 3 times higher. In another part of this study, the skin of 34 out of 38 infants who already had diaper rash or a similar problem cleared up nicely after treatment with the emulsion. The investigators concluded that the allantoin-containing mixture was effective and relatively free from side effects. Allantoin is considered safe and effective for people of all ages when applied in a concentration of 0.5 to 2 percent, as often as needed.

• *ALUMINUM HYDROXIDE GEL:* This white, powdery aluminum compound—also called *aluminum hydroxide* or *aluminum hydrate*—forms a gel when it is kept in contact with water, so it is widely used internally as a nonprescription antacid. It has been marketed as a skin protectant for almost a century, with good consumer acceptance and without reported difficulties. Animal-toxicity tests also attest to its safety.

The effectiveness of aluminum hydroxide gel as a skin protectant is based on two properties: as an astringent, it pulls bacteria and other noxious substances out of sweat, urine, and other excreted body fluids; then it tightly binds and holds these substances so that they cannot re-attach to and thus irritate, damage, or penetrate the skin. This ingredient thus is particularly useful against the irritating wetness found in prickly heat, ringworm, jock itch, and impetigo as well as for the weeping, scaly rashes of poison ivy and similar plant poisons.

Reviewers state that aluminum hydroxide gel can be applied generously whenever necessary to children over 6 months of age and adults. For infants under 6 months, it should be used only under a doctor's orders. The safe and effective concentration is 0.15 to 5 percent.

• *CALAMINE (PREPARED CALAMINE AND CALAMINE LOTION):* A pinkish-colored anodyne, calamine protects the skin by absorbing moisture and chemical irritants; it soothes, too. Calamine is 98 percent zinc oxide, which is white. But it also contains about 0.5 percent—that is, one-half of 1 percent—of the iron compound ferrous oxide. This chemical's red color imparts the pinkish cast, which is wholly "window dressing" according to the experts. The iron contributes nothing to zinc oxide's absorbent and protectant effect, which, like calamine's safety, is principally attested by consumer acceptance and long, trouble-free clinical use. (*See* Zinc Oxide, further on.)

The dosage, for all ages, is a 1 to 25 percent concentration of calamine, applied as often as needed.

• *COCOA BUTTER:* Cocoa butter is a waxy, chocolate-smelling, and chocolate-tasting substance that has the capacity of melting into a soothing, skin-softening oil when warmed by body heat. So it is convenient, as well as quite agreeable, to use cocoa butter both as a lubricant for massages and as a base for medicinal ointments and suppositories.

The ingredient is a fatty extract from the roasted seeds of the cacao plant. The judgments that it is safe and effective are based on long use and wide acceptance rather than on scientific testing.

When applied to sunburned or otherwise injured skin, cocoa

butter prevents evaporation and dryness and keeps the skin soft and pliable, which in turn reduces friction, irritation, and pain. Evaluators say cocoa butter is safe and effective in 50 to 100 percent concentrations. It can be used liberally and as often as needed on the youngest and tenderest to the oldest and toughest of skins.

• DIMETHICONE: An inert, soothing, syrupy silicone, dimethicone is judged to be remarkably free of toxicity. It is chemically similar to simethicone, which is taken internally to relieve symptoms of gas. (*See* ANTI-GAS AGENTS.) Dimethicone clings to the skin and repels water. It will effectively seal a wound against air, wind, and other drying or frictional irritants. Because it can block the ammonia usually produced by bacterial decomposition of urine, this ingredient can be used to treat and prevent diaper rash. Dimethicone also will seal and protect chapped skin and lips against further drying and chapping. It should *not* be used on puncture wounds or infected wounds, however, because some air must reach wound surfaces in order for them to heal; without air they fester.

   Dimethicone is safe and effective in a 1 to 30 percent concentration on the skins of people of all ages. It can be applied in generous amounts and as often as needed.

• GLYCERIN (GLYCERINE AND GLYCEROL): This clear, sweetish, syrupy stuff is highly inert and for the most part innocuous to the human body. Undiluted, as *anhydrous glycerin*, it absorbs water, so it could dry out and irritate the skin. But in a 20 to 45 percent concentration in water—the recommended amount—hydrous glycerin will hold water against the skin so that it stays moist and is not irritated by air, wind, or other drying forces. Glycerin may be applied generously, whenever needed, on persons of all ages *except* infants under 6 months old, for whom you should consult a physician.

• KAOLIN: Also called *China clay, white bole, argilla, and porcelain clay*, kaolin is a powdery, earthy, clay-type material. Technically it is purified and hydrated aluminum silicate. It protects the skin through its ability to avidly absorb moisture and toxic substances dissolved in it.

   Kaolin has been used as an internal and external medication for hundreds of years. There are no reports of toxic reactions following its application to the skin. The substance absorbs perspiration and other moisture, and acts as a dusting powder to dry weepy skin conditions like eczema and the leaky blisters of poison ivy and poison oak. For people of all ages, kaolin is considered safe and effective in concentrations of 4 to 20 percent. It can be applied liberally, when needed.

• *PETROLATUM PREPARATIONS: PETROLATUM AND WHITE PETROLATUM:* These petroleum derivatives can be used to soften, lubricate, and protect the skin. White petrolatum is chemically more refined than yellow or amber petrolatums, but their pharmaceutical properties are the same.

Petrolatum is the base (vehicle) for a variety of internal and external medications, and is regarded as extremely safe. For small, superficial burns, petrolatum by itself (or on a gauze dressing) will keep air out, prevent evaporation of moisture from the wound, and reduce pain. Petrolatum can also be used to relieve sunburn, chapping, and other forms of dry skin, and as an ammonia-blocking agent to prevent diaper rash. It should *not*, however, be used on puncture wounds, lacerated skin, or wounds that have become infected, since the lack of exposure to air retards healing and may cause the wound to form pus.

For persons of all ages, petrolatum preparations are safe and effective in 30 to 100 percent concentrations and can be applied as often as needed.

• *SHARK-LIVER OIL:* This ingredient can be used to cover, soften, and soothe a dry, burned, or otherwise irritated skin surface. It is not scientific, controlled experiments but rather the long-time experience of users, druggists, and doctors that attest to this substance's safety and worth.

Experts recommend this remedy not be used for children under 2 years of age except on a doctor's advice. Otherwise, a 3 percent shark-liver oil preparation is safe and effective when applied generously and as often as needed.

• *SODIUM BICARBONATE:* This white crystalline powder with a salty, somewhat alkaline taste, is a kitchen remedy. It is sometimes called bicarbonate of soda, but is more commonly known as *baking soda*. Sodium bicarbonate fizzes into carbon dioxide gas and water when moistened, leaving behind a paste of sodium carbonate. This soothing residue relieves the itching of bee stings and mosquito bites. It is also helpful in treating *minor* burns. Large acid burns, in particular, should not be treated with sodium bicarbonate because the acid-base chemical reaction can further injure the skin. First aid for large acid burns is cold running water or a cold shower—unlike the still water recommended for other burns—before quick referral for medical attention. (*Also see* the section on Burns in this Unit.)

Persons with widespread itching due to hives, eczema, or similar skin disorders often find relief by bathing in a tub of tepid water that has been well laced with sodium bicarbonate. This relieves the itch and softens and soothes the skin.

The safety and effectiveness of sodium bicarbonate as a skin protectant is largely based on its self-care use, and on consumers' satisfaction with the results. No toxic reaction has ever been reported from its use as a topical drug. Evaluators say that a 1 to 100 percent application of sodium bicarbonate can be used, whenever needed, for persons of any age.

• TOPICAL STARCH (CORN STARCH): This is a powdery, kitchen-cabinet remedy— a food substance, really. Its protective power lies in its ability to absorb huge amounts of liquids when it is dusted on the skin. Topical starch absorbs 25 times more moisture than talc, which also is used for this purpose. Bacteria and their poisonous byproducts, as well as other noxious materials, can be absorbed and held away from the skin by topical starch and thus rendered harmless. Topical starch also smoothes and lubricates body surfaces that have been irritated by friction.

Topical starch feels bland to the skin. This helps explain why no adverse effects have as yet been attributed to dusting it on the body. For adults, children, and infants, the Panel says that a 10 to 98 percent topical starch preparation can safely and effectively be applied to irritated skin as often as needed.

• ZINC ACETATE: An astringent crystalline compound, zinc acetate precipitates bacteria and other proteins out of solution. This neutralizes their harmful effects. Because of this astringent property, zinc acetate sometimes is formulated into deodorant products. A long marketing record, with no reported untoward reactions, attests to zinc acetate's safety as a skin protectant. Wide use and continuing clinical acceptance point to its effectiveness.

While it is not recommended for children under 2 years of age except under medical supervision, for older children and adults a 0.1 to 2 percent preparation is safe and effective. The substance can be applied to the affected skin without restraint and as often as is required.

• ZINC CARBONATE: Zinc carbonate is an inert white powder, insoluble in water. It has been widely used—without reported toxicity—to cover and protect the skin. This substance appears to absorb noxious and irritating substances. Evaluators found no specific studies documenting the effectiveness of zinc carbonate, but they believe it works because of its wide acceptance and because other zinc compounds— like zinc oxide (*see* immediately following)—are recognized as effective for their astringent properties and their ability to soothe and protect irritated skin. The recommended dose of zinc carbonate for persons of all ages is 0.2 to 2 percent as needed.

• *ZINC OXIDE:* This fine, white powdery substance, sometimes known as *flowers of zinc* or *zinc white*, is the basic active ingredient in calamine preparations. Zinc oxide is used to cover the skin to protect it from dryness and other harmful environmental stimuli. It also absorbs toxic substances and serves, too, as a lubricant. Zinc oxide is extremely safe, even when taken internally, and there have been no published reports of complications following its use on the skin. Its effectiveness is established by wide use and acceptance by consumers and doctors; it is the sole or principal ingredient in a wide variety of over-the-counter preparations.

Because of its cooling, slightly astringent, antiseptic, antibacterial, and protective actions, zinc oxide is considered particularly effective in treating diaper rash and prickly heat. It is also useful against eczema, impetigo, and many other itchy conditions. The approved concentration is up to 25 pecent in powders and other formulations, and up to 40 percent in an ointment.

CONDITIONALLY APPROVED SKIN-PROTECTING ACTIVE INGREDIENTS

None.

DISAPPROVED SKIN-PROTECTING ACTIVE INGREDIENTS

• *BISMUTH SUBNITRATE:* This chemical is also known as *basic bismuth nitrate, bismuth oxynitrate, bismuthyl nitrate, white bismuth,* and *Spanish white.*

It is a white, odorless, tasteless powder that has been used as an antiseptic, astringent, and skin protectant. Despite its long use and acceptance, bismuth subnitrate has been found to be lethally toxic when taken internally. Also, because there are no persuasive data to show that it is effective as a skin protectant, evaluators decided that the ingredient is unsafe and ineffective for this purpose.

• *BORIC ACID:* When boric acid, also known as *boracic acid* or *orthoboric acid*, is applied to damaged skin in an ointment, its main constituent, boron, is absorbed into the body. Boron from even a relatively small amount of such an ointment can damage the central nervous system; larger amounts can be fatal. Deaths also have been reported in infants powdered before diapering with a borated talc powder, which indicates that boron can be absorbed through unbroken skin as well as through wounds.

Despite boric acid's wide use and great medicinal popularity in decades past, evaluators judged the ingredient to be unsafe as a topical drug and also ineffective.

Wound Healers

APPROVED WOUND-HEALING ACTIVE INGREDIENTS

None.

CONDITIONALLY APPROVED WOUND-HEALING ACTIVE INGREDIENTS

• LIVE-YEAST-CELL DERIVATIVE: This substance is an alcoholic extract of baker's yeast, the foodstuff that makes bread dough rise. It also is called *skin respiratory factor*, because its purported effect when applied to wounded skin is to increase oxygen uptake. This in turn, claims a manufacturer of live-yeast-cell derivative products, stimulates the growth of new connective tissue and skin.

Some animal tests submitted for review suggest, somewhat equivocally, that live-yeast-cell derivative *does* possess this healing property. But only a single, small experiment on humans (involving 18 patients) was presented to the Panel. They found the study inadequate, so only conditional approval was granted. Efficacy must be proven.

DISAPPROVED WOUND-HEALING ACTIVE INGREDIENTS

None.

Safety and Effectiveness: Active Ingredients in Over-the-Counter Skin Protectants

Active Ingredient	Assessment	Approved Concentration (%)	For Ages
allantoin	safe and effective	0.5-2	all
aluminum hydroxide gel	safe and effective	0.15-5	over 6 months*
bismuth subnitrate	not safe or effective		
boric acid	not safe or effective		
calamine (prepared calamine, calamine lotion)	safe and effective	1-25	all
cocoa butter	safe and effective	50-100	all
corn starch (see topical starch)			
dimethicone	safe and effective	1-30	all
glycerin (glycerine and glycerol)	safe and effective	20-45	over 6 months*
kaolin	safe and effective	4-20	all
live yeast-cell derivatives	safe, not proved effective		
petrolatum preparations: petrolatum and white petrolatum	safe and effective	30-100	all

Safety and Effectiveness: Active Ingredients in Over-the-Counter Skin Protectants (contd)

Active Ingredient	Assessment	Approved Concentration (%)	For Ages
shark-liver oil	safe and effective	3	over 2 years
sodium bicarbonate	safe and effective	1-100	all
topical starch (cornstarch)	safe and effective	10-98	all
zinc acetate	safe and effective	0.1-2	over 2 years
zinc carbonate	safe and effective	0.2-2	all
zinc oxide	safe and effective	1-25	all

* Approved for younger children when under medical supervision.

Unguents and Powders for the Skin: Product Ratings

SINGLE-INGREDIENT PRODUCTS

Product and Distributor	Dosage of Active Ingredients	Rating*	Comment
boric acid			
Boric acid (generic)	**ointment:** 10%	C	not safe or effective
Borofax (Burroughs Wellcome)	**ointment:** 5%	C	not safe or effective
calamine			
Calamine lotion (generic)	**lotion:** 8% calamine + 8% zinc oxide + 2% glycerin	A	
cocoa butter			
Cocoa butter (generic)	**lotion, cream, oil, soap**	A	
cornstarch			
See Topical starch			
glycerin			
Glycerin (generic)	**liquid**	A	
petrolatum preparations			
Vaseline (Chesebrough-Pond's)	**ointment:** white petrolatum, USP	A	

Unguents and Powders for the Skin: Product Ratings (contd)

Product and Distributor	Dosage of Active Ingredients	Rating*	Comment
sodium bicarbonate			
Arm & Hammer Baking Soda (Church & Dwight)	**powder:** bicarbonate of soda, USP	A	a grocery item
Sodium bicarbonate (generic)		A	
topical starch			
Topical starch (generic)	**powder**	A	a grocery item when purchased as cornstarch
zinc oxide			
Zinc oxide (generic)	**ointment:** 20%	A	
	paste: 25% + 25% starch	A	

COMBINATION PRODUCTS

Product and Distributor	Dosage of Active Ingredients	Rating*	Comment
Aveeno Anti-Itch (Rydelle)	**cream:** 3% calamine + 1% pramoxine hydrochloride	A	
Phenolated Calamine (Humco)	**lotion:** 8% calamine + 8% zinc oxide + 2% glycerin + 1% phenol	C	not an approved combination

Resinol (Mentholatum)	ointment: 6% calamine + 12% zinc oxide + 2% resorcinol	A
Schamberg (Paddock)	lotion: 8.25% zinc oxide + 0.25% menthol + 1.5% phenol	A
Schamberg's (C&M)	lotion: zinc oxide + 0.15% menthol + 1% phenol	A

*Author's interpretation of FDA criteria. Based on contents, not claims.

Vitamins and Minerals

Americans spend about $2 billion each year on vitamins, according to surveys published recently in *Chain Drug Review* (January 1, 1992).

The vitamin business first came under federal purview as early as 1906. Yet the safety and efficacy of these products when used for medicinal purposes has never been assessed in a thorough and systematic way.

A major barrier to such systematic assessment—which could guide consumers in deciding if they suffer a vitamin deficiency, and, if so, what they need to do to treat it—has been the resistance by the vitamin industry and by many Americans to the FDA's efforts to formulate rules for the sale and use of these substances. Many Americans fear that such standards might be used to deprive them of their innate right to take highly-concentrated amounts of vitamins and minerals as their friends, health gurus, health-food-store vitamin salespeople, and even the occa-

VITAMINS AND MINERALS is based on the report of the FDA Advisory Review Panel on OTC Vitamin, Mineral and Hemantic Drug Products; the FDA's final order withdrawing this document from its rule-making process; the Recommended Dietary Allowances (10th ed.), published by the National Academy Press (Washington, 1989); the FDA's proposed rule Food Labelling: Reference Daily Intakes (RDI) and Daily Reference Values; and other sources of nutritional information.

sional physician may recommend. These enthusiasts, of whom there are millions, see vitamin supplements as possible *magic bullets* that may prevent or relieve them of a wide range of distressing physical, mental, and emotional conditions. Unfortunately, there are little or no scientific data to confirm the safety and effectiveness of most of these uses.

Some advocacy of vitamins is highly irrational. It also of course is highly profitable for vitamin makers and sellers. The big losers are ordinary, careful consumers, who have denied themselves astute medical and regulatory guidance on the use and misuse of vitamin products. Most thoughtful Americans are grateful that FDA regulates and forbids scientifically unproven claims that a drug makers' medicinal product will prevent or cure serious diseases. But some of the same Americans seem willing, even eager, to allow some of these companies to sell vitamin products for which similarly dramatic but unproven claims are made. This is a puzzling double standard, which the vitamin industry exploits for significant economic advantage.

The FDA's Over-the-Counter Drug Review provides a clear-cut example of this resistance to user-protective standards: The FDA appointed an expert group, the Advisory Review Panel on OTC Vitamin, Mineral and Hemantic Drug Products. It was headed by internist Irwin H. Rosenberg, M.D., of the University of Chicago School of Medicine. After much deliberation, the Panel prepared a report on these products. This was published in the *Federal Register* in 1979.

The Panel's intent was to identify vitamin and mineral *deficiency states* (illnesses or vulnerabilities to illnesses) caused by inadequate intake of vitamins or minerals. The Panel then tried to differentiate those conditions that require professional medical care, *severe anemia*, for example, from milder deficiency states that consumers could self-treat with vitamin supplements. The Panel also proposed specific levels of supplementation that consumers might safely and effectively administer to themselves or family members. This definitional effort came to naught.

The Panel's report created great furor. Vitamin manufacturers and vitamin users united to condemn it. The FDA received thousands of protest letters.

Some objected to the Panel's conservative message that many more vitamins are taken than are needed. Others believed, incorrectly, that the Panel's proposals, if adopted by the FDA, would restrict the over-the-counter marketing of vitamins as nutritional supplements as well as their marketing as drugs.

The result was that FDA, prodded by Congress, withdrew the Panel's recommendations from the OTC Drug Review's rule-making process. This means that the Vitamin Panel's recommendations—unlike those of all other OTC Review Panels—have not been translated into regulations to ensure the safety and effectiveness of this group of products.

In withdrawing the Panel Report from its rule-making process, the FDA stated that its action "does not in any way denigrate the scientific content of the report," and added that the "FDA believes that the information in [it] will provide valuable guidance to both the agency and the industry in the areas of vitamins and minerals."

The Panel's report provided useful information for consumers, and the Panel's recommendations were contained in the first edition of this Guide (VITAMINS AND MINERALS in *The Essential Guide to Nonprescription Drugs* by David R. Zimmerman, New York: Harper & Row, 1983). Since then, however, these recommendations have not been subjected to the rigorous checks and balances of the FDA rule-making process; they also have not been updated by FDA staff people, based on new reports on the medical literature. So the Panel's 14-year-old specific standards and recommendations have not been included here. This author does not know of any similarly astute but contemporary guideline for the self-management of vitamin and mineral deficiency states.

At an FDA hearing in 1991, Dr. Rosenberg, who now is a professor of medicine at the Tufts University Medical School in Boston, testified that his Panel's study "was the first, and as far as I know, only substantive study of its kind . . . and is still perhaps the most comprehensive statement on safety, effectiveness, and fair labeling of vitamins and minerals..."

But the matter is moot.

The result is that consumers who do not wish to put themselves at further risk have only one alternative: If you think that you are suffering from lack of one or more vitamins or minerals, your best—and only—resource is to visit a reputable physician, *not* a "vitamin doctor," and ask that the physical and laboratory tests be done that can confirm or rule out a vitamin deficiency state. If you are deficient, the doctor will help plan and undertake a corrective regimen, which initially may include vitamin injections.

Fortunately, even in these economic hard times, very few ordinary Americans are vitamin deficient because of food deprivation. Those who are, authorities agree, for the most part would do better spending the money that is available to them on wholesome food rather than on vitamin tablets.

Deficiencies are more likely to appear in extreme vegetarians, determined dieters and alcoholics, for all of whom supplements may be advisable. Persons who are chronically ill, chronically medicated, or women who are pregnant or nursing also may need some supplementation; they should consult their doctors.

Regulations for Vitamins as Food Supplements

Most vitamins are sold virtually unregulated as *nutritional supplements*. Nevertheless, the FDA's recent efforts, and those of other public and quasi-public agencies, to set nutritional guidelines for vitamin and mineral products have come under strong attack by opponents of standards and guidelines just as previous efforts to regulate vitamins as drugs did. The current conflict also reflects disagreements among nutritionists and other professionals, and differing understandings about what the standards represent, and how they should be used: a debate that is outside the purview of this Guide.

The FDA experts, like just about everyone else, are confused. One of them said in 1992 that when either the *pro-vitamin* or the *anti-vitamin* advocates are angry, but the other is not, then she worries that the agency is tilting too far to the silent faction's side. But when *both* sides are angry, as at present, she said, then the agency probably is on the right course!

The most recent proposed FDA nutritional guidelines are called the Reference Daily Intakes (RDIs). Their genesis and purpose are briefly explained here.

RDAs and RDIs

For exactly half a century, nutritional guidelines for vitamins, minerals, and other nutritional sources, such as energy, carbohydrates, lipids, and proteins and amino acids, have been prepared by panels appointed by the Food and Nutrition Board of the National Research Council (NRC). The NRC is an arm of the National Academy of Sciences (NAS), a federally charted private organization. These NRC/NAS guidelines are published periodically as the *Recommended Dietary Allowances* (RDA); the tenth edition appeared in 1989.

The RDAs are, unfortunately, confusing. They also have become more and more controversial. But they are the product of careful and meticulous review of the research literature, of significant debate within the Panel that proposes the RDAs, and also of strong debate within the NRC bureaucracy that accepts, changes, or rejects the panelists' proposals.

The RDAs have a significant problem: They ostensibly are *not* intended to serve as nutritional guidelines for individual people, albeit that is the purpose for which many, if not most people use them. They are rather construed as norms for groups of people—adult men, for example, or breast-feeding women—and they are set *high* enough to provide for all, or virtually all, normal, healthy people in the particular group, regardless of an individual's weight, usual rate of exertion, or nutritional idiosyncrasies (such as high- or low-absorption of a particular vitamin or mineral).

The result, according to the FDA, is that the RDAs are too high, in some cases *far* too high for many people in each population group. A person who tries to fulfill the RDA standards thus may be ingesting food, and vitamins and minerals that he or she does not need, in the form of vitamin-enriched food products. What is more, the individual is paying, directly or indirectly, for these unneeded supplements: You may pay more for a vitamin-enriched product at the grocery store compared with the lower cost of a non-enriched product. If you are, say, a high school student, you pay (your parents pay) more, in the school cafeteria, or in taxes, for meals that meet RDA standards through food selection or the purchase of vitamin-enriched products.

This over-supplementation through the RDAs already has been acknowledged by the NRC/NAS, in decisions that are *not* reflected in the tenth edition of its RDA publication. The NRC/NAS now favors *decreases* in the RDAs for vitamin B_{12}, vitamin E, folate, and iron, among others, compared with its earlier standards. The proposed reduction in iron is fueled, at least in part, by research findings that many Americans now are ingesting more iron than they need. This is producing, among other things, an increasing caseload of the iron overload disease *hemochromatosis*—a genetic vulnerability to dietary iron—that afflicts a million American men.

The RDAs had some other significant problems. One is that, based on federal law, the FDA requires that nutritional guidelines that it endorses appear on many food containers. The RDAs have 18 different population categories based on age, sex, and pregnancy and nursing in women—far too much data for any food label.

To resolve these problems, the FDA has proposed a new standard:

The agency's *Reference Daily Intakes*, or *RDIs*, are based on the 1989 RDAs. But they are reduced to 5 age, sex, and reproductive categories instead of 18 categories. More important, the RDIs provide statistically derived *average values* for each nutrient for each of the five demographic groups, rather than the *optimal values* contained in the RDAs.

Vitamins: Comparison of Risk of Deficiency against Risk of Overdose

OTC Vitamin	Deficiency Risk, U.S.Population	Overdose Risk
vitamin A	unclear	moderate
vitamin D	low	moderate
vitamin E	nil	nil
vitamin K	nil	nil
vitamin C	low	low
thiamin	moderate	nil
riboflavin	low	nil
niacin	low	low
vitamin B$_6$	high	low
folic acid	low (except in pregnancy)	nil
vitamin B$_{12}$	low	nil
biotin*	nil	nil
pantothenic acid*	nil	nil

Note: Evaluations reflect author's interpretation of Panel report and NAS/NRC RDAs.
*Nutrients for which there are as yet no Recommended Dietary Allowances (RDAs).

Additional Reference Daily Intakes (RDIs) For Nutrients For Which There Are As Yet No Recommended Dietary Allowances (RDAs)

VITAMINS

Category	Biotin (micrograms)	Pantothenic acid (mg)
Infants under 1	13	2.5
Children ages 1-4	20	3
Children Over 4 and adults	60	5.5

MINERALS

Category	Copper (mg)	Manganese (mg)	Fluoride (mg)	Chromium (micrograms)	Molybdenum (micrograms)
Infants under 1	0.6	0.6	0.5	33	26
Children ages 1-4	0.9	1.3	1	50	38
Children Over 4 and adults	2	3.5	2.5	120	150

Source: FDA, from Federal Register: July 19, 1990, pp. 29481-82.

To facilitate comparisons, the RDIs use the same units of measure as the RDAs.

"FDA elected to establish in its 'Daily Values' proposed adjusted *average* levels for vitamins [and] minerals...recommended for various age/sex groups in the 1989 National Academy's RDA, instead of the highest recommended values," the agency explained in a background paper (BG 92-1, Feb. 12, 1992). "The new averaging approach for all nutrients would give consumers a more current, unified 'measuring stick' to compare the content of all labeled nutrients among different foods."

The RDIs thus tend to be *lower* than previous FDA standards based on the RDAs: an average of 14 percent lower, according to the FDA's calculations.

As indicated previously, vitamin makers and their customers have reacted to this change with anger and rage. Whether they, or the FDA and the scientists who support it, will prevail remains unclear as this book goes to press; the FDA is required to publish its final proposal on this new regulation in the *Federal Register* in November 1992. It is not certain that it will do so, given the huge volume of protests—over 30,000 letters—it has received.

The new regulations originally were to go into effect in May 1993. But the government has postponed them until May 1994. Sooner or later, however, the new standards—in one form or another—are likely to show up on the labels for a wide range of food.

Readers may be able to make up their own minds on the matter by comparing the current RDAs from the National Research Council with the proposed RDIs from the FDA. They appear together in the tables under Comparison of Two Standards for Daily Vitamin and Mineral Intake for Americans of All Ages on pp. 1018-1021.

The FDA has also provided RDIs for several vitamins and minerals (including biotin, pantothenic acid, manganese, and copper) for which NAS/NRC still feels there are too few data to establish RDAs. However, few if any reasonably healthy Americans are believed by either of these agencies to be at significant risk of deficiency of these not-wholly-standardized nutrients.

Uses and Sources of Vitamins and Minerals

Vitamins and minerals are used for a variety of medicinal and nutritional purposes, some of which overlap. The following outline is an effort to separate, simplify, and clarify these uses:

Vitamins and Minerals in Food

Vitamins were discovered no more than a century ago. But humans, and our animal forebears were eating—and living healthy lives—for the preceding millennia without any coaching from nutritionist or vitamin advocates. They ate food and, wholly unaware of it, ingested the vitamins and minerals they needed. It is true that some people, in some food-poor regions, suffered individual or epidemic deficiency states. But the rule is that life thrived.

This means, specifically, that, given the opportunity, people (and other animals) select and eat the foods that their bodies need, including the appropriate vitamins and minerals. It is this natural wisdom of the body that seems to have been lost sight of in the present, shrill debate over vitamins.

For the majority of Americans, even in the current hard times, the available selection of foods and beverages is far wider—and far fresher, thanks to rapid transport by truck, train and airplane—than at any time or in any other place in the history of the world. Therefore, very few Americans are or need to be vitamin-deficient, unless they are practicing some self-restricting dietary regimen, such as extreme vegetarianism. Most healthy Americans do not need vitamin supplements, and, if they do, a simple multi-vitamin, perhaps with added minerals, is likely to more than fulfill their nutritional needs.

Vitamin and Mineral Supplements

As just indicated, very few healthy Americans need supplements, and probably for those who do (or feel that they do) a standard one-a-day multi-vitamin tablet or capsule will more than suffice. The RDAs and RDIs indicate higher-than-normal intakes of some vitamins and minerals for pregnant and breast-feeding women. Most of these increments easily can be obtained through diet. But these needs, and particularly the increase in iron intake during pregnancy also may be more easily obtained through modest supplements.

Despite the arguable need, many Americans take vitamin supplements. Citing survey data, the FDA says over a third of all adults, and between forty and fifty percent of children swallow vitamin pills and capsules.

Only one significant change in the RDAs, based on recent research, argues strongly for a supplement: That is the slightly-more-than-doubling of the folate RDA for pregnant women, in order to prevent severe birth defects in the baby. (*See* Folate, further on for a discussion of these new findings, which could dictate use of a folate supplement during early pregnancy.)

The RDIs are more conservative than the RDAs. The RDI for vitamin A for boys and men, for example, is 875 retinol equivalants, compared with the 1000 such units in the RDA. But the main point is that neither the RDAs nor the RDIs indicate any need for the massive supplementation of several or more vitamins routinely recommended by many vitamin sellers and advocates.

Vitamins and Minerals Administered as Drugs to Correct Deficiency States

People *do* become deficient in vitamins and minerals. Unavailability or poor choice of food is one reason. Genetic predisposition and illness are another. Disease and injuries that arise without genetic predisposition are a third. Pregnancy, old age, and other physiological stress may be others.

When the FDA originally included vitamins and minerals in the OTC Drug Review, it was this limited but medically important realm of usage that it hoped to rationalize, for consumers' benefit. But, as stated previously, this effort has been tabled.

Vitamins and Minerals as Drugs (Pharmacological Uses)

Vitamins are powerful chemicals, which is why only minuscule amounts of them are required to mediate major functions in the body. But far-higher amounts of vitamins are being shown to have beneficial effects as drugs. In some, perhaps most, of these instances—of which only a few have been scientifically confirmed—the pharmacological value appears to be wholly unrelated to the vitamin's nutritional value or to its use to prevent deficiency states. These discoveries are exciting. They may lead to new ways to prevent serious diseases, including some cancers. They may also provide effective new therapies and cures for major diseases. But for most if not all of these pharmacological applications of vitamins, the applicable word still is *may*. Thus, the *New York Times'* excellent and normally level-headed science reporter,

Natalie Angier, has written a rhapsodic account of this research, published under the headline "Vitamins Win Support as Potent Agents for Health" (March 10, 1992). The weasel word *may* appears 20 times in Ms. Angier's story and an accompanying table, which also includes lots of *mights* and *seems* and other such hedges.

Vitamins and Minerals as Rip-off Games (Mind-bending Uses)

A major new fad, as the *New York Times* (June 10, 1992) explained under the headline "'Smart Drugs': Elixir or Snake Oil?," is mega-dosing with mixtures of vitamins, nutrients, and herbs, combined in some instances with (℞) and nonprescription drugs. These combinations are marketed by mail-order companies and health gurus to now-aging hippies, for the ostensible purpose of relieving stress, providing pep, promoting sex, or preventing aging. The huge doses that are used, not surprisingly, *do* have mind-altering effects.

"Something kicks in and you really feel it!" one user told the *Times*. "You feel like you're the center of universe!" another explained.

The FDA, which is investigating "smart drugs," sees risk in this mind-bending fad. So do some doctors. However, it seems unlikely that their cautionary messages will dissuade many turned-on smart-drug users.

May help is not a reason to take any drug or vitamin, unless a disease has been specifically identified and diagnosed, and all of the drugs that "will help" or "probably will help" have been shown not to. Before a "may-help" vitamin can be recommended scientifically, someone must show that it *will* help a reasonable number of people who take it, and that this benefit far exceeds any risk that may be incurred when numbers of people, who may not even be ill, take large amounts of the substance for long periods of time.

So far, this simple test has been met by few if any of the vitamins that are proposed in high doses for drug use. One exception that does seem to work is high dosages of niacin to reduce levels of cholesterol—which *may* prevent heart attacks and other cardiovascular diseases.

In some instances, specific, medicinal forms of vitamins have been shown to be medically effective: Retinoic acid, a form of vitamin A, will relieve severe, cystic acne, for example (*see* ACNE MEDICATIONS). But the form of the vitamin in this case, and in some others, is different from the forms that are available in nutritional supplements. And even comparably large amounts of the oral supplements may fail to provide the anticipated benefit. The NRC/NAS states, in its current RDA publication, described above: "Several nutrients have specific therapeutic uses at high dosages (e.g., vitamin A and other retinoids are used for treating some types of skin disorders), but determinal side effects [can occur] after prolonged use." On the other side of the coin, the NRC/NAS adds: "Chemical analogues of the nutrient that are often most effective pharmacologically may have little or no nutritional activity."

In short, the pharmacological benefits that may result from high dosage therapy with specific vitamin analogues may have nothing to do with taking high doses of nutritional supplements of these vitamins. So, the widespread practice of mega-dosing with vitamins provides little or no health benefit, and it may be harmful.

Sources of Vitamins and Minerals

Internal Contributors

Strictly defined, vitamins are essential organic nutrients that must be obtained from sources *outside* the body. Some vitamins, however, are made internally (even though additional amounts may still be required from external sources). Vitamin D, for example, is manufactured by a fatty biochemical in the skin when it is stimulated by sunlight. Some vitamin A and niacin are also made internally.

Some vitamins—particularly vitamin K and biotin—are not made by the body itself but by bacteria that reside in the intestines. Vitamin B_{12} is synthesized by bacteria in the colon. But these bacteria are probably too far down in the gut for people to absorb and use them; thus each person must rely on external sources for this vitamin.

Diet

Most of the vitamins and minerals people need are available in the food they eat, *if* they eat a balanced diet. Ordinary foods provide remarkably large amounts of the recommended and required nutrients. The product-rating publication *Consumer Reports* once calculated, for example, that one McDonald's 7½ ounce Big Mac sandwich contains the following percentages of the RDAs for an adult woman:

vitamin A	5 percent
thiamin	52 percent
riboflavin	33 percent
vitamin B_6	13 percent
vitamin B_{12}	63 percent
niacin	55 percent
calcium	23 percent
phosphorus	44 percent
iron	23 percent

When the new RDIs are enacted—if they are—consumers are likely to discover from food labels that hamburgers and other common foods provide an even higher percentage of individuals' average daily requirements, since the RDIs are pegged at a moderately lower level than the RDAs, as described previously.

Natural Vitamins

There is no evidence to support the claim that vitamins derived from natural products (like dried plants) have any health advantage over manufactured vitamin products. The designation "natural" on the label implies an advantage that in fact is nonexistent. But the price—and hence the profit—may be significantly higher.

The Panel disapproved of vitamins and minerals from these sources as inappropriate for use in over-the-counter drug products:

acerola	black currants
alanine	bone meal
alfalfa	bone phosphate, edible
algin	brewer's yeast
apricot	buckwheat
arginine	cabbage
aspartic acid	calcium phytate
beet greens	carrot powder
betaine	chaparral
bioflavonoids, mixed	chlorophyll

chlorophyllins

citrus bioflavonoids

cobalamin concentrate

cod-liver oil

comfrey root

cystine

dandelion greens

date powder

desiccated liver

dolomite

dulse

duodenal substance

egg albumin

egg yolk

eggshell

fish-liver oil

glutamic acid

glycine

green buckwheat

green-pepper powder

hesperidin complex

hesperidin

histidine

inositol

isoleucine

kelp

l-lysine monohydrochloride

lecithin

lemon bioflavonoid complex

lemon-grass oil

lettuce

leucine

linoleic acid

linolenic acid

liver fraction

liver fraction, insoluble

liver fractions A and 2

liver substance

liver substance concentrate

liver preparations

lysine

magnesium aluminum hydroxide

malt extract

methionine

molasses

ox-bile extract

oyster shell

p-aminobenzoic acid

pancreatin

papain

papaya

parsley

peas

pepsin

phenylalanine

proline

protein hydrolysate

prune concentrate

red bone marrow

rice bran

rice oil, cold-pressed

rice polishings

rose-hips powder

rutin

serine

soy flower

spinach powder

sulfur

threonine

tillandsia

torula food yeast

torula yeast

tryptophan

turnip greens

tyrosine

unsaturated fatty acids
(vitamin F)

valine

watercress

wheat germ

wheat-germ oil

yeast

Other Ingredients

Besides active agents in vitamins and minerals a number of *inactive* ingredients are used in formulating over-the-counter products and are permissible in reasonable amounts. They include:

alcohol

butyl paraben

corn oil

formic acid

gelatin

lactose

lecithin

pectin

polysorbate

polysorbate 20

safflower oil

silicon dioxide
(silica and silicon)

sodium saccharin

sodium benzoate

sorbitol

soy oil, cold-pressed

soya lecithin

sucrose

vanilla

wild-cherry concentrate

Vitamins Assessed

Vitamins usually are separated into two groups: those that are soluble in fat, and those that are soluble in water.

Fat-soluble Vitamins

• *VITAMIN A:* This vitamin is essential for growth and bone development and for sustaining the membrane structure and function of all body cells. It prevents night blindness—one of the earliest deficiency signs—as well as drying out of the skin and cornea of the eye and other, more serious problems. Most well-nourished people receive adequate amounts of vitamin A in their diets; deficiencies, which develop only very slowly, are rare.

The term *vitamin A* actually describes several biochemicals that are found in rich amounts in whole-milk products, eggs, liver and particularly fish liver, as well as in palm oil and other plant foods. Vitamin A from *carotenoids*—the orange-red plant pigment found in carrots, tomatoes, and other fruits and vegetables—is absorbed less well than vitamin A from animal sources.

Vitamin A is oil-soluble but also can be formulated in emulsions and in water-soluble forms. For over-the-counter use, it does not matter which form is used. However, claims that cod-liver oil and other natural sources of vitamin A in animals are superior to other forms remain unproved.

Excessive use of vitamin A may incur more problems than deficiency! Regular overuse of the vitamin can produce a chronic toxicity characterized by loss of appetite, blurred vision, muscle soreness after exercise, the appearance of reddish pimples on the shoulders and back, and drying out of the skin. Severe liver damage may occur. This chronic syndrome is diagnosed most often in youngsters, and seems to occur when infants are given more than 37,500 retinol equivalents daily. The condition develops more slowly in adults, who can store large amounts of the vitamin in their livers before it begins to cause damage.

Acute toxic reactions have been reported in adults taking 2 to 5 million retinol equivalents of vitamin A, and in infants given much smaller doses. The symptoms of this acute poisoning include severe headache centered in the forehead and eyes, dizziness, drowsiness, nausea, and vomiting. These effects occur within 6 to 8 hours. A few hours later the skin reddens and swells. Later it flakes and peels.

The toxic problems of vitamin A supplements are compounded because the vitamin loses its potency in the bottle. Manufacturers therefore sometimes put more than the labeled amount into their product.

Many spurious claims have been made for vitamin A. It has

not been proven safe or effective as a nonprescription drug for preventing or treating plantar warts, acne, bed sores, respiratory infections, vision problems or eye defects, or dry, scaly, wrinkled, or thickened skin.

• *VITAMIN D:* The "sunshine vitamin" is synthesized from a cholesterol-like substance in the human skin when we are exposed to sunlight. Most people obtain all or almost all of the vitamin D they need in this way. Principal dietary sources of the vitamin are fatty fish, egg yolk, liver, and butter. Vitamin D is added by food processors to milk, breakfast cereals, bread, chocolate, and other foods.

Vitamin D helps the body absorb dietary calcium from the gut. It is required, too, for the formation and replacement of bone, so children—with growing bones—need more than adults. The vitamin D deficiency states, which include *rickets* (defective bone growth) in children and *osteomalacia* (soft bones) in adults, require careful medical care. So vitamin D deficiencies should not be treated with over-the-counter vitamin D supplements.

Vitamin D deficiency diseases are relatively rare in the United States. They are more likely to occur in people who are malnourished, and in dark-skinned persons, who produce less vitamin D of their own in response to sunlight than lighter-skinned persons do. Air pollution and overuse of sunscreens, which both block healthful sun rays, also may lead to low or deficient levels of this vitamin. Vegetarians and people who avoid fatty foods are candidates for vitamin D deficiency, as are very premature infants (who, of course, require medical attention). But vitamin D deficiency is so uncommon in relatively well-nourished populations that some experts think that the practice of fortifying foodstuffs with vitamin D may be unwise.

Conclusive evidence is lacking to support claims that vitamin D supplements will prevent or cure osteoporosis in older people or that it can lower serum cholesterol. Its use is disapproved for these purposes. There is also no evidence that multivitamin preparations containing minerals and vitamin D are better than forms that contain vitamin D without the minerals.

Excess vitamin D is not excreted in the urine to any great extent. Rather, it continues to build up in dangerous amounts in body tissues. Since vitamin D binds and holds calcium in the body, this may result in disorders associated with excess calcium absorption, including kidney stones, mental deficiencies, heart changes, and the buildup of calcium in the kidneys, heart, and blood vessels. Early symptoms include weakness, fatigue, malaise, dry mouth, aches and pains, and a host of other relatively nonspecific complaints.

• *VITAMIN E:* This vitamin is widely used—often in enormous doses—for a variety of disease states for which it has not been proved to be helpful. Its principal virtue seems to be its lack of toxicity. Some people have taken thousands and tens of thousands of units of vitamin E for extended periods of time, even though the RDI for children over 4 years of age and for adults is only 9 *alpha*-tocopherol equivalents daily, and for young children it is lower.

Except in a few premature infants, and a few adult victims of severe illnesses that involve medical management, vitamin E deficiency is rare to nonexistent. So vitamin E was disapproved by the Panel as inappropriate for use by itself. However, they approved it for preventive use only — in combination products sold for the prevention of multiple vitamin deficiencies of the sort that threaten chronic alcoholics, persons with vitamin malabsorption syndromes, and those who get few nutrients because they eat very badly.

Vitamin E is supplied naturally by soybean products, safflower oil, nuts, cereals, and other foods. It appears to contribute to the function of the muscular, vascular, and nervous systems. But, except for *slight* changes in the survival time of red blood cells, the consequences of vitamin E deficiencies have been hard to document.

Claims have been made that large doses of this vitamin enhance fertility or are of benefit against leg cramps, heart and vascular-system diseases, and several rarer disorders that include the finger-curling condition called Dupuytren's contracture. These claims have not been proved.

• *VITAMIN K:* The RDAs—and hence RDIs—for this vitamin have been set only recently, based on research findings. The dietary sources of vitamin K are both plant and animal foods. It also is synthesized in the human intestines. Vitamin K is essential for forming prothrombin and other body proteins that regulate the clotting of blood. Impaired coagulation of the blood, after, say you cut yourself shaving or nick your finger with a kitchen knife, is the only discernible sign of vitamin K deficiency.

Vitamin K deficiency is rare. It occurs in some newborns, who require medical treatment. In older people, the use of drugs — particularly broad-spectrum antibiotics and anticoagulants, can lead to vitamin K deficiency. So can physical stress and illness, and so, too, can excess consumption of vitamin E. Excessive intake of vitamin K has not been shown to be harmful.

Water-soluble Vitamins

• *VITAMIN C (ASCORBIC ACID)*: Other forms of this vitamin are ascorbate calcium and ascorbate sodium.

The reference form of vitamin C is ascorbic acid. The other approved forms are weaker, so that larger doses are required for equivalent results. A milligram of calcium ascorbate, for example, contain only 0.83 as much vitamin C as a milligram of ascorbic acid. A person would need 120 mg of calcium ascorbate to provide the equivalent of 100 mg of ascorbic acid. Similarly, each milligram of sodium ascorbate contains only 0.89 as much vitamin C as a milligram of ascorbic acid. Therefore 110 milligrams of sodium ascorbate will be needed to equal 100 mg of ascorbic acid.

The vitamin C deficiency state is called *scorbutic syndrome*, or more popularly, *scurvy*. Early scurvy symptoms include fatigue, spontaneous bleeding from the gums and other tissues, swollen joints, and aching muscles. Later the teeth loosen and may fall out. New wounds heal slowly, old ones tend to reopen. Emotional changes may also occur. Once a scourge of mariners and others who could not obtain fresh citrus fruit, scurvy is extremely rare today. The body contains a large pool of vitamin C: about 1500 mg in the well-nourished adult. Even if the vitamin is wholly withheld, body stores decrease only by about 3 percent per day. Since scurvy does not appear until body stores drop below 300 mg in an adult, this may take 4 or 5 months. Also, early symptoms are confusing because they may reflect many other disorders. Thus, medical tests are required to confirm the diagnosis.

While vitamin C is required by the body to prevent scurvy, it is also used as a helper or cofactor in the formation of connective tissue. It also helps sustain the internal chemical environment in which certain other life processes occur.

Humans, like some animal species, must replenish their vitamin C stores from external sources. But the vitamin is widely available in food. The average diet provides 30 to 60 mg daily of vitamin C. Even the lower amount, 30 mg, is enough to prevent scurvy in otherwise healthy persons. There are 124 mg of vitamin C in 8 ounces of fresh orange juice and 28 mg in a medium-sized tomato. It is extremely unlikely that essentially healthy, well-fed individuals ever will need vitamin C supplements.

The vitamin C requirement is higher than normal for persons with peptic ulcers, hyperthyroidism, chronic diarrhea, cancer, serious burns, or surgical wounds. Pregnancy and nursing also increase vitamin C needs, as may cigarette smoking, use of oral contraceptives, and heavy ingestion of aspirin and some other drugs. Under none of these conditions, however, does the increased need exceed the amount that can be obtained through a diet that contains citrus fruit or other foods that are rich in vitamin C. There is no evidence to suggest that even people with the problems noted need or would benefit from vitamin C supplements.

Many people consume large—even huge—amounts of vitamin C for reasons unrelated to the prevention and treatment of scurvy. Taking over 1 gram (1000 mg) daily is potentially hazardous: It may prompt the formation of kidney and bladder stones. This risk may be compounded if you eat food with high levels of oxalate, a kidney-stone component; these foods include spinach, rhubarb, chocolate, and tea.

Some users take as many as 16 grams (16,000 mg) of vitamin C each day. Yet ingesting even 4 gm (4000) mg daily can produce upset stomach, nausea, diarrhea, and perhaps more serious complications. Against these risks, there is no evidence that vitamin C, in large or small supplements, will relieve the several other conditions (unrelated to vitamin C deficiency) for which it often is promoted and used. There is no conclusive evidence, for example, that it will prevent or cure the common cold, and it is not approved for this use. It may provide some relief of symptoms. Similarly, vitamin C is not effective against schizophrenia or other mental ills, atherosclerosis or blood clots, or allergies or bed sores. Similarly, it is not safe, not effective or both as a nonprescription drug to combat blood disorders such as idiopathic methmeglobinemia, megaloblastic anemia, capillary fragility unrelated to vitamin C deficiency, iron deficiency, or the side effects of steroid drugs.

• VITAMIN B$_1$ (THIAMIN): Malnutrition and alcoholism are the principal causes of *beriberi*—the severe, sometimes lethal form of vitamin B$_1$ deficiency—but a number of other common conditions, including pregnancy, illness, and old age will produce an asymptomatic deficit state that can be treated and corrected by thiamin supplements.

Thiamin is available in over-the-counter vitamins in two forms: thiamin hydrochloride and thiamin mononitrate.

The RDI for children over 4 years of age and adults is 1.2 mg, principally provided by green vegetables, grains, and meat; some thiamin comes from commercial vitamin fortification of flour and other food sources.

A rich natural source of thiamin is rice hulls, which is why beriberi was first shown to be a dietary deficiency in Oriental peoples: They polished away the hulls because they liked to serve the rice grains gleaming white. They suffered nerve disorders, weakness, paralysis, mental degeneration, heart failure, and death as the result. (Some of these problems are seen in severely debilitated alcoholics, who require emergency thiamin replacement to survive.)

The vitamin's principal physiological role is to help break down sugar for energy. Paradoxically, while poor diets produce thiamin deficiency, it is also true that the more calories you eat, the more thiamin you need.

Contrary to promotional claims, thiamin is not useful against any condition except those related to thiamin deficiency, according to the Panel. False and inaccurate claims have been made that it relieves skin conditions, multiple sclerosis, cancer, impotence, slow-wittedness, and drug toxicity. None of this has been shown to be true. Neither is there any evidence that vitamin B_1 will relieve fatigue or nervous disorders or improve thinking ability—unless of course these conditions were actually caused by thiamin deficiency.

- **VITAMIN B_2 (RIBOFLAVIN):** Riboflavin deficiencies are rare. They tend to occur in alcoholics and in people who eat poorly. Symptoms of vitamin B_2 deficiency include sore mouth and sore throat, pale and cracked lips, swollen tongue, skin disorders, itchy eyes, and cataracts.

This vitamin is available in supplements as riboflavin and as riboflavin-5-phosphate sodium. Both are effective and have a wide margin of safety; no toxic effects have ever been reported. Natural sources of the vitamin include eggs, meat, fish, and liver. The RDI for children over 4 years of age and adults is 1.4 mg. For those whose need for supplements has been determined by a doctor, the Panel said over-the-counter riboflavin supplements are safe and effective for preventing deficiencies in adults and in children over 1 year of age. The preventive dosage is 1 to 2 mg per day.

- **NIACIN:** *Pellagra*, which results from a severe deficiency of niacin, is rare. An early investigator described pellagra as characterized by a "horrible crust" on the skin of the hands and neck; "painful burning of the mouth"; a "perpetual shaking of the body"; and "mania." Once fairly common, this disease has been largely eliminated by the enrichment of commercial flour with niacin supplements. So pellagra now is mostly a problem among some fad dieters, alcoholics, and patients with debilitating illnesses.

However, more modest deficits—manifested by conditions such as loss of appetite, weight loss, and poor milk production in nursing mothers—continue to occur. Also, several recent studies confirmed the popular impression that disadvantaged children suffer some signs of deficient dietary intake of the vitamin. Finally, the cancer drug 6-mercaptopurine and some other drugs have an anti-niacin activity that requires patients to take niacin supplements.

Niacin is a B vitamin, which is also sometimes called *nicotinic acid*. It is water-soluble. Niacin by itself often causes facial flushing, itching, and other side effects when taken as a supplement in standard doses. An alternative form of niacin, called *niacinamide* or *nicotinamide*, is a preferred and approved form of niacin.

Niacin is naturally obtained directly from food, and it is made in the body as a breakdown product of the essential amino acid tryptophan. Both sources are tapped by the ingestion of beef, cow's milk, and eggs, among other foods. Niacin is required for the respiratory activity of all body cells. It also stimulates a number of basic biological processes involving carbohydrates, amino acids, and fats.

Even very large doses of nicotinamide (niacinamide) can be taken safely; nicotinic acid can cause facial flushing and other unpleasant side effects.

• *Vitamin B6 (pyridoxine):* Several large groups of people have a high incidence of vitamin B_6 deficiency, as measured by assays of vitamin B_6 and related biochemicals in the blood and urine. These groups include

> • *People with poor diets.*
>
> • *Pregnant women.* Pregnancy may cause deficiency because B_6 crosses the placenta and becomes concentrated in the fetus. The RDI for pregnant women is 2.2 mg daily.
>
> • *Infants fed heat-sterilized formulas.* Heat may destroy the vitamin.
>
> • *Some women who use oral contraceptives.* As in pregnancy, this low level has not been shown to be dangerous.
>
> • *Alcoholics.* Alcoholics tend to be deficient in vitamin B_6 because they eat poorly, have difficulty absorbing vitamins, and may rapidly excrete B_6 from their damaged livers.
>
> • *Workers exposed to industrial air pollution.* Studies from

Russia suggest that such workers may have a greater need for this vitamin.

Vitamin B_6 has been proposed as a treatment for kidney stones. Conclusive evidence is lacking that it will prevent or relieve this condition, which requires medical management. Neither has it been demonstrated that vitamin B6 will prevent morning sickness during pregnancy, as has been claimed.

Symptoms of B_6 deficiency, which are confusingly close to those for other B vitamin deficits, may (or may not) include inflammation of the tongue and mouth, shakes and seizures, irritability, and mental depression. The similarity of the several B-vitamin deficiency states is why the Panel recommended that nonprescription preventive and B vitamin combinations include all 6 vitamins in the vitamin B group.

The B vitamins:

vitamin B_1 (thiamin)

vitamin B_2 (riboflavin)

vitamin B_6 (pyridoxine)

vitamin B_{12}

folic acid

niacin

Vitamin B_6 occurs in nature in a number of chemical forms, but the commercially available supplemental source is pyridoxine hydrochloride. The vitamin is a cofactor in at least 60 different biological reactions involved in the digestive breakdown of proteins and amino acids, and, to a lesser extent, with the metabolism of fats and carbohydrates and the synthesis of nucleic acid.

Dietary sources that are rich in B_6 include meat, cereals, lentils, nuts, avocados, bananas, and potatoes. Some of the vitamin is destroyed by cooking.

Large amounts—several hundred milligrams—of vitamin B6 daily have been taken without observable ill effects. The much smaller doses of up to 25 mg per day recommended for nonprescription use therefore appear quite safe. Even less is actually needed: The RDI for children and adults is 1.5 mg per day.

• FOLIC ACID: Deficiency in folic acid, a B vitamin, leads to anemia—which can be prevented by supplements. This condition appears to be relatively common and pronounced in pregnant and nursing women and in heavy drinkers.

In normal volunteers, experimental studies show that the liver stores about 7.5 mg of this vitamin. Less than one one-hundredth of this amount, 0.05 mg, is used each day. But because only a fraction of the folic acid that is ingested becomes available to the body, the approved preventive dose is higher.

Women taking oral contraceptives may be helped to maintain normal folic acid levels by supplements of 1 mg daily, but (as with B_{12}) neither the need for nor the efficacy of this treatment has been established. Self-dosing with over-the-counter supplements is *not* approved for the *treatment* of folic-acid deficiency, which requires medical management.

The one relatively clear-cut new use for vitamin supplements in the last decade involves folic acid: A series of careful epidemiological studies conducted in Great Britain has shown that the incidence of spina bifida and other severe spinal cord defects in newborn infants can be reduced by two-thirds or more by giving the mother-to-be large supplements of 4 mg of folic acid, starting before conception and continuing for the first 3 months of pregnancy. Based on these findings, the U.S. Centers for Disease Control (CDC) in Atlanta have issued an interim recommendation for folic acid supplements that applies *only* to women who already have delivered a live or stillborn baby with spina bifida or some other neural tube defect.

In conjunction with their doctors, the CDC says, these women should receive 4 mg of folic acid daily starting one month before planned conception and continuing through the first trimester of pregnancy. This amount of folic acid should be provided on prescription (℞) and should be pure folic acid rather than a component of a multivitamin preparation.

The CDC stipulates that this high dose of folic acid be given only under a physician's supervision, and it is not appropriate for women who have not previously given birth to a spinally defective infant, even if they themselves or a relative suffer from spina bifida or have relatives who have given birth to such a baby. The CDC notes that this use and dosage of folic acid has not yet been approved by the FDA (*Morbidity and Mortality Weekly Report*, Aug. 2, 1991).

Folic acid, one form of the vitamin folacin, is also called pteroylmonoglutamic acid (PGA). It is water-soluble. Natural folacin is provided by a variety of foods—especially liver, leafy vegetables, fruits, and yeast. Only the synthetic folic acid is available in supplements.

All folic-acid sources must be broken down inside the body to be of physiological value. They work, in conjunction with vitamin B_{12}, in the synthesis of DNA and in cell replication. Folic-acid depletion leads to the severe red blood cell deficiency state called *megaloblastic anemia*. Clinical signs include sore mouth, diarrhea, irritability, and forgetfulness—all of which are so nonspecific as to make self-diagnosis difficult.

Toxic reactions to folic acid are extremely rare, even when the vitamin is taken in massively large—and unnecessary—doses.

- **VITAMIN B_{12}:** Vitamin B_{12} is extremely safe. No toxic manifestations have ever been described in people taking as much as 100 micrograms (mcg) per day. Excesses for the most part are excreted in the urine. Vitamin B_{12}, a water-soluble vitamin, is required for the production of DNA, and thus is essential for cell replication. It also plays a number of other important biochemical roles. Animal meat (including liver), and fish, seafood, milk, and eggs all are good sources of the vitamin. Vegetarians who add eggs and milk to their diets can ensure adequate B_{12} intake. Modest supplements may be appropriate for women who are breast-feeding.

Vitamin B_{12} deficiency is extremely uncommon, in part because dietary requirements are low. The daily requirements are in the range of 1 to 2 mcg. In a normal healthy adult, the liver can store 1000 to 1500 mcg of this vitamin: a 3- to 5-year supply.

Deficiencies in vitamin B_{12} occur in rare individuals who lack a gastric biochemical that is required for the vitamin's absorption into the body; this is called *pernicious anemia*. Similarly, deficiency can occur when the segment of the small intestine in which absorption occurs is removed or damaged by surgery or disease. Rare bacterial infections and fish tapeworm infestations of the gut also can lead to vitamin B_{12} deficiencies. All these deficiencies can be treated with B_{12} supplements, but the therapy requires close medical supervision and is much more effective when the vitamin is injected rather than taken orally.

The most commonly used form of vitamin B_{12} is cyanocobalamin.

- **BIOTIN:** Biotin is an extremely potent, water-soluble vitamin that is widely distributed in nature in small amounts. The average diet provides 30 to 40 mcg of biotin daily, which appears to be more than adequate to meet nutritional needs when added to the still-undetermined amount of this vitamin that is formed naturally in the human gut. (*See* Additional Reference Daily Intakes (RDIs) for Nutrients for Which There Are As Yet *No* Recommended Dietary Allowances [RDIs], p. 990.)

The vitamin is a co-factor in many food and energy transformations. These include the digestion and use of carbohydrates, buildup of fatty acids, and interconversions of amino acids.

Little is known about the toxicity of biotin supplements and no upper limit has been set. But the vitamin appears to be relatively harmless.

Deficiency is marked by a red, scaly skin disease that can be relieved by supplements, but this condition is so rare that only two *cases* are known to have occurred in adults, both of whom were being fed with nutrients infused into their bloodstreams. Indeed, the only way to induce the deficiency appears to be by eating enormous quantities of raw eggs—and little else—since uncooked egg white contains a chemical that inactivates biotin. Because biotin deficiency is virtually nonexistent, there is no need for supplements.

• *PANTOTHENIC ACID:* This B-complex vitamin, ubiquitous in plants and animals, was given a Greek name that means "from everywhere." It is abundant in meat, whole grains, and vegetables. (*See* the table Additional Reference Daily Intakes [RDIs] for Nutrients for Which There Are As Yet *No* Recommended Dietary Allowances [RDAs] p. 990.)

Pantothenic acid's ubiquity is matched by its biological importance to humans and other living organisms. It is a precursor of the biochemical coenzyme A, a substance required for a number of biological transformations including energy release and the metabolism of fat, carbohydrate, and protein.

Deficiency of this vitamin is quite rare and has never been produced experimentally by withholding the vitamin from the diet. A nerve disorder called "burning-feet syndrome" that occurs in malnourished prisoners of war and some rural populations in Asia has been attributed to deficit of the vitamin, but these populations well may suffer from other nutritional lacks that are responsible for such symptoms. Similarly, alcoholics may be deficient in this vitamin, but they, too, are likely to be generally malnourished. Most conditions for which pantothenic acid might prove useful require medical management; therefore, the vitamin has a very limited place in nonprescription medication.

Because the vitamin is so widely available in foods, pantothenic acid deficiency is virtually unknown in the United States.

Minerals and Trace Elements

• *CALCIUM:* Because it is a principal skeletal component and is present in all cells, the mineral calcium is one of the most common elements in the human body. Calcium plays a critical role in muscle activity and in the transmission of impulses from nerve ends to muscle cells and other cells. The average adult carries 4 pounds of calcium, 99 percent of it in bone. Many people—of all ages and both sexes—may need calcium supplements.

Calcium supplements within medically approved limits are safe. But higher intakes from excessive use of supplements can very quickly lead to the dangerous calcium-excess state *hypercalcemia.* In some individuals this risk is exacerbated by supplements of vitamin D, which binds to calcium and can enhance its absorption into the body. Hypercalcemia damages the kidneys, heart, blood vessels, and other organs. It can cause painful kidney stones, make the heartbeat dangerously irregular, and impair mental processes. Early signs of this disorder include weakness, fatigue, malaise, dry mouth, vague muscular and skeletal aches and pains, headache, and a metallic taste in the mouth.

In Western countries, the mean daily calcium intake is between about 500 and 1200 mg daily; after age 12 years, males consume more than females. Many women, in fact, ingest less than their calcium RDI, which is 900 mg.

The calcium taken in through food and the calcium the body absorbs are not the same, because a number of factors influence calcium absorption. Children absorb 75 percent of the calcium they consume, for example, whereas adults absorb only 30 to 60 percent of their dietary intake. And while vitamin D enhances calcium uptake, ingestion of foods high in phosphate content—including cocoa, soy beans, kale, and spinach—*decreases* intestinal absorption of calcium.

The intestine compensates to some extent for changes in dietary calcium: the less consumed, the more absorbed. This protective mechanism weakens with age, however, which may be why many older women and some older men suffer from the bone-wasting disease *osteoporosis.*

Milk and dairy products are a principal source of calcium, particularly for youngsters. Many parents properly insist that young children drink lots of milk, but then relax this insistence as the children get older. This may be a mistake, however: A person's greatest need for calcium—whether in milk and other foods or from supplements—

is in the pre-adolescent years, age 10 to 13, when the bones are growing rapidly toward adult proportions.

Pregnant women and nursing mothers also need more calcium
because they are providing it for their babies. So do older people, whose
bodies absorb and use calcium less effectively than younger people do.

Calcium depletion and hypocalcemia require medical management.

• PHOSPHORUS: This mineral is abundantly present in any diet that
includes milk, poultry, fish, and meat. Soft drinks, which Americans
imbibe by the billions, may contain excessive amounts of it in the
form of phosphoric acid. Phosphorus and calcium interact in the
body, and because of the high phosphorus intake achieved by meat-
rich Western diets, the possible consequences of excess phosphorus
intake on calcium excretion are of greater public health concern than
phosphorus depletion, which appears to be virtually nonexistent.
About the only time it is known to occur is in persons who take excessive amounts of certain antacids. Problems of too much phosphorus
fortunately are also rare because the kidneys, unless severely diseased, are capable of quickly removing large excess amounts of it.

• MAGNESIUM: The body contains about an ounce of magnesium, most of
it stored in bone and muscle. It is an important activator for many
enzyme systems involved in the utilization of food for energy. It also
plays a role in protein synthesis and the maintenance of electrical
potentials in the neuromuscular system. Most adult diets provide
between 200 and 330 mg of magnesium daily. About 350 mg per day
are required by an average-sized adult man; women need 280 mg
daily; and more if they are pregnant or nursing. Cereals, nuts,
seafood, peas, beans, corn, and soybeans are rich sources.

The small intestine, through which most of the mineral is
absorbed into the body, controls magnesium levels: the amount
absorbed decreases as intake rises. The body also has a striking ability to conserve this mineral. When magnesium is absent from the diet,
the kidneys retain (rather than excrete) it. Thus less than 12 mg per
day is lost in the urine. But when too much is ingested, the kidneys
rapidly excrete it.

Because magnesium is widely available in food and efficiently
conserved by the body, its deficiency (hypomagnesemia) is essentially
nonexistent in the average American. It occurs in a few malnourished
alcoholics, and in other persons who are ill or who have difficulty
absorbing magnesium. These problems require continuing medical

care, and, when magnesium supplements are required, they usually must be given by injection because such patients rarely respond adequately to oral magnesium.

• IRON: Iron is an essential component of the heme molecule, in the red pigment *hemoglobin* in red blood cells. It is hemoglobin that transports oxygen to all living body cells. The adult body contains some 4 grams of iron in blood, bone marrow, the liver, and the spleen. Although the usual American diet provides 10 to 20 mg daily, many population subgroups appear to be iron deficient. In fact, many of their members may be manifestly anemic. The need for supplements to prevent iron deficiency thus appears to be greater than for any other essential nutrient.

The use of over-the-counter iron supplements was *not* approved for the treatment of iron-deficiency anemia, which is a serious health problem that demands medical attention. The Panel recommended that all iron products carry this

WARNING:

 The treatment of any anemic condition should be under the advice and supervision of a physician.

Iron supplements are sold in a variety of chemical forms, some of which are more readily absorbed than others.

• ZINC: This mineral is required for many body functions, and zinc depletion is reported to occur with a number of serious illnesses. They include retarded growth and sexual development in severe malnutrition, leg ulcers, sickle-cell anemia, and a rare genetic inflammatory disorder of the skin (acrodermatitis enteropathica) that usually occurs in babies. A number of studies indicate many Americans live on diets marginal-to-deficient in zinc, which is cause for concern.

In the Panel's view, zinc deficiencies should be diagnosed and treated by a doctor. Supplements were not approved for self-treating zinc deficiencies because they are extremely difficult even for doctors to diagnose. The Panel warned specifically that self-medication with zinc should not be attempted for leg ulcers or rheumatoid arthritis and also cautioned that zinc depletion associated with sickle-cell disease and other clinical illness requires medical management.

Zinc is an ingredient in more than a dozen of the body's enzymes and coenzymes and contributes to the synthesis of proteins and nucleic acids. It is required for growth and development, wound-healing, and other important physiological processes, including the sense of smell.

Protein-rich foods—including meat, eggs, milk products, and shellfish—tend to be rich in zinc. Unsupplemented vegetarian diets may be deficient in zinc, and diets that are high in fiber and in the chemical *phytate*—which is abundant in grains, nuts, and legumes—appear to specifically reduce the availability of dietary zinc, as do phosphates.

The RDI for zinc is 10 mg in young children and 13 mg daily in older children and adults, except for nursing women, in whom it is higher. The danger levels for acute zinc toxicity are several hundred times higher. The question of whether ongoing, low levels of zinc supplementation may be dangerous has not been fully resolved. Zinc reacts with iron, copper, and other minerals in the body. Thus, too much zinc may cause dangerous imbalances in these substances.

• *IODINE:* Iodine is required for the synthesis of thyroid hormone. Adults need 150 mcg (micrograms) daily, according to the RDIs. But the average American consumes more than 300 mcg each day through tap water, seafood, vegetables, meat, eggs, and dairy products, as well as from iodized salt that has been commercially fortified with this mineral.

Dietary deficiency of iodine can lead to swelling of the thyroid gland, a disease called *goiter*. This disorder was fairly common in the Midwest and Pacific Northwest where the land and its crops are iodine-poor, and seafood was not commonly available. The introduction of iodized salt significantly reduced the incidence of goiter, but recent surveys showed that it continues to occur sporadically (usually in women of childbearing age) in Indiana, Michigan, and Texas and in some other Central States.

Despite the many sources for this mineral, surveys in the mid-1980s showed that Americans' iodine levels have been falling. This may be particularly important in pregnant and nursing women, who provide iodine to their fetuses and babies. The RDAs and RDIs therefore suggest supplements of 25 micrograms daily for pregnant women and 50 micrograms daily for women feeding their babies at the breast.

• *SELENIUM:* People have been taking large, unnecessary, and sometimes dangerous supplements of selenium for years. A pure dietary selenium deficiency has been demonstrated in rats that were fed selenium-poor diets over two generations, but such a dietary deficiency in selenium has never been diagnosed in humans.

Selenium is a catalyst along at least one metabolic pathway in the body, and other possible essential roles are still being explored. Seafood, meat, and particularly organ meat are rich in selenium, as are some grains, but not others, depending in part on the selenium status of the land on which they were grown.

The NRC/NAS recently published its first RDAs for selenium; they range from 45 to 75 micrograms daily in adults. By contrast, some health food advocates take *milligram* amounts of this mineral each day, and more than a few have poisoned themselves as the result. Thickening of the fingernails, a garlic scent to body excretions, nausea, belly pain, and hair loss are among the symptoms that have been reported. The NAS/NRC analysis indicates that no one who eats normal amounts of normal food needs selenium supplements. The Panel had previously proposed to ban such supplements because of their toxic risk.

Other Minerals

According to the Panel, a number of minerals that currently are sold over-the-counter are not safe, not effective or not either for self-medication. In the case of some minerals, the deficiency state requires medical diagnosis. For others, both preventive and therapeutic supplementation must be medically supervised because there is a narrow margin between the useful dose and the toxic dose. What is more, for some minerals, deficiency states are rare to nonexistent, so there is no need for health consumers to self-treat with over-the-counter products. Nevertheless, new data has made it possible to establish RDAs, RDIs, or both for some of these trace elements and minerals, which are described briefly here.

• CHLORIDE: Combined with sodium this mineral—table salt—is the principal negatively charged particle in body fluid. It is essential for maintaining the body's fluid and electrolyte balances. It is an essential, too, as a component of the digestive juices.

Most chloride in the body comes from salt, but except in babies fed poorly produced formulas, dietary chloride deficiency is nonexistent. Chloride and sodium can however be lost, with lethal consequences, through heavy sweating and a variety of illnesses. (*See* SALT SUPPLEMENTS AND SUBSTITUTES: PRELIMINARY REPORT.) There are no RDAs for chloride; the RDI for children over 4 years of age and adults is just over 3 grams daily.

• CHROMIUM: This element is required for the metabolism of glucose (sugar). Low chromium levels are associated with diabetes, the

NAS/NRC says. Chromium supplementation can correct impaired glucose tolerance.

Defining chromium deficiency has been difficult because chromium levels in tissues are hard to measure. Also, chromium is supplied by a wide variety of foods, including calf's liver, American cheese, and wheat germ. The NRC/NAS has not established RDAs for chromium. The FDA's new RDIs do include this element, however, and the chromium RDI for children over 4 years old and adults is 120 mcg (microgram). (*See* p. 990.)

• **COPPER:** Copper, an essential nutrient in trace amounts, is widely available in many foods including nuts, liver, shellfish, kidney, raisins, and dried legumes. The adult body contains 15 to 150 mg of this metal. As a result of the mineral's wide availability, deficiency is extremely rare. (One exception might be in premature infants who have been fed formulas that have little copper.)

The greater danger is excessive intake of copper, which can accumulate in the body and cause a variety of toxic symptoms and can cause death. The early signs of copper intoxication are nonspecific: nausea, vomiting, diarrhea, and headache. These effects may occur even if the intake of copper supplements is relatively low.

For these reasons, the Panel disapproved the use of copper as a nonprescription mineral and recommended that it be removed from over-the-counter products, where it may be present as copper (cupric) gluconate, copper oxide, or copper sulfate. There are no RDAs for copper. The RDI for children over 4 years old and for adults is 2 mg. (*See* p. 990.)

• **FLUORIDE:** The body requires trace amounts of fluoride, but this need is met by the drinking of fluoride in fluoridated and non-fluoridated drinking water and also is supplied by the fluoride that is present in a variety of foods. The fluoridation of community water supplies—intended to prevent dental cavities—provides fluoride and does not appear to be harmful. But reports exist of acne-like skin eruptions, hives, itching, and swelling in persons using fluoride-vitamin products and toothpastes enriched with fluoride. Because of these risks, the Panel disapproved of sodium fluoride or calcium fluoride supplements in over-the-counter vitamin-mineral products. (*See* FLUORIDE TOOTHPASTES AND RINSES FOR CAVITY PREVENTION.) As yet there are no RDAs for fluoride. The RDI is 2.5 mg for children over 4 years of age and adults. (*See* p. 990.)

• **MANGANESE:** This essential mineral is frequently put into mineral supplements and preparations of blood-forming substances. But the need for supplements has yet to be proved.

Manganese is absorbed from the small intestine; carried in the blood; stored in the liver, skin, and skeletal muscles; and excreted in the bile. An adult male has about half an ounce of it in his body. Cereal products, leafy fresh vegetables, nuts, and dried fruits are the richest dietary sources.

A principal medical concern about manganese is *chronic manganism.* This is a manganese-related disorder of the central nervous system that causes tremors and more severe symptoms. It is most prevalent among manganese miners but also could afflict people who ingest high levels of the mineral.

Manganese is required by several of the enzymes that regulate the body's utilization of food. Manganese may be involved in atherosclerosis and other serious illnesses, but no satisfactory evidence has been proposed to explain how manganese therapy might be helpful. More important, from the average consumer's point of view, no overt and unequivocal case of dietary manganese deficiency has ever been found! So there is little if any demonstrable need or value for manganese supplements. (*See* p. 990.)

• **MOLYBDENUM:** This element appears to be required to modulate brain function. Dietary deficiency of molybdenum has not been reported, and the element is widely present in foods, including milk, beans, breads, and cereals. The NRC/NAS is not ready to set RDAs for molybdenum, wanting more data (*see* p. 990). But it says supplements are not needed. The FDA, concurring, did however establish molybdenum RDIs. For children over 4 years old and adults, the RDI is 150 mcg (micrograms).

• **POTASSIUM:** Many body organs require small amounts of potassium for normal function. But excessive amounts of this mineral can lead quickly to cardiac arrest and death.

The kidneys largely control potassium balance in the body and usually are able to rapidly get rid of large excesses. Persons with damaged or malfunctioning kidneys cannot so easily rid themselves of excess potassium, and in fact, large doses of potassium may be hard even for normal kidneys to manage.

There is little if any need for self-dosing with potassium supplements. The mineral is so abundant in animal and vegetable foods that it is difficult to design a diet that provides adequate amounts of calories but does not satisfy the daily potassium requirement. The deficiency state, *hypokalemia,* rarely if ever occurs simply because a person has taken in too little potassium. The usual cause is illness, including diarrhea (the principal cause of hypokalemia in children), severe malnourishment, or perhaps alcoholism. Many alcoholics have low serum potassium levels. So do persons with high blood pressure who routinely take diuretics; this is why doctors often prescribe a supplement for hypertensives on diuretics.

The early symptoms of hypokalemia are common to many illnesses. They include lethargy, irritability, and a decrease in deep tendon reflexes. Laboratory tests are required to establish the diagnosis; thus medical management is clearly required.

Therefore there appears no justification for routine self-medication with over-the-counter potassium supplements. The Panel recommended that nonprescription sale of potassium supplements be banned.

• *OTHER TRACE MINERALS:* More than a dozen other mineral elements have been shown to be essential in animals, but not in humans, or are needed by people in such tiny trace amounts that a normally balanced diet is a sufficient source. The Panel says the following substances should *not* be present in significant amounts in mineral product supplements, since there is no known use for them in this form:

aluminum	*molybdenum*
arsenic	*nickel*
barium	*silicon*
beryllium	*strontium*
cadmium	*tin*
lead	*vanadium*
lithium	

Vitamins and Minerals: Product Ratings

An enormous number of single-ingredient and combination vitamin and mineral products currently are marketed. The majority are labeled as nutritional supplements rather than drugs, which means that no claims for the prevention or treatment of illness are made on the label. Many if not most labels do, however, list the dosages in milligrams or other units of each vitamin or mineral. Consumers therefore can use the two tables under Comparison of Two Standards for Daily Vitamin and Mineral Intake for Americans of All Ages (pp. 1018-1021) to identify the vitamins and minerals that they and family members may need and also can use these tables as a guide for purchasing the appropriate products.

COMPARISON OF TWO STANDARDS FOR DAILY VITAMIN AND MINERAL INTAKE FOR AMERICANS OF ALL AGES

Recommending Dietary Allowances (RDAs)

Issued by the Food and Nutrition Board, National Acadamy of Sciences—National Research Council. Designed for the maintenance of good nutrition of practically all healthy people in the United States.

Category	Age (years) or Condition	Fat-Soluble Vitamins				Water-Soluble Vitamins			
		Vitamin A (retinol equivalents)	Vitamin D (as micrograms cholecalciferol)	Vitamin E (mg alphatocopherol equivalents)	Vitamin K (micrograms)	Vitamin C (mg)	Thiamin (mg)	Riboflavin (mg)	Niacin (mg niacin equivalent)
Infants	0.0–0.5	375	7.5	3	5	30	0.3	0.4	5
	0.5–1.0	375	10	4	10	35	0.4	0.5	6
Children	1–3	400	10	6	15	40	0.7	0.8	9
	4–6	500	10	7	20	45	0.9	1.1	12
	7–10	700	10	7	30	45	1.0	1.2	13
Males	11–14	1000	10	10	45	50	1.3	1.5	17
	15–18	1000	10	10	65	60	1.5	1.8	20
	19–24	1000	10	10	70	60	1.5	1.7	19
	25–50	1000	5	10	80	60	1.5	1.7	19
	51+	1000	5	10	80	60	1.2	1.4	15
Females	11–14	800	10	8	45	50	1.1	1.3	15
	15–18	800	10	8	55	60	1.1	1.3	15
	19–24	800	10	8	60	60	1.1	1.3	15
	25–50	800	5	8	65	60	1.1	1.3	15
	51+	800	5	8	65	60	1.0	1.2	13
Pregnant		800	10	10	65	70	1.5	1.6	17
Lactating									
1st 6 months		1300	10	12	65	95	1.6	1.8	20
2nd 6 months		1200	10	11	65	90	1.6	1.7	20

COMPARISON OF THE STANDARDS FOR DAILY VITAMIN AND MINERAL INTAKE FOR AMERICANS, BY STAGE

[RDAs continued]

					Minerals				
Vitamin B$_6$ (mg)	Folate (micro-grams)	Vitamin B$_{12}$ (micro-grams)	Calcium (mg)	Phosphorus (mg)	Magnesium (mg)	Iron (mg)	Zinc (mg)	Iodine (micro-grams)	Selenium (micro-grams)
0.3	25	0.3	400	300	40	6	5	40	10
0.6	35	0.5	600	500	60	10	5	50	15
1.0	50	0.7	800	800	80	10	10	70	20
1.1	75	1.0	800	800	120	10	10	90	20
1.4	100	1.4	800	800	170	10	10	120	30
1.7	150	2.0	1200	1200	270	12	15	150	40
2.0	200	2.0	1200	1200	400	12	15	150	50
2.0	200	2.0	1200	1200	350	10	15	150	70
2.0	200	2.0	800	800	350	10	15	150	70
2.0	200	2.0	800	800	350	10	15	150	70
1.4	150	2.0	1200	1200	280	15	12	150	45
1.5	180	2.0	1200	1200	300	15	12	150	50
1.6	180	2.0	1200	1200	280	15	12	150	55
1.6	180	2.0	800	800	280	15	12	150	55
1.6	180	2.0	800	800	280	10	12	150	55
2.2	400	2.2	1200	1200	300	30	15	175	65
2.1	280	2.6	1200	1200	355	15	19	200	75
2.1	260	2.6	1200	1200	340	15	16	200	75

COMPARISON OF TWO STANDARDS FOR DAILY VITAMIN AND MINERAL INTAKE FOR AMERICANS OF ALL AGES
(continued)

Reference Daily Intakes (RDIs)

Proposed by the Food and Drug Administration. Average daily values for all persons, based on the RDAs.

Category	Fat-Soluble Vitamins				Water-Soluble Vitamins			
	Vitamin A (retinol equivalents)	Vitamin D (as micrograms cholecalciferol)	Vitamin E (mg alpha-tocopherol equivalents)	Vitamin K (micrograms)	Vitamin C (mg)	Thiamin (mg)	Riboflavin (mg)	Niacin (mg niacin equivalents)
Infants under 1 year	375	9	3.5	7.5	33	0.4	0.5	5.5
Children ages 1–4	400	10	6	15	40	0.7	0.8	9
Children over 4 and adults	875	6.5	9	65	60	1.2	1.4	16
Pregnant Women	800	10	10	65	70	1.5	1.6	17
Lactating Women	1300	10	12	65	95	1.6	1.8	20

Source: FDA, from *Federal Register*: July 19, 1990, pp. 29480–81.

[RDIs continued]

			Minerals						
Vitamin B$_6$	Folate (mg)	Vitamin B$_{12}$ (micrograms)	Calcium (micrograms)	Phosphorus (mg)	Magnesium (mg)	Iron (mg)	Zinc (mg)	Iodine (mg)	Selenium (micrograms)
0.5	30	0.4	500	400	50	8	5	45	13
1	50	0.7	800	800	80	10	10	70	20
1.5	180	2.0	900	900	300	12	13	150	55
2.2	400	2.2	1200	1200	320	30	15	175	65
2.1	280	2.6	1200	1200	355	15	19	200	75

Wart Paints and Plasters

Warts can be unsightly. Some are quite painful. But the more common kinds of warts—those that arise on the hands, feet, face, and some other body surfaces—are not dangerous. They are not early cancers. They do not develop into cancers. They never invade deeper layers of tissues.

Many methods have been developed to remove warts, according to the Panel that assessed over-the-counter drug preparations called *wart paints*. The most successful of these preparations contain the skin-peeling ingredient salicylic acid. This is an aspirin-like drug that was judged not only safe but also effective for wart removal. And while self-treatment with an over-the-counter drug may take several or more weeks, as opposed to having a wart removed surgically in minutes, it is likely to be cheaper.

The evaluators did set one important condition on the self-treatment of warts: Only the two very prevalent and easily identifiable types of warts, common warts and plantar warts, can be self-diagnosed. Therefore, only these two types of warts should be self-treated with

WART PAINTS AND PLASTERS is based on the report "Wart-Remover Drug Products" by the FDA's Advisory Review Panel on OTC Miscellaneous External Products and on the agency's Tentative Final and Final Monographs on these products.

over-the-counter products.

 Claims

Accurate

- "For the removal of common warts. The common wart is easily recognized by the rough 'cauliflower-like' appearance of the surface"
- "For the removal of plantar warts on the bottom of the foot. The plantar wart is recognized by its location only on the bottom of the foot, its tenderness, and the interruption of the footprint pattern"

WARNING:

 Do not use on irritated skin or any area that is infected or reddened, if you are diabetic, or if you have poor blood circulation. If discomfort persists, see your doctor. Do not use on moles, birthmarks, warts with hair growing from them, genital warts or warts on the face or mucous membranes.

What Is a Wart?

A wart is a raised area of skin with underlying tissue that often does not go away or recedes only very slowly. It may be hard or soft. Although it can be the color of normal skin, it also may be gray, tan, or some other hue. A single small wart, or even a cluster of them, on some fairly inconspicuous body surface may be of little concern. But some people develop hundreds of them, and some warts grow into large, bizarre-looking deformities that are the cause of great shame and embarrassment. (This is particularly true of genital warts, which are sexually transmitted and grow on the penis, vagina, rectum, and nearby body surfaces. Genital warts, of course, require medical attention.)

All warts are caused by viruses. They are *papova viruses*, which infect the nucleus and specifically the DNA (the genetic material) of skin cells. These viruses take over the cells' reproductive mechanisms, causing them to produce warty new cells instead of normal ones.

Warts are contagious: One person catches the virus from someone else. But it is difficult, if not impossible, to say from whom because the incubation period—the time before the virus produces a visible wart—may be as long as a year. The virus can also spread from an existing wart to new sites on the body. This risk was demonstrated several years ago by a dermatologist who conducted a two-year study of children with warts, which was described in the Panel report. He found that two-thirds of the originally diagnosed warts disappeared, without treatment, in that period of time. But meanwhile new warts appeared on other body areas in half the children. He blames the reinfection on *auto-inoculation*, which may have occurred when the children scratched or picked at their original warts. Because of this reinfection risk, experts say it is better to treat and remove warts rather than to wait for them to disappear by themselves.

Warts You Can Diagnose

Common Wart

This is a small, hard, grayish wart that is easily recognized by the rough, cauliflower-like texture of its surface. There is a clear margin, or demarcation line, between the elevated wart and the surrounding normal skin. The technical name for common wart is *Verruca vulgaris*.

Plantar Wart

This wart occurs only on the bottom of the feet. It is flat and may be either hard and callused or soft and spongy. A plantar wart, technically called *Verruca plantaris*, can be distinguished from a callus because the normal skin ridges encircle—but do *not* run across—the wart, whereas these footprint ridges continue across the surface of a callus.

Several closely spaced plantar warts may develop into a bumpy, irregularly shaped aggregation called a *mosaic wart*. Individually or in groups, plantar warts can be excruciatingly painful because they are repeatedly compressed by the weight of the body when a person stands. Plantar warts may be so painful that walking becomes impossible.

Warts a Doctor Should Diagnose

All warts that cannot be readily identified from the descriptions just given of common wart and plantar wart should be shown to a dermatologist or another doctor. If there is the slightest doubt about a wart's identity, it must be surgically excised in a manner that does not destroy the wart tissue. This way it can be examined by a pathologist to rule out the possibility that it is not a wart but rather skin cancer.

Treating Warts

A wart may eventually disappear of its own accord. Many folk remedies and rituals have been used through the centuries to cure warts. One scientifically controlled study even has demonstrated that warts respond to hypnotic suggestion. When placebos (dummy drugs) are used on warts in scientific tests, cure rates of about 25 percent are achieved. This response, too, might be attributed to the power of suggestion, or, the fact that warts sometimes disappear of their own accord. "How the mind affects the virus [that causes a wart] is unknown," the Panel's report said.

Medical treatment focuses on destroying the infected cells and the viruses they contain. Surgical methods include removal of the wart by burning, freezing, or cutting out the affected tissue. Drugs that destroy skin tissue can also be used for this purpose, and a number of preparations containing such ingredients are sold without prescription.

Because removal of a wart with over-the-counter drug products may take several weeks or longer, the skin-peeling agent or other active ingredient used to accomplish wart removal must be applied to the wart many times. But nearby skin, which may be damaged by the drug, must be protected. To achieve this, the active ingredient is formulated into a wart paint, a film-like substance that can be applied fairly precisely to just the warty tissue. Some of these preparations are called *collodions*; they contain highly volatile substances like ether or alcohol that evaporate quickly. This action leaves the active drug in a flexible or rigid waterproof film that sticks to the skin. Collodion coverings help hold moisture on the wart, which speeds the action of the wart-removing drugs.

Another delivery system incorporates the active medication into a *wart plaster*, a backing of fabric, plaster, or other material that adheres to the skin, that will remain in place up to two days, after which it should be replaced with a fresh application.

Wart Removers

Reviewers assessed the active ingredients in four wart-removal products submitted for their considerations by pharmaceutical companies. It also evaluated several other ingredients that FDA researchers discovered have been or are being used in such products. Only one ingredient was judged by the Panel to be safe and effective, by itself, for removing common and plantar warts.

APPROVED ACTIVE INGREDIENT

• SALICYLIC ACID: Billions of doses of salicylic acid are sold each year, principally as aspirin tablets for relieving pain, fever, and inflammatory complaints. Applied to the skin, salicylic acid is useful against warts because it acts as a *keratolytic*, or skin-peeling agent. The evaluators were not altogether clear in their explanation of how this occurs. They said that the acid destroys the outer layers of the warty skin by drawing in water, which causes the skin to swell, soften, and slough off. The acid is also said to cause an inflammatory reaction that hastens the wart's disappearance, perhaps by stimulating the body's immune defense system to attack the wart.

Salicylic acid is a standard medical cure for warts. The Panel and the FDA received a number of convincing clinical studies attesting both to its safety and to its effectiveness. However, the process may be slow and is not always wholly effective in curing the wart. In the latter situation, the wart's removal, surgically, by a dermatologist may be required. This is usually a fast and painless procedure. Freezing and destroying the wart with liquid nitrogen is one of the standard methods.

Persons who are treating a wart with a salicylic acid product should continue the treatment as long as the wart continues to shrink in size. But this treatment should not go on longer than 12 weeks. If the wart is not gone by then, consult a doctor.

The approved concentrations of salicylic acid in wart paints, collodion-like preparations and plasters are as follows:
- salicylic acid 12 to 40 percent in a plaster vehicle
- salicylic acid 5 to 17 percent in a collodion-like vehicle
- salicylic acid 15 percent in a karaya gum or a glycol plaster vehicle

CONDITIONALLY APPROVED ACTIVE INGREDIENTS
None.

DISAPPROVED ACTIVE INGREDIENTS
None.

Safety and Effectiveness: Active Ingredients in Over-the-Counter Wart Removers

Active Ingredient	Assessment
salicylic acid	safe and effective

Wart Paints: Product Ratings

Product and Distributor	Dosage of Active Ingredients	Rating*	Comment
SINGLE-INGREDIENT PRODUCTS			
salicylic acid			
Clear Away (Schering-Plough)	medicated disks: 40%	A	
Freezone (Whitehall)	flexible collodion: 13.6%	A	
Maximum Strength Wart-Off Wart Remover (Pfizer Consumer)	flexible collodion: 17%	A	
Mediplast (Beiersdorf)	plaster: 40%	A	
Off-Ezy (Commerce Drug)	flexible collodion: 17%	A	
Trans-Plantar (Tsumura Medical)	transdermal patch: 21%	A	
Trans-Ver-Sal (Tsumura Medical)	transdermal patch: 15%	A	

*Author's interpretation of FDA criteria. Based on contents, not claims.

Worm Killers for
Pinworm Infestation

When a school child awakens to furiously scratch his or her anus during the night and complains of intense itchiness, the cause may well be pinworms. In girls, the itching may extend to the vulva. Adults, too, may be afflicted. In fact, every member of a family with one pinworm victim will need to be treated with a worm-killing drug. But children are the usual sufferers of these infestations.

Pinworms are the most common parasite that afflicts human beings. They are found in all areas of the United States, rural and urban, and in all socioeconomic groups. These worms can be extremely disturbing: Children cannot sleep. They wet the bed, and they may develop bacterial infections if their persistent scratching breaks the skin. Fortunately, pinworm infestations can be successfully treated with a nonprescription drug. It is extremely effective: A single dose will destroy the worms in most cases.

WORM KILLERS FOR PINWORM INFESTATION is based on the report "Anthelmintic Drug Products" by the FDA's Advisory Review Panel on OTC Miscellaneous Internal Drug Products and the FDA's Tentative Final and Final Monographs on these products.

Claims

Accurate
• "For the treatment of pinworms"

WARNING:

 Abdominal cramps, nausea, vomiting, diarrhea, headache, or dizziness sometimes occur after taking this drug. If any of these conditions persist, consult a doctor. If you are pregnant, do not take this drug unless directed by a doctor.

Pinworms

How to Detect Them

A standard procedure to detect pinworms, performed by a technician or a doctor, is to press a short length of Scotch tape against the area just below the anus of the child or adult who is complaining of a suddenly itchy anus. The tape is then inspected under a microscope, which is the only way the worm's eggs can be spotted. A second, do-it-yourself detective method involves inspecting the anus and adjacent skin with a flashlight. Look for movement of a female pinworm as she lays her 11,000 eggs. The pinworm is ¼ to ½ inch in length and can be seen with the naked eye, or, more clearly, with a magnifying glass. If a child is the sufferer it is a good idea to wait an hour or so after he or she has gone to sleep to make this inspection.

How They Spread and Symptoms of the Infestation

Pinworms live in the intestinal tract; they have a life span of 4 to 6 weeks. When the time comes to reproduce, the female travels out through the anus to deposit her eggs on the nearby skin. It is this activity that causes the itching.

The eggs are extremely light, and can float through the house in the air. They may be picked up on the hands from clothes, bedding, or bathroom fixtures and then swallowed. Unfortunately, these eggs are resistant to household disinfectants. Children may reinfect themselves by scratching, which transfers the eggs to their fingernails. The eggs then may be dropped onto food, water, or other substances children put into their mouths.

Besides the intense perianal itching, pinworms produce few other symptoms. Nausea and other vague gastrointestinal complaints may occur. Surprisingly, most such infestations cause no symptoms at all, not even itching. So many people have pinworms without knowing it.

Treatment

All members of the family—except children under 2 years of age or those who weigh less than 25 pounds—should be treated if one family member has an infestation. The decision of whether and how to treat small children should be made by a pediatrician.

Only one treatment should be given. If an additional treatment seems needed, consult a doctor.

The drug that can be used effectively to treat pinworms is also effective against other, more serious parasitic infestations, including the large roundworm (*Ascaris lumbricoides*). However, these worms are more difficult to diagnose and pose a greater health risk. So roundworm infestations should be treated by a physician. *Pinworms are the only parasites that can be self-diagnosed and then self-treated with nonprescription drugs.*

The Pinworm-Killing Drug

APPROVED ACTIVE INGREDIENT

While the Panel initially approved two compounds, the FDA disagreed about one of them. Only the following drug meets both of their criteria.

• PYRANTEL PAMOATE: This is a relatively new drug that was approved for prescription use in 1972 under rigorous FDA licensing standards. There have been no reports of significant toxicity resulting from accidental overdosage. In therapeutic doses, even minor side effects, such as nausea, diarrhea, and cramps, are rare.

The drug acts on the worm by paralyzing muscles it uses to hold on to the intestinal wall. So it is swept away in the stool. In one large study of 1506 persons, most of them children, a single dose of 5 mg of pyrantel pamoate per pound of body weight eliminated the worms in 97 percent of subjects. Other studies have produced comparably impressive results.

Dosage Table for Pyrantel Pamoate

Body Weight	Dosage (taken as a single dose)
Less than 25 lb or under 2 years old	Do not use unless directed by a doctor
25-37 lb	125 mg
38-62 lb	250 mg
63-87 lb	375 mg
88-112 lb	500 mg
113-137 lb	625 mg
138-162 lb	750 mg
163-187 lb	875 mg
188 lb and over	1000 mg (1 gram)

Conclusion: Pyrantel pamoate is a safe and effective pinworm-killing drug *for one-time use only* at the recommended dosage of 5 mg per pound of body weight. A 50-pound child requires a 250-mg dose; a 100-pound child requires 500 mg, as indicated in the Dosage Table. Do not take a second dose unless directed to do so by a doctor. If symptoms persist, consult a doctor.

CONDITIONALLY APPROVED ACTIVE INGREDIENTS
None.

DISAPPROVED ACTIVE INGREDIENTS
None.

Safety and Effectiveness:
Active Ingredient in Pinworm Products

Active Ingredient	Assessment
pyrantel pamoate	safe and effective

Worm Killers for Pinworm Infestation: Product Ratings

Product and Distributor	Dosage of Active Ingredients	Rating*	Comment
pyrantel pamoate			
Pin-Rid (Apothecary)	capsules: 180 mg liquid: 144 mg per ml	A	℞ to OTC switch
Reese's Pinworm Medicine (Reese)	liquid: 50 mg per ml	A	℞ to OTC switch

*Author's interpretation of FDA criteria. Based on contents, not claims.

'Yeast' Killers for Feminine Itching

Many women suffer from time to time from intense inflammation and itching of the vagina, vulva, and surrounding skin surfaces. According to the Antimicrobial Panel II reviewers, one very common cause of this extreme itching is infection by organisms of the species called *Candida*—particularly *Candida albicans*. Over 20 million of these infections are diagnosed in the United States each year, according to drug industry data. Many women come to recognize yeast infections and can differentiate them from other kinds of *vaginitis* or *vulvovaginitis*, because *C. albicans* also produces a characteristic white, malodorous vaginal discharge.

Candidiasis

Yeast infections due to *C. albicans* and related yeasts are known as

'YEAST' KILLERS FOR FEMININE ITCHING is based on the report on vaginal drug products by the FDA's Advisory Review Panel on OTC Contraceptives and Other Vaginal Drug Products and on the report "Topical Antifungal Drug Products for OTC Human Use" by the FDA's Advisory Review Panel on OTC Antimicrobial Drug Products (the Antimicrobial II Panel). It also is based on FDA-approved manufacturers' information on anti-candidiasis drugs recently switched from prescription (℞) to nonprescription marketing.

candidiasis or *moniliasis* (from the alternative technical term, *monilia*), or just plain "yeast." The organism thrives on warm, moist areas of the body. It produces itchy, bright-red runny patches with numerous pus-filled pimples along the well-defined outer edge. The entire vulva may become moist, red, and raw. This itching may become so intense that the patient must seek emergency medical treatment.

Yeast also causes eruptions elsewhere on women's bodies, and in the groin and at other body sites on men, too (*see* the section on Candidiasis in JOCK ITCH, ATHLETE'S FOOT, AND RINGWORM CURES). But it can be mistaken for other itchy conditions, particularly by women who are unfamiliar with its symptoms. Initially, the FDA had doubts about whether candidiasis could be self-diagnosed and self-treated.

Prodded by the Panel, and by manufacturers, the FDA eventually decided that yeast infections *can* be self-diagnosed and successfully managed on the second and subsequent occasions on which a woman may suffer this condition, but *not* on the first such episode. The agency's rationale is that until a woman has experienced a yeast infection that has been professionally—and correctly—diagnosed by a physician, she might make an incorrect self-diagnosis when she suffers genital itching, burning, and discomfort and so might treat the condition with the wrong drug. Once the itching and the diagnosis have been put together, according to this thinking, then the woman will be able to care for herself safely and effectively the next time the infection recurs, if it does. Of course, if you are in doubt, or is certain yeast is *not* the cause of the problem, then seek medical help.

The decision that yeast is self-treatable came in the context of efforts by the Panel, and by drug makers, to switch several rather new, highly effective drugs with solid records as prescription (℞) drugs into the nonprescription category. These ℞ to OTC switches have now been made for one effective itch-reliever, hydrocortisone, in concentrations of up to 1 percent, and two drugs that effectively cure yeast infections: clotrimazole and miconazole nitrate. A lively competition has developed between the two makers and their ad and public relations agencies, which has led to some unusually frank but delicate Television advertising, with messages such as, "It's important that now most women can cure their own recurrent vaginal yeast infections."

Candidiasis is by no means the only source of vaginal itching. Another less common cause is the protozoa *Trichomonas vaginalis*, which is called "tric." In one study published in the *Journal of the American Medical Association* (vol. 162, pp. 268-71), several gynecológists reported that among women whom they treated in their offices for vaginitis and vaginal discharge, yeast infections outnumbered tric

---

Will Yogurt Stop Yeast?

The answer is, "Well, maybe!"

Yogurt has become the great folk remedy for controlling *C. albicans.* Some women eat lots of yogurt. Some swallow capsules or tablets that contain the yogurt-making bacteria *Lactobacillus acidophilus.* Some place the yogurt or the tablets in their vaginas. Many swear by these methods.

An experiment reported in the *Annals of Internal Medicine* (vol. 116, pp. 353-57, 1992) by infectious disease specialist Eileen Hilton, M.D., and her colleagues at Long Island Jewish Medical Center in New Hyde Park, N.Y., now provides some scientific support for these practices: The doctors put 33 women with recurring yeast infections on one of two diets: with yogurt, or without, for six months, and then tried to switch them to the alternate.

The yogurt used in the study was a commercial brand that had a high proportion of *L. acidophilus,* which may be, but is not necessarily present in commercial yogurt. These bacteria make yogurt that is high in lactic acid. It changes the acid-base balance of the vagina, which, it is conjectured, renders it inhospitable to yeast.

Women on the yogurt diet had only a third as many yeast infections as those who were not: about 0.4 attacks per six months for those who ate 8 ounces of yogurt daily, compared to 2.5 attacks per six months in those who did not. Most women on the yogurt diet were so pleased with it that they refused to be switched to the no-yogurt diet. Dr. Hilton and her colleagues conclude that 8 ounces of *L. acidophilus*-rich yogurt daily "decreased candidal colonization and infection."

One problem with this approach, a commentator says in the *Archives* is that some commercial yogurts contain *L. acidophilus,* but others do not. Some yogurts are pasteurized, which kills the *L. acidophilus* and may negate the yogurt's medicinal value, while others are not pasteurized. The next step, this commentator says, might be to re-run the experiment, comparing pasteurized and non-pasteurized *L. acidophilus* yogurts.

infections 7 to 1 among women who were not pregnant and 15 to 1 among women who were pregnant.

The Panel believes that with tric, as with yeast, the first time a woman has the infection it should be diagnosed by a doctor but subsequently can be self-diagnosed. However, the FDA thus far has not approved any nonprescription drug specifically for curing trichomoniasis.

 Claims

Accurate

For clotrimazole and miconazole nitrate:

• "Cures most vaginal yeast (Candida) infections"

For hydrocortisone and hydrocortisone acetate:

• "For temporary relief of external genital itching"

WARNING:

 The warnings that regard use of these approved ingredients are summarized in the 3 entries given here.

APPROVED ACTIVE INGREDIENTS

• *CLOTRIMAZOLE 1 PERCENT IN CREAM, OR 100 MG IN VAGINAL INSERTS:* This drug is effective against a number of fungal disorders. (*See* JOCK ITCH, ATHLETE'S FOOT, AND RINGWORM CURES.) It is quite effective against yeast infections and was switched to nonprescription status for this purpose early in the present decade. Side effects are rare and mild; they include rashes, itching, and irritation.

Clotrimazole's record of use over a decade and a half convinced the FDA that it is safe and effective and can be used successfully by women to self-treat recurrent candidiasis or initial infections that have been diagnosed by a doctor. The drug is supplied as a vaginal cream, with an applicator, or as vaginal tablets, for use once daily at bedtime. The course of treatment is seven days; if treatment is interrupted earlier, the infection may return. The itching, burning discomfort should begin to abate by the third day.

WARNING:

 Do not use if you have abdominal pain, a fever, or a foul-smelling vaginal discharge. You may have a condition that is more serious than a yeast infection. Consult your doctor. Do not use this product if this is your first experience with vaginal itch and discomfort. See your doctor. If there is no improvement within three days, you may have a condition other than a yeast infection. Stop using the drug and consult your doctor. If symptoms recur within a two-month period, contact your doctor. Do not use during pregnancy, except under the advice and supervision of a doctor. For vaginal use only.

- *HYDROCORTISONE AND HYDROCORTISONE ACETATE (0.25 TO 1 PERCENT):* Dramatic relief from external feminine itching and inflammation—from yeast and a variety of other causes—can be obtained quickly with over-the-counter hydrocortisone preparations. (*See* pp. 571-572.) The Antimicrobial II Panel noted, however, that these preparations usually do not kill the yeast or other causative organism, if there is one. So treatment with an anti-candidal or other specific drug may well be necessary. For fast, overnight relief of an itching emergency, this might be the nonprescription drug to try.

    For women and girls over two years of age, apply to the affected area not more than 3 or 4 times daily.

WARNING:

 For hydrocortisones:
Do not use inside the vagina.

- *MICONAZOLE NITRATE (TWO PERCENT CREAM, OR 100 MG VAGINAL INSERTS):* This anti-candidal agent first was approved by the FDA as a prescription drug two decades ago, in 1973, under the strict guidelines for safety and effectiveness that are applied to all new prescription products. The Antimicrobial II Panel recommended that it be switched to non-prescription status for yeast infections, which was done in 1991.

    In one Belgian study, cited by the Panel, 147 out of 165 women treated with miconazole nitrate for vulvovagininitis caused by *C. albicans* were clinically cured and found to be free of the yeast after treatment ended. The most successful dosage was 2 percent miconzole cream twice daily for two weeks. In three later studies, this formulation yielded cure rates of 76 percent, 90 percent, and 93 percent. Side effects included temporary worsening of vaginal itching, burning, and discomfort; cramping, headache, and hives also were reported.

The recommended dosage is one vaginal insert (suppository) once daily at bedtime, plus some of the cream if needed for external application, for one week. The symptoms should abate before the week has passed, but self-treatment should continue for the full week.

WARNING:

 Do not use, or stop using if you have fever (over 100° F. orally); pain in the lower abdomen, back, or shoulder; or a vaginal discharge with a bad, fishy smell. In these circumstances, contact your doctor: You may have a more serious illness. If there is no improvement, or infection worsens within three days, or complete relief is not obtained within seven days, or symptoms return within two months, you may have something other than a yeast infection. Consult your doctor. Do not use tampons while taking this medication. Do not use if you are under 12 years of age. If you are pregnant, or think you may be, do not use except with a doctor's advice and supervision.

CONDITIONALLY APPROVED INGREDIENTS

None.

DISAPPROVED INGREDIENTS

None.

When Further Relief Is Needed

Doctors can prescribe more potent steroids and other itch-relievers. They also can prescribe other, possibly more effective anti-candidal drugs.

Safety and Effectiveness: Active Ingredients
in Topical Drugs to Relieve or Cure Yeast Infections

Active Ingredient	Assessment: For Relieving Symptoms	Assessment: Kills Yeast
clotrimazole	safe and effective	yes
hydrocortisone	safe and effective	no
hydrocortisone acetate	safe and effective	no
miconazole nitrate	safe and effective	yes

'Yeast' Killers for Feminine Itching: Product Ratings

Product and Distributor	Dosage of Active Ingredients	Rating*†	Comment
clotrimazole			
Gyne-Lotrimin (Schering-Plough)	cream: 1% vaginal tablets: 100 mg	A	℞ to OTC switch
FemCare (Schering-Plough)	cream: 1% vaginal suppositories: 100 mg	A	generic version—less expensive; ℞ to OTC switch
Mycelex-7 (Miles)	cream: 1% vaginal tablets: 100 mg	A	℞ to OTC switch
miconazole nitrate			
Monistat 7 (Ortho)	cream: 2% vaginal suppositories: 100 mg	A	℞ to OTC switch

*Author's interpretation of FDA criteria. Based on contents, not claims.
†For hydrocortisone and hydrocortisone acetate products, see pp. 571-572.

Advisory Review Panels and Their Members

The Advisory Review Panel on OTC Antacid Drugs included:

Franz J. Ingelfinger, M.D., Chairman, editor of the *New England Journal of Medicine*, Boston, MA; Howard C. Ansel, Ph.D., *Professor of Pharmacy and Head of School of Pharmacy, University of Georgia*, Athens, GA; Morton I. Grossman, M.D., *Internist, Veterans Administration Center*, Los Angeles, CA; Stewart C. Harvey, Ph.D., *Associate Professor of Pharmacology, University of Utah College of Medicine*, Salt Lake City, UT; Edward W. Moore, M.D., *Professor of Medicine, Medical College of Virginia*, Richmond, VA; John F. Morrissey, M.D., *Professor of Medicine, University of Wisconsin School of Medicine*, Madison, WI; Howard M. Spiro, M.D., *Professor of Medicine, Yale University School of Medicine*, New Haven, CT.

The Advisory Review Panel on OTC Antimicrobial Drug Products for Repeated Daily Human Use (Antimicrobial I Panel) included:

Harvey Blank, M.D., Chairman, *Professor of Dermatology, University of Miami School of Medicine*, Miami, FL; Frank B. Engley, Jr., Ph.D., *Professor and Chairman, Department of Microbiology, University of Missouri School of Medicine*, Columbia, MO; William L. Epstein, M.D., *Chairman of the Department of Dermatology, University of California San Francisco Medical Center*, San Francisco, CA; Wallace L. Guess, Ph.D., *Dean, School of Pharmacy, University of Mississippi*, University, MS; Florence K. Kinoshita, Ph.D., Northbrook, IL; Mary Marples, M.D., D.T., M. & H., Old Woodstock, Oxfordshire, England; Paul D. Stolley, M.D., *Johns Hopkins School of Hygiene and Public Health*, Baltimore, MD.

The Advisory Review Panel on OTC Antimicrobial Drug Products (Antimicrobial II Panel) included:

Wallace L. Guess, Ph.D., Chairman, *Dean, School of Pharmacy,*

University of Mississippi, University, MS; W. Kenneth Blaylock, M.D., *Assistant Dean for Graduate Medical Education, Medical College of Virginia*, Richmond, VA; Ruth E. Brown, R. Pharm., *Director of Pharmacy, Retired, Group Health*, Seattle, WA; Frank B. Engley, Jr., Ph.D., *Professor and Chairman, Department of Microbiology, University of Missouri School of Medicine*, Columbia, MO; Zenona W. Mally, M.D., *Dermatologist*, Washington, DC; James E. Rasmussen, M.D., *Department of Pediatrics, Buffalo Children's Hospital*, Buffalo, NY; William F. Schorr, M.D., *Director, Dermatologic Residency Training Program, Marshfield Clinic*, Marshfield, WI; E. Dorinda Loeffel Shelley, M.D., *Assistant Professor of Dermatology, University of Illinois Medical Center*, Chicago, IL; Paul D. Stolley, M.D., M.P.H., *Johns Hopkins School of Hygiene and Public Health*, Baltimore, MD; Anne N. Tucker, Ph.D., *Department of Pharmacology, Medical College of Virginia*, Richmond, VA; George B. Youngstrom, M.D., *Dermatologist and Allergist*, Everett, WA.

The Advisory Review Panel on OTC Antiperspirant Drug Products included:

E. William Rosenberg, M.D., Chairman, *Professor and Chairman, Department of Dermatology, University of Tennessee College of Medicine*, Memphis, TN; J. Wesley Clayton, Ph.D., *Director, Toxicology Program, The University of Arizona*, Tucson, AZ; Charles Evans, M.D., Ph.D., *Professor, Department of Microbiology, University of Washington*, Seattle, WA; Zenona W. Mally, M.D., Dermatologist, Washington, DC; Jane Rosenzweig, M.D., *Clinical Instructor, The Permanent Medical Group*, San Francisco, CA; Robert Scheuplein, Ph.D., *Principal Associate in Biophysics, Department of Dermatology, Massachusetts General Hospital*, Boston, MA; Eli Shefter, Ph.D., *Associate Professor of Pharmaceutics, School of Pharmacy, State University of New York at Buffalo*, Buffalo, NY.

The Advisory Review Panel on OTC Cold, Cough, Allergy, Bronchodilator, and Antiasthmatic Products included:

Francis C. Lowell, M.D., Chairman, *Chief, Allergy Unit, Massachusetts General Hospital*, Boston, MA; Hylan A. Bickerman, M.D., *Associate Clinical Professor of Medicine, College of Physicians and Surgeons, Columbia University*, New York, NY; Halla Brown, M.D., *Chief, Allergy Unit, George Washington University Hospital*, Washington, DC; Robert K. Chalmers, Ph.D., *Associate Dean for Professional Education Program, School of Pharmacy and Pharmacal Science, Purdue University*, Lafayette, IN; Mary Jo Reilly, M.S., *Assistant Executive Director, American Society of Hospital Pharmacists*, Washington, DC; James R. Tureman, M.D., *Professor of Pharmacology, Department of Pharmacology, College of Medicine, Howard University*, Washington, DC; Colin R. Woolf, M.D., *Director, Tri-Hospital Respiratory Service, Toronto General Hospital*, Toronto, Ontario, Canada.

The Advisory Review Panel on OTC Contraceptives and other Vaginal Drug Products included:

Elizabeth B. Connell, M.D., Chairman, *Associate Director for Biomedical Sciences, The Rockefeller Foundation*, New York, NY; Evelyn M. Benson, R.Ph., *Pharmacist, Mission Pharmacy*, Seattle, WA; Cynthia W. Cooke, M.D., *Obstetrician-Gynecologist*, Bryn Mawr, PA; Myron Gordon, M.D., *Associate Professor of Obstetrics and Gynecology, New York Medical College*, New York, NY; William A. MacColl, M.D., *Pediatric Allergist*, Berkeley, CA; William H. Pearlman, Ph.D., *Professor of Pharmacology, University of North Carolina School of Medicine*, Chapel Hill, NC; Louise B. Tyrer, M.D., *Vice President for Medical Affairs, Planned Parenthood World Population*, New York, NY.

The Advisory Review Panel on Dentifrice and Dental-Care Drug Products included:

Louis P. Gangarosa, Ph.D., D.D.S., Chairman, *Professor of Oral Biology, Medical College of Georgia*, Augusta, GA; Joseph J. Aleo, Ph.D., *Assistant Dean, Temple University Dental School*, Philadelphia, PA; Arthur N. Bahn, Ph.D., *Department of Microbiology, Southern Illinois University*, Edwardsville, IL; Howard H. Chauncey, D.M.D., Ph.D., *Veterans Administration Outpatient Clinic*, Boston, MA; Valerie Hurst, Ph.D., *Associate Professor of Microbiology, University of California School of Dentistry*, San Francisco, CA; Joy B. Plein, Ph.D., *Associate Professor of Pharmacy, University of Washington College of Pharmacy*, Seattle, WA; Delos E. Raymond, D.D.S., *Dentist*, Inkster, MI; Roger H. Scholle, D.D.S., M.S., *Assistant Secretary, Council of Dental Therapeutics, American Dental Association*, Chicago, IL; Lawrence E. Van Kirk, Jr., D.D.S., M.P.H., *Department of Restorative Dentistry, University of Detroit School of Dentistry*, Detroit, MI.

The Advisory Review Panel on OTC Hemorrhoidal Drug Products included:

Claude E. Welch, M.D., Chairman, *Senior Consulting Surgeon, Massachusetts General Hospital*, Boston, MA; Leon Banov, Jr., M.D., *Colonic and Rectal Surgeon*, Charleston, SC; Eugene A. Castiglia, M.D., *Gastroenterologist*, Albuquerque, NM; Winston H. Gaskin, R.Ph., *Veterans Administration Hospital*, Syracuse, NY; Jean Dace Golden, M.D., *General and Plastic Surgeon*, East Stroudsburg, PA; Thaddeus S. Grosicki, Ph.D., *Professor of Pharmaceutics, School of Pharmacy, University of Arkansas*, Little Rock, AR; Judith Karen Jones, M.D., Ph.D., *Internist and Clinical Pharmacologist*, San Francisco, CA.

The Advisory Review Panel on OTC Internal Analgesic, Antipyretic, and Antirheumatic Products included:

Henry W. Elliott, M.D., Ph.D., Chairman, *Professor and Chairman,*

Department of Medical Pharmacology and Therapeutics, Orange County Medical Center, Orange, CA; J. Weldon Bellville, M.D., Chairman, *Department of Anesthesiology, University of California School of Medicine*, Los Angeles, CA; William H. Barr, Ph.D., *Department of Pharmacy, Medical College of Virginia*, Richmond, VA; Julius M. Coon, M.D., Ph.D., *Professor of Pharmacology, Thomas Jefferson University*, Philadelphia, PA; Ninfa I. Redmond, Ph.D., *Department of Pharmacology, Faculty of Medicine, University of Montreal*, Montreal, Quebec, Canada; Naomi F. Rothfield, M.D., *Chief, Arthritis Section, Professor of Medicine, University of Connecticut School of Medicine*, Farmington, CT; George Sharpe, M.D., Kensington, MD.

The Advisory Review Panel on OTC Laxative, Antidiarrheal, Emetic and Antiemetic Drug products included:

Nicholas C. Hightower, Jr., M.D., *Director of Research and Education, Scott and White Memorial Hospital*, Temple, TX; Carol R. Angle, M.D., *Professor of Pediatrics, University of Nebraska*, Omaha, NE; James C. Cain, M.D., *Gastroenterologist and Internist, Mayo Clinic*, Rochester, MN; Ivan E. Danhof, M.D., Ph.D., *Associate Professor of Physiology, University of Texas Medical School*, Dallas, TX; James W. Freston, M.D., Ph.D., *Chairman, Division of Gastroenterology, University of Utah Medical Center*, Salt Lake City, UT; Albert L. Picchioni, Ph.D., *Head, Department of Pharmacology and Toxicology, University of Arizona*, Tucson, AZ; Sheila West, Pharm. D., *Program Director, Pharmacy Studies, Johns Hopkins Medical Institutions*, Baltimore, MD.

The Advisory Review Panel on OTC Miscellaneous External Drug Products included:

William E. Lotterhos, M.D., Chairman, *Director, Montgomery Family Practice Program*, Montgomery, AL; George C. Cypress, M.D., *Pediatrician*, Private Practice, Newport News, VA; Rose Dagirmanjian, Ph.D., *Professor of Pharmacology, University of Louisville*, Louisville, KY; Vincent J. Derbes, M.D., *Dermatologist*, Private Practice, New Orleans, LA; J. Robert Hewson, M.D., *Department of Family Practice, University of South Carolina School of Medicine*, Columbia, SC; Yelva L. Lynfield, M.D., *Chief, Dermatology Section, Veterans Administration Hospital*, Brooklyn, NY; Harry E. Morton, Sc.D., *Professor Emeritus of Microbiology, University of Pennsylvania School of Medicine*, Philadelphia, PA; Marianne N. O'Donoghue, M.D., *Dermatologist*, Private Practice, River Forest, IL; Chester L. Rossi, R.Ph., D.P.M., *Podiatrist, Torno Medical Clinic*, Pasadena, TX.

The Advisory Review Panel on OTC Miscellaneous Internal Drug Products included:

John W. Norcross, M.D., Chairman, *Internist*, Belmont, MA; James L. Tullis, M.D., Chairman, *Department of Hematology, New England-Deaconess*

Hospital, Boston, MA; William R. Arrowsmith, M.D. *Department of Internal Medicine, Ochsner Clinic,* New Orleans, LA; Elizabeth C. Gablin, N.N., Ed.D., *Professor of Physiological Nursing, University of Washington,* Seattle, WA; Richard D. Harshfield, M.D., *Associate Professor of Pharmacology, University of Illinois,* Rockford, IL; Theodore L. Hyde, M.D., *General Surgeon,* The Dalles, OR; Diana F. Rodriguez-Calvert, Pharm. D., *Pioneer Pharmacy,* Wagoner, OK; Claus A. Rohweder, D.O., *Director of Medical Education, Kirksville College of Osteopathic Medicine,* Kirksville, MO.

The Advisory Review Panel on OTC Ophthalmic Drug Products included:

Philip Ellis, M.D., Chairman, *Chairman of Ophthalmology, University of Colorado Medical School,* Denver, CO; Donald E. Cadwallader, Ph.D., *Professor of Pharmacy, University of Georgia School of Medicine,* Athens, GA; Calvin Hanna, Ph.D., *Department of Pharmacology, University of Arkansas Medical Center,* Little Rock, AR; William H. Havener, M.D., *Chairman of Ophthalmology, Ohio State University,* Columbus, OH; James F. Koetting, O.D., *Professor of Optometry, University of Houston College of Optometry,* Houston, TX; Pearl A. Watson, M.D., *Ophthalmologist,* Washington, D.C.

The Advisory Review Panel on OTC Oral-Cavity Drug Products included:

Lawrence Cohen, M.D., Ph.D., D.D.S., Chairman, *Emergency Medicine Specialist,* Wilmette, IL; John Adriani, M.D., *Clinical Professor of Anesthesiology, Charity Hospital,* New Orleans, LA; Arthur N. Bahn, Ph.D., *Microbiologist, Southern Illinois University,* Edwardsville, IL; Roy C. Darlington, Ph.D., Washington, DC; Martin J. Goldberg, D.D.S., *Dentist,* Kensington, MD; Valarie Hurst, Ph.D., *Professor of Microbiology, School of Dentistry, University of California,* San Francisco, CA; Walter E. Loch, M.D., *Associate Professor of Otolaryngology, School of Medicine, Johns Hopkins University,* Baltimore, MD.

The Advisory Review Panel on OTC Sedative, Tranquilizer, and Sleep-Aid Drug Products included:

Karl E. Rickels, M.D., Chairman, *Professor of Psychiatry and Pharmacology, Department of Psychiatry, University of Pennsylvania,* Philadelphia, PA; Carleton K. Erickson, Ph.D., *School of Pharmacy, University of Kansas,* Lawrence, KS; Helen Dun Goiun, R.Ph., M.S., Arlington, VA; Ernest L. Hartmann, M.D., *Professor of Psychiatry, Tufts University School of Medicine,* Boston, MA; Sumner M. Kalman, M.D., *School of Medicine, Stanford University,* Stanford, CA; Lester C. Mark, M.D., *Professor of Anesthesiology, College of Physicians and Surgeons, Columbia University,* New York, NY; Frances S. Norris, M.D., *Medical Director, Division of Licensing and Certification, Maryland Department of Health,* Baltimore, MD.

The Advisory Review Panel on OTC Topical Analgesic, Antirheumatic, Otic, Burn, and Sunburn Prevention and Treatment Drug Products included:

Thomas G. Kantor, M.D., Chairman, *Associate Physician, New York University Medical Center*, New York, NY; John Adriani, M.D., *Clinical Professor of Anesthesiology, Charity Hospital*, New Orleans, LA; Col. William A. Akers, M.C., U.S.A., *Commander, Letterman Army Institute of Research*, San Francisco, CA; Maxine E. Bennett, M.D., *Professor of Otolaryngology, University of Wisconsin Hospitals*, Madison, WI; Minerva S. Buerk, M.D., *Dermatologist*, Wynnewood, PA; Walter L. Dickison, Ph.D., *Dean, School of Pharmacy, Southwestern Oklahoma State University*, Weatherford, OK; Jerry M. Shuck, M.D., *Associate Professor of Surgery, University of New Mexico School of Medicine*, Albuquerque, NM.

The Advisory Review Panel on OTC Vitamin, Mineral, and Hemantic Drug Products included:

Irwin H. Rosenberg, M.D., Chairman, *Chief, Gastroenterology Section, University of Chicago School of Medicine*, Chicago, IL; Louis V. Avioli, M.D., *Director, Metabolic Clinic, Washington University School of Medicine*, St. Louis, MO; George M. Briggs, Ph.D., *Professor of Nutrition, University of California*, Berkeley, CA; Robert S. Goodhart, M.D., *Executive Secretary, Committee on Medical Education, The New York Academy of Medicine*, New York, NY; Mary Anne Kimble, Pharm. D., *Assistant Clinical Professor of Pharmacy, University of California*, San Francisco, CA; Carroll M. Leevy, M.D., *Director, Division of Hepatic Metabolism, College of Medicine and Dentistry of New Jersey*, Newark, NJ; Mary Susanne Roscoe, M.D., *Emergency Medicine Specialist*, Aurora, IL.

In addition to the Panel members listed here, the Advisory Panels included a number of non-voting liaisons, some of whom represented the interests of consumer organizations, and some, the nonprescription drug industry.

Sources

The fundamental source of this Guide is the Over-the-Counter (OTC) Drug Review that is being conducted by the Food and Drug Administration (FDA), an agency of the federal government. The official documents generated in this Review are published in the *Federal Register*. Some two hundred of these documents, ranging in length from a page or two to over two hundred of the *Register*'s tight-packed three-column pages, have appeared so far. I have read these documents, in order to distill their essence here.

For readers who wish to delve further into the OTC Drug Review, a list of these documents follows this section. This list includes all reports of the 17 Advisory Review Panels that initially assessed the status of most active ingredients in the Review. The FDA's initial responses to these proposals, which are called *Tentative Final Monographs*, or *TFM*s also are listed. The TFMs now have been published for all but a handful of OTC drug classes. What is more, for some of these classes of drugs, two or more *TFM*s have already resulted from new pharmacological developments, jockeying between drug makers and the agency, and the legal and administrative complexities of the FDA's regulatory process.

The *Final Monographs* (*FM*s), of which 45 have thus far been published, present and briefly explain the rules that will govern marketing of the particular drugs of each class. The *FM*s become effective within one year after publication in the *Federal Register*. The monographs also are published in the *Code of Federal Regulations (CFR)*, which is widely accessible in libraries.

In the list of sources, only the date of each *Federal Register* citation is given. Multiple listings indicate that the FDA has published more than one *Panel Report, TFM,* or *FM* on the drugs covered in a Unit; additional FDA amendments can of course be anticipated as new drugs become available and rules are changed to accommodate them. All *CFR* entries are in volume 21 of the Code (21 *CFR*).

In preparing this Guide, I consulted several standard drug reference sources. In the FDA's *Approved Drug Products* (the "Orange Book"), which is published annually with monthly updates, there is an "OTC Drug Product List" containing ℞-to-OTC switches (drugs that were previously available only by prescription but have been changed to nonprescription availability) and new OTC drugs approved on the basis of New Drug Applications (NDAs). In the Product Ratings that conclude most Units in this Guide, an effort has been made to include at least one example of each drug on the OTC Drug Product List as of March 1992.

Two FDA working summaries, "Milestone Status of OTC Drug Review Documents," through June 1, 1992, and "OTC Drug Review Ingredient Status Report," updated to December 2, 1991, which is the most recent update, have been quite helpful.

Among non-governmental sources, the American Medical Association's *Drug Evaluations* (Chicago: AMA), now published annually, is an authoritative source. It is fairly selective in its coverage of over-the-counter drugs. For information directly from drug manufacturers, the annual *Physicians' Desk Reference* (PDR) *for Nonprescription Drugs* (Montvale, New Jersey: Medical Economics), is useful because it consists exclusively of manufacturers' information on their products; most if not all of this information has been approved by the FDA for use on product labels and package inserts.

Pharmacists use a sister publication from Medical Economics, *Drug Topics Red Book* (1992) to shop wholesale for drug products. For reference purposes, the pharmacists' professional society, the American Pharmaceutical Association, periodically publishes a large *Handbook of Nonprescription Drugs*, which now is in its 9th edition (Washington, D.C.: APA, 1990). It covers most, if not all classes of OTC drugs, and through the years has come more and more to reflect decisions in the OTC Drug Review.

Physicians, pharmacologists, and pharmacists turn to the loose-leaf *drug facts and comparisons* (St. Louis, Missouri: Facts and Comparisons) for current information that combines FDA and drug makers' information. It contains monographs on a wide number of ℞ and OTC drugs, and is updated monthly.

For news about the drug industry and the FDA, the most complete file is the weekly newsletter called "The Pink Sheet" or *F-D-C Reports*, published in Chevy Chase, Maryland. For a far more austere and critical look at drugs, physicians in particular consult the fortnightly *Medical Letter on Drugs and Therapeutics*, published in New Rochelle, New York. It mostly covers ℞ drugs, but occasionally reports on OTCs.

All of these sources have been consulted in preparing this Guide.

Below are the *Federal Register* and *Code of Federal Regulations* citations for the Units in this Guide:

Acne Medications: *PR* 3/23/82; *TFM* 1/15/85, 8/7/91; *FM* 8/16/91; *CFR* 333. Allergy Drugs: *PR* 9/9/76; *TFM* 10/26/82, 10/19/83, 1/15/85, 8/24/87, 8/12/88, 11/14/88, 7/6/89,10/29/89. Antacids: *PR* 4/5/73; *TFM* 11/12/73, 7/3/88, 11/16/88, 12/24/91; *FM* 6/4/74; *CFR* 331. Anti-Gas Agents: *PR* 4/5/73; *TFM* 11/12/73, 1/29/88; *FM* 6/4/74. Antiperspirants *PR* 10/10/78; *TFM* 8/20/82; *CFR* 332. Aphrodisiacs: *PR* 10/1/82; *TFM* 1/15/85; *FM* 7/7/89; *CFR* 310. Asthma Drugs: *PR* 9/9/76; *TFM* 10/26/82, 1/15/85, 8/24/87, 8/12/88, 11/14/88; *FM* 10/2/86.

Bleaches for Skin Blemishes: *PR* 11/3/78; *TFM* 9/3/82. Boil Ointments: *PR* 6/9/82; *TFM* 1/26/88.

Camphor: Special Note: *PR* 9/26/80; *TFM* —; *FM* 9/21/82; *CFR* 310.526. Cold And Cough Medicines: *PR* 9/9/76; *TFM* 7/9/82, 10/26/82, 10/19/83, 1/15/85, 8/24/87, 8/12/88, 11/14/88, 7/6/89, 10/2/89; *FM* 11/8/85, 10/2/86, 8/12/87, 2/28/89, 7/6/90, 10/3/90, 6/30/92; *CFR* 310.533, 341, 343, 357, 369. Cold-Sore Balms: *PR* 9/7/82; *TFM* 1/31/90; *FM* 6/30/92. Contraceptives: *PR* 12/12/80. Corn and Callus Removers: *PR* 1/5/82; *TFM* 2/20/87; *FM* 8/14/90; *CFR* 358f. Cradle-Cap Removers: *PR* 12/3/82; *TFM* 7/30/86; *FM* 12/4/91; *CFR* 358h.

Dandruff and Seborrheic Scale Shampoos and Other Treatments: *PR* 12/3/82; *TFM* 7/30/86; *FM* 12/4/91; *CFR* 358h. Deodorants For Incontinence and Ostomies: *PR* 1/5/82; *TFM* 6/17/85; *FM* 5/11/90; *CFR* 357i. Diaper-Rash Relievers: *PR* 9/7/82; *TFM* 6/20/90. Diarrhea Remedies: *PR* 3/21/75; *TFM* 4/30/86. Digestive Aids: *PR* 1/5/82; *TFM* 1/29/88. Douches And Other Vaginal Drugs: *PR* 10/13/83.

Ear-Care Aids: *PR* 12/16/77; *TFM* 7/9/82, 7/30/86; *FM* 8/8/86; *CFR* 344. Eye Drops and Ointments: *PR* 5/6/80; *TFM* 6/28/83; *FM* 3/4/88; *CFR* 349. Eyes: Artificial Tears: *PR* 5/60/80; *TFM* 6/28/83; *FM* 3/4/88; *CFR* 349. Eyes: Corneal Edema: *PR* 5/60/80; *TFM* 6/28/83; *FM* 3/4/88; *CFR* 349. Eyewash: *PR* 5/60/80; *TFM* 6/28/83; *FM* 3/4/88; *CFR* 349.

First-Aid Antiseptics: *PR* 9/13/74, 1/5/82, 5/21/82; *TFM* 1/6/78, 7/22/91; *FM* 12/11/87, 5/25/88, 3/15/90, 10/3/90, 12/5/90; *CFR* 333, 444, 448. First-Aid Antibiotics: *PR* 4/1/77; *TFM* 1/6/78, 7/9/82, 8/18/89, 5/11/90, 6/8/90, 7/23/91. Fluoride Toothpastes and Rinses for Cavity Prevention: *PR* 3/28/80; *TFM* 9/30/85, 6/15/88.

Germ-Killing Soaps: *PR* 1/7/72, 9/13/74; *TFM* 1/6/78, 7/22/91; *FM* 9/27/72.

HAIR-GROWTH STIMULANTS AND BALDNESS PREVENTIVES: *PR* 11/17/80; *TFM* 1/15/85; *FM* 7/7/89; *CFR* 310. HANGOVER AND OVERINDULGENCE RELIEVERS: *PR* 10/1/82; *TFM* 12/24/91; *FM* 7/19/83. HEMORRHOID MEDICATION AND OTHER ANORECTAL APPLICATIONS: *PR* 5/27/80; *TFM* 8/15/88; *FM* 8/3/90; *CFR* 310, 346, 369. HORMONE SKIN CREAMS AND OILS: *PR* 1/5/82; *TFM* 10/2/89.

INGROWN-TOENAIL RELIEVERS: *PR* 10/17/80; *TFM* 9/3/82. INSULIN FOR DIABETICS: (Not Part Of OTC Drug Review). ITCH AND PAIN REMEDIES APPLIED TO THE SKIN: *PR* 12/4/79; *TFM* 2/8/83, 7/30/86, 8/25/88, 2/27/90.

JOCK ITCH, ATHLETE'S FOOT, AND RINGWORM CURES: *PR* 3/23/82; *TFM* 12/12/89.

KIDNEY AND BLADDER DRUGS: *PR*—.

LAXATIVES: *PR* 3/21/75; *TFM* 1/15/85, 10/1/86. LOUSE POISONS: *PR* 6/29/82; *TFM* 4/3/89. LINIMENTS AND POULTICES FOR ACHES AND PAINS: *PR* 12/4/79; *TFM* 2/8/83, 7/30/86, 8/25/88, 2/27/90.

MEDICAMENTS FOR SORE GUMS, MOUTH & THROAT: *PR* 11/2/79, 3/28/80, 5/25/82; *TFM* 7/26/83, 1/27/88, 9/24/91, 5/13/92. MENSTRUAL DISTRESS PREPARATIONS: *PR* 12/7/82; *TFM* 11/16/88. MOTION-SICKNESS MEDICINES: *PR* 3/21/75; *TFM* 7/13/79; *FM* 4/30/87; *CFR* 336. MOUTHWASH FOR ORAL HYGIENE: *PR* 5/25/82.

NAIL-BITING AND THUMB-SUCKING DETERRENTS: *PR* 10/17/80; *TFM* 9/3/82.

PAIN, FEVER AND ANTI-INFLAMMATORY DRUGS TAKEN INTERNALLY: *PR* 7/8/77; *TFM* 11/16/88, 12/24/91. PANCREATIC ENZYME SUPPLEMENTS: *PR* 12/21/79; *TFM* 11/8/85, 7/15/91. PHENOL: SPECIAL NOTE: *PR* 9/13/74; *TFM* 1/6/78, 7/22/91. POISON IVY-OAK-SUMAC PREVENTIVES AND PALLIATIVES: *PR* 12/4/79, 9/7/82; *TFM* 10/3/89. POISONING ANTIDOTES: *PR* 3/21/75, 1/5/82; *TFM* 9/5/78. PREMATURE EJACULATION RETARDANTS: *PR* 9/7/82; *TFM* 10/2/85. PSORIASIS LOTIONS: *PR* 12/3/82; *TFM* 7/30/86; *FM* 12/4/91; *CFR* 358h.

QUININE FOR LEG CRAMPS: *PR* 7/8/77, 10/1/82; *TFM* 11/8/85.

REDUCING AIDS: *PR* 2/26/82; *TFM* 10/30/90; *FM* 8/8/91.

SALT SUPPLEMENTS AND SUBSTITUTES: PRELIMINARY REPORT: *PR* —. SLEEP

AIDS: *PR* 12/8/75; *TFM* 6/13/78; *FM* 2/14/89; *CFR* 338. SMELLING SALTS: PRELIMINARY REPORT: *PR* —. SMOKING DETERRENTS: *PR* 1/5/82; *TFM* 7/3/85. STIMULANTS: *PR* 12/8/75; *TFM* 6/13/78; 12/24/91 *FM* 2/29/88; *CFR* 340. STYPTIC PENCILS AND OTHER ASTRINGENTS: *PR* 9/7/82; *TFM* 4/3/89. SUNSCREENS: *PR* 8/25/78.

TEETH DESENSITIZERS: *PR* 5/25/82; *TFM* 9/24/91. TEETH: ANTI-PLAQUE PRODUCTS: *PR* —. TEETHING EASERS *PR* 5/25/82; *TFM* 9/24/91. THYROID PROTECTORS FOR NUCLEAR EMERGENCIES: FINAL RECOMMENDATION: (Not Part of OTC Drug Review) *TFM* 6/29/82. TOOTHACHE RELIEVERS: *PR* 5/25/82; *TFM* 9/24/91.

UNGUENTS AND POWDERS TO PROTECT THE SKIN: *PR* 8/4/78; *TFM* 2/15/83.

VITAMINS AND MINERALS: *PR* 3/16/79; *TFM* 7/19/90; *FM* 11/27/81; *CFR* 345.

WART PAINTS AND PLASTERS: *PR* 10/30/80; *TFM* 9/3/82, 3/27/87; *FM* 8/14/90; *CFR* 358. WORM-KILLERS FOR PINWORM INFESTATION: *PR* 9/9/80; *TFM* 8/24/82; *FM* 8/1/86; *CFR* 357b.

YEAST KILLERS FOR FEMININE ITCHING: *PR* 3/23/82, 10/13/83; *TFM* 12/12/89.

---

*PR = Panel Report(s); *TFM* = Tentative Final Monograph(s); *FM* = Final Monograph(s); *CFR* = Code of Federal Regulations, Volume 21 (Parts). Incomplete Regulations May Not Be Listed.

General Index

A

A and D, 296t
A-Caine Rectal, 517t
A/K Rinse, 403t
A-200, 659t
Abdomen, upper, burning distress in, 51
Abdominal bloating, 318
Abdominal bloating and pain, 711
Abdominal cramps, 298
Abortion, spontaneous, and douching, 333
Abrasives, in anti-plaque products, 932, 935-936; in toothpaste, 439
Abscess, *see also* Boils; perianal, 480; staphylococcal, on eyelid, 367

Absorbents, in skin protectants, for diaper rash, 276
Accutane, for severe acne, 7
Acetaminophen or APAP, 795t
Acetaminophen, adult's dosage of, 767, 769t; child's dosage of, 768, 770t; claims for, 771; equivalent dosages of, 766-768; for hangover, 471, 473; for menstrual distress, 714; in overindulgence remedies, 468; as pain reliever, 768; product ratings for, 795t-796t; vs. acetanilide, 785
Acetaminophen with codeine elixir, 799t
Acetanilide, disapproved for pain relief, 785

• a 't' appearing next to a page number denotes table
• bold type indicates a brand name or generic product
• bold numbers are unit references

Avobenzone, 911; claims for, 902-903; as UVA-blocking sunscreen, 916

Avobenzone (Parsol 1789), and UVA light rays, 908

B

B vitamins, 1007, *see also* under specific B vitamin

Babee Teething, 947t

Baby, *see* Infant

Baby Anbesol, 947t

Baby Orajel, 947t

Baciguent, 411t

Bacia, 226t

Bacitracin, 411t

Bacitracin, 408, 409t, 411t; zinc, 408, 409t

Bacteria, and bad breath, 743; body odor and, 85; in diaper rash, 273; gram-negative, 410t, 448; gram-positive, 410t, 448; inhibition of, to relieve bad breath, 744-745; in mouth, 741; and underarm wetness, 86

Bacterial infection, diaper rash and, 286; vs. fungal infection, 578

Bacterial plaque, 435, 922-933, *see also* Dental plaque

Bactine, 428t

Bactine Antiseptic Anesthetic, 433t

Bactine First Aid Antibiotic Plus Anesthetic, 412t

Bactine Hydrocortisone, 571t

Bactrim, 307

Bad breath, 739, 742-743; elimination of, 743-744; severe, 750

Bag Balm, 971

Baker's yeast, and insulin production, 544

Baking soda, 352t, 826t, 982t, *see also* Sodium bicarbonate; alkalinity of,

692; in anti-plaque products, 935-936; for cleaning sore mouth, 692-693; for diaper rash, 282, 292t; in douches, 339, 343; as gargle, 690; and insect bites, 975-976; for poison ivy-oak-sumac, 819; as skin protectant, 975-976

Baldness, male pattern, 458; medical care for, 463

Baldness preventives, **456-465**; disapproved active ingredients in, 460; estrogenic, 461; inactive ingredients in, 463; lack of product ratings for, 464; nonprescription, FDA ban on, 456; product claims for, 459; safety and effectiveness of, 464t

Balm, definition of, 639

Balnetar, 267t, 850t

Balsam, Peruvian, for diaper rash, 282

Banalg Hospital Strength Lotion, 651t

Banalg Lotion, 651t

BanSmoke, 885t

Bantron, 885t

Bar soaps, 447

Barc, 659t

Basaljel, 67t

Basement, child-proofing of for poison prevention, 832

Basic fuchsin, as antifungal, 590

Bathroom, child-proofing of for poison prevention, 832

Bayer Children's Aspirin, 797t

BC Cold Powder Non-Drowsy Formula, 190t

BC Powder, 800t

BC Tablets, 800t

Bedding disinfection for lice, 654

Bedroom, child-proofing of for poison prevention, 832

Beef insulin, 544

Beeswax, disapproved as temporary filling, 958

Behavior modification, and dieting, 864-865; and nail-biting, 755

Behçet's syndrome, 664

Belching, 316, 467

Beline sulfate, as smoking deterrent, 883

Belix, 45t, 182t

Ben-Aqua 10, 17t

Ben Gay Lotion, 651t

Ben Gay Original Ointment, 650t

Ben Gay Ultra Strength Cream, 650t

Ben-Gay Warming Ice, 649t

Benadryl, for allergy, 45t; as itch-pain remedy, 571t; for poison ivy-oak-sumac, 826t

Benadryl 25, 45t, 182t, 737t

Benadryl Cold Liquid, 201t

Benadryl Decongestant, 195t

Benadryl Degongestant Elixir, 187t

Benhydryl piperazines, for motion sickness, warning about, 734

Benoxyl 5, 17t

Benoxyl 10, 17t

Benylin, 45t, 183t

Benylin Cough Syrup, 180t, 737t; diphenhydramine hydrochloride in, 144-145

Benylin Expectorant Liquid, 207t

Benza, 430t

Benzalkonium chloride, as antiseptic, 430t, *see* Quaternary ammonium compounds; for diaper rash, 292t; in douches, 334, 345t; in eyewash, 402; for oral care, 678; for oral hygiene, 746

Benzalkonium chloride HVS 1 + 2, 224t

Benzalthonium chloride, in cold sore products, 214

Benzedrex, 48t, 186t

Benzene, in coal-tar shampoos, 257

Benzethonium, in douches, safety and effectiveness of, 345t

Benzethonium chloride, as antifungal, 590; as antiseptic, 430, *see* Quaternary ammonium compounds; for diaper rash, 288; in douches, 334; for oral hygiene, 746

Benzocaine, 220t, 825t, 866t; in acne preparations, 15t; as appetite suppressant, 861; in boil ointments, 122t; for cold sores, 215; for diaper rash, 292t; in douches, 334, 345t; in hemorrhoid medications, 490; for itch-pain relief, 557-558, 571t; nonabsorption of, 556; as premature ejaculation retardant, 841-842, 843t; for sore gums, mouth, or throat, 671, 705t; for teething pain, 946; as toothache reliever, 959

Benzocaine in polyethylene, for hemorrhoids, 512t

Benzocaine Topical, 844t

Benzodent, 706t

Benzodiazepines, as prescription sleep aids, 875

Benzoic acid, 462; in acne preparations, 15t; as antifungal, 590; for oral care, 679

Benzoic acid compounds, as pain-relief adjuvants, 787

Benzoin, as gingival protectant, 707t

Benzoin compound, 708t

Benzoin preparations, as mucosal protectants, 697-698; for sore throat and mouth, 707t

Benzoin tincture, 697-698

Benzophenone-3, and UVA and UVB light rays, 908

Benzoxiquine, *see* Oxyquinolines

Benzoyl peroxide, 17t

Butacaine sulfate, for sore gums, mouth, or throat, 672; as toothache reliever, 959

Butamben picrate, 283t, 571t; for itch-pain relief, 558-559

Butesin Picrate, 571t

Butter, discouraged for burns, 969

Butter of zinc, for oral health care, 689

C

Cacao plant, 973

Caffedrine, 891t

Caffeine, 891t; as adjuvant, 714-715; in pain relievers, 786-787; in cold-cough remedies, 169; dependency on, 889; for hangover, 471; mechanism of, 887; for menstrual distress, 714-715; as only approved OTC stimulant, 887-888, 888t; in overindulgence remedies, 468; as pain-relief adjuvant, 786-787; for premenstrual edema, 719; restoration of alertness vs. prevention of fatigue and, 889; warnings about, 890

-*caine* drugs, 217, 669; absorption of, 556

Cake alum, as astringent, 895

Caladryl, 826t

Caladryl Cream, 575t

Caladryl Lotion, 129t; as itch-pain remedy, 575t

Calamine, 825t, 981t; for diaper rash, 275t, 278, 292t; in hemorrhoid medications, 497, 501-502; as skin protectant, 973

Calcidrine Syrup, 206t

Calcilac Tablets, 70t

Calcium, 1010-1011; absorption of, 1010; and Vitamin D, 1000

Calcium aspirin, soluble, 777

Calcium carbonate, 68t

Calcium carbonate, 68t

Calcium compounds, as antacids, 65t, 61

Calcium hydroxide, for diarrhea, 305

Calcium phosphate, in anti-plaque products, 935

Calcium polycarbophil, for diarrhea, 305

Calcium polysulfide, for acne, 15t

Calcium pyrophosphate, 439

Calcium thiosulfate, for acne, 15t

Calcium undecylenate, *see* Undecylenic acid; for diaper rash, 288, 292t

Calcium undecylenic acid, and diaper rash, disapproved, 285

Calculus, professional dental care needed for, 936

CaldeCort, 572t

CaldeCort Anti-Itch, 572t

Caldesene, 296t

CaldoCort, 515t

Calicylic Creme, 246t, 267t

Calluses, causes of, 240; definition of, 240; treatment of, warnings about, 240-241

Calomel, as antiseptic, 424

Cama Arthritis Pain Reliever, 797t

Camalox, 55t

Camalox Suspension, 73t

Campho-Phenique Liquid, 129t, 432t, 433t, 812t; as itch-pain remedy, 574t

Campho-Phenique Antibiotic Plus Pain Reliever Ointment, 412t

Campho-Phenique Cold Sore Gel, 224t

Camphor, 124-127, 283t; for acne, 15t; approved uses of, 128; for colds, 167; for diaper rash, 293t; disapproved as antifungal, 594; disapproved for oral health care,

Citrate of magnesia, as laxative, 632t

Citrates, as antacids, 62

Citric acid, in douches, 338, 346t; as overindulgence reliever, 470; warning about, 470

Citric acid + sodium citrate in poloxamer 407, for dental hypersensitivity, 941

Citro-Nesia, 632t

Citrocarbonate, 76t

Citronella, oil of, 531, 533

Citrucel, 628t

Cleaning fluid, poisoning with, 830

Clear Away, 1028t

Clear Eyes, 385t

Clear Eyes ACR, 385t

Clearasil, 20t

Clearasil Antibacterial Soap, 21t

Clearasil Double Clear, 18t

Clearasil Maximum Strength Acne Treatment, 18t

Clearasil 10%, 18t

Climax, sexual, and premature ejaculation, 839-841

Clinical Care Wound Cleanser, 428t

Clioquinol, as antifungal, 586, 599t; warnings about, 586

Cloflucarban, 426; as germ killer, 452

Clomipromine hydrochloride, and nail-biting, 755

Clor-pheniramine, 44t

Clor-Trimeton Repetabs, 44t

Clothing disinfection for lice, 654

Clotrimazole, 1042t; as antifungal, 587, 599t; warnings about, 1039; for yeast infections, 1038-1039, 1041t

Clove oil, in toothache reliever, 960

Clycofed Tablets, 194t

Cnicus benedictus, disapproved for menstrual distress, 723

CNS, *see* Central nervous system

Coal tar, disapproved as antifungal, 594; safety and effectiveness of, in acne preparations, 16t

Coal-tar lotions and bath preparations, product ratings for, 850t

Coal-tar lotions and shampoos, for psoriasis, 847-848

Coal-tar preparations, 264t; safety and effectiveness of, 263t; for scalp care, 266t; for seborrheic dermatitis and long-term use of, 258

Coal-tar shampoos, 255

Coco-glycerides, hydrogenated, *see* Hard fat

Cocoa butter, 515t

Cocoa butter, 283t, 981t; for diaper rash, 281; in hemorrhoid medications, 497; as skin protectant, 973

Cod-liver oil, for diaper rash, 275t, 278, 293t; in hemorrhoid medications, 497

Codamil Tablets, **Capsules**, 200t

Codeine, 139; in combination form, 193t; disapproved for pain relief, 785-786; recommended dosage for, 144; and terpin hydrate elixir, 196t

Codeine preparations, 142-143

Coenzyme A, and pantothenic acid, 1009

Coenzymes, and zinc, 1012

Coffee, caffeine in, 888t, 889

Cola drinks, caffeine in, 888t, 889

Colace, 634t

Cold, dental hypersensitivity to, 939

Cold and cough medicines, **130-209**, *see also*; Allergy drugs; Antihistamines; Cough medicines; Nasal decongestants; *See also* by individual ingredient or brand name; alcohol in, 138; amount sold

Sinus Caplets, 190t
Contac Severe Cold & Flu Hot Medicine Powder, 202t
Contac Severe Cold Formula Caplets, 202t
Contact lenses, and corneal edema, 397; and polyvinyl alcohol, 392; and povidone, 392; and vasoconstrictors, 369
Contraception, and douching, 231, 327
Contraceptives, **227-238**; approved active ingredients in, 232-233; claims for, 228; combination products, 232; conditionally approved active ingredients in, 234; disapproved active ingredients in, 235; vaginal, 228-231
Control, 866t
Cool Mint Listerine, 748, 752t, 933
Coolants, 642
Cope, 800t
Copper, 1015; reference daily intake for, 990t
Copper undecylenate, *see* Undecylenic acid
Coricidin 'D' Decongestant Tablets, 198t
Coricidin Demilets Tablets, 198t
Coricidin Max Strength-Sinus Headache Tablets, 199t
Coricidin Tablets, 191t
Corn, causes of, 240; definition of, 240
Corn and callus removers, **239-246**; claims for, 239-240; forms of treatment for, 241; warnings about, 240
Corn silk, disapproved for menstrual distress, 723
Corn starch, *see* Topical starch; as skin protectant, 976
Cornea, 365; scratched, and vasocon-

strictors, 369; and Vitamin A, 999
Corneal edema, 364-365, **396-399**; causes and treatment of, 397, *see also* Hypertonicity agents; claim for, 396; doctor's supervision for, 396; warnings about, 397
Corneas, 401
Corns, 239; treatment of, 240-241; warnings about treating, 240-241; types of, 240
Corrective Mixture with Paregoric, 313t
Correctives, in pain relievers, 788
Correctol, 635t
Corrosive acid, poisoning with, 830
Corrosive alkali, poisoning with, 830
Cortaid, 515t
Corticosteroids, *see also* Hydrocortisone preparations; in hemorrhoid medications, 506-508, 512t; for minor skin conditions, 550-551
Cortisol, *see* Hydrocortisone
Cortizone-5, 514t, 571t, 572t
Cortizone-10, 514t, 572t
Cortril, 514t
Coryanthe johimbe, 99, *see also* Yohimbine
Cosmetics, and antiperspirants, 83; astringents as, 892; claims made for, 523; cover-up, for acne, 8; douches as, 326-327; and hair, 459; and hormone preparations, 520; mouthwashes as, 739, 742; promotion of, 523; sunless tanners as, 919; toothpastes as, 932; vs. drugs, 417, 457
Cotton tips, misuse of, 354
Couch grass, disapproved for menstrual distress, 723
Cough, during colds, 131t; dry, and asthma, 102; duration of, 135; and sore throat, 666; types of, 134

Cough-cold-allergy drugs, as single category, 25

Cough Formula Comtrex Liquid, 209t

Cough medicines, *see also* Cold and cough medicines; active ingredients in, 173t-175t

Cough suppressors, 134, 139-143, 180t; approved active ingredients in, 140-147; claims for, approved, 140; classification of, 139; disapproved active ingredients in, 147; oral, recommended dosages for, 144t; testing methods for, 140

Coughing, 134; and asthma, 103; causes of, 134; purpose of, 134

Counterirritants, *see also* Liniments and poultices; absorption of, 639; active ingredients in, safety and effectiveness of, 648t; approved active ingredients in, 643-647; claims for, 638-639; combination, 642-643; and how they work, 639; and pain, 640-641; product ratings for, 649t-651t; types of, 641-642; warnings about, 640

Counterirritation, and toothache, 957, 961-962

Cow balm, 971

Cows, insulin from, 544

CPR, *see* Cardiopulmonary resuscitation

Crabs, 652, 654

Cradle cap, 247; unavailability of drugs for, 247; white petrolatum for, 247

Cradle-cap removers, **247-250**

Cramping pain, 301

Cramps, abdominal, 298, 318; of "growing pains," 853; menstrual, 720, 780; nighttime, in legs, 852; runners', 852; severe, 725

Creams, *see also* Skin protectants

Creosote, as toothache reliever, 959

Cresol, disapproved for oral health care, 686; disapproved for oral hygiene, 748-749; for sore gums, mouth, or throat, 676; as toothache reliever, 959

m-Cresol, 809; as antifungal, 591-592

Cresols, 809; as antifungals, 591-592

Cruex, as antifungal, 600t

Cut, minor, 415

Cuticura Acne, 17t

Cyanobalamin, 1004

Cyclizine hydrochloride, for motion sickness, 737t, warning about, 734

Cysteine hydrochloride, for diaper rash, 282, 293t

Cystic fibrosis, 803-804

Cytostatic agents, *see also* Pyrithione zinc; Selenium sulfide; for psoriasis, 847; for scalp care, 254-255

D

D-S-S, 634t

D-S-S plus, 635t

d-Seb Gel Skin Cleanser, 21t

Dairy products, as source of calcium, 1010

Dandelion, as diuretic, 717

Dandelion root, disapproved for menstrual distress, 723

Dandruff, 251; cause of, 252; classes of drugs used for, 254; flake traits of, 253t

Dandruff and seborrheic-scale shampoos, **251-264**; approved active ingredients in, 255-261; combination products for, 262t; conditionally approved active ingredients in, 261-262; dandruff-control products, 252; medicated hair dressings, 266t; safety and effec-

Dramamine, 737t

Dri/Ear, 361t

Dristan—AF Tablets, 199t

Dristan Long Lasting, 47t, 184t; **Dristan Nasal**, 50t, 187t; **Dristan Sinus Caplets**, 181t

Dristan Tablets, 199t

Driving, and eye dryness, 388

Drixoral Sustained-Action Tablets, 194t

Drixoral Syrup, 197t

Drops, eye, *see* Eye drops

Drowsiness, and antihistamines, 151; and diphenhydramine hydrochloride, 144-145; and motion-sickness medicines, 734, 735

Drug interactions, *see* Monoamine oxidase (MAO) inhibitors; Warnings under specific drug; and caffeine, 890

Drugs, *see also* specific drug; and antiperspirants, 83; astringents as, 892; and hormone preparations, 520; mouthwashes as, 739, 742; sunless tanners as, 919; toothpastes as, 932; vitamins and minerals as, 993-994; vs. candy, 696; vs. cosmetics, 417

Dry and Clear, 17t

Dry cough, 134

Dry eye, 388-389; in older people, 389; and outdoor activities, 389; severe, 390

"Dry eye," 362

Dry mouth, 467

Dryness, of eye, 387; of skin, acne preparations and, 3; vaginal, 344

Drytex Lotion, 21t

Ducolax, 631t

Duodenum, and ulcers, 57

Duratears Naturale, 385t

Duration, 47t, 184t, 185t

Dusting powders, *see* Skin protec-

tants

Dyclonine hydrochloride, 221t; in hemorrhoid medications, 491; for itch-pain relief, 560; for sore gums, mouth, or throat, 672-673

Dye, triple, as antiseptic, 425

Dysmenorrhea, 710; symptoms of, 711

E

Ear, blocked feeling in, 356; cleaning of, 354; drainage of fluid from, 353; ringing in, 353; swimmer's, 353

Ear care, aids for, **353-361**

Ear wax, 354-356; misconceptions about, 354

Ear wax removal of, softening agent for, 355; approved active ingredients in, 355; claims for, 355; warnings about, 355

Earache, 353, 354

Eardrum, perforated, warnings about, 355, 358

Eating, to relieve bad breath, 744

Eccrine glands, effect of antiperspirants on, 87; and sweat secretion, 84-85

Ecotrin Tablets and Caplets, 796t

Ectopic pregnancy, and douching, 328

Eczema, 281, 974, 977; kaolin for, 279

Edema, 711; corneal, 364-365; premenstrual, 717

Edetate disodium, in douches, 335, 346t

Edetate sodium, in douches, 335, 346t

Edetate sodium + sodium fluoride + strontium chloride, disapproved for dental hypersensitivity,

Fingernails, 755-756

First aid, antibiotics for, **404-413**; antiseptics for, **414-433**; basic, 415; for burns, 969; for eyes, 401, 403; for wounds, 405, 415

Fish-poison tree extract, disapproved for menstrual distress, 723

Flakes on scalp, 251-253

Flatulence, 58

Flatulex, 81t

Flatus, 77, 316, 318, 479

Fleet Babylax, 633t

Fleet Laxative, 631t

Fleet Relief Anesthetic Hemmorrhoidal, 513t

Flex-all 454, 694t

Flocculation, of insulin vials, 541

Flora, vaginal, 337

Flossing, to relieve bad breath, 744

Flowers of zinc, *see* Zinc oxide; as skin protectant, 977

"Flu relief", cold-cough products for, 133

Flu symptoms, acetaminophen safe for, 771; danger of aspirin for, 771; late-winter, danger of aspirin for, 771

Fluid and electrolyte balances, and chloride, 1014

Fluidex with Pamabrom, 729t

Fluids, body, loss of in diarrhea, 299-301

Fluorapatite, 436

Fluoridation, effectiveness of, 437; by percentage of state population, 445; of water supply, 434, 436

Fluoride, disapproved in vitamin-mineral products, 1015; dosage forms of, 438-440; professional application of, 437, 438; reference daily intake for, 990t; risk factors for, 439; toxicity of, 439

Fluoride preparations, in products for dental hypersensitivity, 941-942

Fluoride supplementation, of water supply, 434, 436-438

Fluoride toothpastes and rinses, **434-446**

Fluorides, 435-443, *see also* Anticavity preparations; action of, 941; effectiveness of, 437; in prevention of tooth decay, 436; product ratings for, 446t; products containing, 439-444; sources of, 436

Fluorine compounds, *see* Fluorides

Fluorosalan, 426

Foams, aerosol, as vaginal contraceptives, 229; for hemorrhoids, 484

Foille Plus, 574t

Folacin, 1004

Folic acid, 1006-1008; and reduction in birth defects, 1004-1005

Fontanels, 247

Food, and acne, 4; and anal itching, 481; and bad breath, 743; bran as, 608; digestion of, 51; and drink, overindulgence in, 466; and dry mouth, 668; flatuogenic, and gas, 77-78; and gas, 316; nitrates in, 940; overindulgence in, 320t; passage of through digestive system, 319; and RDA labeling, 988; sodium-rich, and water retention, 711; spicy, and heartburn, 58; spicy, and and sweating, 85; sweet, and tooth decay, 436; vitamins in, 995-996

Food additive, guar gum as, 860

Food pipe, 59

Food supplements, as product classification, 456; vitamins as, 987

Foot, athlete's, *see* Athlete's foot

Foot salves, 241, 244

Foreign body in eye, 365, 402; doctor's care for, 402; sensation of, in

combination, 451-452; disapproved active ingredients in, 454; effectiveness of, 450; efficacy of, 447; Panel and FDA assessment of, 448; product ratings for, 455t; safety and effectiveness of, 454t; warning about, 451

Gin and tonic, 854

Gingiva, *see* Gums

Gingival infections, 661

Gingival protectants, product ratings for, 707t-708t

Gingivitis, 661, 662-663; definition of, 662; and plaque, 932

Ginseng, as aphrodisiac, 98; safety and effectiveness of, 100t

Glaucoma, 365, 367, 369; and antihistamines, 872; and corneal edema, 397

Glucose metabolism, chromium and, 1014-1015

Gly-Oxide, 708t

Glycate Tablets, 71t

Glycerides, *see* Hard fat

Glycerin, 221t, 380t, 392t, 981t; anhydrous for fluoride gel, 443; anhydrous for swimmer's ear, 359, 360t; aqueous, in hemorrhoid medications, 497-498; for diaper rash, 282, 293t; hydrous, as skin protectant, 974; as laxative, 619, 633t; as oral soother, 695

Glycerin, USP, 633t

Glycerine, *see also* Glycerin; as skin protectant, 974

Glycerol, *see also* Glycerin; as skin protectant, 974

Glyceryl aminobenzoate, as waterproof UV-blocking sunscreen, 918-919

Glycine, as antacid, 65, 62

Glycofed Tablets, 205t

Glycol monosalicylate, *see* Glycol salicylate

Glycol salicylate, 221t; for itch-pain relief, 565-566; as pain reliever, 216

Glycotuss, 181t

Glycyrrhiza, 99

Glycyrrhiza glabra, 721-722

Glytuss, 181t

Goiter, 1013

Golden seal, as aphrodisiac, 98; safety and effectiveness of, 100t

Goldenseal, disapproved for menstrual distress, 723

Gonococcal sore, of the mouth, 664

Gonorrhea infections, and contraceptive sponge, 230

Goose grease, discouraged for burns, 969

Gotu kola, as aphrodisiac, 98; safety and effectiveness of, 101t

Gout, 765, 791

Grain alcohol, *see* Ethyl alcohol

Gram-negative, definition of, 410t

Gram-negative bacteria, 410t, 448

Gram-positive, definition of, 410t

Gram-positive bacteria, 410t, 448

Gram's stain, 410t

Granulated eyelid, anti-infectives for, 377

Granulated eyelids, 366

Grass, and allergy, 23

Greasy substances, discouraged for burns, 969

Groin, fungal infection of, 578; yeast infection of, 581

Growth inhibitor, *see* Cytostatic agent

Guaifenesin, 181t

Guaifenesin, 137, 181t; clinical study of, 149; dosage of, 149-150; as expectorant, 149-150; FDA assessment of, 148; safety and effectiveness of, 174t

Guar gum, FDA ban on, 860

Guiatuss-AC Syrup, 206t

Guiatuss-DM Liquid, 207t

Guiatuss Syrup, 196t

Gum, chewing, and tooth decay, 436; medicated, 705t; sugarless, and dry mouth, 668

Gum chewing, 316

Gum infections, 661

Gums, 661-663; inflammation of, 662; sore, see Sore gums

Gyne-Lotrimin, 1042t

Gynol II Contraceptive, 237t

H

Habit, nail-biting, 755

Habit Reversal procedure, and nail-biting, 755

Hair, length of, and lice, 654

Hair dressings, medicated, 266t

Hair growth, cycle of, 458; and estradiol, 462; research of, 457

Hair-growth stimulants, **456-465**

Hair loss, 458, see Hair-growth stimulants; causes of, 458; medical care for, 464

Hair transplants, 463

Hairline, receding, 458

Halcion, as prescription sleep aid, 875

Haley's M-O, 636t

Halfprin, 797t

Halitosis, 742-743

Halls Mentho-Lyptus Spearmint, 188t

Hamamelis virginiana, 485, 502

Hamamelis water, NF XI, as astringent, 895-896; claims for, 894

Hamamelis water NF XI, 485; in hemorrhoid medications, 502; for hemorrhoids, 516t

Hangover minimizer, 473

Hangover relievers, **466-477**; claims for, 472; combination products, 471; product ratings for, 476t-477t

Hard corn, 240

Hard fat, in hemorrhoid medications, 498

Hard pimples, in fungal infection, 580

Hay fever, see Allergy

Head & Shoulders, 265t

Head lice, 652, 653-654

Headache, and caffeine withdrawal, 762, 889; during colds, 133; and diarrhea, 298; dysmenorrhea and, 711; from fever, 762; from hangover, 762; hangover and, 467; hypertensive, 762; and hypoglycemia, 540; inflammatory, 763; migraine, 762; and PMS, 711; in rhinitis, 135; sinus, 763; of sinusitis, 135; tension, 762-763; traction, 763; vascular, 762

Hearing loss, 353, 356; aspirin and, 773

Heart, caffeine and, 887

Heart attack, aspirin in prevention of, 790-791

Heart disease, and sodium-restricted diet, 868

Heart problems, and ephedrine sulfate, 493

Heartbeat, rapid, and hypoglycemia, 540

Heartburn, 54, 58, 79, 319, 467; and gas, 58; hangover and, 467, 470; mild, treatment of, 59; overindulgence and, 467

Heat, dental hypersensitivity to, 939; for earache, 353

Heat lamps, 641

Heet Liniment, 129t, 651t

Heet Spray, 129t, 651t

Ileostomy, and odor, 268; chlorophyllin copper complex for, 269
Immune reaction, 24
Immune system, and fungal infections, 579
Imodium A-D, 312t; for diarrhea,
299
Impetigo, 281, 977
Impotence, 96
Incontinence, fecal, 268-269; and
odor, 268; urinary, 268-269
Indigestion, 51, 59, 79
Infants, and absorption of external
analgesics, 556; and antibiotics,
406; and antifungal agents, 577;
and cradle-cap, 247; and dangerous compounds, 287; diarrhea in,
danger of, 298, 299; and
germ-killing soaps, 451; and hexachlorophene, 449; mineral oil
restricted for, 622; and phenol,
warnings about, 275; and resorcinol, warning about, 564; and
teething, 945; and tooth decay,
435; and toxic absorption of phenol, 453; and toxic absorption of
triclocarban, 453
Infection, bacterial vs. fungal infection,
578; diaper rash and, 286; due to
nail-biting, 755; of eye, 367; fungal,
578-579; and germ-killing soaps,
450; and red eye, 365; of tear duct,
368; upper-respiratory, and bad
breath, 743
Inflammation, of airways, 145;
anorectal, 480, 483t; around toenail, 525; of boil, 119; of gums,
662; of nasal tissues, 163; of
scalp, in cradle cap, 247; of sinus
membranes, 135; of sinuses, 763;
of urethral tissues, 841
Ingrown toenail, pedicure in prevention of, 526

Ingrown toenail relievers, conditionally approved active ingredients in
527-528, 528t; claims for,
525-526; drugs in treatment of,
526-529; and pain killers, 527;
warnings about, 526
Ingrown-toenail relievers, **525-529**;
product ratings for, 529t
Inhibitors, monoamine oxidase, *see*
Monoamine oxidase inhibitors
Injections, desensitizing, for allergy,
24
Injectors, needle-less, for insulin, 546
Injury, minor, pain relief for, 418;
serious, first aid for, 415
Insect bites, and sodium bicarbonate,
975-976
Insect repellents, **530-537**, 531
Insect venom, drugs to neutralize,
532; sensitivity to, 530, 534
Insects, deet for, 534
Insomnia, 875
Insulin, nondiabetic production of,
539; normal production of,
538-539
Insulin for diabetics, **538-549**;
administration of, 541; claim for,
539; concentration of, 543-544;
makers of, 540-541; mixing of,
restrictions on, 545; OTC availability of in U.S., 547t-549t; premixed, 545; purity of, 542-543;
source of, 544-545; storage and
handling of, 541-542; and travel,
543; types of, 540-541; warnings
about, 539
Insulin reaction, 540
Intercept Contraceptive Inserts,
237t
Intermediate-acting insulin, 545
Intestine, and calcium absorption,
1010; gas in, 316; and magnesium
levels, 1011; and ulcers, 57-59

Jock itch, **576-601**, 580, *see also* Antifungal agents; causes of, 580; cures for, product ratings for, 599t-601t; fungal molds of, 577

Juniper oil, disapproved for menstrual distress, 724

Juniper tar, 221t; for diaper rash, 294t; in hemorrhoid medications, 504; for itch-pain relief, 562

K

K-Pek, 311t

Kaolin, for diaper rash, 275t, 279, 293t; for diarrhea, 305-306; in hemorrhoid medications, 498-499; as skin protectant, 974

Kaolin with pectin, 312t

Kaopectate Advanced Formula, 311t

Kaopectolin, 314t

Kaopectolin with paregoric, 313t

Karaya, as laxative, 609-610

Kasof, 633t

Keratin, 755; and fungal molds, 577

Keratoconjunctivitis sicca, 389

Keratolytic agents, 239, *see also* Skin peelers; for hemorrhoids, 482, 510t; for psoriasis, 847; for scaling of the scalp, *see* Salicylic acid; Sulfur preparations

Keratolytics, for scalp care, 254-255

Kerosene, poisoning with, 830

Ketoconazole, prescriptive, for dandruff, 254

KI, *see* Potassium iodide

Kidneys, adverse effects of aspirin on, 773

Kidney disease, and ammonium chloride, 719; upper-respiratory, 743

Kidney drugs, **602-603**

Kidney function, bicarbonate compounds and, 61

Kidney irritation, 602

Kidney problems, and aluminum-containing antacids, 60-61; and ibuprofen, 780; and magnesium compounds, warnings about, 62; and salt substitutes, 868; and sodium compounds, in antacids, 63

Kidneys, and potassium balance, 1016

Kitchen, child-proofing of for poison prevention, 832

Komed Mild, 20t

Kondremul Plain, 635t

Kondremul with Phenolphthalein, 636t

Konsyl-D, 629t

Korean ginseng, *see* Ginseng

Kôromex, 237t

L

L-Lysine, 226t

Lacri-Lube S.O.P. Ointment, 385t

Lacril, 394t

Lacrimal glands, 389

Lactic acid, and cramps, 852; in douches, 338, 346t

Lactic acid + sodium lactate, in douches, 347t

Lactinex, 226t

Lactobacilli, 336-337; for cold sores, 226t

Lactobacillus acidophilus, 1037; for cold sores, 219; safety and effectiveness of, 223t

Lactobacillus bulgaricus, for cold sores, 219; safety and effectiveness of, 223t

Lactose intolerance, and gas, 78

Lactril, 394t

Lanacaine, 575t

Lanacort 5, 515t, 572t

Poloxamer iodine complex, as antiseptic, 425

Polycarbophil, 312t; for diarrhea, 299, 304; as laxative, 610, 628t; in vaginal moisturizers, 344

Polydine, 431t

Polyethylene glycol 300, 381t, 392t

Polyethylene granules, and acne treatment, 8

Polymer, 390

Polymixin B sulfate, 408, 409t

Polyps, rectal, 481

Polysorbate 80, 381t, 393t

Polyvinyl alcohol, 381t, 393t; as demulcent, 391-392

Polyvinylpyrrolidone-vinyl Acet, disapproved for poison ivy, 815-816, 821

Pontocaine, 513t, 573t

Porcelain clay, 279; as skin protectant, 974

Porcelana, 118t

Porcelana with Sunscreen, 118t

Porcine insulin, 544

Postprandial distress, definition of, 318

Potassium, 1016-1017

Potassium alum, as antifungal, 590

Potassium aluminum sulfate, in douches, 347t; for oral health care, 688-689

Potassium bicarbonate, as antacid, 61

Potassium carbonate, for diarrhea, disapproved, 306

Potassium chlorate, disapproved for oral health care, 687

Potassium compounds, as antacids, 63; safety and effectiveness of, 66t

Potassium hydroxide, poisoning with, 830

Potassium iodide, claims for, 952; dosage of, vs. dosage for bronchial asthma, 952; FDA licensing of,

951; for nuclear emergencies, 948, 950-952; OTC availability of, 953; safety and effectiveness of, 954t; shelf life of, 951; sources of, 951; time factor in use of, 948, 949

Potassium nitrate, for dental hypersensitivity, 940-942; for extreme dental hypersensitivity, 943

Potassium salicylate, 784

Potassium-sodium-copper chlorophyllin, for sore gums, mouth, or throat, 675

Poultice, definition of, 639

Poultices, *see* Liniments and poultices; mouth, warning for, 667; for toothache, warnings about, 957

Povidone, 373, 381t, 393t; as demulcent, 391-392; disapproved for poison ivy, 815-816, 821

Povidone-Iodine, 431t; as antifungal, 599t

Povidone-iodine, as antifungal, 588; as antiseptic, 423, 431t; in douches, 351t; for oral care, 684; for scalp care, 264t; safety and effectiveness of, in acne preparations, 16t

Powders, *see also* Skin protectants; tooth, 434-435

Pramocaine, *see* Pramoxine hydrochloride

Pramoxine hydrochloride, 573t

Pramoxine hydrochloride, 221t; for diaper rash, 294t; in hemorrhoid medications, 491; for hemorrhoids, 512t; for itch-pain relief, 563-564

Prax, 573t

Pregnancy, *see also* under specific drug or ingredient for restrictions on use during pregnancy; and camphor poisoning, 127; danger

798t, 856t; side effects of, 854

Quinphenol-8-hydroxyquinoline, *see* Oxyquinoline sulfate

R

R + C, 659t

RA, 20t

Race, and acne, 5

Racemethionine, for diaper rash, 294t

Racephedrine hydrochloride, for asthma, *see* Ephedrine preparations

Radiation, and nuclear emergencies, 948-950; solar, and sunburn, 907

Radiation blocking, in U.S., 950-951

Radioactive fallout, description of, 949

Ramses Extra, 237t

Rash, bright red, irritating, 273; and cough, 140; diaper, causes of, 273; in fungal infection, 580; itching of, 551; of poison-ivy-oak-sumac, 813; of seborrheic dermatitis, 259

Rashes, and external analgesics, 556

Rebound congestion, caused by nasal decongestants, 163; nasal decongestants and, 24-25, 32

Rebound effect, of vasoconstrictors, 369

Recombinant DNA insulins, 544

Recommended Daily Allowances (RDA), vs. Reference Daily Intakes (RDI), 991, 993, 1018t-1021t

Recommended Dietary Allowances (RDA), 987-991; and FDA food labeling requirements, 988; as norms for groups of people vs. individuals, 988; NRC/NAS decreases in, 988

Rectagene II, 519t

Red eye, 365

Red peppers, 644, 645

Red petrolatum, as waterproof UVB/UVA-blocking sunscreen, 921

Reducing aids, **857-867**; approved active ingredients in, 861-864, 865t; claims for, 858; combination, 859, 865t; product ratings for, 866t-867t; warnings about, 858

Reese's Pinworm Medicine, 1034t

Reference Daily Intakes (RDI); for nutrients lacking RDAs, 990t; as replacement for RDA, 988-989; vs. Recommended Daily Allowances (RDA), 991, 993, 1018t-1021t

Regular insulin, 545

Reguloid, 629t

Regutol, 634t

Rehydralyte, 300

Rehydration, oral, formula for, 300

Relaxants, muscle, for menstrual distress, 712, 720-721

Relief, 386t

Removal, debris, *see* Debris removers/wound cleansers

Removers, corn and callus, *see* Corn and Callus Removers; cradle-cap, *see* Cradle-cap removers

Repellents, insect, *see* Insect repellents

Reporal Tablets, 184t

Res-Q, 838t

Resinol, 983t

Resins, cation + anion exchange, for poison ivy-oak-sumac, 820

Resorcinol, 221t, 809; for diaper rash, 295t; disapproved active ingredients in, 289; disapproved as antifungal, 594; in hemorrhoid medications, 505; for itch-pain relief, 564; warning about, 564

Resorcinol + resorcinol monoacetate, for acne, 10

resorcinol, safety and effectiveness of, in acne preparations, 16t

Respiratory allergy, *see* Allergy

Resporal Tablets, 194t

Resuscitation, mouth-to-mouth, 415

Retin-A, 115-116

Rezamid, 20t

Rheaban Maximum Strength, 311t

Rheum officinale, 306

Rheum rhubarbarum, 306

Rheumatoid arthritis, 765

Rhinall, 48t, 186t

Rhinitis, 135; allergic, 135; drugs for, 136; vasomotor, 136

Rhinosyn Syrup, 197t

Rhubarb fluid extract, for diarrhea, disapproved, 306

Rhuli Cream, 128t, 827t

Rhuli Gel, 827t

Rhuli Spray, 128t, 827t

Rhynchosia pyramidalis, 99

Riboflavin (Vitamin B2), 1008

Rice hulls, removal of, and beriberi, 1008

Rickets, and Vitamin D, 1000

Ricola Cherry Mint Herb Throat Drops, 189t

Ricola Menthol-Eucalyptus Herb Throat Drops, 189t

Rid-A-Pain, 705t

RID Shampoo, 659t

Ringing in the ears, aspirin and, 773

Ringworm, **576-601**, *see also* Antifungal agents; cures for, product ratings for, 599t-601t; as fungal infection, 580; nail, 581; scalp, 581

Rinses, antimicrobials in, safety and effectiveness of, 751t; and children, restrictions on, 674; fluoride, 434, 439, 442-444; mouth, 434, 437

Riopan, 55t, 68t

Riopan Extra Strength, 69t; acid-neutralizing capacity of, 55t

Riopan Plus Suspension, 74t

Riopan Plus Tablets, 72t

Robitussin, 179t

Robitussin A-C Syrup, 206t

Robitussin-PE Liquid, 205t

Robitussin Pediatric, 180t

Rolaids, 54, 68t

Roundworm, 1031

Ru-tuss Expectorant Liquid, 208t

Rub, definition of, 639

Rubbers, *see* Condoms

Rutgers 6-12, 533

Ryna-C Liquid, 204t

Ryna-CX Liquid, 208t

Ryna Liquid, 197t

S

Safeguard, 455t

Sage oil, 744

Salicyl alcohol, for sore gums, mouth, or throat, 674-675

Salicylamide, 784; for menstrual distress, 715; as pain-relief adjuvant, 787

Salicylates, 670, *see also* Aspirin; for arthritis relief, 765; dosages of, 765; labeling of, 765; in overindulgence remedies, 468

Salicylic Acid, 246t, 267t, 851t

Salicylic acid, 850t-851t, 1028t; for acne, 6, 10, 18t-19t; as antifungal, 593; for corns and calluses, 242-243; as keratolytic agent, 239; for psoriasis, 848, 849t; for scalp care, 265t; for seborrheic dermatitis, 259-260; for warts, 1022, 1026, 1027t; and water, 241

Salicylic Acid Soap, 19t

Salicylic Acid and Sulfur, 21t

Salicylic acid + sulfur, for scalp care,

255

Salicylsalicylic acid, 784-785

Saligel Acne Gel, 19t

Saline solutions, sterile, for corneal edema, 397

Salinity, of eyewash, 401

Saliva, 741; fluoride in, 436; and mouthwashes, 667

Saliva substitutes, 668; product ratings for, 709t

Salivart Saliva Substitute, 709t

Salivation, inadequate, 668

Salol, *see* Phenyl salicylate

Salsalate, 784-785

Salt, chloride in, 1014

Salt supplements and substitutes, **868-869**

Salt water, salt, 690; sterile, for corneal edema, 396

Salts, body, loss of in diarrhea, 299-301

Sandarac, disapproved as temporary filling, 958

Sanguinaria, as antimicrobial, 935

Sarcoptes scabiei, z0

Sarsaparilla, as aphrodisiac, 98; safety and effectiveness of, 101t

Sastid, 21t

Scabies, 657

Scales, 251, 252

Scalps, of babies, 247; sores on, 654

Schamberg, 983t

Sclera, 365, 402

Scope, 753t

Scopolamine patch, 736

Scorbutic syndrome, *see* Scurvy

Scrubs, abrasive, in acne treatment, 8; to treat acne, 6

Scurvy, 1002

Sealants, for teeth, 445

Seasickness, 732

Seasons, and allergy, 24

Sebaceous glands, in acne, 5; and

hair loss, 460

Sebaquin, 265t

Seborrhea, 252

Seborrheic dermatitis, 251; cause of, 252, 253; coal-tar preparations for, 258; drugs used for, 254-255; flake traits of, 253t; of infant, 257

Sebucare, 265t

Sebulex, 265t

Sebum, in acne, 5; excess, 253; and hair loss, 460; progesterones and, 523; and scalp flaking, 253

Secondary amyltricresols, 809; as antifungals, 591-592; for oral care, 684-685

Secondary amyltricresols + mercufenol chloride, as antiseptics, 425

Sedation, *see* Sleep aids

Seed corn, 240

Selenium, 1013-1014

Selenium sulfide, 267t

Selenium sulfide, for scalp care, 265t, 267t; for seborrheic dermatitis, 260-263; warning about, 260

Selsun Blue, 267t

Senecio aureus, disapproved for menstrual distress, 723

Senexon, 630t

Senile lentigines, 115

Senna Black-Draught, 630t

Senna preparations, as laxatives, 612, 630t

Sennosides A and B, calcium salts of, 630t

Senokot, 630t

Senokot S, 636t

Senolax, 630t

Sensitive teeth, 939-940

Sepp Antiseptic, 429t, 433t

SeptiSoft, 432t, 455t

Serum, and astringents, 893; and mercurial antiseptics, 419